Periodontal Medicine

Periodontal Medicine

Louis F. Rose, DDS, MD
Professor of Surgery and Medicine
MCP Hahnemann School of Medicine
Philadelphia, Pennsylvania
and Clinical Professor of Periodontics
University of Pennsylvania
School of Dental Medicine
Philadelphia, Pennsylvania

Robert J. Genco, DDS, PhD
Distinguished Professor and Chair of Oral Biology
State University of New York
Buffalo, New York

D. Walter Cohen, DDS
Chancellor-Emeritus
MCP Hahnemann University of Health Sciences
Dean-Emeritus
University of Pennsylvania School of Dental Medicine
Philadelphia, Pennsylvania

Brian L. Mealey, DDS, MS
Chief of Periodontics
Chief of Dental and Professional Services
US Air Force Hospital
Eglin Air Force Base
Fort Walton Beach, Florida

2000
B.C. Decker Inc.
Hamilton • London • Saint Louis

B.C. Decker Inc.
4 Hughson Street South
P.O. Box 620, L.C.D. 1
Hamilton, Ontario L8N 3K7
Tel: 905-522-7017; 1-800-568-7281
Fax: 905-522-7839
e-mail: info@bcdecker.com
website: http://www.bcdecker.com

00 01 / PC / 9 8 7 6 5 4 3 2 1
ISBN 1-55009-120-4

SALES AND DISTRIBUTION

United States
B.C. Decker Inc.
P.O. Box 785
Lewiston, NY 14092-0785
Tel: 800-568-7281
e-mail: info@bcdecker.com

Canada
B.C. Decker Inc.
4 Hughson Street South
P.O. Box 620, L.C.D. 1
Hamilton, Ontario L8N 3K7
Tel: 905-522-7017; 800-568-7281
Fax: 905-522-7839
e-mail: info@bcdecker.com

Japan
Ishiyaku Publishers Inc.
7–10, Honkomagome 1-Chome
Bunkyo-ku, Tokyo 113
Japan
Tel: 03 5395-7631
Fax: 03 5395-7633

U.K., Europe, Scandinavia, Middle East
Harcourt-Brace & Company Ltd.
24–28 Oval Road
London, NW1 7DX
United Kingdom
Tel: 71-267-4466
Fax: 71-482-2291

India
K.M. Varghese Company
Hind Rajasthan Building
Dadasaheb Phalke Road, Dadar
Bombay 400 014 India
Tel: 91 22 414 6904
Fax: 91 22 414 9074
e-mail: km.varghese@pobox.com

Foreign Rights
John Scott & Co.
International Publishers' Agency
P.O. Box 878
Kimberton, PA 19442
Tel: 610-827-1640
Fax: 610-827-1671

Notice: The authors and publisher have made every effort to ensure that the patient care recommended herein, including choice of drugs and drug dosages, is in accord with the accepted standard and practice at the time of publication. However, since research and regulation constantly change clinical standards, the reader is urged to check the product information sheet included in the package of each drug, which includes recommended doses, warnings, and contraindications. This is particularly important with new or infrequently used drugs.

Contributors

James D. Beck, PhD
Kenan Professor
Department of Dental Ecology
University of North Carolina at Chapel Hill
Chapel Hill, North Carolina

Sebastian G. Ciancio, DDS
Professor and Chair, Department of
    Periodontics and Endodontics
Clinical Professor of Pharmacology, State
    University of New York at Buffalo School
    of Dental Medicine
Buffalo, New York

D. Walter Cohen, DDS
Chancellor-Emeritus, MCP Hahnemann
    University of Health Sciences
Dean-Emeritus, University of Pennsylvania
    School of Dental Medicine
Philadelphia, Pennsylvania

Joel Epstein, DDS, MSD
Faculty of Dentistry, University of
    British Columbia
Department of Oral Medicine,
    University of Washington, Seattle
Department of Dentistry,
    Vancouver General Hospital
Dentistry, B.C. Cancer Agency
Vancouver, Canada

Robert J. Genco, DDS
Distinguished Professor and Chair of
    Oral Biology, School of Dental Medicine,
    State University of New York at Buffalo
University Dental Associates
Buffalo General Hospital
Buffalo, New York

Michael Glick, DMD
Professor, Department of Oral Medicine
Director, Programs for Medically Complex
    Patients, University of Pennsylvania
Philadelphia, Pennsylvania

Sara G. Grossi, DDS, MS
Clinical Director, Periodontal Disease
    Research Center
Department of Oral Biology
School of Dental Medicine
State University of New York at Buffalo
Buffalo, New York

Carl W. Haveman, DDS, MS
Staff, University Hospital
Assistant Professor
Department of General Dentistry
The University of Texas Health Science
    Center
San Antonio, Texas

Palle Holmstrup, PhD, DrOdont
Professor of Periodontology
University of Copenhagen
School of Dentistry
Department of Periodontology
Copenhagen, Denmark

Marjorie Jeffcoat, DMD
University of Alabama School of Dentistry
University of Alabama at Birmingham
Birmingham, Alabama

Kenneth S. Kornman, DDS, Ph.D.
University of Texas Health Science Center
    at San Antonio
San Antonio, Texas
Harvard University
Boston, Massachusetts

Brian Mealey, DDS, MS
Chief of Periodontics
Chief of Dental Professional Services
US Air Force Hospital
Eglin Air Force Base, Florida
Clinical Assistant Professor
Department of Periodontics
University of Texas Health Science Center
San Antonio, Texas

Robert E. Mecklenburg, DDS, MPH
Coordinator, Tobacco and Oral Health
    Initiatives, Tobacco Control Research
    Branch, National Cancer Institute
Potomac, Maryland

Michael G. Newman, DDS
University of California School of Dentistry
Section of Periodontics
Pacific Palisades, California

Steven Offenbacher, DDS
Professor and Director
Center for Oral and Systemic Diseases
University of Carolina School of Dentistry
Chapel Hill, North Carolina

Spencer W. Redding, DDS, MEd
Staff, University Hospital
Professor, Department of General Dentistry
The University of Texas Health Science
    Center at San Antonio
San Antonio, Texas

Louis F. Rose, DDS, MD
Professor of Surgery and Medicine
MCP Hahnemann School of Medicine
Clinical Professor of Periodontics
University of Pennsylvania School of
    Dental Medicine
Philadelphia, Pennsylvania

Terry D. Rees, DDS, MSD
Periodontics Department
Baylor College of Dentistry
Dallas, Texas

Frank A. Scannapieco, DMD, PhD
Department of Oral Biology
School of Dental Medicine
Associate Professor
State University of New York at Buffalo
Buffalo, New York

Harold C. Slavkin, DDS
Director, National Institute of Dental and
    Craniofacial Research Laboratory
Chief, Craniofacial Developmental Biology
National Institute of Arthritis,
    Musculoskeletal, and Skin Disease
Bethesda, Maryland

Barbara J. Steinberg, DDS
Professor of Surgery and Medicine
MCP Hahnemann School of Medicine
Clinical Assistant Professor of Oral Medicine
University of Pennsylvania
School of Dental Medicine
Philadelphia, Pennsylvania

Edwin J. Zinman, DDS, JD
Former Lecturer, University of California
    at San Francisco
San Francisco, California

To my beautiful granddaughter, Cameron Sara, who has brought so much love and joy into my life. To my mother-in-law, Helen Aberbach, whose love and kindness will remain with me forever. And to my wife, Claire, and children, Michael, David, and Hedy, whose unconditional love and support have allowed me to pursue my professional dreams.

Louis F. Rose

To D. Walter Cohen, Henry Goldman, Nicholas Marfino, James English, Fred Karush, and Art Ellison. These mentors instilled in me their intense appreciation for the role of the host in modulating oral diseases, and for the effect of oral disease on the rest of the body.

Robert J. Genco

To the late Russell Ross, DDS, PhD, one of the most distinguished scientists of the Twentieth Century.

D. Walter Cohen

To my loving wife Carla, who has supported me in every endeavor and has given me the most beautiful family a man could ever have. I also devote this undertaking to the honor of my mother, Jeanne C. Mealey, who taught me the value of a challenge, who showed through her personal example the gains derived from sacrifice, and who demonstrated that love and devotion overcome all difficulties.

Brian L. Mealey

Preface

Over the past 70 years, a number of astute clinicians in the field of dental medicine have observed and recorded the relationship between periodontopathies and systemic manifestations of disease. The influence of systemic conditions on the oral environment, and especially the periodontium, has long been recognized and supported by scientific evidence. However, an evidence base for the influence of periodontal diseases on overall systemic health has only recently begun to be established. Fascinating research has eroded the tradition-bound concept that oral infections such as periodontitis are simply local entities whose effects are limited to the oral tissues. While the clinical observations of many practitioners have long suggested that periodontal diseases can have widespread systemic effects, only recently has rigorous scientific investigation supported this concept. The information in this text has not been collected in this format previously, and one of the goals of the authors is to offer the material to physicians, dentists, and other health-care professionals collaborating in treatment of patients with periodontal disease who may also have systemic involvement. This will allow the practicing clinician to enhance the medical-dental interface when evaluating a patient and will contribute to a continuing dialogue between the dentist and physician. We are hopeful that this information will stimulate new collaborations between physicians and dentists and serve as a basis for further studies to help improve the total health of our society. This effort should also prove useful to medical and dental students as well as those in residency training and post-doctoral studies.

Bridging the gap between the dental and medical professions will provide better education, research and patient care. Our purpose is to provide existing evidence that supports and strengthens the association and relationships between periodontal diseases and systemic diseases/conditions. The information presented will demonstrate the practical application in day to day practice.

Our sincere gratitude to the many excellent contributors to this volume and sincere appreciation to their families who sacrificed to make this a timely and valuable publication. We applaud Mr. Brian Decker for inspiring the authors to assemble this material in an effective and expeditious manner and the support provided by his excellent editorial staff. Our heartfelt thanks to the various federal agencies, corporations and foundations, who had the courage and creativity to support the numerous studies that are reported in this volume.

Dr. Genco would like to thank his colleagues at the University of Buffalo, School of Dental Medicine, who have supported and contributed to our efforts in this emerging science, particularly Lou Goldberg for unfailing support of our efforts in periodontal medicine. He thanks his wife, Sandra, for her patience with his hectic schedule which intensified during the editing of the text. She was a wonderful sounding board for ideas about the importance of good health. He also wishes to thank Rose Parkhill for her unceasing efforts in preparing materials, editing, and performing other tasks that are so essential in making such a book possible.

The Editors
August, 1999

Contents

CHAPTER 1

PERIODONTAL DISEASE AND SYSTEMIC DISEASE

D. Walter Cohen, DDS
Harold C. Slavkin, DDS

Health sciences are in the midst of major transitions. The scientific and technologic paradigms of dentistry, medicine, nursing, and pharmacy are changing as well as the management and financing of health care, the demographics of the United States, the patterns of disease, and even the public's expectations for "quality of life." Marked variations in disease occurrence and survival exist among different subgroups of the population of the United States. Some of these are attributable to factors such as age, gender, ethnicity, sexual orientation, geographic locations, and socioeconomic status. This chapter describes the scientific advances and responsibilities for health professionals, to help them revisit how we address the connections between a number of oral microbial infections and major systemic diseases and how we manage the oral complications of systemic diseases.

On a macro level, scientific and technologic advances are defining new paradigms for dentistry, medicine, nursing, and pharmacy to which traditional theory may not apply. Improved understanding of human biology at the molecular level is rapidly advancing and may make invasive surgery, intensive care units, and long-term home care, for example, far less necessary in the not too distant future. Costly and often clinically inadequate interventions may soon be replaced by the postgenomic products of gene-based diagnostics and therapeutics, innovations from bioengineering and biomaterials, and progress toward understanding individual, family, and community behaviors.

Advances over infectious diseases have been hindered by changes in the patient population. Increasingly older and medically compromised patients, including immunosuppressed ones, now constitute a significant proportion of the seriously infected population. Health professionals use immunosuppressive drugs in patients to prevent the rejection of transplants, and patients can become immunosuppressed as a consequence of many of the treatments for neoplastic and inflammatory diseases. Some infections, most notably those caused by the human immunodeficiency virus (HIV), immunocompromise the host in and of themselves. Lesser degrees of immunosuppression are associated with many other infections, such as influenza, viral meningitis, and a number of sexually transmitted diseases, such as syphilis. The microenvironment of immunosuppression can induce the prominence of once obscure microbes, such as *Pneumocystis carni, Cryptosporidium parvum, Mycobacterium avium,* and *Candida albicans.*

There is growing evidence that a number of complex human diseases are caused or profoundly influenced by opportunistic infections, such as in Legionnaire's disease, Lyme disease, gastric ulcer and gastric cancers, a number of other malignancies, cardiovascular disease, low-birth-weight premature babies, and osteoarthritis. As a consequence, there has been a resurgence of interest in oral microbial ecology, so-called "biofilms," mucosal immunity, and systemic diseases throughout the human lifespan. This renewed interest is taking place at a time when advances in epidemiology, microbiology, immunology, molecular biology and cell biology have enabled meaningful questions regarding oral infections and systemic diseases to be addressed.

This chapter introduces the theme of oral infection associated with systemic diseases and highlights the rapidly expanding understanding of microbial ecology, mucosal immunity, and complex human diseases.

ORAL INFECTION AND SYSTEMIC DISEASE: A PARADIGM SHIFT

The adult human body consists of 10^{13} somatic cells, and 10^{14} normal or commensal mirobes. These commensal bacteria reside on the surfaces of teeth and/or prosthetic implants within complex ecosystems termed "biofilms," and they reside on the surfaces of the mucosal epithelia that line the oral cavity, respiratory tract, esophagus, gastrointestinal tract, and urinary tract. Under a variety of conditions, some of these microorganisms become opportunistic and are associated with local or systemic infections, such as *Hemophilus influenza, Streptococcus pneumonia, Neisseria meningitis,* and *Staphylococcus aureus* infection.

The oral cavity contains almost half the commensal bacteria in the human body; approximately 6 billion microbes representing 300 to 500 species reside in the oral cavity. The oral microbial ecosystem is remarkably dynamic. During human development, viruses, bacteria, and yeast are transmitted from mother to child and, in addition, microbes are transmitted from caretaker to child, from spouse to spouse, and can be also acquired from the environment.

The oral microbial ecology is extremely sensitive to the potential insults that confront the human hosts throughout their lifespan. From fetal life through senescence, the oral cavity is continuously challenged by opponunistic infections on the one hand and the oral complications of systemic diseases and disorders on the other. These dynamic interactions between hosts and pathogens are the essence of a paradigm shift in oral medicine. There is growing evidence that oral bacteria contribute to systemic disease. One of the best documented examples is the involvement of the gram-positive *Streptococcus sanguis* and *Streptococcus oralis* in infective endocarditis.

An association between oral infections and systemic diseases has been suspected for centuries. The effect of oral health on the rest of the human body was proposed by the Assyrians in the seventh century BC. In the 18th century, a Pennsylvania physician named Benjamin Rush was quoted as remarking that arthritis could be treated in some people after they had infected teeth extracted. Over the past decade, a growing body of scientific evidence suggests an exquisite association between oral infection (eg, viruses, bacteria, yeast) and systemic diseases (eg, atherosclerosis, cardiovascular disease, cerebrovascular disease, prematurity and low birth weight, and pulmonary diseases and disorders) and also between systemic diseases (eg, arthritis, diabetes, HIV infection, and osteoporosis) and oral, dental, and craniofacial diseases and disorders.

Transmissible and opportunistic microorganisms are responsible for dental caries. Transmissible and opportunistic microorganisms are also responsible for periodontal diseases. In the case of periodontal diseases, the microbial-induced infection presents a substantial infectious burden to the entire body. Further, specific microorganisms within the microbial ecology associated with the disease process release toxins that invoke an inflammatory response. Bacteria, bacterial toxins, localized tissue response cytokines, and other inflammatory mediators enter the vascular circulation and may activate a systemic response. The subsequent pathogenesis of the disease process reflects gene–gene and gene–environment interactions. Nested in a complex interaction of host susceptibility, external exposures, and life-style behaviors, the management of health and disease will require interdisciplinary education, strategies, and health-care delivery. These scientific and technologic advances are creating new paradigms.

ANATOMIC PRIMER OF THE PERIODONTIUM

The following provides an anatomic primer of the periodontium to facilitate the reader's understanding of this chapter and those to follow. The periodontium includes those tissues that invest and support the tooth—the gingiva, the cementum covering the root surfaces of each tooth, the periodontal ligament that attaches the tooth root surface to the adjacent alveolar bone process that supports each tooth, and the alveolar bone. The gingiva covers the structures that comprise the attachment apparatus (cementum, ligament, and adjacent alveolar bone). The gingiva is divided into free and attached gingiva. The free gingiva extends from the base of the gingival sulcus to the gingival margin. The tissues extending from the bottom of the sulcus to the mucogingival junction are those that comprise the attached gingiva. Apical to the mucogingival junction, the alveolar mucosa is continuous with the mucous membrane of the lip, cheek, and the floor of the mouth.

The adult dentition presents the gingival margin located on the enamel surface approximately 0.5 to 2.5 mm coronal to the cervical line of each tooth. The gingival margin is rounded and is adjacent to the opening of the gingival sulcus, which is normally 2 to 4 mm in depth. Placing of a calibrated instrument, such as a periodontal probe, into the gingival sulcus provides the clinician with a measurement referred to as the probing depth.

The term "pocket" is used to describe the histopathology in the soft and possibly the underlying bony tissues, reflecting an inflammatory response to oral infection. "Pocket" is used to differentiate from the healthy gingival sulcus. The gingival sulcus contains fluid. The gingival sulcus fluid in disease reflects inflammation as measured by the levels of cytokines and tissue necrosis factor. Pocket depth and pocket levels of cytokine biomarkers can be used to monitor health and disease.

There are two major forms of periodontal disease (Table 1–1). One is gingivitis, in which the most apical portion of the junctional epithelium is on the enamel, or at or near the cementoenamel junction (Table 1–2). Periodontitis occurs when the periodontal ligament, the connective tissues that attach the tooth to the Alveolar Bone is destroyed by the inflammatory process. This is associated with apical migration of the junctional epithelium onto the root surface beyond the cementoenamel junction. Periodontal disease occurs in the presence and absence of systemic conditions (Table 1–3). For example, gingivitis may occur simply associated with dental plaque, in which case it is called marginal gingivitis. It may also occur as a result of systemic involvement such as gingivitis in AIDS patients and hyperplastic gingival conditions associated with intake of drugs such as phenytoin, cyclosporine, nifedipine, and the dihydropyridines.

Periodintitis occurs as two major forms: adult and juvenile or early onset. The adult form may occur in the presence or absence of systemic complications. Juvenile forms are usually associated with abnormalities in neutrophil functions.

Structure of the Periodontium

The gingival tissues are covered with keratinized and parakeratinized epithelia. The gingival epithelium has three components: oral, sulcular, and junctional. The underlying dermis or connective tissue beneath the gingival epithelium connects the gingiva to the tooth root cementum and the adjacent alveolar process (Figure 1–1). The gingiva is firm and is tightly attached to the tooth and the alveolar process by the supra-alveolar connective tissue fibers. The gingival tissues are covered with oral epithelium which is usually keratinized.

The lining of the gingival sulcus is sulcular epithelium which resembles the oral epithelium but is not keratinized. The base of the sulcus is formed by the junctional epithelium, which consists of a thin layer of epithelium that joins the gingival connective tissue to the tooth surface (Figure 1–1). In recently erupted teeth, the junctional epithelium extends from the bottom of the gingival sulcus to the apical border of the enamel tooth surface. The thickness of epithelial tissue varies from 15 to 30 cells in the vicinity of the gingival sulcus to as few as 1 cell at its apical extension. The junctional epithelim is not keratinized. The sulcular and junctional epithelia form the critical anatomic location at which bacterial biofilms of the subgingival microbiota interact with host defense mechanisms.

Supra-alveolar Connective Tissue

The dermis of the gingiva coronal to the alveolar crest comprises the supra-alveolar connective tissue and consists of fibers, cells, blood vessels, and nerves, in a rich dense connective tissue. The principal cell is the gingival fibroblast, which produces the main elements of the connective tissue. There are also undifferentiated mesenchymal cells, macrophages, and mast cells. Types I and III collagen, elastin, and fibronectin, along with proteoglycans, assemble into the reticular fibers that are observed beneath the basement membrane adjacent to the epithelium, and they are also seen in the connective tissue stroma associated with blood vessels. The greatest part of the gingival connective tissue are the collagen fibers; some are arranged in distinct bundles with a definite orientation. There are bundles that run around the tooth in a ring-like pattern and are referred to as circular fibers. Interdentally, there are bundles that run from the cementum of one tooth to another and are called the trans-septal fibers. Other fibers may not be in a distinct pattern. The dentogingival fibers are bundles that arise from

---

TABLE 1–1. Diseases of the Periodontal Tissues

I. Gingival diseases and conditions
   A. Gingivitis (no systemic involvement)
   B. Gingivitis and gingival changes with systemic involvement

II. Periodontal Diseases and Conditions
   A. Periodontitis in adults (no systemic involvement)
   B. Periodontitis in juveniles
   C. Periodontitis with systemic involvement
   D. Occlusal traumatism

TABLE 1–2. Gingival Diseases and Conditions

A. Gingivitis
1. Marginal gingivitis
2. Acute necrotizing ulcerative gingivitis (ANUG)
B. Gingivitis and other gingival changes with systemic involvement
1. Gingival changes associated with sex hormones
   a. "Pregnancy" gingivitis
   b. Gingivitis associated with oral contraceptives
   c. Gingivitis associated with other hormonal alterations (eg. Polycystic ovaries, puberty, and menopause)
2. Gingival changes associated with diseases of the skin and mucous membranes
   a. Pemphigus
   b. Cicatrical pemphigoid
   c. Bullous pemphigoid
   d. Lichen planus
   e. Psoriasis
   f. Desquamative gingivitis
   g. Lupus erythmatosus
   h. Erythma multiforme
   i. Idiopathic gingival fibromatosis
   j. Recurrent aphthous stomatitis
3. Gingivitis in generalized systemic diseases
   a. Diabetes
   b. Acute leukemia
   c. Thrombocytopenia
   d. Hemophilia
   e. Sturge-Weber syndrome
   f. Wegener's granulomatosis
   g. Sclerosis
   h. Hypodrenocorticism
   i. Vitamin C deficiency
   j. AIDS
   k. Sarcoidosis
4. Infective gingivostomatitis
   a. Herpetic gingivostomatitis
   b. Herpes zoster
   c. Herpangina
   d. Syphilis
   e. Candidiasis
   f. Actinomycosis
   g. Histoplasmosis
5. Drug-associated gingival changes
   a. Systemic medications
      i. Phenytoin (Dilantin)
      ii. Sodium valproate
      iii. Cyclosporine
      iv. The dihydropyridines: nifedipine (Prodardia) and nitrendipine
   b. Compounds with local effects
      i. Caustic compounds
      ii. Heavy metals

the cementum and run parallel to the sulcus. Another group runs at right angles to the root surface; yet another group emerges from the cementum, passes over the alveolar crest, and blends with the mucoperiosteum of the gingiva, and these fibers are called dento-peristeal fibers.

Blood Supply of Gingiva

The gingival tissues are rich in blood vessels, which have their origins from the supraperiosteal vessels originating from the lingual, mental, buccinator, and palatine arteries. These vessels give off branches along the facial and oral surfaces of the alveolar process. Branches of the alveolar arteries may penetrate the interdental septa or from the coronal parts of the periodontal ligament. Numerous capillaries are seen immediately below the basement membrane of the sulcular, junctional, and oral epithelium.

Clinical Criteria of Healthy Gingiva

Healthy gingiva is usually pink in color, well adapted to the teeth, with a stippled surface texture, and bound tightly to the underlying alveolar process and the roots of the dentition (Figure 1–2). The gingival sulcus varies in depth from 1 to 3 mm and shows no signs of bleeding when probed. Histologically, it has been shown that a small number of lymphocytes and plasma cells are observed in the connective tissue of the gingiva under the sulcular epithelium in health gingiva as elsewhere in the gastrointestinal tract.

Attachment Apparatus

Attachment of the tooth to the alveolus consists of numerous bundles of collagenous tissue (principal fibers) arranged in groups in between, which is loose connective tissue together with blood vessels, lymph vessels, and nerves. This attachment apparatus functions as the investing and supporting mechanism for the tooth. It comprises the cementum of the tooth, the periodontal ligament, and the alveolar process. The periodontal ligament is the tissue that surrounds the roots of the tooth and attaches it to the bony alveolus. Cementum is the hard tissue covering the anatomic roots of the teeth. The alveolar process is made up of the alveolar bone and supporting bone and the outer cortical bone. The alveolar bone that lines the tooth socket is termed the lamina dura. In addition to its supportive function, the dentoalveolar unit has sensory, nutritional, and formative roles to play.

Cementum

Cementum is the calcified tissue that covers the roots of the teeth and is deposited during tooth formation. There are two types of root cementum: acellular and cellular. The acellular type is clear and structureless and is formed by cementoblasts, which do not become embedded in it as they do when the cellular type is formed. Those collagen fibers that become embedded in the cementum are known as Sharpey's fibers (Figure 1–3). Most of the root is covered by acellular cementum, with cellular cementum forming on the apical portions of the root. Cellular cementum is bone-like, with the cementocytes embedded in it. Cementum is unlike bone in that it does not remodel throughout life. Incremental lines of cementum deposition are seen with the aging of the individual. These dark-staining lines also reflect the activities or function of the tooth, with cementoblasts continuing to line the cemental surface throughout life and compensating for the physiologic movements of the tooth within the attachment apparatus.

Alveolar Process

The alveolar process consists of osseous tissue, and the alveolar bone is the portion that lines the tooth socket. It is thin compact bone containing small openings through which blood vessels, nerves, and lymphatics pass. The alveolar bone contains the embedded ends of the connective tissue fibers of the periodontal ligament known as Sharpey's fibers (see Figure 1–3). The supporting bone is the cancellous bone between the alveolar bone and the cortical plates. This supporting bone or spongiosa makes up the greatest part of the interdental septum but is much more active than cementum, showing areas of resorption and deposition. It is composed of a network of osteocytes and extracellular matrix. The calcified portion consists of apatite crystals. Alveolar bone is deposited next to the periodontal ligament by the osteoblasts and is reinforced by the supporting bone. Larger vessels are found in the inter-radicular bony process and branches from them to enter the periodontal ligament through the numerous openings in the cribiform plate.

Periodontal Ligament

The fibers of the periodontal ligament that attach the tooth to the alveolar bone are arranged in groups according to their direction, with the alve-

TABLE 1–3. Periodontal Diseases and Conditions

A. Periodontitis in adults
   1. AAP Classification I, II, III, IV
   2. Epidemiologic; moderately and rapidly progressing periodontitis
   3. Clinical based on treatment; refractory and recurrent
   4. Clinical based on history; recurrent acute necrotizing ulcerative periodontitis and postlocalized juvenile periodontitis
B. Periodontitis in juveniles
   1. Localized juvenile periodontitis
   2. Generalized juvenile periodontitis
C. Periodontitis with systemic involvement
   1. Periodontitis in primary neutrophil disorders
      a. Agranulosytosis
      b. Cyclic neutropenia
      c. Chediak-Higashi syndrome
      d. Neutrophil adherence abnormalities
      e. Job's syndrome
      f. "Lazy leukocyte" syndrome
      g. Neutrophil functional syndrome
   2. Periodontitis in systemic diseases with secondary or associated neutrophil impairment
      a. Diabetes mellitus type I
      b. Diabetes mellitus type II
      c. Papillon-LeFevre syndrome
      d. Down's syndrome
      e. Inflammatory bowel disease: Crohn's disease
      f. Preleukemic syndrome
      g. Addison's Disease
      h. AIDS
   3. Other systemic diseases associated with changes in the structures of the periodontal attachment apparatus
      a. Ehlers-Danlos syndrome (VIII)
      b. Histiocytosis (Cosinophilic granuloma)
      c. Sarcoidosis
      d. Scleroderma
      e. Hypophosphatasia
      f. Hypoadrenocorticism
      g. Hyperthyroidism
D. Miscellaneous conditions affecting the periodontium
   1. Periodontal abscesses
   2. Periodontal cysts
   3. Ankylosis
   4. Root resorption
   5. Periodontal-pulpal communicating lesions
   6. Pericoronal abscesses
   7. Dentinal hypersensitivity
   8. Retained roots
   9. Bony sequestration
   10. Infections associated with fractured roots, or anatomic defects
   11. Neoplasms of the attachment apparatus
E. Occlusal traumatism

olar crest fibers running from the alveolar crest to the cementum. The horizontal fibers pass in a perpendicular fashion from tooth to bone. Most of the fibers are in the oblique group, which run from the alveolus in an apical direction to the cementum. The apical fiber group surrounds the apex of the root. In multirooted teeth, the fibers running from the inter-radicular crest to the furcation are called the inter-radicular fibers.

The ligament is made up of collagen fibers, which are arranged in bundles (see Figure 1–3). Research suggests that there is a high turnover of

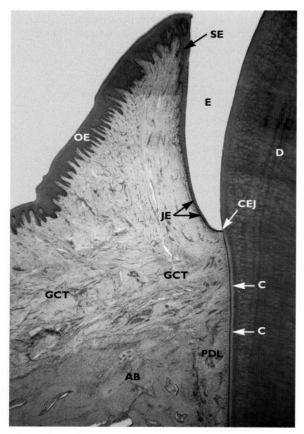

Figure 1–1. Histology of the healthy periodontium. E = enamel; C = cementum of the root surface; CEJ = cemento-enamel junction; D = dentin; OE = oral epithelium; SE = sulcular epithelium; JE = junctional epithelium; GCT = gingival connective tissue; AB = alveolar bone; PDL = periodontal ligament. In health, the junctional epithelium forming the base of the sulcus termiantes at or near the cemento-enamel junction (CEJ). Gingival connective tissue fibers and the fibers of the periodontal ligament insert into root surface cementum. In inflammatory periodontal disease, the connective tissue attachment is destroyed, allowing the juctional epithelium to migrate apically. Alveolar bone is also destroyed. The overall effect is a deepening of the gingival sulcus ("pocket") and a loss of support for the tooth.

collagen in the ligament. It has been observed that the fibers on the cementum side are numerous and relatively thin; they tend to spread out and are interwoven into a network that makes up the greatest width of the ligament. On the bone side, the fiber bundles are fewer in number and are of greater diameter than on the cementum side.

The ligament contains a network of blood vessels and lymph vessels as well as nerve bundles. These vessels are closer to the alveolar side of the ligament and connect with larger vessels in the marrow spaces through the perforations in the alveolar bone.

The cellular components of the periodontal ligament include fibroblasts, cementoblasts, osteoblasts, osteoclasts, and epithelial cell rests.

Regenerative Capacity

The attachment apparatus has been shown to regenerate in certain surgical therapies. The periodontal ligament behaves as a double periosteum, giving rise to the cells that form cementum, bone, and connective tissue as well as numerous growth factors. This capability is of great value to the clinician who is seeking to restore lost supporting tissues.

ORAL INFECTION, SYSTEMIC DISEASE, AND THE GENETIC PARADIGM

The host's reaction to invading microbes (viruses, bacteria, yeast) involves a rapidly amplifying polyphony of signals and responses that may spread beyond the invaded tissue. Fever or hypothermia, tachypnea, and tachycardia often herald the onset of the systemic response to microbial invasion and may be described as bacteremia (viable bacteria in the blood), fungemia (viable yeast in the blood), or septicemia (systemic illness caused by the spread of microbes in the blood).

Commensal bacteria living on tooth and mucosal epithelial cell surfaces create an interactive system, in which the host synthesizes and secretes various immunoglobulins and antibacterial peptides that control this remarkable eucaryotic/procaryotic ecosystem.

Molecular medicine and dentistry are defined as the use of genotypic analysis (DNA testing) to enhance the quality of health care, including presymptomatic identification of predisposition to disease, preventive interventions, selection of pharmacotherapy, and the design and fabrication of gene-based diagnostics and therapeutics.

Genomic progress continues to change the practice of dentistry and medicine. Gene-based diagnostics for viral, bacterial, and yeast infections as well as the numerous clinical applications throughout the human lifespan are continuing to enhance health care. Gene testing for inherited diseases as well as for predisposition to diseases or disorders has enormous potential benefits to improve health care. During 1998, more than 30,000 human genes were isolated, sequenced, and mapped to specific locations on one of the 23 pairs of human chromosomes. By the year 2003, the complete nucleotide sequence of the approximately 100,000 structural and regulatory genes that comprise the human genetic lexicon will be completed. In tandem, the genomes of many significant microbes and animals are also being deciphered, including those of viruses, bacteria, yeast, parasites, plants, animals (eg, fruit fly, zebrafish, mouse, rat), and data from these genomes are being used to revolutionize our thinking about biology, health, and disease. Completion of the microbial genomes of opportunistic viral, bacterial, and yeast species (putative pathogens) as well as the human genome may provide even faster progress in the diagnostics and therapeutics related to oral infections, systemic diseases, and the oral complications of systemic diseases.

Perhaps with the sole exception of trauma, essentially all human diseases are genetic. Genetic dentistry and medicine are based on the paradigm that changes or mutations in individual genes or alleles result in inherited diseases. For example, mutations in the amelogenin gene located on the human X and Y chromosomes can produce X-linked dominant or recessive amelogenesis imperfecta; mutations in the fibroblast growth factor receptor 2 gene can produce Crouzon syndrome as well as other craniofacial syndromes with craniosynostosis; or mutations in a number of transcription factors that regulate development can produce craniofacial malformations. These and other scientific discoveries are rapidly defining single-gene mutations, mapping these individual genes in their precise positions on human chromosomes, and are being used to diagnose inherited clinical phenotypes throughout the human lifespan. Moreover, these advances in human molecular genetics are identifying candidate genes for developing targeted gene-mediated therapeutic approaches to many clinical problems.

Gene mutations define not only the virulence of microbes (viruses, bacteria, yeast, and parasites) but also the fidelity of the human immune system. Of course, microbial as well as human genes are

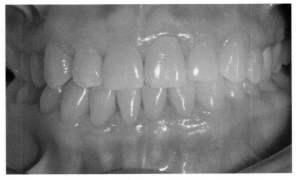

Figure 1–2. Clinical appearance of healthy gingival tissue in a 60 year old female. The gingival tissues are pink and firm. No areas of redness or inflammation are seen. The depth of the gingival sulcus ranges approximately from 1 to 3 mm and does not bleed following probing.

extremely sensitive to environmental "stress" and can and do mutate or change resulting in multidrug and/or antibiotic resistance. The genetic variance within microbial genomes, such as that of *Candida albicans*, may be closely aligned with the host changes associated with immunologically compromised patients. The HIV viral genome is another particularly useful model for considering viral mutation frequency within the human population.

Moreover, genes are also the foundation of even more complex human diseases. First, multiple mutations that are acquired can produce cancers. We now appreciate that all cancers are genetic and that most cancers are not inherited but rather result from acquired multiple mutations. Oropha-

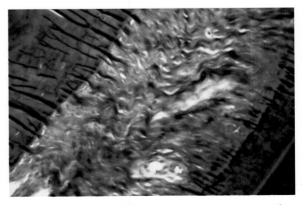

Figure 1–3. Periodontal ligament between the root surface and the alveolar bone. Collagen fibers of the periodontal ligament are arranged in bundles. These fibers (Sharpey's fibers) connect the cementum on the root surface to the alveolar bone. The collagen fibers are destroyed by proteases during inflammatory periodontal disease, allowing the epithelium of the pocket to migrate apically.

ryngeal cancer is the sixth most common neoplastic disease; one American dies every hour of oral cancer. The major "risk factors" for oral cancer are tobacco products and alcohol.

Second, we are beginning to understand that variations or polymorphisms in multiple genes confer susceptibility or resistance to chronic and disabling diseases and disorders, such as osteoporosis, periodontal diseases, and temporomandibular diseases and disorders. In these examples, multiple genes and multiple gene–environment and gene–gene interactions are associated with the molecular pathophysiology of the disease process. For example, single nucleotide polymorphisms (SNPs) in such genes as IL-1α, IL-1β, IL-1 receptor, IL-2, IL-6, IL-10, IL-12, and TNF α in various combinations and in juxtaposition to a number of risk factors may explain genetic susceptibility to periodontal diseases and/or associations with cardiovascular diseases.

The human genome consists of 100,000 genes, and each gene is likely to be represented in the population with 10 variant alleles. To comprehensively cover the entire human genome and have the capacity to identify SNPs, 1 million SNPs will be required. The recent consortia by the federal government and the private sector in SNPs, sufficient to cover the entire human genome, will significantly accelerate the progress toward defining the multiple genes associated with complex human diseases.

These microbial and human genomic databases will provide remarkable opportunities for the identification, design, and production of a new generation of biomarkers for diagnostics and for the development of innovative therapeutics such as drugs and vaccines to improve human health and advance periodontal medicine.

SUMMARY

There is growing evidence that a number of complex human diseases are associated with opportunistic infections in periodontal medicine. As a consequence, there has been a resurgence of interest in oral microbial ecology, mucosal immunity, and associations with systemic conditions, such as prematurity and low birth weight, pulmonary diseases, cardiovascular diseases, and cerebrovascular diseases. This renewed interest in periodontal medicine is taking place at a time when dramatic advances in the fields of microbiology, immunology, molecular biology, and cell biology have allowed in-depth exploration of microbial genomics, oral infections, the human genome project, host immunity, and a variety of systemic diseases and disorders. The following chapters will highlight the many advances and opportunities for improved health care in the 21st century.

SELECTED REFERENCES

Oral Infections and Systemic Disease: A Paradigm Shift

Andrews WW, Goldenberg RL, Hauth JC. Preterm labor: emerging role of genital tract infections. Infect Agent Dis 1995;4(4):196–211.

Drangsholt MT. A new causal model of dental diseases associated with endocarditis. Annals of Periodontology 1998;3(1):184–196.

Davenport ES, Williams ECS, Sterne JAC, Sivanpathasundram V, Fearne JM, Curtis MA. The east london study of maternal chronic periodontal disease and preterm low birth weight infants: study design and prevalence data. Annals of Periodontology 1998;3(1)213–221.

Herzberg MC, Meyer MW. Dental plaque, platelets, and cardiovascular diseases. Annals of Periodontology 1998;3(1):151–160.

Kinane DF. Periodontal diseases' contributions to cardiovascular disease: an overview of potential mechanisms. Annals of Periodontology 1998;3(1):142–150.

Limeback H. Implications of oral infections on systemic diseases in the institutionalized elderly with a special focus on pneumonia. Annals of Periodontology 1998;3(1)262–275.

Loesche WJ, Schork A, Terpenning MS, Chen YM, Kerr C, Dominguez BL. The relationship between dental disease and cerebral vascular accident in elderly united states veterans. Annals of Periodontology 1998;3(1):161–174.

Mealey BL. Periodontal implications: medically compromised patients. Annals of Periodontology 1996;1(1)256–321.

Nishimura F, Takahashi K, Kurihara M, Takashiba S, Murayama Y. Periodontal disease as a complication of diabetes mellitus. Annals of Periodontology 1998;3(1)20–29

Offenbacher S. Periodontal disease: pathogenesis. Ann Periodontol 1996;1(1):821–78.

Page RC, Beck JD. Risk assessment for periodontal disease. Int Dent J 1997;47:61–87.

Petit MDA, Van Steenbergen TJM, Degraaff J, et al. Transmission of *Actinobacillus actinomycetemcomitans* in families of adult periodontitis patients. J Periodontal Res 1996;28:335–45.

Salvi GE, Beck JD, Offenbacher S. Pge₂, Il-1α, and TNF-α responses in diabetics as modifiers of periodontal disease expression. Annals of Periodontology 1998;3(1)40–50.

Scannapieco FA, Papandonatos GD, Dunford RG. Associations between oral conditions and respiratory disease in a national sample survey population. Annals of Periodontology 1998;3(1):251–256.

Slavkin HC. Infection and immunity. J Am Dent Assoc 1996;127:1792–6.

Slavkin HC. Emerging and re-emerging infectious disease. J Am Dent Assoc 1997;128:108–13.

Slavkin HC. And we all lived happily ever after: understanding the biological controls of aging. J Am Dent Assoc 1998;129:629–33.

Slavkin HC. Chronic disabling diseases and disorders. J Am Dent Assoc 1997;128:1583–9.

Slavkin HC. Diabetes, clinical dentistry and changing paradigms. J Am Dent Assoc 1997;128:638–44.

Slavkin HC. Notes on a silent disease. J Am Dent Assoc 1996;127:801–5.

Slavkin HC. An update on HIV/AIDS. J Am Dent Assoc 1996;127:1401–4.

Slavkin HC. The war on oral cavity and pharyngeal cancer. J Am Dent Assoc 1996;127:517–20.

Slavkin HC. First encounters: transmission of infectious oral diseases from mother to child. J Am Dent Assoc 1997;128:773–8.

Soskolne WA. Epidemiological and clinical aspects of periodontal diseases in diabetics. Annals of Periodontology 1998;3(1):3–12.

Von Troil-Linden F, Alahuusua S, Wolf J, et al. Periodontitis patient and the spouse: periodontal bacteria before and after treatment. J Clin Periodontol 1997;2:893–9.

Winn DM, Diehl SR, Horowitz AM, et al. Scientific progress in understanding oral and pharyngeal cancers. J Am Dent Assoc 1998;129:713–8.

Yuan A, Luh KT, Yang PC. Actinobacillus actinomycetemcomitans pneumonia with possible septic embolization (letter). Chest 1994;105:646.

Zijlstra EE, Swart GR, Godfroy FJM, Degener JE. Pericarditis, pneumonia and brain abscess due to a combined actinomyces-actinobacillus actinomycetemcomitans infections. J Infect 1992;25: 83–87.

Anatomic Primer of the Periodontium

Armitage GC. Periodontal diseases: diagnosis. Annals of Periodontology 1996;1(1)37–215.

Genco RJ, Goldman HM, Cohen DW. Contemporary periodontics. St. Louis, MO: The C.V. Mosby Company; 1990.

Page RC. The pathobiology of periodontal diseases may affect systemic diseases: inversion of a paradigm. Annals of Periodontology 1998;3(1)108–120.

Oral Infections, Systemic Disease, and the Genetic Paradigm

Amer A, Singh G, Darke C, Dolby AE. Association between HLA antigens and periodontal disease. Tissue Antigens 1988;31:53–58.

Backman B. Inherited enamel defects. In: Chadwick DJ, Cardew G, editors. Dental enamel. London: John Wiley & Sons Ltd; 1997. p. 175–96.

Baum BJ, Atkinson JC, Baccaglini L, et al. The mouth is a gateway to the body: gene therapy in 21st century dental practice. CDA J 1998;25:455–60.

Bodmer W, McKie R. The book of man: the Human Genome Project and the quest to discover our genetic heritage. New York: Scribner Publishers; 1995.

Boughman JA, Halloran SL, Roulston D, Schwartz S, Suzuki JB, Weitkamp LR, Wenk RE, Wooten R, Cohen MM. Autosomal dominant form of juvenile periodontitis: it's localization to chromosome 4 and linkage to dentinogenesis imperfecta and Gc. Journal of Craniofacial Genetic Development Biology 1986;6:341–350.Porter R. The greatest benefit to mankind. New York: W.W. Norton & Company; 1997.

Chambers DA. DNA: the double helix: 40 years, prospective and perspective. New York: New York Academy of Sciences; 1995.

Cohen MM Jr. Molecular biology of craniosynostosis with special emphasis on fibroblast growth factor receptors. In: Cohen MM Jr, Baum BJ, editors. Studies in stomatology and craniofacial biology. Amsterdam: IOS Press; 1997. p. 307–30.

Field MJ. Dental education at the crossroads. Washington, D.C.: National Academy Press; 1995.

Finch CE, Pike MC. Maximum lifespan predictions from the Gompertz mortality model. J Gernotol 1996;51(3):3183–94.

Hart TC, Marazita ML, McCanna KM, Schenkein HA, Diehl SR. Reevaluation of the chromosome 4q candidate region for early onset periodontitis. Human Genetics 1993;91:416–422.

Kevles BH. Naked to the bone. New Brunswick, New Jersey: Rutgers University Press; 1997.

Kornman KS, Page RC, Tonetti MS. The host response to microbial challenge in periodontitis: assembling the players. Periodontology 2000 14:33–53, 1997

Kornman KS, di Giovine FS. Genetic variations in cytokine expression: a risk factor for severity of adult periodontitis. Annals of Periodontology 1998;3(1)325–338.

Mealey BL. Periodontal implications: medically compromised patients. Ann Periodontol 1996;1(1): 256–321.

Schwartz WB. Life without disease. Berkeley: University of California Press; 1998.

Slavkin HC. Possibilities of growth modification: nature versus nurture. In: MacNamara R, editor. Ann Arbor, Michigan: University of Michigan Press. 1999. [In press]

Slavkin HC. Understanding human genetics. J Am Dent Assoc 1996;127:266–7.

Slavkin HC. Clinical dentistry in the 21st century. Compendium 1997;18(3):212–8.

Slavkin HC. Basic science is the fuel that drives the engine of biotechnology: a personal science transfer vision for the 21st century. Tech Health Care 1996; 4:249–53.

Slavkin HC. Advice to coaches of students in one of the youngest sciences. J Dent Edu 1998;62:226–9.

Toteson DC, Adelstein SJ, Carver ST. New pathways to medical education. Cambridge, Massachusetts: Harvard University Press; 1994.

CHAPTER 2

RISK FACTORS FOR PERIODONTAL DISEASE

Robert J. Genco, DDS, PhD

Periodontal diseases, now recognized as bacterial infections, are among the most common, chronic diseases of humans, affecting 5 to 30% of the adult population in the age group of 25 to 75+ years. Periodontal diseases are also among the most important causes of pain, discomfort, and tooth loss in adults.[1–3] While a significant portion of the population is susceptible to periodontitis, there are those that are relatively resistant to the severe forms of periodontal disease. This leads to the hypothesis that there are susceptibility factors or risk factors that modulate susceptibility or resistance of individuals to destructive periodontal disease.

In addition to being a major cause of discomfort, disfigurement, and tooth loss in the population, emerging evidence suggests that periodontitis increases the risk for certain systemic diseases such as heart disease,[4] low birth weight,[5] respiratory disease,[6] and possibly other conditions.[7] It is clear then that prevention and treatment of periodontal disease are necessary to maintain periodontal health; without periodontal health, general health is often compromised. Present day concepts of management of periodontal disease include primary and secondary prevention, treatment of existing disease to resolve the periodontal infection, and modification of adverse risk factors which increase susceptibility to initial or re-infection with periodontal organisms. The goals of this chapter, therefore, are to provide the reader with (1) an understanding of the microbial etiology and pathogenesis of periodontal infection, (2) detailed knowledge of factors which increase the risk of periodontal disease, and (3) information to be used in assessing individual patients to determine their risk profile or risk level for development of periodontal infection. Information on modification of risk is found in other chapters of this book.

ETIOLOGY

Concepts of the etiology of periodontal disease have changed markedly in the last four decades. Several specific subgingival oral bacteria including *Porphyromonas gingivalis, Actinobacillus actinomycetemcomitans, Prevotella intermedia, Bacteroides forsythus,* and perhaps others such as *Campylobacter rectus, Fusobacterium nucleatum,* and spirochetes are associated with severe forms of periodontal disease.[8] In addition, a group of pathogens not normally found in the oral cavity, except as transients, has been associated with periodontal disease, including *Enterobacteriaceae, Pseudomondacea, Klebsiella* spp and *Acinetobacter* as well as others such as *Staphylococcus aureus,* and *Candida albicans.*[9] Periodontal diseases, therefore, are infections in which severe forms of the disease are often associated with specific bacteria that colonize the subgingival area in spite of the host's protective mechanisms. Many of these bacteria have potent virulence factors such as cytotoxins for mammalian phagocytes produced by *A. actinomycetemcomitans,* a potent array of proteases produced by *P. gingivalis,* and the ability to invade epithelial cells exhibited by *A. actinomycetemcomitans* and *P. gingivalis.*[10] Recently, *P. gingivalis* has also been shown to invade the endothelial cells which may explain, in part, the link between periodontal disease and heart disease.[11]

Studies have linked specific therapies to specific infections in periodontal disease. For example, van Winkelhoff[12] found that amoxicillin with metronidazole was useful in controlling periodontal infection when *A. actinomycetemcomitans* was found in plaque samples. Further, microbiologic tests have been developed and are useful in the assessment of periodontal infection and the selection of appropriate therapies.

PATHOGENESIS

The periodontal pathogens have virulence factors which cause direct damage. However, it appears that a significant contribution to tissue destruction in periodontal disease comes from an imbalance in host protective and destructive mechanisms induced by periodontal infection.[13] Host hyper-responsiveness or reactivity is induced by periodontal infection and includes activation of neutrophils, which migrate to the area of periodontal infection, and induction of antibodies, both of which appear to be protective. On the other hand, extracellular matrix components of the gingiva and periodontal ligament are destroyed and alveolar bone is resorbed mainly through induction of matrix metalloproteinases.[14] This leads to connective tissue destruction and production of proinflammatory cytokines, such as IL-1,[15] resulting in alveolar bone resorption. These cytokines can cause activation of fibroblasts, which then produce major metalloproteinases that destroy the extracellular matrix. In addition, proinflammatory cytokines such as IL-1, IL-6, and TNF-α lead to activation of osteoclasts, which leads to bone resorption. A full description of cytokines and prostaglandins in immune hemostasis and tissue destruction in periodontal disease is reviewed by Gemmell and colleagues.[16]

Briefly, the pathogenesis of periodontal disease could be thought of as a pathway, including direct toxic effects on cells from proteases and toxins produced by bacteria, to triggering of cells by mitogens and antigens. This initially results in a wave of neutrophil chemotaxis and antibody production, which is protective, leading to reduction of the infecting flora. However, several of the periodontal bacteria can evade the neutrophil-protective response by killing neutrophils, inhibiting their function, or digesting antibody and complement. The next wave is the induction of mononuclear cells such as resident macrophages and fibroblasts to produce matrix metalloproteinases, reactive oxygen species, and proinflammatory cytokines, which results in connective tissue destruction and bone resorption. The organisms then eventually appear to be controlled by antibodies that neutralize the toxins and by phagocytes that remove them from the site of infection causing the disease to go into remission. Episodes of periodontal disease exacerbation and remission follow blooms of the organism once the immune response subsides and allows the organism to propagate again, resulting in a repeat of the cycle and recurrence of periodontitis.

It is clear then that host factors play a major role in the pathogenesis of periodontal disease. Exogenous factors such as smoking, which alter immune function and tissue repair, or endogenous or intrinsic factors such as genetic predisposition to hyperproduction of cytokines, low production of antibody, or depressed neutrophils can lead to marked changes in the disease process. These factors then modify the host response to periodontal infection, altering susceptibility to infection by periodontal organisms.

ASSESSMENT OF RISK FACTORS

A risk factor for periodontal disease is a characteristic, an aspect of behavior, or an environmental exposure that is associated with destructive periodontitis.[17] Numerous factors are modifiable while others cannot be easily modified. The term "risk factor" often implies a modifiable condition; however, this is not always the case. Those risk factors that cannot be modified are often called determinants or background factors. The term "risk indicator" is used to describe a possible or putative factor associated with the disease often identified from case-control or cross-sectional studies. True risk factors that are associated with disease are confirmed in longitudinal and interventional studies and by the existence of a biologically plausible mechanism for their actions.[18]

There are several study designs that are useful in the assessment of risk factors for diseases that are considered multifactorial diseases, such as periodontitis. Table 2–1[19] presents a series of study designs ranging from anecdote, to case reports, to case series, to randomized controlled trials that constitute evidence of increasing strength for risk factors. The anecdotes, case reports, and case series provide the weakest evidence for association of risk with disease; however, they are important because they often provide the basis for generating important hypotheses.

The next line of evidence concerning the association between a potential risk factor or risk indicator and disease is provided by case-control studies. Case-control studies can identify risk indicators but often are not able to assess the role of important confounding factors. For this, cross-sectional, population-based studies are necessary because they describe large populations and allow a more rigorous assessment of confounders or co-risk factors by multivariate statistical analysis. Cross-sectional studies are important because they can

TABLE 2–1. Hierarchy of Evidence for Risk Factors*

Study Design	Hypothesis Generating	Hypothesis Testing	Interpretation and Health Policy Implication

1. Anecdote
   case report
   case series
	X		Suggests a relationship

2. Case control	X	X	Evidence for risk indicator
3. Cross-sectional	X	X	Evidence for risk indicator
4. Longitudinal (cohort)		X	Evidence for risk factor

5. Interventional
   • RCT of treatment effects in
     high vs. low risk groups
		X	Evidence for risk factor modulation

• RCT in which risk factor is modified		X	Strongest evidence for specific interaction to apply to population

*Adapted from Ibrahim M. Epidemiology and health policy. Rockville (MD): Aspen Systems Corporation; 1985.
RCT = randomized controlled trial.
Table reprinted with permission from the *Journal of Periodontology*.

lead to identification of risk indicators that are reasonable or plausible correlates of disease.

Longitudinal studies are necessary to provide strong evidence that a risk indicator or a putative risk factor is indeed a true risk factor. Risk indicators are not always confirmed as risk factors in longitudinal studies. Although longitudinal studies provide strong evidence, they are often difficult to carry out for periodontal disease because periodontitis is a slowly progressing disease, and the definition of a new case is by no means clear. However, longitudinal studies are necessary to resolve the temporal sequence of putative risk factors as they are associated with disease. A true risk factor should precede the development of disease.

Analysis of risk is ultimately directed to improving the health of the population. Evidence for efficacy of the elimination or suppression of a risk factor in modulating or reducing disease often is gained from randomized controlled trials in which intervention is rigorously tested. It is important that the mechanism of action of risk factors is biologically plausible to understand how the risk factor exerts its influence on the disease. Also, knowing the mode of action may allow development of effective risk intervention strategies that intercept or modulate the effects of the risk factor on disease.

Accurate and precise measurement of periodontitis can be carried out by assessing several surrogate variables for periodontal disease, such as estimate of alveolar bone destruction by measurement of radiographs, clinical attachment loss, and gingival inflammation including bleeding on probing and probing pocket depth. In large scale clinical epidemiologic studies, relative attachment levels are often measured from an arbitrary but fixed point, such as the cemento-enamel junction, and are better indicators of destructive periodontitis than probing depths.[20] Ideally, both attachment loss and radiographic measurement of alveolar bone loss in epidemiologic studies are carried out. Measurement of alveolar bone loss may be more sensitive than attachment loss in assessing risk factors. This, in fact, has been observed by Grossi and co-workers.[21,22]

Establishment of a definition for a periodontal case is often arbitrary. Various cut-off points for attachment loss, bone loss, and pocket depth have been suggested but none is universally agreed upon. Perhaps the best approach would be to assess the extent and severity of disease in the population and determine cut-off points or case definitions appropriate for the population. Lack of a clear-cut definition of a case of periodontitis has hindered longitudinal studies that attempt to define incidence or occurrence of new cases, and often progression of periodontal disease is used. For example, the rate of periodontal attachment loss using repeated measures and the establishment of step-wise thresholds—based on factors that contribute to error including pocket depth, tooth type, and tooth location—for each individual patient and for examiners have also been used with success to assess risk factors.[23]

RISK ASSESSMENT STUDY DESIGN AND ANALYSIS OF DATA

Correlation or univariate analysis is often seen in older studies of risk, especially in case-control or small cross-sectional studies. The weakness of such analysis resides in the inability of a single correlation analysis to develop comprehensive models of disease since only one or, at most, a few potential risk factors can be analyzed at one time. Also, univariate analysis does not allow for adjustments for confounding or co-risk variables or factors. Powerful, modern statistical analyses using multiple regression models, linear discriminate analysis, and multivariate logistic regression have provided the necessary tools to assess the role of risk factors in periodontal disease. These analyses often make adjustments for confounding factors and are useful in assessing risk. The unit of study in epidemiologic assessment of risk is necessarily the patient. However, data often come from multiple sites in the same patient and hence lead to complex statistical issues. For example, there is often a lack of independence of multiple observations in the same patient, and several approaches to the assessment of relationships between site-specific variables and statistical models assessing risk of periodontal disease have been described.[24–26] Recently, general estimating equations that allow the use of a broad range of regression models that take into account and adjust for the dependence between observations in the same individuals have been described and are in wide use.[27]

Ultimately, however, association studies for risk usually require that there be a concordance of several well-executed studies on different populations. In addition, it is important that the risk factor show some type of dose response; the more the exposure to the risk factor, the worse is the disease. Furthermore, it is important that longitudinal studies show that there is a logical occurrence of the risk factor prior to the development of disease. Finally, for decisions on the clinical importance of the risk factor, it is necessary for the intervention studies to show that modification of the risk factor will result in modification of the disease. It is the confluence of these multiple experimental approaches that leads to confidence in assigning a risk factor to a disease and thereby taking the next step, which is implementation of risk factor modification in practice and in public health.

BACKGROUND FACTORS OR DETERMINANTS

Age

Studies of periodontal disease prevalence, extent, and severity show more disease in older age groups compared with younger groups.[1,21,22,27–29] Several studies also show that there is greater dental plaque and more severe gingivitis in elderly persons compared with younger individuals, suggesting age-related effects.[29] Most studies, however, show that periodontal disease is more severe in the elderly because of the cumulative destruction over a lifetime, rather than an age-related intrinsic deficiency or abnormality that affects susceptibility to periodontal infection. For example, an analysis of the epidemiologic data from the National Health and Nutrition Surveys (NHANES) in the United States concluded that when oral hygiene status was considered, age was not an important factor in determining periodontal disease.[29]

A longitudinal study addressing the cumulative nature of periodontal attachment loss suggests that, at least up to age 70 or 75 years, the rate of periodontal destruction has been the same throughout adulthood.[30] Several other longitudinal studies came to the same conclusion.[31–33] However, Ismail and colleagues[34] from the Tecumseh study found that age was a significant factor in a multivariate model relating greater attachment loss to age. However, it is instructive to note that in this study, the age range of individuals was >65 or 70 years, the maximum age in most of the other studies. It appears that age, per se, is not an intrinsic risk factor, at least until the age of 70 or 75 years. It is still unknown whether the deterioration of host-protective mechanisms or the acceleration of host-destructive mechanisms affects susceptibility to periodontal disease beyond age 70 or 75 years. Indeed, there may be an increased risk of periodontal disease associated with advanced age; per se, however, this does not appear to be manifested before age 70 or 75 years. Further work is needed to resolve this issue.

Race

Assessment of risk factors related to race, socioeconomic status, and poverty have been unsuccessful in making associations with periodontal disease. For example, in recent studies where periodontal status was adjusted for oral hygiene and smoking, the association between lower socioeconomic status and more severe periodontal disease was not seen.[21,22]

In a study of risk indicators for African American and Caucasian Americans, there were more indicators related to socioeconomic status for the former than for the latter. For example, *Prevotella intermedia* was a risk indicator for African Americans, but not for Caucasian Americans. However, when persons from both races belong to the same socioeconomic group, differences in periodontal disease often disappeared.[21,22,35] Further studies are necessary to look at the relative role of race and ethnicity, which may be tied to genetic factors in Asians, Native Americans, Hispanics, and other racial and ethnic groups in the American population.

Gender

Periodontal disease is regularly reported to be more prevalent or more severe in men than in women at comparable ages.[1,21,22,36] Men exhibit poorer oral hygiene and report fewer visits to the dentist than do women.[37] However, when correcting for oral hygiene, socioeconomic status, visits to the dentist, and age, being male is still associated with more severe disease when either attachment loss or bone height is used as a measure of periodontal disease.[21,22]

Assessment of the effects of hormones, particularly the female hormone estrogen, which likely protect against destructive periodontal bone loss, may help us understand the small but definite increase in periodontal disease seen in men.

SYSTEMIC RISK FACTORS AND RISK INDICATORS

Two groups of systemic factors are associated with periodontal disease.[38] One group includes smoking and diabetes mellitus, for which there is considerable evidence based on cross-sectional, longitudinal, intervention, and mechanism studies, and it is reasonable to call these true risk factors. Certainly, modification of these factors is important in the management of periodontal disease.

The second set of factors associated with periodontal disease is related to an earlier stage of development and understanding and are probably best called risk indicators at this point. These include osteopenia and osteoporosis; stress, distress, and coping; dietary factors including calcium and vitamin C; and genetic factors. There are also a group of immune system diseases such as AIDS; primary and secondary neutrophil disorders, such as congenital neutropenia and drug-related agranulocytosis; and diseases affecting host response, such as Papillon-Lefèvre syndrome, Ehlers-Danlos syndrome, and hypophosphatasia, which are associated with more severe disease in juveniles and likely significantly increase the risk for periodontal disease.

Tobacco Use

In spite of the long history of the association between tobacco smoking and periodontal disease,[39–41] the observation that greater levels of plaque and calculus in smokers may have accounted for the association failed to convince the community of the importance of smoking and periodontal disease risk. However, in 1983, Ismail and co-workers analyzed smoking and periodontal disease and found that smoking remained a major risk indicator for periodontal disease after adjusting for potential confounding variables, such as age, oral hygiene, and socioeconomic status.[42]

In recent studies,[21,22] smoking was shown to be a strong risk indicator for periodontal disease with an odds ratio of 2.0 to 5.0 when using clinical attachment loss as a measurement. Odds ratios of 1.5 to 7.0 were achieved when using alveolar bone loss as a measure of periodontal disease in these studies. These studies were adjusted for age, gender, socioeconomic status, plaque, and calculus, and hence strongly implicate cigarette smoking per se as a major risk indicator for periodontal disease. Grossi and co-workers[21,22] also found a direct and linear dose response between level of smoking (pack years) and destructive periodontitis, supporting the contention that smoking is a risk factor for periodontal disease (Figure 2–1). Longitudinal studies have confirmed that current smokers exhibited greater disease progression as compared with nonsmokers.[43] Attachment loss is also directly related to serum cotinine levels.[44] A longitudinal study of the association between smoking and tooth loss over a 10-year period was carried out in 273 individuals.[45] Younger individuals who smoked more than 15 cigarettes per day had the highest risk. In this study, the odds ratio for association of smoking with periodontitis, adjusted for age and gender, for current smokers relative to

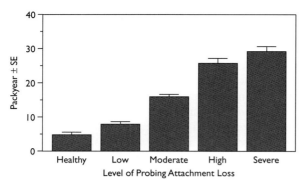

Figure 2–1. The relationship of more severe periodontal disease as assessed by increasing levels of probing attachment loss, with increasing exposure to cigarette smoking (expressed as packyears) is depicted. (Figure is reprinted with permission from Grossi SG, Zambon JJ, Ho AW, et al. Assessment of risk for periodontal disease. I. Risk indicators for attachment loss. J Periodontol 1994; 65:260–7.)

those who never smoked, was 3.3, and for former smokers versus those who never smoked, the odds ratio was 2.1. These longitudinal studies provide convincing evidence, along with other lines of evidence, that tobacco use is a major risk factor for periodontal disease.

Although direct intervention studies of periodontal disease in smokers who have quit smoking have not been carried out, other studies show that periodontal therapies are less effective in smokers than in nonsmokers, and recurrence of disease is more likely in smokers after periodontal therapy.[44–53] Also, smoking cessation appears to yield clinical benefits.[21,22,52,54–56] In these reports, the periodontal status of former smokers is comparable with that of nonsmokers. In the study by Grossi and colleagues,[52] there was no relationship to time of cessation of smoking (although cessation times of less than 1 year were not observed), which suggests that smoking cessation for as little as 1 year results in healing after periodontal therapy comparable with that in a nonsmoker.

The mechanisms by which cigarette smoking affects the periodontal tissues are quite diverse. Smoking causes constriction of the blood vessels of the gingiva[57] and has deleterious effects on leukocyte function.[58] Smoking also has been shown to suppress serum antibody levels to certain periodontal bacteria.[59–60] The effect may be specific since smoking suppresses production of the IgG_2 class of immunoglobulin both in patients with periodontitis and in those with normal periodontium.[59–60] Smoking also may have direct effects on tissues. For example, cytotoxic substances can penetrate the

epithelium and may exert deleterious effects on fibroblasts.[61] Smoking also decreases intestinal absorption of calcium and may thereby affect osteoblast function and increase bone loss in otherwise healthy postmenopausal women.[62,63] Postsurgical healing may be interfered with by absorption of the toxic substances in tobacco smoke by the root surfaces.[51,64] Recently, two studies have shown the adverse effects of smoking on the subgingival flora.[65,66] While there is no evidence that the use of smokeless tobacco increases susceptibility to periodontal disease, smokeless tobacco may affect gingival inflammation by affecting levels of IL-1β and PGE in gingival tissues.[67,68] Although there is no direct evidence, it is likely that cigar and pipe smoking will have effects similar to cigarette smoking if the exposures are comparable. It is clear that there are many mechanisms by which the components of tobacco smoke can deleteriously affect periodontal tissues.

Diabetes Mellitus

There is a large body of evidence supporting the association between diabetes mellitus and periodontal diseases. There is remarkable consistency in finding either greater prevalence, severity, or extent of at least one manifestation of periodontal disease in the overwhelming majority of these studies. Studies of children and adolescents with type 1 diabetes and a group of similar ages without diabetes found greater periodontal disease in the diabetics as compared to the controls.[69–77] However, Goteiner and colleagues[78] did not find such a relationship. In another group of studies, subjects between the ages of 15 and 35 years with type 1 diabetes were assessed and, essentially, all the studies found greater periodontal disease in the diabetics.[79–84] A set of studies of insulin-dependent diabetics, presumably mostly type 1, in adults 20 to 70 years of age, also found greater periodontal disease in diabetics as compared with controls.[85–88]

A series of studies of type 2 diabetic subjects also has been reported, and the investigators reported greater periodontal disease in the diabetics than in the controls.[89–95] In a longitudinal study,[89] the increased relative risk of advanced periodontal disease in the diabetics was found to be 2.6 (95% CI 1.0 to 6.6). A further study of the same population by Taylor and colleagues[96] showed that type 2 diabetes was a significant risk factor for progression of alveolar bone loss with an odds ratio of 4.2 (95% CI 1.8 to 9.9).

There are a series of studies that do not separate type 1 and type 2 diabetes and, in general, these also support an association of diabetes with periodontal disease.[21,97,98] In the study by Grossi and colleagues,[21] the estimates of association between diabetes and attachment loss severity had an odds ratio of 2.3 (95% CI 1.2 to 4.6). Hence, it is clear from case-control, cross-sectional, and longitudinal studies that diabetes is a significant risk factor for periodontal disease.

Randomized controlled trials of the effects of therapy on both periodontal disease and diabetes status have also provided evidence that treatment of periodontal disease can be successfully carried out in diabetics. Furthermore, resolution of periodontal infections in diabetics can contribute to the management of glycemic control in type 1 or type 2 diabetes (see Chapter 8).[52,99,100] The study by Aldridge and colleagues[99] did not show a beneficial effect but the two studies by Grossi and colleagues[52,100] did show a beneficial effect. Perhaps it is significant that in the Grossi studies, systemic doxycycline was used. Miller and colleagues[101] also used systemic doxycycline and mechanical therapy and found an effect on glycemic control, pointing to the possible effect of antibiotics in this beneficial response.

Further rigorous, controlled studies of treatment of periodontal disease in diabetics are needed to confirm the extent to which treatment not only resolves periodontal infection but enhances glycemic control. Further studies also are needed to assess the extent to which control of the diabetes status is related to control of periodontal disease status. Case reports as well as clinical experience do support this contention. However, randomized controlled trials are needed to fully assess the extent to which glycemic control in diabetics will prevent or minimize periodontal destruction.

Acquired Immune Deficiency Syndrome and Other Immunodeficiencies

Systemic diseases, especially those that compromise the host's ability to fend off infections, often lead to more severe periodontal disease. There are studies that describe severe forms of destructive periodontal disease in acquired immune deficiency syndrome (AIDS) patients, resulting in necrotizing ulcerative lesions, often affecting the alveolar bone. Furthermore, a "linear" form of gingivitis has also been described in AIDS patients. A wide variety of oral lesions have been described in persons infected with HIV,[102] the etiologic agent for AIDS. Several reviews of the oral manifestations of HIV infection have been published recently.[103–105]

Oral Candidiasis

Oral candidiasis is an infection of the oral tissues by yeasts of the genus *Candida*, and its association with severe underlying disease has been noted for many years.[106] Oral candidiasis is rarely seen in previously healthy individuals[107] and is often seen as part of the acute HIV syndrome.[108] It can also be a common problem when CD4 lymphocyte counts fall.[109] There are four clinical variants of oral candidiasis including pseudomembranous, erythematous, hyperplastic, and angular cheilitis.[110] Both the pseudomembranous and erythematous forms of candidiasis appear to be important predictors of progression of HIV infection.[107–111]

Oral Hairy Leukoplakia

Oral hairy leukoplakia is an oral lesion that was first reported in the early days of the AIDS epidemic.[112–113] In HIV-positive persons, oral hairy leukoplakia predicts more rapid progression to AIDS.[109] Oral hairy leukoplakia is associated with the Epstein-Barr virus and generally occurs infrequently among immunocompetent individuals.[114–115]

Non-Hodgkin's Lymphoma

Non-Hodgkin's lymphoma and Kaposi's sarcoma are two AIDS-associated malignancies that can occur in the mouth. Because it involves the gingivae, non-Hodgkin's lymphoma is frequently mistaken for common periodontal or dental infections.[116]

Linear Gingival Erythema

Periodontal disease in AIDS patients often presents in several forms. A gingival lesion known as linear gingival erythema (formerly known as HIV-gingivitis) has been described in HIV-infected individuals.[117–118] It is characterized by a red band on the marginal and attached gingiva, and does not resolve with routine dental curettage and prophylaxis.[109]

Necrotizing Ulcerative Periodontitis

Necrotizing ulcerative periodontitis (formerly known as HIV periodontitis) also can occur in HIV-infected individuals. It is characterized by painful, ulcerative, bleeding lesions of the gingiva which often are rapidly destructive and involve the deep periodontal tissues and alveolar bone.[109–119] Necrotizing ulcerative periodontitis may be generalized or localized and may lead to tooth loss and bone sequestration.

Neutrophil Disorders

Severe periodontal disease may also occur in patients with neutrophil abnormalities, and many of these conditions are reviewed by Van Dyke and colleagues.[120] Patients with neutrophil defects that are either quantitative (neutropenia) or qualitative (adherence, chemotaxis, microbicidal functional activity) often suffer from oral mucosal ulcerations, gingivitis, and periodontitis. Severe oral disease occurs with both primary and secondary neutrophil abnormalities. The primary neutrophil disorders characterized by severe periodontal disease include neutropenia (chronic or cyclic), leukocyte adhesion deficiency (LAD), and Chédiak-Higashi syndrome. Neutrophil abnormalities that occur secondary to underlying systemic disease and those that are also associated with severe periodontal disease include diabetes, Papillon-Lefèvre syndrome, Down syndrome, hyperimmunoglobulin-E recurrent infection syndrome (HIE or Job's syndrome), inflammatory bowel disease, Crohn's disease, preleukemic syndrome, AIDS, and acute myeloid leukemia.[121] Drugs which induce agranulocytosis, including some drugs used to treat cancer, can result in mucositis or periodontal disease. Other conditions such as acatalasia, alpha-1 antitrypsin deficiency, and Ehlers-Danlos syndrome are also described in which periodontal disease is more severe, some of which may well involve neutrophil abnormalities.

Hence, it appears that neutrophil disorders that are either primary neutrophil dyscrasias, secondary to systemic diseases, or result from chemotherapy are often associated with severe periodontal disease. Hence, neutrophil dysfunction is a risk factor for periodontitis, most likely as it lowers the host resistance to periodontal infection by subgingival microflora.

Osteoporosis

Osteoporosis is one of the most important health concerns in the United States. It affects over 20 million people, most of whom are women, and causes nearly two million fractures per year. Osteoporosis is a physiologic, gender-, and age-related condition resulting from bone mineral content loss. It is a disease characterized by low bone mass and fragility, which in turn may lead to increase in fractures. Primary osteoporosis includes postmenopausal osteoporosis, age-related osteoporosis, and idiopathic osteoporosis. Secondary osteoporosis is that caused by an identifiable agent or disease. The rate of bone mineral density (BMD) loss is approximately two times greater in women than in men, and postmenopausal osteoporosis is a heterogeneous disorder that begins after natural or surgical menopause and leads to fractures within 15 to 20 years from the cessation of ovarian function.

Cortical bone loss is, on average, 0.3 to 0.5% per year until menopause. At menopause, 2 to 3% loss per year occurs for the next 8 to 10 years. Trabecular bone is lost at a greater rate, with 4.8% being lost per year in the 5 to 8 years following menopause. This loss occurs when an imbalance is caused by more bone resorption than formation. Calcium balance, vitamin D metabolism, estrogens, and aging are interrelated factors in the causation of osteoporosis.

Osteoporosis has long been suspected as a systemic risk factor for loss of oral bone, including loss of the alveolar process associated with periodontal infection. From assessment of osteoporosis in the jaws by dual photon absorptiometry,[122–126] it was found that reduction in total skeletal mass is directly related to reduction in mandibular density in osteoporotic women.[127–128] Studies by Kribbs and Chesnut[129] and Henrikson and Wallenius[130] showed that mandibular BMD correlated with skeletal BMD. Ortman and colleagues[131] found a significantly higher percentage of women with severe alveolar ridge resorption than men, which may be related to the findings of Humphries and colleagues[132] showing that age-related loss of BMD in an edentulous adult mandible is important in females but not in males.

As shown by Daniell[133] and Krall and colleagues,[134] who conducted a study of estrogen replacement after menopause and tooth retention in 488 women, osteoporosis is clearly related to tooth loss. Estrogen users had more teeth than did nonusers, and the duration of estrogen use independently predicted the number of remaining teeth.

Several studies have shown a relationship between periodontal disease and osteoporosis. For example, Von Wowren,[124] in a case control study of 12 female patients with osteoporotic fractures compared with 14 normal women, found significantly more loss of periodontal attachment in osteoporotic women than normal women. Groen and colleagues[135] found edentulism and severe periodontal disease among 38 patients, who exhibited severe radiographic evidence of osteoporosis. Wactawski-Wende and colleagues[136] found a relationship between alveolar crestal bone height as a measure of periodontal disease and skeletal osteopenia. It appears that osteopenia, measured as BMD of the trochanter and total femur, was related to both greater probing attachment loss and greater alveolar crestal height loss. Although these studies point to the possibility that osteopenia may be a risk factor for periodontal disease, further studies are clearly needed, especially large-scale studies in which multiple risk factors affecting both osteoporosis and periodontal disease are taken into consideration. Furthermore, longitudinal studies are necessary to establish if skeletal bone loss and mandibular BMD precede the development of periodontal disease. Finally, intervention studies are needed to evaluate the extent to which reduction or prevention of osteopenia—through nutritional supplements, estrogen use, or use of bone-sparing agents such as alendronate—will affect periodontal disease.

Dietary Factors

Studies of diet and periodontal disease, based on our knowledge of the pathogenesis of periodontal disease and the role of bone metabolism in inflammatory responses, may well lead to uncovering other important dietary factors that increase the risk for periodontal disease or decrease the ability of the periodontal tissues to heal. Clinical recommendations regarding diet or use of nutritional supplements must be based on randomized controlled trials of diet or nutritional supplements, and these have not yet been done with respect to periodontal disease for calcium, vitamin C, or other nutrients.

Calcium

Nishida and co-workers evaluated the role of dietary calcium intake as a contributing factor to the risk for periodontal disease.[137] They evaluated a large study of the United States population from NHANES data. In the NHANES III data set, which involved subjects assessed from 1988 to 1992, it was found that both men and women in the younger age group (20 to 39 years) and men in the middle-age group (40 to 59 years) who ingested lower levels of calcium in their diet showed increased risk for periodontal disease. The odds ratio for increased risk for periodontal disease associated with lower dietary levels of calcium for those 20 to 39 years of age was 1.84 (95% CI 1.36 to 2.48); for women aged 20 to 39 years, it was 1.99 (95% CI 1.34 to 2.97). For middle-aged men, the odds ratio was 1.9 (95% CI 1.4 to 2.54). These odds ratios were obtained after adjusting for gingival bleeding, tobacco consumption including smoking cigarettes or cigars and chewing tobacco, and alcohol consumption. Nishida and colleagues[137] also showed that women in the younger age group (20 to 39 years) had lower total

serum calcium levels and that those with the lower serum calcium levels showed a significantly higher risk of periodontal disease (odds ratio 6.1; 95% CI 2.35 to 15.84). These analyses of over 12,000 subjects representative of the United States population suggest that reduced dietary calcium intake and reduced total serum calcium levels are associated with increased risk for periodontal disease. Further studies on other populations carried out in a longitudinal fashion, with consideration for dietary calcium supplementation, as well as intervention studies, are necessary to fully determine if low dietary calcium is indeed a true risk factor for periodontal disease.

Vitamin C

Several studies suggest that vitamin C plays a role in maintaining the health of the gingiva.[138] In fact, severe forms of vitamin C deficiency can cause a gingivitis known as "scorbutic" gingivitis.

A recent analysis of the NHANES III (1988 to 1992) study assessed the relationship between dietary vitamin C and periodontal disease.[139] In this study, a representative sample of 12,419 individuals in the United States, 20 to 90+ years of age, were analyzed. Those taking less dietary vitamin C showed an increased risk of periodontal disease, especially among current tobacco users (odds ratio 1.28; 95% CI 1.04 to 1.59); the odds ratio for former users was 1.21 (95% CI 1.02 to 1.43) compared with those who did not smoke. These results suggest that reduced dietary vitamin C intake, especially in smokers and former smokers, increases the risk for periodontal disease. Further studies are needed, especially longitudinal studies, to determine if lower dietary intake of vitamin C precedes the development of periodontal disease.

Stress and Psychological Disorders

Stress and psychological disorders have been suggested to be related to oral diseases including temporomandibular disorders, dental caries, salivary dysfunction, and periodontal disease in HIV infection. Little definitive data exist, however, with respect to the role of stress on oral diseases. An evaluation of mental health, family interaction, and life events of infants and toddlers with caries by Wendt and colleagues[140] found that there was considerable stress in most of the families. However, there was not a typical family pattern in which infants developed caries.

In studies of acute necrotizing ulcerative gingivitis, stress and emotional factors have been identified as risk indicators since the early 1950s.[141–142] Recently, the role of psychosocial factors in adult periodontitis has been assessed. For example, Marcenes and Sheiham[143] showed that among the 135 subjects studied, those who faced greater work-related mental demand had greater periodontal disease as assessed by probing depth. Monteiro da Silva and colleagues[144] carried out a case-control study comparing 50 patients with severe periodontitis, 50 patients with chronic adult periodontitis, and 50 controls. They found that the subjects with severe periodontitis had higher levels of psychosocial maladjustment than the other two groups. Specifically, the severe periodontitis group presented increased depression and loneliness compared with the other groups. Linden and colleagues[145] studied 23 dental patients over 5 years. They found that loss of periodontal attachment was greater in those with increasing age, lower socioeconomic status, lower job satisfaction, and type A personalities, suggesting a relationship between progression of periodontitis and psychosocial measures. These studies are interesting in that they suggest the hypothesis that periodontal disease is associated with psychological stress.

Recently, in a cross-sectional epidemiologic study, 1,426 adults were evaluated for stress, distress, and coping as related to periodontal disease severity.[146–147] The large study group allowed for adjustment for presently known confounders, such as age, gender, smoking status, systemic health, dental care, and oral hygiene practices. Furthermore, this study addressed not only stress but also measures of distress and coping. To estimate stress, the Life Events Scale[148] and the Daily Strain Scale[149] were used. To measure distress, the Brief Symptom Inventory of Derogatis and Cleary was used.[150] Coping styles were assessed using the COPE Inventory.[151]

The associations between psychosocial factors and periodontal disease status were evaluated, and it was found that individuals who suffered from high levels of clinical attachment loss had higher scores on the financial strain scales compared with periodontally healthy individuals, after adjusting for age, gender, and cigarette smoking ($p = .008$). A similar significant difference was found for individuals with high levels of financial strain and greater loss of alveolar bone height compared with those in the low financial strain group. Stepwise ordinal logistic regression analysis showed that financial strain was associated with significantly greater clinical attachment loss (odds ratio 1.70; 95% CI 1.09 to 2.65), and with alveolar bone loss (odds ratio 1.68; 95% CI 1.20 to 2.37), after adjusting for age, gender, and cigarette smoking. Hence, it appears that stress, likely chronic stress as would be associated with financial strain, is a risk indicator for periodontal disease.

When coping behaviors were evaluated for those with high financial strain, it was found that those who were high emotion–focused copers, a form of inadequate coping, had a higher risk of having more severe attachment loss and alveolar bone loss compared with those with low levels of financial strain. However, subjects with high levels of financial strain and reported high levels of problem-focused coping, a form of adequate or good coping, have no more periodontal disease than those with low levels of financial strain. From this study, it appears that psychosocial measures of stress associated with financial strain are significant risk indicators for periodontal disease in adults. Furthermore, this study suggests that adequate coping behaviors may reduce stress-associated risk for periodontal disease. Adjustment for oral hygiene status and previous dental care did not change the associations significantly, suggesting that other at-risk health behaviors did not account for the findings.

The mechanism(s) by which stress may moderate periodontal disease is presently unknown. However, there are at least two pathways that stress can affect in infectious disease: the biologic model and the behavior model.[147] Stress effects on periodontal disease may be biologically moderated through the hypothalamic-pituitary-adrenal (HPA) axis to promote the release of corticotropic-releasing hormone from the hypothalamus and glucocorticoids from the adrenal cortex. Glucocorticoids may inhibit or reduce periodontal destruction. The effects of psychosocial stress also may occur through behavioral changes which affect at-risk health behaviors such as smoking, poor oral hygiene, and poor compliance with dental care. Any evaluation of the role of stress in periodontal disease should take into consideration at-risk health behaviors as well as the biologic effects transmitted through the HPA axis.

Genetic Factors

Genetic factors affect most oral conditions. These will be discussed as (1) abnormalities of the teeth, affecting size, shape, and number of teeth, defects in enamel and dentin, and abnormalities in the dental pulp; (2) genetic abnormalities affecting the orofacial complex; and (3) genetic factors associated with periodontal disease.

Orofacial genetic abnormalities include cherubism, osteoporosis, osteogenesis imperfecta, cleidocranial dysplasia, craniofacial dysostosis, mandibulofacial dysostosis, Pierre-Robin syndrome, Marfan's syndrome, Ehlers-Danlos syndrome, Down syndrome, trisomy 21, hemifacial hypertrophy, clefts of the lip and palate, and the fragile X syndrome. In some of these conditions, such as Ehlers-Danlos syndrome and Down syndrome, severe periodontitis may occur.

Genetic Aspects of Localized Periodontal Disease

Localized juvenile periodontitis (LJP) has a familial aggregation and hence has been long thought to be a genetically determined condition. Melnick and colleagues[152] suggested an X-linked transmission; however, Saxén,[153] Long and colleagues,[154] and Beaty and colleagues[155] proposed an autosomal mode of inheritance of juvenile periodontitis. Hart and colleagues[156] and Saxby[157] also proposed autosomal modes of transmission. Hart points out, however, that juvenile periodontitis may be a heterogeneous group of diseases and, indeed, some rare X-linked forms may exist. Hart and colleagues[158] convincingly argue that the predominance of evidence suggests that most cases of juvenile periodontitis are inherited in an autosomal manner. Additional studies are needed to provide definitive evidence of the specific genetic contributions to juvenile periodontitis.

Specific traits associated with juvenile periodontitis that may have genetic backgrounds include abnormalities in neutrophil function. For example, Van Dyke and colleagues[159] studied 22 families in which the probands suffered from localized juvenile periodontitis. The families included a total of 44 affected individuals: 25 female and 19 male patients, including the probands. Among the siblings, exclusive of probands, the proportion of affected females (0.41) was the same as that of males (0.41). In 19 of the 22 families, neutrophil abnormalities were observed while in the other 3 families, there were no subjects with neutrophil abnormalities, suggesting heterogeneity. However, the predominant number of cases of juvenile periodontitis appear to have neutrophil chemotactic and possibly other disorders. Others have also reported neutrophil chemotactic disorders in families with juvenile periodontitis, in which the affected children have the neutrophil defect, but not the unaffected children.[160]

Recent studies have shown genetic polymorphisms to be associated with neutrophil function in subjects with juvenile periodontitis.[161–162] For example, Gwinn and colleagues[161] found a polymorphism in the f-met-leu-phe receptor, a receptor for chemotactic factors produced by bacteria. This polymorphism is found in most juvenile periodontitis patients and few normal controls. Wilson and Kalmar[162] found Fc receptor polymorphisms also associated with poor binding of IgG_2 Fc to neutrophils to be much more common in LJP patients than in matched controls.

The search for genetic polymorphisms in candidate genes has been successful in the two studies, reported above, in neutrophil chemotactic receptors and Fc opsonic receptors. Further studies of candidate genes for polymorphisms may explain some of the subjects' increased susceptibility to periodontal infection in LJP.

Attempts to associate human leukocyte antigens (HLA) with juvenile periodontitis are conflicting. For example, Cullinan and colleagues[163] showed that the segregation patterns of HLA in LJP were not conclusive. Similar findings were reported by Saxén and Koskimies.[164] However, in a population-based study, Reinholdt and colleagues[165] showed that LJP patients have a higher prevalence of HLA-A9, HLA-A28, and HLA-BW15 than the general population, suggesting an association between HLA markers and the gene(s) for localized juvenile periodontitis.

Genetic Aspects of Adult Periodontitis

Periodontal diseases are common, with mild forms affecting 75% of adults in the United States,[1] and bacteria are generally thought to be the initiating etiologic agents. However, the host response triggered by pathogenic bacteria largely determines the course and severity of the disease. Host responses may affect initial colonization and infection and the growth of the organisms. They may also affect the immune and inflammatory response to the periodontopathic bacteria, which, in turn, determines the severity and rate of progression of the disease.[166]

Three approaches to the study of genetic influences have been carried out in adult periodontitis. One approach is linkage analysis, that is, to associate periodontal disease with inherited disease markers, such as blood groups or HLA. The second approach is through twin studies, and the third and most recent approach is to assess genetic polymorphisms in candidate genes.

Human Leukocyte Antigen Associations

Early studies showed negative association of adult periodontal disease with HLA-A2.[167–169] Klouda and colleagues[170] and Amer and colleagues[171] showed an increase in HLA-A9 in patients with periodontal disease, which may be related to the reported increased frequency of HLA-A9 as well as other HLA types by Reinholdt and colleagues[165] in juvenile periodontitis. Further studies of HLA linkage are needed to resolve the issue of HLA association in adult periodontal disease.

Twin Studies

Twin studies were carried out on 26 sets of twins aged 12 to 17 years, in which 7 pairs were monozygotic and 19 dizygotic.[172] No differences were found in gingival recession, gingival crevice depth, gingival bleeding, calculus, or plaque. Michalowicz and colleagues[173] studied 120 pairs of adult twins, including 62 pairs of monozygotic twins reared together, 25 pairs of same-sex dizygotic twins reared together, and 33 pairs of monozygotic twins reared apart. They found that alveolar bone height was significantly affected by genetic factors. A second study from this group[174] studied 110 pairs of adult twins, including 66 monozygotic and 33 dizygotic twins reared together and 14 monozygotic twin pairs raised apart. They found a genetic influence on gingivitis, probing depth, attachment loss, and plaque. These studies are provocative, leading to hypotheses relating to genetic factors in periodontal disease. However, the authors point out that the data must be viewed cautiously. For example, changes in alveolar bone height may be genetic due to anatomic variation and may or may not be related to periodontal disease per se.

Corey and colleagues[175] studied 116 monozygotic and 233 dizygotic pairs and compared their periodontal disease history. They found that the proband-wise concordance rates were 0.38 for monozygotic twins, and only 0.16 for dizygotic twins. These results provide further evidence that genetic factors make an important contribution to adult periodontal disease.

Genetic Polymorphisms

Genetic polymorphisms have been associated with adult periodontitis. For example, Kornman and colleagues[176] studied genetic polymorphisms in the proinflammatory cytokines interleukin-1 (IL-1) and tumor necrosis factor-alpha (TNF-α). They report a specific periodontitis-associated IL-1 genotype, comprising a variant in the IL-1B gene associated with high levels of IL-1 production. This genotype was associated with severe periodontitis only in nonsmokers. In smokers, severe periodontal disease was not correlated with any of the tested genotypes. Tests for this combined genotype are commercially available and may be of value in understanding risk for periodontal disease, especially in nonsmokers. Further studies with larger populations including controls with no periodontal disease as well as populations of various racial and ethnic groups are needed to fully evaluate polymorphisms.

Van Schie and colleagues[177] report an Fcγ receptor polymorphism pattern associated with periodontitis. They compared 105 adults with moderate to severe periodontitis with 132 age- and race-matched controls without periodontitis. The FcγRIIA-H/H131 and FcγRIIIB-NA2/NA2 genotype was elevated in patients compared with controls (18.8% versus 3.8%) while the combined FcγRIIA-R/H131 and FcγRIIIB-NA2/NA2 genotype was reduced in the periodontitis group (6.3%) compared with the controls (22.9%). This association observed between the combined FcγRIIA and FcγRIIIB genotype and moderate to severe periodontitis suggests that reduced opsonization associated with this combined genotype impairs phagocytosis of pathogenic bacteria in individuals carrying these receptors. This may be an important risk factor in adult periodontitis. However, further studies with different racial populations and with larger populations are needed to better account for possible confounding factors to fully assess the role of this risk indicator.

Hence, it appears that candidate gene polymorphisms are a useful approach in assessing genetic factors in both adult and juvenile forms of periodontal disease. Future efforts along these lines may reveal a set of important genes in periodontitis in which genetic polymorphisms affect the function of the molecules encoded for by these genes and thereby increase susceptibility or resistance to periodontal infections. It is likely that genetic polymorphisms will explain risk for periodontal disease in subsets of the population. In the future, a larger battery of such polymorphisms may be useful to understand genetic influences on risk for periodontal disease.

EFFECTS OF MEDICATIONS AND PERIODONTAL DISEASE

Phenytoin

Sodium 5,5-phenylhydantoin has been used for 50 years in the treatment of grand mal epilepsy and also has been used for management of other neurologic disorders. Overgrowth of the gingiva is one of the most troublesome side effects of phenytoin.[178] A gross increase in gingival size is due to a dramatic expansion of the connective tissue component. The growth is not a true fibrosis but a gingival overgrowth since it results from neither hypertrophy nor hyperplasia. Treatment consists of replacing phenytoin with an alternative drug such as carbamazepine or sodium valproate, conservative periodontal therapy to reduce the inflammatory component of enlargement, and surgery, if necessary.

Cyclosporine

Cyclosporine has been used in the United States since 1984 for the prevention of rejection phenomena following solid organ and bone marrow transplantation. It is also used in other countries in the treatment of type 2 diabetes mellitus, rheumatoid arthritis, psoriasis, multiple sclerosis, malaria, sarcoidosis, and some other diseases with an immunologic basis. Cyclosporine selectively suppresses subpopulations of T lymphocytes interfering with production of interleukins, especially interleukin-1. Gingival overgrowth has been associated with cyclosporine.[179] Histopathologically, cyclosporine-induced gingival overgrowth is associated with apparent fibroplasia, redundant collagenous elements, epithelial thickening as well as secondary inflammation. Reduction of dental plaque and low drug dosages may discourage the gingival overgrowth associated with the use of cyclosporine. Furthermore, cyclosporine substitute drugs appear to have little or no effect on the gingivae.

Dihydropyridines: Nifedipine and Nitrendipine

Nifedipine (Procardia) is a substituted dihydroprolidine widely used since 1978 in the treatment of angina pectoris and postmyocardial syndrome. Nifedipine is a calcium ion blocker which induces gingival overgrowth.[180] Histologically, there is thickened epithelium, elongation of epithelial rete ridges, redundant connective tissue, and abundant fibroblasts. Inflammation may be reduced with good plaque control, and scaling and root planing; however, often periodontal surgery is required for treatment.

Another commonly used calcium antagonist in cardiology is verapamil hydrochloride (Calan). Verapamil hydrochloride has not been associated with gingival enlargement or fibrosis elsewhere in the body.

Heavy Metals

Pigmentation of the gingiva or other mucosa results when heavy metals, primarily heavy metal sulfides, are present in the body. Oral manifestations of mercury, lead, and bismuth intoxication are well described; however, the presence of such manifestations has decreased significantly as exposure to heavy metals by way of occupational hazards and metal-containing drugs has declined. Bismuth line is seen as a blue-black, easily discernible, diffuse pigmentation of marginal gingiva. Lead poisoning results in a line with grayish pigmentation typically located a few millimeters apical to the gingival margin. A mercury line on the gingiva resulting from deposition of mercurial salts, mainly mercuric sulfide, may be deposited in the gingiva. Cases of true allergy to mercury present in the silver amalgam dental restorations are rare.[181] The role of lead and other heavy metals in the risk for periodontal disease has not been studied but is possible since these metals have major biologic effects, and their ingestion is increasing in our society.

LOCAL RISK FACTORS: PERIODONTAL MICROFLORA

There are over 400 genera and species of microorganisms that have been identified in the oral flora of man. Only a few members of the subgingival periodontal microflora, however, have been identified as candidate pathogens for the initiation and progression of periodontal disease. In a large epidemiologic study, Grossi and co-workers[21,22] tested a panel of candidate pathogen microorganisms, many of which have been implicated as periodontal pathogens from animal, virulence, and case-control human studies. This panel included *Actinobacillus actinomycetemcomitans*, *Bacteroides forsythus*, *Campylobacter rectus*, *Capnocytophaga* species, *Eubacterium saburreum*, *Fusobacterium nucleatum*, *Porphyromonas gingivalis*, and *Prevotella intermedia*. Of this panel, only two, *P. gingivalis* and *B. forsythus*, were associated with increased risk for attachment loss as a measure of periodontal disease, after adjustment for age, plaque, smoking, and diabetes.[21] The same two organisms were also identified as risk indicators for periodontal alveolar bone loss.[22] Epidemiologic studies of Beck and co-workers[182] suggested that specific bacteria such as *P. gingivalis* and *P. intermedia* play a role in periodontal disease in older adults. They found in their study of older adults that the difference in the prevalence of periodontal disease between African Americans and Caucasian Americans is explained in part by the prevalence of *P. gingivalis* and *P. intermedia*. In a longitudinal study of 886 patients,

Wolff and colleagues[183] found that *P. gingivalis*, *A. actinomycetemcomitans*, *P. intermedia*, *Eikenella corrodens* and *F. nucleatum* were found in higher numbers in areas of increasing probing depths with relative risks between 2.7 and 4.0. A very strong association has been found between the presence of *A. actinomycetemcomitans* and periodontal disease in localized juvenile periodontitis.[184–185]

The presence and level of spirochetes have been associated with increased risk of periodontal disease;[186] however, this finding has to be tempered by the observation that spirochetes are also elevated when patients have poor oral hygiene.[187] Haffajee and co-workers[188] found that *P. intermedia, C. rectus, B. forsythus,* and *Peptostreptococcus micros* were predictors of future periodontal progression in patients who were already affected by adult periodontitis. Listgarten[189] found that the absence of *A. actinomycetemcomitans, P. intermedia,* and *P. gingivalis* served as an indicator of periodontal health to a greater extent than their presence being a marker for future disease. He suggests that they have a high negative predictive value. The importance of specific bacteria in periodontal destruction is highlighted by the finding that the quantity of total plaque accumulation is only correlated weakly with destructive periodontal disease.[21,22,190] Further studies are necessary to determine the extent to which other organisms (eg, *A. actinomycetemcomitans*) may play a role in juvenile forms of periodontal disease.

Oral Hygiene, Plaque, and Calculus

Microbial dental plaques have been strongly associated as causative agents for gingivitis; however, the association of supragingival plaque with periodontitis is not clear. For example, in the studies by Grossi and colleagues,[21,22] they are not found to be risk factors for periodontal disease. In treatment studies, such as that by Axelsson and colleagues,[191] it was shown that patients who maintain excellent hygiene measures and who undergo scaling and root planing every 2 to 3 months for 9 years, and twice annually for an additional 6 years, had very little clinically detectable periodontal disease. Thus, it is clear that periodontitis can be prevented and established periodontitis arrested by control of microbial deposits. Supragingival plaque may provide a favorable environment for colonization with specific subgingival flora and indirectly affect the pathogenic subgingival flora.[192–193] Therefore, the association that has been documented above for the specific flora is a direct one in terms of risk factors.

Calculus and its relationship to periodontitis is complex. Calculus developing in certain sites, such as the lower incisal areas, in patients receiving regular dental care does not result in significant periodontal disease.[194] On the other hand, studies report a high correlation between measures of calculus and measures of periodontal disease and since they coexist, it is difficult to determine that calculus per se is a risk factor for periodontal disease. Calculus is likely a deposit that forms after periodontal disease develops and likely contributes to progression of periodontitis by providing a nidus for microbial plaque accumulation and persistence.

Bleeding on Probing

Surprisingly, gingival bleeding on probing appears to have weak predictive value for future periodontal breakdown.[195–196] However, the repeated absence of bleeding upon probing is associated with no disease progression.[197–198] In these studies, it was found that setting level of bleeding upon probing at 50% is predictive for future periodontal disease with a relative risk of 3, after adjusting for smoking, microbial dental plaque accumulation, diabetes, and baseline flora.

Preexisting Periodontal Disease

Perhaps one of the most strongly associated risk factors for future periodontal breakdown is presence and severity of periodontal disease assessed by attachment loss or alveolar bone loss at baseline.[32,34,188–189,199–203] In a study of 79 patients with established periodontitis who were monitored every 3 months for 1 year, Machtei and co-workers[203] found that individuals with baseline pocket depth ≥3.2 mm were at greater risk for future bone loss 1 year later (relative risk: 2.97; 95% CI 1.02 to 8.70). A multivariate analysis of this study also found that smokers were at increased risk for further attachment loss when compared to nonsmokers (relative risk: 5.41; 95% CI 1.50 to 19.5) and that subjects who harbored *B. forsythus* at baseline were at seven times greater risk for increased pocket depth (relative risk: 7.84; 95% CI 1.74 to 35.3). This study confirms that pre-existing periodontal disease is among the true risk factors for development of periodontal disease.

Lack of regular dental therapy has also been suggested as a risk factor for periodontal disease in studies using univariate analyses. However, with multivariate analysis, most studies showed that previous dental therapy is not a risk factor when one considers existing levels of disease, such as existing pocket depth or existing gingivitis in the model.[21,22]

Individual Tooth Risk Factors

Several factors have been proposed to affect the risk of further periodontal disease on individual teeth. These include

1. occlusion, especially functional malocclusion such as bruxism;
2. excessive occlusal stress, which may be primary if the tooth has excessive stress with inadequate support, or secondary if the tooth is under even normal stress and has inadequate support; and
3. teeth with pulpal infections that show periapical lesions; these have greater chance of future loss of attachment than those with no pulpal

infection. More study of the role of occlusion in periodontal disease is needed.

CLINICAL APPLICATION OF RISK FACTOR ANALYSIS

Table 2–2 lists important risk indicators and risk factors for periodontal disease and summarizes their strength of association. On the basis of the strength of the association, those factors that appear to be true risk factors for periodontal disease in adults include the subgingival periodontal pathogens *P. gingivalis* and *B. forsythus*, diabetes mellitus, male gender, smoking, and pre-existing periodontal disease. Putative risk factors or risk indicators at this time include genetic factors; osteoporosis; stress, distress, and coping; and dietary factors such as low calcium intake. Further studies are necessary to determine the extent to

TABLE 2–2. The Strength of Association of Local and Systemic Factors with Destructive Periodontal Disease

Factor	Case Report Studies	Case-Control Studies	Cross-Sectional Studies	Longitudinal Studies	Intervention Studies
Specific bacteria					
P. gingivalis	Yes	Yes	Yes	Yes	Yes
B. forsythus	Yes	Yes	Yes	Yes	Yes
P. intermedia	Yes	Yes	Yes	Yes	Yes
Gender					
Male	Yes	NR	Yes	NR	NR
Age	Yes	Yes	Yes	No (to 7th decade)	NR
Diabetes mellitus					
Type 2	Yes	Yes	Yes	Yes	Yes (treatment reduces glycosylated hemoglobin)
Type 1	Yes	Yes	Yes	NR	NR
Smoking	NR	Yes	Yes	Yes	Yes (smokers heal poorly)
Osteoporosis	Yes	Yes	Yes	NR	NR
Stress, distress, coping	Yes	Yes	Yes	NR	NR
PMN disorders	Yes	Yes	NR	Yes (case series)	NR
Genetic factors (IL-1 polymorphisms)	NR	Yes	NR	NR	NR
Dietary calcium	NR	Yes	Yes	NR	NR
Preexisting periodontal disease	Yes	Yes	Yes	Yes	Yes

NR = not reported, or not relevant; PMN = polymorphonuclear.
Adapted from Genco RJ. Current view of risk factors for periodontal diseases. J Periodontal 1996;67(Suppl):1041–9.

which these risk indicators are true risk factors for periodontal disease.

DETERMINING A PATIENT'S RISK PROFILE

Determination of patient-based as well as site-based risk factors for periodontal disease is a necessary component of the evaluation and diagnosis of our patients. Identification of risk factors for each patient, and their management should be part of the treatment plan.

RISK FACTOR MODIFICATION IN CLINICAL MANAGEMENT

Periodontal diseases are infections and, by and large, are treated with anti-infective therapy, and residual defects are restored by regenerative therapy. The third mode of therapy, modification of risk, is becoming more and more important as indicated by studies that show that if risk factors are not modified, periodontal healing is compromised, especially in patients who smoke.[52,204] It would seem that smoking cessation is indicated for optimal periodontal healing as well as for other general health reasons. Diabetics who respond successfully to periodontal therapy also have a reduction in glycated hemoglobin, particularly if they are treated with tetracycline.[100] Several other studies have shown similar results. Hence, management of periodontal disease, that is, modification of risk factors, is part of contemporary treatment of periodontal disease and is supported by intervention studies.

SUMMARY

In this chapter, those factors associated with increased risk for periodontal disease, functioning as systemic factors or as local factors, are described, and data supporting these factors as true risk factors are provided. A model for the assessment of risk for the development of periodontal disease in patients with no or moderate periodontal disease is provided. Furthermore, the concept of risk management, that is, modification of risk factors as part of periodontal therapy, in those at high risk is presented.

REFERENCES

1. Miller AJ, Brunelle JA, Carlos JP, et al. Oral Health of United States Adults: National Findings. Bethesda, MD: National Institute of Dental Research; 1987. NIH Publication No. 87-2868.
2. Hugoson A, Jordan T. Frequency distribution of individuals aged 20–70 years according to severity of periodontal disease. Commun Dent Oral Epidemiol 1982;10:187–92.
3. Brown LJ, Löe H. Prevalence, extent, severity and progression of periodontal disease. Periodontol 2000 1993;2:57–71.
4. Genco RJ. Periodontal disease and risk for myocardial infarction and cardiovascular disease. Cardiovasc Rev Rep 1998;19(3):34–40.
5. Offenbacher S, Katz V, Gertik G, et al. Periodontal infection as a possible risk factor for preterm low birth weight. J Periodontol 1996;67:1103–13.
6. Scannapieco FA, Papandonatos GD, Dunford RG. Associations between oral conditions and respiratory disease in a national sample survey population. Annals Periodontol 1998;3:251–6.
7. Scannapieco FA. Periodontal disease as a potential risk factor for systemic diseases [position paper]. J Periodontol 1998;69:841–50.
8. Haffajee AD, Socransky SS. Microbial etiological agents of destructive periodontal diseases. Periodontol 2000 1994;5:78–111.
9. Slots J, Feik D, Rams TE. Age and sex relationships of superinfecting microorganisms in periodontitis patients. Oral Microbiol Immunol 1990;5:305–8.
10. Njoroge T, Genco RJ, Sojar HT, et al. A role for fimbriae in *Porphyromonas gingivalis* invasion of oral epithelial cells. Infect Immun 1997;65:1980–4.
11. Genco CA, Odusanya BM, Potempa J, et al. A peptide domain on gingipain R which confers immunity against *Porphyromonas gingivalis* infection in mice. Infect Immun 1998;66:4108–14.
12. van Winkelhoff AJ, Tijhof CJ, de Graaff J. Microbiological and clinical results of metronidazole plus amoxicillin therapy in *Actinobacillus actinomycetemcomitans*-associated periodontitis. J Periodontol 1992;63:52–7.
13. American Academy of Periodontology. The pathogenesis of periodontal diseases [informational paper]. J Periodontol 1999;70:457–70.
14. Reynolds JJ, Meikle MC. Mechanisms of connective tissue matrix destruction in periodontitis. Periodontol 2000 1997;14:144–57.
15. Honig J, Rordorf-Adam C, Siegmund C, et al. Increased interleukin-1β concentration in gingival tissue from periodontitis patients. J Periodontal Res 1989;24:362–7.
16. Gemmell E, Marshall R, Seymour G. Cytokines and prostaglandins in the immune hemostasis and tissue destruction in periodontal disease. Periodontol 2000 1997;14:112–43.

17. Last JM. A dictionary of epidemiology, 2nd ed. New York, NY: Oxford University Press; 1988.

18. Beck JD. Methods of assessing risk for periodontitis and developing multi-factorial models. J Periodontol 1994;65:468–78.

19. Ibrahim M. Epidemiology and health policy. Rockville, MD: Aspen Systems Corporation; 1985.

20. Goodson JM. Selection of suitable indicators of periodontitis. In: Bader JD, editor. Risk assessments in dentistry. Chapel Hill, NC: University of North Carolina Dental Ecology; 1990. p. 69.

21. Grossi SG, Zambon JJ, Ho AW, et al. Assessment of risk for periodontal disease. I. Risk indicators for attachment loss. J Periodontol 1994;65:260–7.

22. Grossi SG, Genco RJ, Machtei EE, et al. Assessment of risk for periodontal disease. II. Risk indicators for alveolar bone loss. J Periodontol 1995;66:23–9.

23. Carlos JP, Wolfe MD, Kingman A. The extent and severity index: a simple method for use in epidemiologic studies of periodontal disease. J Clin Periodontol 1986;13:500–5.

24. DeRouen TA. Statistical methods for assessing risk of periodontal disease. In: Bader JD, editor. Risk assessments in dentistry. Chapel Hill, NC: University of North Carolina Dental Ecology; 1990. p. 239–44.

25. Hujoel PP, Loesche WJ, DeRouen TA. Assessment of relationships between site-specific variables. J Periodontol 1990;61:368–72.

26. DeRouen TA, Mancl L, Hujoel P. Measurement of association in periodontal diseases using statistical methods for dependent data. J Periodontal Res 1991;26:218–29.

27. Marshall-Day CD, Stevens RG, Quigley LF Jr. Periodontal disease prevalence and incidence. J Periodontol 1955;26:185–203.

28. Schei O, Waerhaug J, Lövdal A, Arnö A. Alveolar bone loss as related to oral hygiene and age. J Periodontol 1959;30:7–16.

29. Abdellatif HM, Burt BA. An epidemiological investigation into the relative importance of age and oral hygiene status as determinants of periodontitis. J Dent Res 1987;66:13–8.

30. Machtei EE, Dunford R, Grossi SG, Genco RJ. Cumulative nature of periodontal attachment loss. J Periodontal Res 1994;29:361–4.

31. Papapanou PN, Wennström JL, Grondahl K. A 10-year retrospective study of periodontal disease progression. J Clin Periodontol 1989;16:404–11.

32. Albandar JM, Rise J, Gjermo P, Johansen JR. Radiographic quantification of alveolar bone level changes. A 2-year longitudinal study in man. J Clin Periodontol 1986;13:195–200.

33. Wennström JL, Serino G, Lindhe J, et al. Periodontal conditions of adult regular dental care attendants. A 12-year longitudinal study. J Clin Periodontol 1993;20:714–22.

34. Ismail AI, Morrison EC, Burt BA, et al. Natural history of periodontal disease in adults: findings from the Tecumseh periodontal disease study. 1959–1987. J Dent Res 1990;69:430–5.

35. Russell AL. Geographical distribution and epidemiology of periodontal disease. Geneva: World Health Organization; (WHO/DH/33/34), 1960.

36. U.S. Public Health Service. National Center for Health Statistics. Periodontal disease in adults, United States 1960–1962. PHS Publication No. 1000, Series 11, No. 12, Washington, DC: Government Printing Office; 1965.

37. U.S. Public Health Service. National Center for Health Statistics. Basic data on dental examination findings of persons 1–75 years; United States, 1971–1974. DHEW Publication No. (PHS) 79-1662, Series 11, No. 214, Washington, DC: Government Printing Office; 1979.

38. Genco RJ. Current view of risk factors for periodontal diseases. J Periodontol 1996;67(Suppl): 1041–9.

39. Pindborg JJ. Tobacco and gingivitis. I. Statistical examination of the significance of tobacco in the development of ulceromembranous gingivitis and in the formation of calculus. J Dent Res 1947;26:261–4.

40. Frandsen A, Pindborg JJ. Tobacco and gingivitis. III. Difference in action of cigarette and pipe smoking. J Dent Res 1949;28:464–5.

41. Solomon HA, Priore RL, Bross IDJ. Cigarette smoking and periodontal disease. J Am Dent Assoc 1968;77:1081–4.

42. Ismail AI, Burt BA, Eklund SA. Epidemiologic patterns of smoking and periodontal disease in the United States. J Am Dent Assoc 1983;106: 617–23.

43. Machtei EE, Hausmann E, Dunford R, et al. Longitudinal study of predictive factors for periodontal disease and tooth loss. J Clin Periodontol 1999;26:374–80.

44. Gonzalez YM, De Nardin A, Grossi SG, et al. Serum cotinine levels, smoking and periodontal attachment loss. J Dent Res 1996;75:796–802.

45. Holm G. Smoking as an additional risk for tooth loss. J Periodontol 1994;65:996–1001.

46. Preber H, Bergström J. Occurrence of gingival bleeding in smoker and nonsmoker patients. Acta Odontol Scand 1985;43:315–20.

47. Preber H, Bergström J. The effect of non-surgical treatment on periodontal pockets in smokers

and nonsmokers. J Clin Periodontol 1985;13:319–23.

48. Preber H, Bergström J. Effect of cigarette smoking on periodontal healing following surgical therapy. J Clin Periodontol 1990;17:324–8.

49. Kaldahl WB, Kalkwarf KL, Patil KD, Molvar MP. Relationship of gingival bleeding, gingival suppuration and supragingival plaque to attachment loss. J Periodontol 1990;61:347–51.

50. Tonetti MS, Pini-Prato G, Cortellini P. Effect of cigarette smoking on periodontal healing following GTR in infrabony defects. A preliminary retrospective study. J Clin Periodontol 1996;22:229–34.

51. Preber H, Linder L, Bergström J. Periodontal healing and periopathogenic microflora in smokers and non-smokers. J Clin Periodontol 1996;22:946–52.

52. Grossi SG, Skrepcinski FB, DeCaro T, et al. Responses to periodontal therapy in diabetics and smokers. J Periodontol 1996;67(Suppl):1094–102.

53. Kaldahl WB, Kalkwarf KL, Patil KD, et al. Long-term evaluation of periodontal therapy. II: Incidence of sites breaking down. J Periodontol 1996;67:103–8.

54. Bergström J, Eliasson S, Preber H. Cigarette smoking and periodontal bone loss. J Periodontol 1991;62:242–6.

55. Haber J, Wattles J, Crowley M, et al. Evidence for cigarette smoking as a major risk factor for periodontitis. J Periodontol 1993;64:16–23.

56. Haber J, Kent RL. Cigarette smoking in a periodontal practice. J Periodontol 1992;63:100–6.

57. Baab DA, Oberg PA. The effect of cigarette smoking on gingival blood flow in humans. J Clin Periodontol 1987;14:418–24.

58. Palmer RM. Tobacco smoking and oral health: review. Br Dent J 1988;164:258–60.

59. Haber J, Brinnell C, Crowley M, et al. Antibodies to periodontal pathogens in cigarette smoking. J Dent Res 1993;72(Special Issue): Abstract 1126.

60. Tew JG, Zhang J-B, Quinn S, et al. Antibody of the IgG$_2$ subclass, *Actinobacillus actinomycetemcomitans*, and early-onset periodontitis. J Periodontol 1996;67(Suppl):317–22.

61. Raulin L, MacPherson J, McQuade M, Hanson B. The effect of nicotine on the attachment of human fibroblasts to glass and human root surfaces in vitro. J Periodontol 1988;59:318–25.

62. Krall EA, Dawson-Hughes B. Smoking and bone loss among postmenopausal women. J Bone Min Res 1991;6:331–7.

63. Daniell HW. Osteoporosis of the slender smoker. Arch Intern Med 1976;136:298–304.

64. Cuff MJ, McQuade MJ, Scheidt MJ, et al. The presence of nicotine on root surfaces of periodontally diseased teeth in smokers. J Periodontol 1989;60:564–9.

65. Zambon JJ, Grossi SG, Machtei EE, et al. Cigarette smoking increases the risk for subgingival infection with periodontal pathogens. J Periodontol 1996;67(Suppl):1050–4.

66. MacFarlane G, Herzberg M, Wolff L, Hardie N. Refractory periodontitis associated with abnormal polymorphonuclear leukocyte phagocytosis and cigarette smoking. J Periodontol 1992;63:908–13.

67. Poore TK, Johnson GK, Rheinhardt RA, Organ CC. The effects of smokeless tobacco on clinical parameters of inflammation and gingival crevicular fluid prostaglandin E$_2$, interleukin-1α, and interleukin-1β. J Periodontol 1995;66:177–83.

68. Johnson GK, Poore TK, Rayne JB, Organ CC. Effect of smokeless tobacco extract on human gingival keratinocyte levels of prostaglandin E$_2$ and interleukin-1. J Periodontol 1996;67:116–24.

69. Ringelberg ML, Dixon DO, Francis AO, Plummer RW. Comparison of gingival health and gingival crevicular fluid flow in children with and without diabetes. J Dent Res 1977;56:108–11.

70. Faulconbridge AR, Bradshaw WC, Jenkins PA, Baum JD. The dental status of a group of diabetic children. Br Dent J 1981;151(8):253–5.

71. Cianciola LJ, Park BH, Bruck E, et al. Prevalence of periodontal disease in insulin-dependent diabetes mellitus (juvenile diabetes). J Am Dent Assoc 1982;104:653–60.

72. Harrison R, Bowen WH. Periodontal health, dental caries, and metabolic control in insulin-dependent diabetic children and adolescents. Pediatric Dent 1987;9:283–6.

73. Novaes AB Jr, Pereira ALA, de Moraes N, Novaes AB. Manifestations of insulin-dependent diabetes mellitus in the periodontium of young Brazilian patients. J Periodontol 1991;62:116–22.

74. de Pommereau V, Dargent-Pare C, Robert JJ, Brion M. Periodontal status in insulin-dependent diabetic adolescents. J Clin Periodontol 1992;19 (Pt. 1):628–32.

75. Pinson M, Hoffman WH, Garnick JJ, Litaker MS. Periodontal disease and type 1 diabetes mellitus in children and adolescents. J Clin Periodontol 1995;22:118–23.

76. Firatli E, Yilmaz O, Onan U. The relationship between clinical attachment loss and the duration of insulin-dependent diabetes mellitus (IDDM) in children and adolescents. J Clin Periodontol 1996;23:362–6.

77. Firatli E. The relationship between clinical periodontal status and insulin-dependent diabetes mellitus. Results after 5 years. J Periodontol 1997;68:136–40.

78. Goteiner D, Vogel R, Deasy M, Goteiner C. Periodontal and caries experience in children with insulin-dependent diabetes mellitus. J Am Dent Assoc 1986;113:277–9.

79. Kjellman O, Henriksson CO, Berghagen N, Andersson B. Oral conditions in 105 subjects with insulin-treated diabetes mellitus. Svensk Tandlakaretidskrift 1970;63:99–110.

80. Sznajder N, Carraro JJ, Rugna S, Sereday M. Periodontal findings in diabetic and nondiabetic patients. J Periodontol 1978;49:445–8.

81. Galea H, Aganovic I, Aganovic M. The dental caries and periodontal disease experience of patients with early onset insulin dependent diabetes. Intl Dent J 1986;36:219–24.

82. Rylander H, Ramberg P, Blohme G, Lindhe J. Prevalence of periodontal disease in young diabetics. J Clin Periodontol 1987;14:38–43.

83. Guven Y, Satman I, Dinccag N, Alptekin S. Salivary peroxidase activity in whole saliva of patients with insulin-dependent (type 1) diabetes mellitus. J Clin Periodontol 1996;23:879–81.

84. Cohen MM. Transforming growth factor beta and fibroblast growth factors and their receptors: role in structural biology and craniosynostosis. J Bone Min Res 1997;12:322–31.

85. Glavind L, Lund B, Löe H. The relationship between periodontal state and diabetes duration, insulin dosage and retinal changes. J Periodontol 1968;39(6):341–7.

86. Hugoson A, Thorstenson H, Falk H, Kuylenstierna J. Periodontal conditions in insulin-dependent diabetics. J Clin Periodontol 1989;16:215–23.

87. Thorstenson H, Hugoson A. Periodontal disease experience in adult long-duration insulin-dependent diabetics. J Clin Periodontol 1993; 20:352–8.

88. Tervonen T, Karjalainen K. Periodontal disease related to diabetic status. A pilot study of the response to periodontal therapy in type 1 diabetes. J Clin Periodontol 1997;24:505–10.

89. Nelson RG, Shlossman M, Budding LM, et al. Periodontal disease and NIDDM in Pima Indians. Diabetes Care 1990;13:836–40.

90. Shlossman M, Knowler WC, Pettitt DJ, Genco RJ. Type 2 diabetes and periodontal disease. J Am Dent Assoc 1990;121:532–6.

91. Emrich LJ, Shlossman M, Genco RJ. Periodontal disease in non-insulin dependent diabetes mellitus. J Periodontol 1991;62:123–30.

92. Morton AA, Williams RW, Watts RLP. Initial study of periodontal status in non-insulin-dependent diabetics in Mauritius. J Dent 1995;23:343–5.

93. Novaes AB Jr, Gutierrez FG, Novaes AB. Periodontal disease progression in type II non-insulin-dependent diabetes mellitus patients (NIDDM). Part I. Probing pocket depth and clinical attachment. Brazilian Dent J 1996;7:65–73.

94. Taylor GW, Burt BA, Becker MP, et al. Non-insulin dependent diabetes mellitus and alveolar bone loss progression over two years. J Periodontol 1998;69:76–83.

95. Taylor GW, Burt BA, Becker MP, et al. Glycemic control and alveolar bone loss progression in type II diabetes. Ann Periodontol 1998;3(1):30–9.

96. Taylor GW, Burt BA, Becker MP, et al. Severe periodontitis and risk for poor glycemic control in subjects with non-insulin-dependent diabetes mellitus. J Periodontol 1996;67:1085–93.

97. Dolan TA, Gilbert GH, Ringelberg ML, et al. Behavioral risk indicators of attachment loss in adult Floridians. J Clin Periodontol 1997;24:223–32.

98. Szpunar SM, Ismail AI, Eklund SA. Diabetes and periodontal disease: analyses of NHANES I and HHANES [abstract 1605]. J Dent Res 1989; 68(Special Issue):383.

99. Aldridge JP, Lester V, Watts TL, et al. Single-blind studies of the effects of improved periodontal health on metabolic control in type 1 diabetes mellitus. J Clin Periodontol 1995;22:271–5.

100. Grossi SG, Skrepcinski FB, DeCaro T, et al. Treatment of periodontal disease in diabetics reduces glycated hemoglobin. J Periodontol 1997;68:713–9.

101. Miller LS, Manwell MA, Newbold D, et al. The relationship between reduction in periodontal inflammation and diabetes control: a report of 9 cases. J Periodontol 1992;63:843–8.

102. Clearinghouse on oral problems related to HIV infection and WHO Collaborating Centre on Oral Manifestations of the Immunodeficiency Virus. Classification and diagnostic criteria for oral lesions in HIV infection. J Oral Pathol Med 1993;22(7):289–91.

103. Greenberg MS. HIV-associated lesions. Dermatol Clin 1996;14:319–26.

104. Greenspan D, Greenspan JS. HIV-related oral disease. Lancet 1996;348(9029):729–33.

105. Phelan JA. Oral manifestations of human immunodeficiency virus infection. Med Clin North Am 1997;81:511–31.

106. Samaranayake LP, Holmstrup P. Oral candidiasis and human immunodeficiency virus infection. J Oral Pathol Med 1989;18:554–64.

107. Klein RS, Harris CA, Small CB, et al. Oral candidiasis in high risk patients as the initial manifestation of the acquired immunodeficiency syndrome. N Engl Med J 1984;311(6):35–48.

108. Tindall B, Carr A, Cooper DA. Primary HIV infection: clinical, immunologic, and serologic aspects. In: Sande MA, Volberding PA, editors. The medical management of AIDS. Philadelphia: WB Saunders; 1995. p. 105–29.

109. Glick M, Muzyka BC, Lurie D, Salkin LM. Oral manifestations associated with HIV-related disease as markers for immune suppression and AIDS. Oral Surg Oral Med Oral Pathol 1994; 77:344–9.

110. Daniels TE. Oral candidiasis and HIV infection. In: Greenspan JS, Greenspan D, editors. Oral manifestations of HIV infection. Chicago, IL: Quintessence; 1995. p. 80–4.

111. Dodd CL, Greenspan D, Katz MH, et al. Oral candidiasis in HIV infection: Pseudomembranous and erythematous candidiasis show similar rates of progression to AIDS. AIDS 1991;5(11): 1339–43.

112. Greenspan D, Greenspan JS, Conant M, et al. Oral "hairy" leukoplakia in male homosexuals: evidence of association with both papillomavirus and a herpes-group virus. Lancet 1984;2:831–4.

113. Greenspan D, Greenspan JS, Lennette ET, et al. Oral viral leukoplakia—a new AIDS-associated condition. Adv Exp Med Biol 1985;187:123–8.

114. Eisenberg E, Krutchkoff D, Yamase H. Incidental oral hairy leukoplakia in immunocompetent persons. A report of two cases. Oral Surg Oral Med Oral Pathol 1992;74:332–3.

115. Felix DH, Watret K, Wray D, Southam JC. Hairy leukoplakia in an HIV negative, nonimmunosuppressed patient. Oral Surg Oral Med Oral Pathol 1992;74(5):563–6.

116. Epstein JB, Silverman S Jr. Head and neck malignancies associated with HIV infection. Oral Surg Oral Med Oral Pathol 1992;73:193–200.

117. Lamster I, Grbic J, Fine J, et al. A critical review of periodontal disease as a manifestation of HIV infection. In: Greenspan JS, Greenspan E, editors. Oral manifestations of HIV infection. Chicago, IL: Quintessence; 1995. p. 247–56.

118. Winkler JR, Robertson PB. Periodontal disease associated with HIV infection. Oral Surg Oral Med Oral Pathol 1992;73:145–50.

119. Winkler JR, Grassi M, Murray PA. Clinical description and etiology of HIV-associated periodontal diseases. In: Robertson PB, Greenspan JS, editors. Perspectives on oral manifestations of AIDS: diagnosis and management of HIV-associated infections. Littleton (MA): PSG Publishing; 1988.

120. Van Dyke TE, Levine MJ, Genco RJ. Neutrophil function in oral disease. J Oral Pathol 1985;14: 95–120.

121. Sofaer JA. Genetic approaches to the study of periodontal disease. J Clin Periodontol 1990;17(7 Pt. 1):401–8.

122. Phillips HB, Ashley FP. Relationship between periodontal disease and a metacarpal bone index. Br Dent J 1973;134:237–9.

123. Von Wowren N. Dual-photon absorptiometry of mandibles: in vitro test of a new method. Scand J Dent Res 1985;93:169–77.

124. Von Wowren N, Klausen B, Kollerup G. Osteoporosis: a risk factor in periodontal disease. J Periodontol 1994;65:1134–8.

125. Von Wowren N, Kollerup G. Symptomatic osteoporosis: a risk factor for residual ridge reduction of the jaws. J Prosthet Dent 1992;67:656–60.

126. Von Wowren N, Storm TL, Olgaard K. Bone mineral content by photon absorptiometry of the mandible compared with that of the forearm and the lumbar spine. Calcif Tissue Int 1988; 42:157–61.

127. Kribbs PJ, Smith DE, Chesnut CH. Oral findings in osteoporosis. Part I: Measurement of mandibular bone density. J Prosthet Dent 1983; 50:576–9.

128. Kribbs PJ, Smith DE, Chesnut CH. Oral findings in osteoporosis. Part II: Relationship between residual ridge and alveolar bone resorption and generalized skeletal osteopenia. J Prosthet Dent 1983;50:719–24.

129. Kribbs PJ, Chesnut CH, III. Osteoporosis and dental osteopenia in the elderly. Gerodontology 1984;3:101–6.

130. Henrikson P, Wallenius K. The mandible and osteoporosis—a qualitative comparison between the mandible and the radius. J Oral Rehab 1974;1:67–74.

131. Ortman LF, Hausmann E, Dunford RG. Skeletal osteopenia and residual ridge resorption. J Prosthet Dent 1989;61:321–5.

132. Humphries S, Devlin H, Worthington H. A radiographic investigation into bone resorption of mandibular alveolar bone in elderly edentulous adults. J Dent 1989;17:94–6.

133. Daniell H. Postmenopausal tooth loss. Contributions to edentulism by osteoporosis and cigarette smoking. Arch Intern Med 1983;143:1678–82.

134. Krall EA, Dawson-Hughes B, Hannan MT, et al. Postmenopausal estrogen replacement and tooth retention. Am J Med 1997;102:536–42.

135. Groen JJ, Menczel J, Shapiro S. Chronic destructive periodontal disease in patients with presenile osteoporosis. J Periodontol 1968;39:19–23.

136. Wactawski-Wende J, Grossi SG, Trevisan M, et al. The role of osteopenia in oral bone loss and periodontal disease. J Periodontol 1996;67:1076–84.

137. Nishida M, Grossi SG, Dunford RG, et al. Role of dietary calcium and the risk for periodontal disease. J Periodontol 1999. [Submitted]

138. Rubinoff AB, Latner PA, Pasut LA. Vitamin C and oral health. J Canadian Dent Assoc 1989;55:705–7.

139. Nishida M, Grossi SG, Dunford RG, et al. Dietary vitamin C and the risk for periodontal disease. J Periodontol 1999. [Submitted]

140. Wendt LK, Svedin CG, Hallonsten AL, Larsson IV. Infants and toddlers with caries. Mental health, family interaction, and life events with infants and toddlers with caries. Swed Dent J 1995;19(1-2):17–27.

141. Moulton R, Ewen S, Thieman W. Emotional factors in periodontal disease. Oral Surg Oral Med Oral Pathol 1952;5:833–60.

142. Melnick SL, Roseman JM, Engel JD, Cogen RB. Epidemiology of acute necrotizing ulcerative gingivitis. Epidemiol Rev 1988;10:191–211.

143. Marcenes WS, Sheiham A. The relationship between work stress and oral health status. Soc Sci Med 1992;35:1511–20.

144. Monteiro da Silva AM, Oakley DA, Newman HN, et al. Psychosocial factors in adult onset rapidly progressing periodontitis. J Clin Periodontol 1996;23(8):789–94.

145. Linden GJ, Mullally BH, Freeman R. Stress and the progression of periodontal disease. J Clin Periodontol 1996;23(7):675–80.

146. Genco RJ, Ho AW, Grossi SG, et al. Relationship of stress, distress, and inadequate coping behaviors to periodontal disease. J Periodontol 1999. [In press]

147. Genco RJ, Ho AW, Kopman J, et al. Models to evaluate the role of stress in periodontal disease. Ann Periodontol 1998;3(1):288–302.

148. Dowrenwend BS, Drasnott L, Ashenasj AR, Dowrenwend BP. Exemplification of a method for scaling life events: the PERI life events scale. J Health Soc Beh 1978;19:205–9.

149. Pearlin LI, Schooler C. The structure of coping. J Health Soc Behav 1978;19:2–21.

150. Derogatis LR, Cleary PA. Confirmation of the dimensional structure of the SCL-90: a study in construct validation. J Clin Psychol 1977;33:981–9.

151. Carver CS, Scheier MF, Weintraub JK. Assessing coping strategies: a theoretically based approach. J Pers Soc Psychol 1989;56:267–83.

152. Melnick M, Shields ED, Bixler D. Periodontosis. A phenotypic and genetic analysis. Oral Surg Oral Med Oral Pathol 1976;42:32–41.

153. Saxén L. Heredity of juvenile periodontitis. J Clin Periodontol 1980;7:276–88.

154. Long JC, Nance WE, Aring P, et al. Early onset periodontitis. A comparison and evaluation of two proposed modes of inheritance. Genet Epidemiol 1987;4:13–24.

155. Beaty TH, Boughman JA, Yang P, et al. Genetic analysis of juvenile periodontitis in families ascertained through an affected proband. Am J Hum Genet 1987;40:443–52.

156. Hart TC, Marazita ML, Gunsolley JA, et al. No female preponderance in juvenile periodontitis after correction of ascertainment bias. J Periodontol 1991;62:745–9.

157. Saxby MS. Juvenile periodontitis: an epidemiological study in West Midlands of the United Kingdom. J Clin Periodontol 1987;14:594–8.

158. Hart TC, Marazita ML, Schenkein HA, Diehl SR. Re-interpretation of the evidence for X-linked dominant inheritance of juvenile periodontitis. J Periodontol 1992;63:169–73.

159. Van Dyke TE, Schweinebraten M, Cianciola LJ, et al. Neutrophil chemotaxis in families with localized juvenile periodontitis. J Periodontal Res 1985;20:503–14.

160. Page RC, Vandesteen GE, Ebersole JL, et al. Clinical and laboratory studies of a family with a high prevalence of juvenile periodontitis. J Periodontol 1985;56:602–10.

161. Gwinn MR, Sharma A, De Nardin E. Sequence analysis of chemotactic receptor DNA in LJP [abstract 130]. J Dent Res 1998;77(Special Issue B):648.

162. Wilson ME, Kalmar JR. FcgRIIa (CD32): a potential marker defining susceptibility to localized juvenile periodontitis. J Periodontol 1996;67:323–31.

163. Cullinan MP, Sachs J, Wolf E, Seymour GJ. The distribution of HLA-A and -B antigens in patients and their families with periodontitis. J Periodontal Res 1980;15:177–84.

164. Saxén L, Koskimies S. Juvenile periodontitis—no linkage with HLA-A antigens. J Periodontal Res 1984;19:441–4.

165. Reinholdt J, Bay I, Svejgaard A. Association between HLA-antigens and periodontal disease. J Dent Res 1977;56:1261–3.

166. Kornman KS, Page RC, Tonetti MS. The host response to the microbial challenge in periodontitis: assembling the players. Periodontol 2000 1997;14:33–53.

167. Kaslick RS, West TL, Chasens AI. Association between ABO blood groups, HL-A antigens and periodontal diseases in young adults: a follow-up study. J Periodontol 1980;51:339–42.

168. Kaslick RS, West TL, Chasens AI, et al. Association between HL-A2 antigen and various periodontal diseases in young adults. J Dent Res 1975; 54(2):424.

169. Teraski PI, Kaslick RS, West TL, Chasens AI. Low HL-A2 frequency and periodontitis. Tissue Antigens 1975;5:286–8.

170. Klouda PT, Porter SR, Scully C, et al. Association between HLA-A9 and rapidly progressive periodontitis. Tissue Antigens 1986;28(3):146–9.

171. Amer A, Sing G, Drake C, Dolby AE. Association between HLA antigens and periodontal disease. Tissue Antigens 1988;31:53–8.

172. Ciancio SC, Hazen SP, Cunat JJ. Periodontal observations in twins. J Periodontal Res 1969;4:42–5.

173. Michalowicz BS, Aeppli DP, Kuba RK, et al. A twin study of genetic variation in proportional radiographic alveolar bone height. J Dent Res 1991;70:1431–5.

174. Michalowicz BS, Aeppli D, Virag JG, et al. Periodontal findings in adult twins. J Periodontol 1991;62:293–9.

175. Corey LA, Nance WE, Hofstede P, Schenkein HA. Self-reported periodontal disease in a Virginia twin population. J Periodontol 1993;64:1205–8.

176. Kornman KS, Crane A, Wang H-Y, et al. The interleukin-1 genotype as a severity factor in adult periodontal disease. J Clin Periodontol 1997; 24:72–7.

177. Van Schie RC, Grossi SG, Dunford RG, et al. Fcγ receptor polymorphisms are associated with periodontitis [abstract 129]. J Dent Res 1998; 77(Special Issue B):648.

178. Hassell T. Epilepsy and oral manifestations of phenytoin therapy. Basel, Switzerland: S. Karger; 1981.

179. Adams D, Davies G. Gingival hyperplasia induced by cyclosporine-A. A report of two cases. Brit Dent J 1984;157(3):89–90.

180. Lucas RM, Howell LP, Wall BA. Nifedipine-induced gingival hyperplasia: a histochemical and ultrastructural study. J Periodontol 1985; 56:211–5.

181. Finne K, Goransson K, Winckler L. Oral lichen planus and contact allergy to mercury. Intl J Oral Surg 1982;11(4):236–9.

182. Beck JD, Koch GG, Zambon JJ, et al. Evaluation of oral bacteria as risk indicators for periodontitis in older adults. J Periodontol 1992;63:93–9.

183. Wolff LF, Aeppli DM, Pihlstrom BL, Anderson L. Natural distribution of five bacteria associated with periodontal disease. J Clin Periodontol 1993;20:699–706.

184. Dzink JL, Tanner ACR, Haffajee AD, Socransky SS. Gram-negative species associated with active destructive periodontal lesions. J Clin Periodontol 1985;12:648–59.

185. Mandell RL. A longitudinal microbiological investigation of *Actinobacillus actinomycetemcomitans* and *Eikenella corrodens* in juvenile periodontitis. Infect Immun 1984;45:778–80.

186. Listgarten MA, Levin S. Positive correlation between the proportions of subgingival spirochetes and motile bacteria and susceptibility of human subjects to periodontal deterioration. J Clin Periodontol 1981;8:122–38.

187. Dahlén G, Manji G, Baelum V, Fejerskov O. Putative periodontopathogens in "diseased" and "non-diseased" persons exhibiting poor oral hygiene. J Clin Periodontol 1992;19:35–42.

188. Haffajee AD, Socransky SS, Dzink JL, et al. Clinical, microbiological, and immunological features of subjects with refractory periodontal diseases. J Clin Periodontol 1988;15:390–8.

189. Listgarten MA, Slots J, Nowotny AH, et al. Incidence of periodontitis recurrence in treated patients with and without cultivable *Actinobacillus actinomycetemcomitans*, *Prevotella intermedia*, and *Porphyromonas gingivalis*. A prospective study. J Periodontol 1991;62:377–86.

190. Haffajee AD, Socransky SS, Dzink JL, et al. Clinical, microbiological, and immunological features of subjects with destructive periodontal diseases. J Clin Periodontol 1988;15:240–6.

191. Axelsson P, Lindhe J, Nystrom B. On the prevention of caries and periodontal disease: results of a 15-year longitudinal study in adults. J Clin Periodontol 1991;18:182–9.

192. Smulow JB, Turesky SS, Hill RG. The effect of supragingival plaque removal on anaerobic bacteria in deep periodontal pockets. J Am Dent Assoc 1983;107:737–42.

193. Müller H-P, Hartmann J, Flores-de-Jacoby L. Clinical alterations in relation to the morphological composition of the subgingival microflora following scaling and root planing. J Clin Periodontol 1986;13:825–32.

194. Anerud A, Löe H, Boysen H. The natural history and clinical course of calculus formation in man. J Clin Periodontol 1991;18:160–70.

195. Claffey N, Nylund K, Kiger R, et al. Diagnostic predictability of scores of plaque, bleeding, suppuration and probing depth for probing attachment loss. J Clin Periodontol 1990;17:108–14.

196. Badersten A, Nilveus R, Egelberg J. Scores of plaque, bleeding, suppuration, and probing depth to predict probing attachment loss. 5 years observation following nonsurgical therapy. J Clin Periodontol 1990;17:102–7.

197. Lang NP, Adler R, Joss A, Nyman S. Absence of bleeding on probing is an indicator of periodontal stability. J Clin Periodontol 1990;17:714–21.

198. Lang NP. Clinical markers of active periodontal disease. In: Johnson NW, editor. Risk markers for oral diseases, Vol. 3. Periodontal Disease, Cambridge: Cambridge University Press; 1991. p. 179–202.

199. Grbic JT, Lamster IB, Celenti RS, Fine JB. Risk indicators for future clinical attachment loss in adult periodontitis. Patient variables. J Periodontol 1991;62:322–9.

200. Haffajee AD, Socransky SS, Lindhe J, et al. Clinical risk indicators for periodontal attachment loss. J Clin Periodontol 1991;18:117–25.

201. Axelsson P, Lindhe J. Effect of controlled oral hygiene procedures on caries and periodontal disease in adults. J Clin Periodontol 1978;5:133–51.

202. Haffajee AD, Dzink JL, Socransky SS. Effect of modified Widman flap surgery and systemic tetracycline on subgingival microbiota of periodontal lesions. J Clin Periodontol 1988;15:255–62.

203. Machtei EE, Dunford R, Hausmann E, et al. Longitudinal study of prognostic factors in established periodontitis patients. J Clin Periodontol 1997;24:102–9.

204. Grossi SG, Zambon JJ, Machtei E, et al. Effects of smoking and smoking cessation on healing after mechanical periodontal therapy. J Am Dent Assoc 1997;128:599–607.

CHAPTER 3

CLINICAL HISTORY AND LABORATORY TESTS

Louis F. Rose, DDS, MD
Barbara J. Steinberg, DDS

PATIENT EVALUATION

Medical emergencies can occur in any patient; however, they are most prevalent in geriatric or medically compromised patients. There is a rapidly growing segment of the population whose physical or psychosocial problems may complicate dental treatment. The elderly or medically compromised patient who is frequently taking one or more medications such as steroids, anticoagulants, cardiac drugs, or immunosuppressive agents may require special consideration before undergoing dental treatment. As ever-increasing numbers of such individuals seek dental care, it becomes the responsibility of the dentist to avoid adverse therapeutic interactions and to deal with medical emergencies when they occur.[1–5]

Careful study has shown that the compromised patient is actually in the majority, with more than 50% of 4,365 patients recently surveyed giving a history of more than one significant medical problem.[6] Sophisticated surgical manipulation and medical intervention have made possible the ambulatory treatment of patients with cardiovascular, endocrine, and degenerative diseases-disorders that just a few years ago would have meant confinement or death. Medical advances, along with increasing public awareness of dental health, probably explain the increased numbers of elderly and chronically ill patients seeking dental treatment.

With an increasing likelihood of medical emergencies in this population, the practising dentist and auxiliary staff are responsible for identifying patients with a potential for medical risk by obtaining a comprehensive pretreatment physical evaluation.[7–9] This evaluation is performed to determine patients' physical and emotional status and how well they will tolerate a specific dental procedure.[5]

Little and King, in 1971,[10] presented the reasons for an evaluation of general health in the dental office, and these are summarized as follows:

1. To identify patients with undetected systemic disease that could be a serious threat to the life of the patient or whose condition could be complicated by dental treatment
2. To identify patients who are taking drugs or medications that could adversely interact with drugs prescribed, that would complicate dental therapy, or that may serve as a clue to an underlying systemic disease the patient has failed to mention
3. To provide information for the dentist to modify the treatment plan for the patient in light of any systemic disease or potential drug interactions
4. To enable the dentist to select and communicate with a medical consultant concerning the patient's possible systemic problems
5. To help establish a good patient-doctor relationship by showing patients the clinician's interest in them as individuals and concern for their overall well-being

Information obtained from a comprehensive health evaluation may prevent a medical emergency. A well-conceived evaluation of the patient includes the following: (1) recording a complete medical history; (2) recording appropriate findings on physical examination; (3) when indicated, ordering and interpreting necessary laboratory studies; and (4) initiating medical consultation or referral as needed.[5]

In addition, to detect changes in general health that may affect dental treatment, the medical evaluation must be updated every time the patient is seen during maintenance therapy (eg, every 3 to 6 months) and at appropriate intervals during protracted active therapy.

MEDICAL HISTORY

History-taking is a technique for eliciting subjective information. These data are organized logically to portray the patient's physical and emotional status. Diagnosis of a specific medical disorder may require consultation. Medical history puts physical examination into perspective by supplying information that should alert the examiner to suspected abnormalities.[3] Even in a life-threatening situation, once the immediate threat has been contained, a history should be obtained from the patient, if possible, or from a relative or friend if the patient is unable to respond.

Two basic methods for obtaining a medical history are the questionnaire and the personal interview. At first, it might seem that a great deal of time and trouble could be saved if we were to have each patient complete a printed questionnaire and then have the answers coded. There are, however, several problems with this approach. For instance, a "no" answer may mean the patient never had the symptoms or the disease or that the question is not understood or is thought to be irrelevant since the patient only wants to have a tooth restored or extracted. On the other hand, a personal history elicited through dialogue allows for observation of patients and their reactions to questions. This often provides more important information than the answer itself. The personal dialogue allows the practitioner to evaluate the patient's mental status in a nonthreatening atmosphere. The patient who is afraid or uninterested will respond quite differently from the one who is self-confident and truly concerned about oral health.

A questionnaire can be used in conjunction with the dialogue to obtain a more complete medical history. The questionnaire may help a patient recall frequently used medications and various symptoms that indicate disease. It can also assist the dentist in determining which areas to emphasize and further explore when conducting the dialogue. The questionnaire completed by the patient in privacy can also alleviate embarrassment in answering questions concerning habits, addictions, or sexually transmitted diseases, all of which are important components of a complete medical history.

A comprehensive medical history helps the dentist evaluate present health status, past medical history, allergies, medications, and pertinent familial and social history as well as conduct a review of body systems. The following information may be elicited under each area of the medical history.[1,11,12]

Present Health Status

The patient should be asked the date and results of the last complete physical examination. If the patient states, for example, that they have diabetes, it is important to determine the date of the initial diagnosis, the degree of success in controlling the disease, and the therapeutic regimen as well as the date, type, and results of the last blood glucose study. If the patient has not had a recent physical examination, it may be advisable to make a recommendation for an examination, especially if the patient is in a high-risk group. The patient's perception of their present health status may be an important indication of their psychological makeup and potential compliance with treatment.

Past Medical History

The date, diagnosis, and treatment rendered at significant hospitalizations for illnesses during childhood and adult life will help evaluate the patient's past medical history and clearly indicate whether their average state of health has been one of normal vigor or chronic illness.

Allergies

The patient should be asked about allergies or reactions to any foods, medications, or environmental factors. Specifically, aspirin, local anesthetics, antibiotics, and any other potential allergens that may be used in dental therapy should be mentioned.

Medications

In questioning about medications, it is imperative to determine the brand and/or generic name of the drug, why and by whom it was prescribed, the dosage, and the length of time the medication has been taken. Patients may not include medications used for allaying anxiety or for inducing sleep, such as tranquilizers and sedative-hypnotic drugs. An effective way of obtaining this information is to ask patients if they ever have to take anything to help them rest, relax, or sleep. Also, some women will not include oral contraceptives or supplemental hormones, either of which may affect oral tissues.

Review of Systems

The review of body systems (see Table 3–1) is the main component of the interview approach to history-taking. It provides additional data about each system and reveals symptoms not already elicited that may indicate a previously treated or undiagnosed disorder. The review of systems helps to refresh the patient's memory, thus preventing any inadvertent oversight.

Family History

Family history is taken to determine if there is a familial predisposition to diseases or if there are diseases in which inheritance is an important factor. For example, a patient with a strong family history of diabetes mellitus, with no apparent signs or symptoms of the disease, should be evaluated periodically since clinical manifestations may appear later in life. Also, those with a history of diabetes may have a greater risk for developing infections such as periodontal disease. The dentist should inquire specifically about a family history of diabetes, cancer, heart disease, high blood pressure,

seizure disorders, mental disorders, and other diseases that may be familial.

Social History

Social history may assist in determining the patient's response to the demands and conflicts of modern society. In addition, it may help explain untoward reactions to health problems and to the therapeutic recommendations. For example, the alcoholic patient may be unwilling to follow recommendations about diet and oral hygiene. Also, the alcoholic patient is an anesthetic risk and may develop prolonged and profound hypotensive episodes secondary to certain anxiety and pain-control drugs. Social history should include the patient's occupation and any associated health hazards, marital status, diet, and use of alcohol, tobacco, or other drugs. Possible exposure to various infectious diseases, such as hepatitis B, herpes, or acquired immunodeficiency syndrome (AIDS), should be determined. Social history is therefore important in assessing whether a patient is in a high-risk group, for example, those with alcoholism, drug addiction, or contagious infections such as herpes, hepatitis, tuberculosis, or

TABLE 3–1. Review of Systems

Skin	Itching, rash, ulcers, excessive dryness, pigmentary change, changes in hair or nails, hair loss
Eyes	Vision, inflammation, diplopia, blurring
Ears, nose, throat	Hearing, earache, epistasis, sore throat, hoarseness, sinus pain
Respiratory system	Cough, sputum (describe quantity, color, odor, blood), wheezing, infections, exposure to tuberculosis, prior chest radiographic examination
Heart	Chest pain, palpitation, dyspnea, orthopnea, swelling of ankles, history of rheumatic fever, rheumatic heart disease, "heart attack," high blood pressure, murmur
Gastrointestinal system	Appetite, nausea, vomiting, dysphagia, heartburn, indigestion, food intolerance, abdominal pain, jaundice, hepatitis
Genitourinary system	Dysuria, nocturia, polyuria, hematuria, frequency, difficulty starting stream, sexually transmitted diseases, kidney infection For women: • Menstrual history: last menstrual period and previous menstrual periods, dysmenorrhea • Menopause: age of occurrence, hot flashes • Obstetric history: pregnancies, miscarriages, living children
Extremities	• Vascular: varicose veins, phlebitis • Joints: pain, stiffness, swelling of joints • Muscles: weariness, pain, tenderness, cramps
Nervous system	Syncope, convulsions, headache, lightheadedness, vertigo, tremor, paralysis, paresthesias, anesthesia
Psychiatric	"Nervousness," irritability, depression, history of previous "nervous breakdown," family history of mental illness
Blood	Bleeding tendency, excessive bruising, anemia, known exposure to radiation or toxic agents

AIDS. Direct confirmation of these conditions often requires testing and consultation.

Medical Summary and Recommendations

Positive findings should be summarized and recommendations recorded. This will enable the dentist and the dental staff to quickly review a patient's medical status at each visit and facilitate the diagnosis and treatment of any medical emergency that may arise.

Initially, the medical history form described here represents one of the most accurate methods for determining the physical and emotional status of the patient, the patient's tolerance for specific procedures, and the presence of any medical risk factors. In essence, this form aids in the decision to proceed with dental treatment with relative safety or to seek medical consultation before beginning therapy.[13,14]

In conclusion, a comprehensive medical history is an important procedure that dentists must adopt and routinely use to ensure that their patients are receiving the optimum benefit from all available health resources. A form for recording the medical history has been suggested by the American Dental Association. (Figure 3–1)

INTERPRETATION OF CLINICAL LABORATORY STUDIES

On occasion, the patient's medical history and physical examination warrant laboratory tests to confirm a diagnosis or to uncover incidental findings separate from the chief complaint.[15–17] Depending on the dentist's background and experience in interpreting such tests, the patient will be referred directly to either a clinical laboratory or a physician for appropriate examination, tests, and opinion. With the first alternative, the dentist assumes responsibility for the interpretation and then refers the patient to a physician for confirmation and treatment, if indicated. With the second alternative, the physician assumes all responsibility for preparing the patient and evaluating the findings. Table 3–2 lists some commonly used clinical laboratory tests.

Complete Blood Count

The complete blood count (CBC) will routinely include hemoglobin (HgB), hematocrit (Hct), red blood cell (RBC) count, and white blood cell (WBC) count, with a differential WBC count and a statement on the adequacy of platelets.

Hemoglobin

Hemoglobin is the oxygen carrier of the blood. It is decreased in hemorrhage and anemias and increased in hemoconcentration and polycythemia. The normal range is 14 to 18 g/dL of blood in men and 12 to 16 g/dL of blood in women.

Hematocrit

Hematocrit reflects the relative volume of cells and plasma in the blood. In anemias and after blood loss, it is lowered and is elevated in polycythemia and dehydration. The normal Hct range is 40 to 54% for men and 37 to 47% for women, or roughly three times the HgB value.

RBC Count

The RBCs contain HgB. An increase in RBCs may indicate hemoconcentration or polycythemia. A decrease in the number of RBCs may be indicative of blood loss or one of the anemias.

WBC Count

White blood cells are important in the bodily defense against invading microorganisms. An increase in the WBC count is seen in leukemias, bacterial infections, infectious mononucleosis, and certain parasitic infections as well as after exercise and emotional stress. A decrease in the WBC count is seen in aplastic anemia, lupus erythematosus, acute viral infections, and drug and chemical toxicity. A normal WBC count is 5000 to 10,000/mm^3.

There are several kinds of WBCs that can be identified microscopically; such identification is called the differential. It is important to know whether the proportions of these cells have changed since they may be indicative of a particular type of ailment.

1. Neutrophils (50 to 70%) are increased in most bacterial infections. An increase in the number of immature neutrophils is frequently found in acute infections. This is the so-called "shift to the left."
2. Eosinophils (1 to 4%) are increased in allergic conditions and parasitic infections.
3. Basophils (0 to 1%) may be increased in some blood dyscrasias.
4. Lymphocytes (25 to 40%) are noted to be increased in measles and in several bacterial or chronic infections.
5. Monocytes (4 to 8%) may be increased during recovery from severe infections and Hodgkin's disease.

Medical History Form

Date _____

Name _____ Home Phone (_____) _____
     Last   First   Middle

Address _____ Business Phone (_____) _____
      Number, Street

City _____ State _____ Zip Code _____

Occupation _____ Social Security No. _____

Date of Birth ___/___/___ Sex M F Height _____ Weight _____ Single _____ Married _____
       mo. day yr.

Name of Spouse _____ Closest Relative _____ Phone (_____) _____

If you are completing this form for another person, what is your relationship to that person? _____

Referred by _____

For the following questions, *circle yes or no*, whichever applies. Your answers are for our records only and will be considered confidential. Please note that during your initial visit you will be asked some questions about your responses to this questionnaire and there may be additional questions concerning your health.

1. Are you in good health? . . . . Yes   No
2. Has there been any change in your general health within the past year? . . . . . . Yes   No
3. My last physical examination was on _____
4. Are you now under the care of a physician? . . . . Yes   No
   If so, what is the condition being treated? _____
5. The name and address of my physician(s) is _____
   _____
   _____

6. Have you had any serious illness, operation, or been hospitalized in the past 5 years? . . . . Yes   No
   If so, what was the illness or problem? _____
7. Are you taking any medicine(s) including non-prescription medicine?. . . . . Yes   No
   If so, what medicine(s) are you taking? _____
8. Do you have or have you had any of the following diseases or problems?
   a. Damaged heart valves or artificial heart valves, including heart murmur or rheumatic heart disease . . . . Yes   No
   b. Cardiovascular disease (heart trouble, heart attack, angina, coronary insufficiency, coronary occlusion, high blood
      pressure, arteriosclerosis, stroke) . . . . Yes   No
      1. Do you have chest pain upon exertion? . . . . Yes   No
      2. Are you ever short of breath after mild exercise or when lying down?. . . . . . Yes   No
      3. Do your ankles swell? . . . . Yes   No
      4. Do you have inborn heart defects? . . . . Yes   No
      5. Do you have a cardiac pacemaker? . . . . Yes   No
   c. Allergy . . . . Yes   No
   d. Sinus trouble . . . . Yes   No
   e. Asthma or hay fever . . . . Yes   No
   f. Fainting spells or seizures . . . . Yes   No
   g. Persistent diarrhea or recent weight loss . . . . Yes   No
   h. Diabetes . . . . Yes   No
   i. Hepatitis, jaundice or liver disease . . . . Yes   No
   j. AIDS or HIV infection . . . . Yes   No
   k. Thyroid problems . . . . Yes   No
   l. Respiratory problems, emphysema, bronchitis, etc. . . . . Yes   No
   m. Arthritis or painful swollen joints . . . . Yes   No
   n. Stomach ulcer or hyperacidity . . . . Yes   No
   o. Kidney trouble . . . . Yes   No
   p. Tuberculosis . . . . Yes_   No
   q. Persistent cough or cough that produces blood . . . . Yes   No
   r. Persistent swollen glands in neck . . . . Yes   No
   s. Low blood pressure . . . . Yes   No
   t. Sexually transmitted disease . . . . Yes   No
   u. Epilepsy or other neurological disease . . . . Yes   No
   v. Problems with mental health . . . . Yes   No
   w. Cancer . . . . Yes   No
   x. Problems of the immune system . . . . Yes   No

(over)

Figure 3–1. Medical history form, side 1.

		Yes	No
9.	Have you had abnormal bleeding?.	Yes	No
	a. Have you ever required a blood transfusion?	Yes	No
10.	Do you have any blood disorder such as anemia?	Yes	No
11.	Have you ever had any treatment for a tumor or growth?	Yes	No
12.	Are you allergic or have you had a reaction to:		
	a. Local anesthetics	Yes	No
	b. Penicillin or other antibiotics	Yes	No
	c. Sulfa drugs	Yes	No
	d. Barbiturates, sedatives, or sleeping pills	Yes	No
	e. Aspirin	Yes	No
	f. Iodine	Yes	No
	g. Codeine or other narcotics	Yes	No
	h. Other _____		
13.	Have you had any serious trouble associated with any previous dental treatment?	Yes	No
	If so, explain _____		
	_____		
14.	Do you have any disease, condition, or problem not listed above that you think I should know about?	Yes	No
	If so, explain _____		
	_____		
15.	Are you wearing contact lenses?	Yes	No
16.	Are you wearing removable dental appliances?	Yes	No

Women

		Yes	No
17.	Are you pregnant?	Yes	No
18.	Do you have any problems associated with your menstrual period?	Yes	No
19.	Are you nursing?	Yes	No
20.	Are you taking birth control pills?	Yes	No

Chief Dental Complaint _____

_____

I certify that I have read and understand the above. I acknowledge that my questions, if any, about the inquiries set forth above have been answered to my satisfaction. I will not hold my dentist, or any other member of his/her staff, responsible for any errors or omissions that I may have made in the completion of this form.

_____
Signature of Patient

For completion by the dentist.
Comments on patient interview concerning medical history: _____
_____
_____
_____

Significant findings from questionnaire or oral interview: _____
_____
_____
_____

Dental management considerations: _____
_____
_____
_____

_____   _____
(Date)   Signature of Dentist

Medical history update:

Date	Comments	Signature
_____	_____	_____
_____	_____	_____
_____	_____	_____
_____	_____	_____
_____	_____	_____

S500   © American Dental Association 1988

Figure 3–1. Medical history form, side 2.

Blood Glucose

Blood glucose tests are performed to evaluate glucose metabolism. Basic tests for disorders of blood glucose are the fasting blood sugar test, the glucose tolerance test, and the random blood sugar test. The normal range for blood glucose is 70 to 100 mg/dL of serum.

Blood Urea Nitrogen

Blood urea nitrogen (BUN) is used as a screening test for kidney function; however, it is not entirely specific. An increased value may be seen in extensive kidney disease, congestive heart failure, and dehydration. Protein intake may also directly affect BUN values. If renal disease is suspected, a more reliable assessment is the serum creatinine test. The ratio of BUN to creatinine is 10:1. The normal range for BUN is 8 to 23 mg/dL of blood.

Serology

There are a variety of serologic tests for the screening of syphilis. All are nonspecific tests and may give both false-positive and false-negative results. Interpretation of these serologic tests requires correlation with the patient's history and clinical findings. Normally, results of these tests are negative; if results are positive, confirmation with the fluorescent treponemal antibody-absorption test (FTA-abs) or the microhemagglutination treponemal pallidum test (MHA-tp) is indicated.

Screening Tests for Hemorrhagic Disorders

Bleeding Time
Bleeding time is the time required for hemostasis to occur in a standard wound of the capillary bed. Bleeding time varies with vascular and platelet abnormalities. The normal range is 1 to 7 minutes.

Platelet Count
Platelets are decreased in thrombocytopenic purpura. In myeloproliferative disease, platelets are increased. The normal platelet count is 150,000 to 400,000/mm^3.

Prothrombin
The prothrombin (PT) test is an indirect test of the clotting ability of the blood. This test gives an indication of prothrombin deficiency arising from liver disease, fibrinogen deficiency, and lack of or

TABLE 3–2. Normal Values

Test	Normal Values*
Blood chemistry	
Albumin	3.8–5.0 g/dL
Bilirubin	
• direct	<0.3 mg/dL
• indirect	0.1–1.0 mg/dL
• total	0.1–1.2 mg/dL
Calcium	9.2–11.0 mg/dL
	4.6–5.5 mEq/L
Creatinine	0.6–1.2 mg/dL
Glucose	70–110 IU/L
Lactate dehydrogenase	25–100 IU/L
Phosphatase, alkaline	
• child	20–150 IU/L at 30°C
• adult	20–90 IU/L at 30°C
Transferases	
• aspartate amino (SGOT)	16–60 U/mL at 30°C
• alanine amino (SGPT)	8–50 U/mL at 30°C
Urea nitrogen	8–23 mg/dL
Hematology	
Leukocyte count (WBC)	5000–10,000/mm^3
	5–10 × 10^3/μL
• neutrophils	
– segmented	50–70%
– band	0–5%
• lymphocytes	25–40%
• monocytes	4–8%
• eosinophils	1–4%
• basophils	0–1%
Erythrocyte count (RBC)	
• male	4.5–6.2 million/mm^3
	4.6–6.2 × 10^6/μL
• female	4.2–5.4 million/mm^3
	4.2–5.4 × 10^6/μL
Hemoglobin	
• male	13.5–18.0 g/dL
• female	12.0–16.0 g/dL
Hematocrit	
• male	40–54%
• female	37–47%
RBC indices	
• mean corpuscular hemoglobin	27–31 pg
• mean corpuscular volume	80–96 μm^3
• mean corpuscular hemoglobin concentration	32–36%
Platelet count	150,000–400,000/mm^3
	150–400 × 10^3/μL
Bleeding time (Ivy)	1–7 min
Partial thromboplastin time	≤ 45 sec (variable)
Prothrombin time	12–14 sec

*There may be interlaboratory variations.

inability of the body to use vitamin K. The normal range is 12 to 14 seconds, depending on the type of thromboplastin used. In treatment with Coumadin, the physician will attempt to keep the prothrombin time at 2 to 2 1/2 times the normal value (see "Test to Monitor Oral Anticoagulants").

Partial Thromboplastin Time

The partial thromboplastin time (PTT) test is designed to help the clinician recognize mild to moderate deficiencies of the intrinsic clotting factors. This test is necessary because PT entirely bypasses the intrinsic clotting system. Another use for PTT is to demonstrate a circulating anticoagulant in plasma. The normal PTT is 45 seconds or less; however, because there are wide variations in technique, the normal range for PTT varies somewhat between laboratories.

Test to Monitor Oral Anticoagulants

The international normalized ratio (INR) is the ratio of a patient's PT to the mean PT value determined by using a given thromboplastin, and this ratio is raised to the power of the international sensitivity index (ISI) that is provided by the reagent manufacturer. By using the INR, the degree of anticoagulation achieved by warfarin therapy may be compared, regardless of the thromboplastin used. Use of the INR allows PT results to be compared among clinical laboratories around the world, resulting in better patient man-

agement. It must be emphasized that the purpose of the INR is to monitor patients taking oral anticoagulants; it is not intended to be used for initial evaluation of the hemostatic system or thrombotic conditions. Anticoagulation to a target INR of 3.0 should be made before patients with cardiac valve prosthesis undergo dental procedures involving the risk of bleeding.

MEDICAL RISK ASSESSMENT

Having completed all the components of the physical evaluation and a thorough oral examination, the dentist must gather all the information and determine if the patient is capable, physiologically and psychologically, of tolerating in relative safety the stresses involved in the proposed dental treatment. Is there a greater risk (of morbidity or mortality) than normal during the dental therapy? If the patient decides to go ahead with the treatment in spite of the risk of being medically compromised, then appropriate modifications in the planned dental treatment must be considered to minimize the risk.[18]

To categorize dental patients from the standpoint of medical status, each patient should be assigned an appropriate medical risk category recommended by the American Society of Anesthesiologists. This is commonly referred to as the ASA physical status classification system and is summarized in Table 3–3.

TABLE 3–3. Medical Risk Categories*

ASA Classification	Dental Consideration
Physical status 1 A patient without systemic disease; a normal healthy patient	Routine dental therapy without modification
Physical status 2 A patient with mild systemic disease	Routine dental therapy with possible treatment limitations or special considerations (eg, duration of therapy, stress of therapy, prophylactic consideration, possible sedation, and medical consultation)
Physical status 3 A patient with severe systemic disease that limits activity but is not incapacitating	Dental therapy with possible strict limitations or special considerations
Physical status 4 A patient with incapacitating systemic disease that is a constant threat to life	Emergency dental therapy only with severe limitations or special considerations

*Adopted in 1962 by the American Society of Anesthesiologists (ASA)

DENTAL HISTORY

Significant items of the past dental history that should be recorded at this visit include previous restorative, periodontic, endodontic, or oral surgical treatment; reasons for loss of teeth; untoward complications of dental treatment; attitudes toward previous dental treatment; experience with orthodontic appliances and dental prostheses; and radiation or other treatment for oral or facial lesions.[19] General features of past treatment, rather than specific, detailed, tooth-by-tooth descriptions are needed at this time. In the case of radiation or other treatment for oral or facial lesions, exact information regarding the date and nature of the diagnosis, the type and anatomic location of treatment, and the name, address, and telephone number of the physicians and/or dentists involved as well as the facility (hospital, clinic) where the treatment was given, must be recorded. Likewise, clear details of any previous untoward complications of dental treatment must be recorded.

REFERENCES

1. Genco R, Goldman H, Cohen DW. Contemporary periodontics. St Louis, MO: The CV Mosby Publishing Co.; 1990.
2. Rose LF. Diagnosis and management of medical emergencies in the dental office. Univ PA School Dent Med 1977;3.
3. Rose LF. Medical history as a dental procedure. Dent Dimens 1977; Jan–March;13.
4. Rose LF, Hendler BH. Medical emergencies in dental practice. Chicago: Quintessence Publishing Co.; 1981.
5. Rose LF, Steinberg BJ, Hendler BH. Physical evaluation. Alpha Omegan 1984;77(4):17.
6. Colton JA, Kafrawy, AH. Medications and health histories; a survey of 4,365 dental patients. J Am Dent Assoc 1979;98:713.
7. Hendler BH, Rose LF. Common medical emergencies; a dilemma in dental education. J Am Dent Assoc 1975;91:575.
8. Malamed SF. Handbook of medical emergencies in the dental office. St. Louis, MO: The CV Mosby Publishing Co.; 1982.
9. McCarthy FM. Emergencies in dental practice. 2nd ed. Philadelphia: W.B. Saunders Company; 1972.
10. Little JW, King OR. The significance of physical diagnosis, patient history, data and medical screening in the dental office. Am Dent 1972;3:31.
11. Bates G. A guide to physical examination. Philadelphia: J.B. Lippincott Co.; 1974.
12. Halsted CL, et al. Physical evaluation of the dental patient. St. Louis, MO: The CV Mosby Publishing Co.; 1982.
13. Brasher WJ, Rees TD. The medical consultation: its role in dentistry. J Am Dent Assoc 1977;95:961.
14. Redding SW, Rose LF. The consultation: a means of communication between dentists and physicians. Gen Dent 1979;Sept/Oct p.54.
15. Rose LF. Hospital dental practice. Dent Clin North Am 1975;19(4).
16. Sonis ST, Sandinski JJ. Physical and laboratory diagnosis. Dent Clin North Am 1974;18(1).
17. Zambito RF. Hospital dental practice: a manual. New York: Medical Examination Publishing; 1978.
18. Little JW, et al. Dental management of the medically compromised patient. 5th ed. St. Louis, MO: The CV Mosby Publishing Co.; 1997.
19. Kerr DA, Ash MM, Millard DH. Oral diagnosis. 6th ed. St. Louis, MO: The CV Mosby Publishing Co.; 1983.

CHAPTER 4

Role of Genetics in Assessment, Risk, and Management of Adult Periodontitis

Kenneth S. Kornman, DDS, PhD
Michael G. Newman, DDS

PERIODONTAL DISEASE

Periodontitis, a chronic multifactorial disease in adults, is caused mainly by gram-negative microorganisms, such as *Porphyromonas gingivalis, Prevotella intermedia,* and *Actinobacillus actinomycetemcomitans.* The most common form of periodontitis is adult periodontitis, which has been reported to affect more than 30% of the population, with severe disease reported in 7 to 13%.[1] Adult periodontitis is characterized by an interaction between the host immunoinflammatory response and gram-negative bacteria. With periodontal disease, plaque microorganisms adjacent to the gingiva stimulate host cells, resulting in the production of molecules that play an important role in activating and regulating the immunoinflammatory response. Microbial substances such as lipopolysaccharide (LPS) activate host cells (ie, fibroblasts, macrophages, and polymorphonuclear leukocytes [PMNs]) to secrete proinflammatory cytokines such as interleukin-1 beta (IL-1β) and tumor necrosis factor alpha (TNF-α).[2]

Clinical evidence has demonstrated that not all individuals have the same response to similar amounts of plaque accumulation. There are patients with moderate and advanced disease who have very little plaque while other patients with little disease have large amounts of plaque. Most importantly, large studies that have assessed the relationship of plaque quantity, as well as the presence of specific bacteria, to the severity of periodontitis indicate that a substantial part of the variation in clinical severity of disease may be explained by factors other than the bacterial challenge. It should be emphasized that this statement in no way means that bacterial plaque is unimportant—in fact, it is quite the contrary. Bacterial plaque is absolutely essential for the initiation and progression of periodontitis. However, it now appears that once the bacteria are present, the amount of periodontitis that a patient develops is due to factors related to the body's response to the bacterial challenge. One reason for the differences in how patients respond to plaque, manifest disease, and respond to treatment is that there are different types of plaque. Some types of plaque are more virulent than others.[3–5] Although a few laboratories have offered microbial analysis of subgingival plaque samples for many years, the value of plaque sampling in nonresponding patients is of growing interest as some research groups have started to clarify how the resulting information can be integrated into clinical practice.

The presence of bacteria is necessary for periodontal disease to occur; however, this presence alone does not predict the presence or severity of periodontitis. The differences in disease severity observed among individuals cannot be explained solely by the presence of different quantities or types of bacteria.[6] For the presence, absence, or level of specific microbes believed to be periodontal pathogens, the correlation coefficients are in the range of 0.3 to 0.4 in current multivariate models of periodontitis that incorporate microbial factors. These findings indicate that less than 20% of the variability in periodontal disease expression can be explained by the levels of specific microbes. It has been shown that specific elements of host susceptibility, such as an individual's systemic disease state and immune response, are important factors in disease expression.[7,8]

Genetics and Clinical Presentation of Periodontal Disease

It has long been observed that unusual forms of periodontitis, such as disease affecting young individuals (early onset periodontitis), "run in families." The evidence for a genetic influence on early-onset periodontitis has been well reviewed in recent years.[7,9,10] Since it was believed that adult periodontitis was totally determined by bacterial plaque, less effort was devoted to exploring a genetic influence. In addition, the genetic influence in an adult-onset chronic disease is difficult to study since so many factors change during the course of the disease and it is more difficult to study families with adult-onset disorders than those with diseases affecting children.

Early studies reported significant differences in gingivitis among different ethnic groups.[9] However, the finding of familial aggregation or ethnic differences in a disease does not prove a genetic component because a common familial environment or the variable environments of different ethnic groups may bring about these findings.[11] However, in recent years, new studies demonstrated substantial genetic influences on adult periodontitis. In particular, studies in twins indicate that a significant part of the variance in clinical and radiographic measures of adult periodontitis may be explained by genetic factors.[12–14] The combination of two observations—(1) the recognition that much of the clinical expression of periodontitis was not explainable solely by the bacterial parameters, and (2) studies in twins—led to renewed interest in finding specific genetic factors that influence the severity and therapeutic responses of the most common form of periodontitis.

Types of Genetic Disorders

Genetic diseases can be divided into three major categories: chromosomal disorders, Mendelian disorders, and non-Mendelian disorders.

Congenital Chromosomal Disorders

Congenital chromosomal disorders are caused by an abnormal dose of normal genes (not abnormal genes) because of a deficiency or excess of chromosomal material. Chromosomal abnormalities occur in approximately 1 per 160 live births.[15] The majority of these abnormalities are sporadic, involving an extra chromosome due to nondisjunction of meiosis during egg or sperm formation. A minority of abnormalities result from chromosomal rearrangements (ie, translocation), which may be inherited or sporadic. Down syndrome (trisomy 21), which is caused by the presence of an extra chromosome 21, is a classic example of a chromosome abnormality.[15]

Mendelian Disorders

Mendelian disorders are caused by a mutation in a single gene and, therefore, are also referred to as single-gene (or major gene effect) disorders. The inheritance patterns of Mendelian disorders may be described in terms of the classic patterns of how certain traits, such as autosomal dominant or autosomal recessive disorders, are transmitted through successive generations. An autosomal dominant disorder is caused by a mutation of a gene located on one of the autosomes (chromosomes 1 to 22). Individuals usually have two alleles (copies) of each autosomal gene. With autosomal dominant disorders, individuals may have one "normal" copy of a gene and one "abnormal" copy of the same gene. In dominant disorders, if one of the two copies of the gene is abnormal that is sufficient to cause disease. There is a 50% chance that each offspring of an affected individual will receive the dominant gene from an affected parent. Offspring who receive a normal copy of the gene (and also have a normal copy from the other parent) will not develop the disease or pass it on to their offspring.[15]

There are several general features of autosomal dominant disorders that may disguise the inheritance pattern, such as delayed age of onset, pleiotropism, and variable expression (Table 4–1).[15] Genetic disorders are not necessarily clinically evident at birth, and delayed age of onset is found in the majority of common adult diseases. Pleiotropism refers to the multiple effects of a single gene. Several common disease associations may be explained by pleiotropism, such as the increased incidence of both insulin-dependent diabetes mellitus (IDDM) and autoimmune thyroid disease in the same patient and family, suggesting a common immunogenetic basis for both disorders. Variable expression refers to the differences in the severity and/or extent of disease manifestation among affected individuals.[15]

With autosomal recessive disorders, two alleles of an abnormal gene are necessary for disease expression. Affected individuals are homozygous for the disease gene (homozygotes). Individuals that have a single dose of the normal gene and a single dose of the abnormal gene (heterozygotes) are considered carriers. Although autosomal recessive disorders can occur at any time during an individual's life, they more frequently occur during infancy or childhood.[15]

A mutation at a single gene locus can produce a gene product that predisposes an individual to a disease. A single dose of a mutant allele (heterozygote) is often associated with disease susceptibility whereas a double dose of a mutant allele (homozygote) is associated with direct development of a more severe form of the disease.[15]

Some single-gene disorders occur with enough frequency to make a significant contribution to a common disease or a subgroup of a common disease. For example, the heterozygous state for familial hypercholesterolemia occurs with a frequency of approximately 1 per 500 in the population. Gene carriers have a high probability of developing atherosclerosis. In addition, this gene is found in the heterozygous state in 5 to 10% of men age 60 years or younger who experience myocardial infarcts.[15]

Non-Mendelian Disorders

Most common adult-onset diseases have a genetic component that cannot be explained by either a chromosomal abnormality or a major gene effect. In particular, the genetic influence of non-Mendelian disorders does not fit the typical inheritance patterns within families. For example, in cardiovascular disease, there is an unusual major gene disorder called hypercholesterolemia. Individuals with this Mendelian disorder will have severe cardiovascular disease at a very early age. Most cardiovascular diseases, however, do not involve hypercholesterolemia but seem to be familial and to have genetic influences. These non-Mendelian disorders are undoubtedly multifactorial; they are caused by a combination of genetic and environmental factors. The genetics of these disorders is complicated by several factors: (1) a similar clinical condition may be the result of different disorders and different genetics (genetic heterogeneity); (2) the clinical condition may be polygenic—many additive genes, each of which produces a small effect; and (3) the clinical condition may not be evident unless two different genetic factors are present (multilocus).

Table 4–1. Autosomal Dominant Disorders

Common Autosomal Dominant Disorders
  Familial hypercholesterolemia
  Familial combined hyperlipidemia
Features that may disguise this inheritance pattern
Delayed age of onset
  Adult polycystic kidney disease: cysts are not evident until the second or third decade of life
Pleiotropism
  Marfan syndrome: a single abnormal gene can produce changes in the great vessels, eyes, heart, and skeleton: probably through an alteration in a structural protein common to these tissues
Variable Expression
  Mitral valve prolapse: in a single family, affected members may have significant rhythm disturbances or mitral insufficiency whereas other family members have only an audible click on physical examination with no other symptoms

COMMON DISEASES GENERALLY INVOLVE BOTH GENETIC AND ENVIRONMENTAL FACTORS

From a population genetics point of view, a common disease is defined as an arbitrary frequency of approximately 1 affected individual per 1,000 in the population.[15] King and associates defined the genetic basis of a common disease as "the presence of a genetically susceptible individual, an individual who may or may not develop the disease, depending on the interaction of factors such as other genes, diet, activity, environmental exposures, or even some degree of random biologic variation such as occurs in the immune system and may be operative during development."[15]

There is no absolute distinction between common and single-gene diseases because a single-gene mutation may not cause disease until the carrier of the gene is exposed to a specific environmental agent. For example, an individual with the β-globulin gene polymorphism that leads to sickle cell anemia will have different clinical disease experiences at sea level and at high altitudes, where the oxygen is more limited. The actions of several genes are involved in most common diseases, and sometimes a few genes can be identified as playing a major role in susceptibility. Individuals with different genetic backgrounds have different susceptibilities; therefore, the etiologies of common diseases are usually genetically heterogeneous, that is, different genetic mechanisms lead to the same clinical endpoint. In addition, not everyone who is genetically susceptible will develop the disease. These points suggest that some individuals may have increased susceptibility whereas others will have reduced susceptibility.

The majority of common diseases fall between having a purely genetic cause and a purely environmental cause; they are the result of an interaction between genetic and environmental factors. In addition, some mechanisms of genetic susceptibility involve the actions of genes that control environmental response, such as the histocompatibility (human leukocyte antigen [HLA]) complex on chromosome 6. The involved HLA genetic pattern identifies individuals who will have a specific immunologic response when exposed to various environmental agents.

The clinical manifestation of the gene(s) that an individual possesses is called "the phenotype." Complex phenotypes, such as cardiovascular disease, cluster in certain families but they do not exhibit simple Mendelian inheritance patterns and may have many genetic and environmental causes. By this definition, most chronic, common disorders are considered to be complex. The complexity originates from the fact that multiple genetic and environmental factors may interact with each other in unpredictable ways; the association between the phenotype and any single factor by itself may not be perceptible. With nonlinear interactions (including genotype by environment interactions), clinical expression may not be accurately predicted from understanding the individual effects of each of the component factors considered alone, no matter how well the separate components are understood.[16]

Common Genetic Variations (Polymorphisms)

Gene polymorphisms are a mechanism by which individuals may have variations within the biologically normal range. In a population, a genetic polymorphism is present when variant forms of a gene at a given locus exist with a frequency of more than 1 to 2%. One of the more well-studied examples of gene polymorphisms relates to enzymes involved in normal metabolism. Estimates indicate that approximately 30% of all enzyme gene loci are polymorphic, and approximately 7% of the population is heterozygous at each enzyme locus.[15] Polymorphisms in enzyme genes produce alternative active forms of an enzyme that are shown to differ from the standard enzyme, using electrophoresis,

isoelectric focusing, or other methods of separation. There are frequently subtle differences in enzyme activities between products of different alleles of the polymorphic genetic factor. These differences may result in subtle differences in genetic susceptibility to a disease.

Studies have shown that stable immune phenotypic characteristics, including cytokine production, antibody titer, and monocyte function, may result from specific genetic polymorphisms. For example, studies have focused on the role of genetics in an individual's susceptibility to disease by showing that individuals with an unusual genetic variant in the chemokine receptor CCR5 demonstrate a striking resistance to human immunodeficiency virus (HIV) infection.[7]

Influence of Genetic Susceptibility on Different Characteristics of a Disease

The underlying genetic characteristics of a patient's immune system (a patient's "resistance") determine, in part, how a patient will react to bacterial challenges. Individuals are not equally susceptible to many common diseases, mainly due to differences in their genetic constitutions. Genetic variation is important for classifying diseases, diagnosing and managing patients with common disorders, defining the etiology of common diseases, and evaluating family members of patients. The genetic basis of common diseases, including coronary artery disease, obstructive lung disease, and periodontitis, has several similar factors. These factors include clinical appearance in midlife, a family component, and onset of the underlying pathogenesis, which may begin as early as adolescence.[17] Almost all common disorders have a familial component, which suggests that the distribution of these diseases is not random, and certain individuals are at high risk.[15]

There are different types of genetic susceptibility—susceptibility to a disease, differences in the natural history of a disease, and different therapeutic responses. Susceptibility to the disease itself is the most direct type and may be considered the most important type because it puts an individual and some family members at increased risk of developing the disease. The advantages of assessing this type of susceptibility include being able to identify individuals at risk before disease onset and the potential benefits of preclinical intervention. Susceptibility is usually a complex issue with common diseases. The actions of several genes are usually involved with common diseases but few genes can be identified as playing a major role in the disease. Different genetic backgrounds create different susceptibilities, encouraging the opportunity for different etiologies to lead to the same clinical expression of a disease (ie, different species of bacteria can cause pneumonia or periodontal disease).

Individuals may have susceptibility to differences in the natural history of a disease; they may be more likely to follow a particular clinical course for a disease. After initiation of the disease process, the genetic make-up of the affected individual can influence the course of the disease in terms of severity and complications. Clinicians with the ability to identify these susceptibilities can, in turn, identify individuals at risk for specific complications and apply specific interventions or different therapies. A single genetic factor that significantly changes the clinical course of a disease may have great practical importance for the clinical management of the disease.

Individuals may also exhibit susceptibility to different therapeutic responses, which is commonly found to exist as a genetic subtype of the disease. In addition, individuals may exhibit genetic susceptibility to complications of a specific therapy or variations in their response to therapy. Reductions in poor therapeutic responses or unwanted drug complications could be achieved by an improved ability to recognize this type of susceptibility.

Host Immune Response to Microbial Infection

There are many genetic loci that have been associated with the immune response of the host to microbial infection. Certainly, the most well-studied genetic factor is the major histocompatibility complex (MHC) on chromosome 6, which defines the HLA system that is involved in many interactions between the cells of immune response. The MHC genetics have been associated with increased susceptibility to various microbial infections, including tuberculosis, HIV, and certain parasitic diseases. Recently, a polymorphism in the gene that produces a specific receptor (chemokine receptor CCR5) on the surface of monocytes has been shown to produce strong resistance to HIV-1 infection, even with frequent exposure to the virus.[18,19]

Both CD32 and CD16 are receptors on immunoinflammatory cells for the Fc fragment of immunoglobulin G (Fc-gamma). Variants of genes that code for the Fc-gamma receptor produce a receptor that results in reduced phagocytic capacities, which provide a mechanism for heritable susceptibility to microbial infections. Genetic variants in Fc-gamma receptors have been associated with both early-onset periodontitis[20] and recurrent adult periodontitis.[21]

ROLE OF GENETICS IN PERIODONTAL DISEASE

Periodontal diseases have many of the characteristics of complex diseases, such as the temporal nature of the disease, difficulty in measuring and classifying disease phenotypes, and complex interactions between the host and microbial, environmental, and genetic factors, which make genetic studies difficult.[7]

Several immune response traits have been associated with clinical forms of periodontitis, and the underlying genetic determinants are known for some of these factors. It will be important to identify the genetic factors that imply significant clinical risk. A gene can be considered as possibly having a causative or modifying role in periodontitis if the physiologic processes determined by the gene have been associated with disease presence or severity.[7]

As previously mentioned, some mechanisms of genetic susceptibility involve the actions of genes that control environmental response, such as the HLA complex on chromosome 6. The chromosome 6 HLA region contains several genes involved in the immune response, and the TNF-α gene maps to this region. It has been shown that genetic polymorphisms in the 5' region of the TNF-α gene are involved in the response to an infectious challenge; these polymorphisms may be important in some forms of periodontitis.[7]

As previously discussed, the initiation of periodontitis requires the accumulation of specific bacteria. However, studies of the quantity and types of bacteria have not fully explained the differences in disease severity seen among adults. After disease initiation, there is a correlation between some markers of periodontitis and the host immunoinflammatory response; yet, none of these markers could be used to predict in advance an individual's susceptibility to disease. In addition, there has not been a reliable mechanism for determining the course of the disease to identify patients who require more aggressive therapy.[1]

Why are there clinical differences in the prevalence and severity of adult periodontitis? The answer is that there is a strong genetic component to the disease. A patient's resistance to periodontal disease is influenced by genetics, and this has been determined from a variety of sources: studies of twins, laboratory studies of antibodies, natural history studies, and cytokine genetics studies.[17]

For many years, clinical and laboratory studies found substantial variability in the severity of periodonitits, even with high plaque challenges. Löe and colleagues conducted a study on the natural history of periodontal disease in man over a 15-year period.[22] The study group consisted of Sri Lankan men (age range 14 to 31 years) who did not follow any conventional oral hygiene measures. They exhibited large amounts of plaque, calculus, and stain on their teeth, and almost all the gingival units were inflamed. Among this group, three sub-populations were identified on the basis of interproximal loss of attachment and tooth mortality rates: (1) individuals with rapid progression of periodontal disease (approximately 8%), (2) those with moderate progression of periodontal disease (about 81%), and (3) individuals with no progression of periodontal disease beyond gingivitis (approximately 11%) (Figure 4–1). The group exhibiting rapid progression had a mean loss of attachment of approximately 9 mm at age 35 years, which increased to approximately 13 mm at age 45 years, with an annual rate of destruction of 0.1 to 1.0 mm. In individuals exhibiting moderate progression, the mean loss of attachment was approximately 4 mm at age 35 years and 7 mm at age 45 years, with an annual rate of destruction between

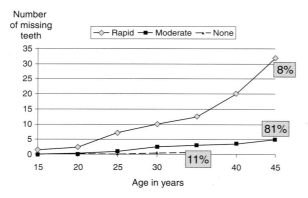

Figure 4–1. Sri Lanka: tooth loss. (Data from Löe H, Anerud A, Boysen H, Morrison E. Natural history of periodontal disease in man. Rapid, moderate, and no loss of attachment in Sri Lankan laborers 14 to 46 years of age. The curves show the number of teeth lost in each of the three groups that were based on the rate of disease progression. The numbers in boxes (8%, 81%, 11%) show the percentage of the study population in that specific disease-progression group. J Clin Periodontol 1986;13:431–45.)

0.05 and 0.5 mm. The mean loss of attachment in individuals with no progression of disease was 1 mm at age 35 years, with an annual rate of destruction between 0.05 and 0.09. Most in the study group were caries free; therefore, essentially all the missing teeth were the result of periodontal disease. Based on modern views of susceptibility, the results of this study show that there may be individuals who are less susceptible to disease.

Studies of Twins

The most convincing demonstration of a genetic influence on adult periodontitis came from studies of twins. Comparison of concordance rates of disease (ie, if both twins in a pair are affected, the concordance rate is 100%) in monozygotic or dizygotic twins is the classic method for determining whether familial patterns of disease are the result of common genetic or common environmental factors. Monozygotic twins are genetically identical whereas dizygotic twins are no more genetically alike than siblings. When the concordance rate is higher in monozygotic twins compared with dizygotic twins, especially same-sex dizygotic twins, a significant part of the familial agreement is caused by genetic factors. When the concordance rate is equal, the familial agreement is mainly determined by environmental factors. With monozygotic twins, it is sometimes difficult to separate heredity from environment as these twins tend to select similar environments, probably because of their genetic identity. Examples of diseases in which the concordance rate is higher in monozygotic twins compared with dizygotic twins include coronary heart disease, diabetes, and peptic ulcer disease. The concordance rate in monozygotic twins is rarely 100%, suggesting an environmental or random component to these disorders, in addition to a genetic component. When 100% concordance is observed in monozygotic twins, genetic factors are of great importance in the specific environment in which the twins were studied.[15]

Michalowicz and colleagues conducted a study to examine the relative contribution of environmental and host genetic factors to the clinical factors of periodontal disease in adult twins.[12] The study group included 77 monozygous twins (63 pairs were reared together and 14 pairs were reared apart) and 33 dizygous twins. Probing depth, clinical attachment loss, gingivitis, and plaque were assessed from the Ramfjord index teeth, and bootstrap sampling was used to estimate and provide confidence limits of between-pair and within-pair variances, heritability, and intraclass correlations. A significant genetic component was identified for plaque, gingivitis, probing depth, and attachment loss based on ratios of within-pair variances or heritability estimates. Heritability estimates showed that between 38 and 82% of the population variance for the clinical factors of disease studied can be attributed to genetic factors.[12] Another study by Michalowicz and colleagues estimated the genetic variance for alveolar bone height in adult twins.[13] Panoramic radiographs were obtained from 62 pairs of reared-together monozygous twins, 25 pairs of same-sex, reared-together dizygous twins, and 33 pairs of reared-apart monozygous twins. Mesial and distal bone heights were determined as a proportion of tooth length. By averaging these proportions from all measurable teeth, a full-mouth bone score was determined for each twin. Calculations of the between-pair and within-pair variances were made for each twin group. Results showed that the population variances (between-pair and within-pair) of the monozygous and dizygous twins were similar, validating a basic assumption of the twin model. In addition, intraclass correlations and heritability estimates were calculated for the reared-together monozygous (0.70) and dizygous twins (0.52), as well as the reared-apart monozygous twins (0.55). The results of this study indicate that there is significant genetic variance for proportional alveolar bone height in the population.[13] In addition, comparisons of reared-together and reared-apart adult monozygous twins showed that early family environment had no substantial influence on probing depth and attachment loss measures in adults.[23]

Although there was strong evidence for some genetic influence on the severity of adult periodontitis, there was not, until the past few years, clear evidence of a specific genetic factor that may explain genetic susceptibility to periodontitis. Increased understanding of the biology of periodontal disease and new understandings of genetic factors that influence responses to bacterial challenges guided the search for candidates that may explain the genetic influences on periodontitis.

Candidate Genes in Adult Periodontitis

Recent reviews have discussed some of the key candidate genes that may be of value, given current knowledge, in the search for genetic influences on periodontitis.[7] The key is to identify genetic factors that are strong enough to significantly influence the clinical outcomes of disease. In general, a gene may be considered a candidate for a significant modifying role in periodontitis if the physiologic processes determined by the gene have been associated with the presence or severity of disease. It should be emphasized that genetic variations that dramatically alter major protective mechanisms are unlikely to be involved in common chronic diseases such as periodontitis. Patients with such major defects are likely to suffer serious childhood problems and complications from various infectious diseases. The most likely candidates for a genetic influence in adult periodontitis are, therefore, genetic variants that produce a subtle change in the magnitude of biologic processes.

The most prominent candidates for a genetic influence on adult periodontitis include factors that produce variations in the relative ability of antibodies and PMNs to kill bacteria and factors that change the relative magnitude of inflammatory processes.

Genetic variations in the quantity of antibody and in the magnitude of PMN binding of antibody (Fc-gamma receptors) have been described and have been associated with early-onset periodontitis. One study associated genetic factors involved in Fc-gamma receptors with recurrence of adult periodontitis in Japanese patients.[21] Studies in U.S. adults have not supported these observations.[24]

The strongest biochemical associations with the severity of periodontitis have been reported for prostaglandin E$_2$ (PGE$_2$), IL-1 and TNF-α, and the enzymes that destroy collagen (matrix-metalloproteinases). Genetic variations in these components should be reasonable candidates for influences on adult periodontitis. There are currently no data to indicate that variations in the genes for PGE$_2$ or for matrix-metalloproteinases influence the severity of periodontitis. Variations in the TNF-α genes were tested for association with severity of periodontitis and showed no association with disease.[1] At present, data indicate that IL-1 gene variations are involved in the clinical severity of periodontitis in adults.

Role of IL-1 in Adult Periodontitis

Chemicals in the tissues that provide communications between cells are generally referred to as cytokines. One cytokine, IL-1, plays a critical signaling role in many different systems in the body and has been strongly implicated in the progression and severity of adult periodontitis.

The cytokines IL-1α, IL-1β, and TNF-α are important mediators of inflammatory responses and appear to play a central role in the pathogenesis of many chronic inflammatory diseases.[25,26] It is now well documented that their biologic activities in vivo are sufficient to produce local inflammation and destruction of connective tissue and bone.[27] The cytokine IL-1 is one of the first chemical mediators activated following any external stimulus, such as a bacterial challenge. As an early response factor, it activates other nonspecific and protective mechanisms, including recruitment of PMNs and activation of blood clotting. It also activates specific protective mechanisms and is involved in wound healing and bone and connective tissue metabolism.

Higher production of these cytokines has also been associated with response to infection, where local induction of IL-1 and TNF facilitates the elimination of the microbial invasion. However, classic studies also report that in some infectious conditions very high levels of monocytic cytokines are produced and initiate a cascade of concomitant events, such as tissue catabolism, vascular reactivity, and hypercoagulation, with damaging effects on the host.[28,29]

Elevated tissue and gingival fluid levels of IL-1β in particular have been repeatedly associated with the severity of periodontitis.[30–35] The relationship between IL-1 and periodontitis has been extensively reviewed by Offenbacher.[8] Although the inflammatory process automatically increases the local tissue levels of IL-1, stable differences between people in cytokine production rates have been reported.[36,37]

Genetic Variations in the IL-1 Genotype and Increased Levels of IL-1

Three IL-1 genes (IL-1A, IL-1B, and IL-1RN) cluster on chromosome 2q13. Interleukin-1A and IL-1B encode the proinflammatory proteins IL-1α and IL-1β, and IL-1RN encodes IL-1ra, a related protein that functions as a receptor agonist. Several genetic polymorphisms have been identified in the genes of the IL-1 cluster. In recent studies, severe adult periodontal disease in nonsmokers[38] was correlated with a composite genotype in the IL-1 gene cluster that includes at least one copy of allele 2 of the IL-1A-889 polymorphism and at least one copy of allele 2 of the +3953 polymorphism of the IL-1B gene. The IL-1A (–889) locus is in > 99% linkage disequilibrium (eg. the two are inherited together) with a polymorphism at the IL-1A (+4845) locus which is currently used in the laboratory in place of IL-1A (–889) in the composite genotype test for severity of adult periodontitis.

A study by di Giovine and colleagues showed that peripheral blood monocytes from individuals with at least one copy of allele 2 at IL-1B (+3953) produced up to four times more IL-1 in response to the same bacterial challenge than those who were genotype negative.[39] Individuals inherit one copy of the IL-1 gene from each parent. Individuals who had two copies (homozygous) of the most common IL-1B (+3953) polymorphism (allele 1) produced a certain amount of IL-1β (5.2 ng/mL) when stimulated by the bacterial component LPS. Individuals who were homozygous for the polymorphism associated with periodontitis (allele 2) produced approximately four times more IL-1β than normal (19.9 ng/mL) (Figure 4–2). And individuals with one copy of allele 1 and one copy of allele 2 of the IL-1B (+3953) polymorphism (heterozygous), produced approximately twice as much IL-1β (12.4 ng/mL).[39]

Patients with the composite IL-1 genotype have higher levels of IL-1 in the gingiva than those observed in genotype-negative patients. Recent studies have determined the levels of IL-1α and IL-1β in gingival biopsies and the levels of IL-1β in gingival crevicular fluid (GCF).[40] The IL-1 genotype positives had higher levels of IL-1β in GCF, with the greatest differences between genotype-positive and genotype-negative patients in sites of minimal probing depth (Figure 4–3). Tissue levels of IL-1β were also higher and levels of IL-1α were marginally higher in genotype-positive patients. These findings were dramatic and indicate that IL-1 genotype-positive patients will have higher levels of IL-1 in periodontal tissues when there is a bacterial challenge. Related observations were made in a pilot study by Jotwani and colleagues who examined the response of periodontally healthy patients to plaque accumulation. This study found that IL-1 genotype-positive patients, but not the genotype-negative patients, had a significant increase in GCF IL-1β after 3 days without oral hygiene.[41]

Genetic Variations in IL-1 Genotype and Increased Severity of Adult Periodontitis

The first report of an association between the IL-1 genotype and severity of adult periodontitis was published in 1997.[1] Since that time, other studies that confirm these findings have been reported.

In the first report the study population included only adults with no known history of early-onset disease and most likely included patients with both adult periodontitis and refractory periodontitis. The association between severe periodontitis and the genetic polymorphism in the IL-1 genes was present only when smokers were excluded, which confirmed the importance of smoking as a risk factor for periodontitis. This was the first study that identified a genetic polymorphism that corresponds with a phenotypic immune response variable (IL-1 production) in adult periodontitis patients.[1] The IL-1 genotype identified in this study appears to be a marker of a strong biologic change that results in severe periodontitis, without regard to the amount of bacterial challenge. This does not mean that bacteria are not important in the disease process—quite the contrary. The first findings indicate that the significant association between the IL-1 genotype and severity of periodontitis did not require any adjustments for the amount of bacterial plaque. The combination of having either the specific genotype or smoking accounted for the majority (86%) of severe cases of periodontitis. The IL-1 genotype was a very strong predictor of severe periodontitis in nonsmokers age 40 to 60 years (odds ratio 18.90) (Figure 4–4). Among similar-aged individuals with mild periodontitis, 84% were genotype negative.[1]

It is noteworthy that the association between the genetic polymorphism in IL-1 genes with severe periodontitis was only evident when smokers are excluded. These data support the importance of other environmental factors, such as smoking, as a risk factor for periodontitis.[34,103] The association of severe periodontitis with smoking and the IL-1 genotype suggests that both factors play an important role in the pathogenesis and clinical course of adult periodontitis.

Other studies have confirmed these early observations. McDevitt and colleagues found similar associations between the IL-1 genotype and adult periodontitis (Figure 4–5).[42] McGuire and Nunn have reported an increased susceptibility to tooth loss after periodontal therapy in IL-1 genotype-positive patients.[43] Recently, Gore and colleagues (1998) reported a significant association between the IL-1β polymorphism and severity of disease.[44] In this study, the composite genotype (IL-1A plus IL-1B) did not offer advantages over just the IL-1B markers. Such differences among the studies are not surprising as genetic studies usually have small numbers of subjects.

The above studies were performed primarily in Caucasians. One obvious question is, what is the role of the IL-1 genotype in other ethnic groups? In most of the populations that have been tested, this genotype occurs in approximately 30% of individuals.[1] Although it is expected that the IL-1 geno-

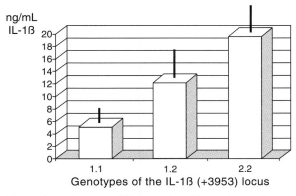

Figure 4–2. Amount of IL-1 produced by patients who are homozygous (2.2) or heterozygous (1.20 for the allele for adult periodontitis . (Data from diGiovine FS, Cork MJ, Crane A, et al. Novel genetic association of an IL-1β gene variation a + 3953 with IL-1β protein production and psoriasis [abstract]. Cytokine 1995;7:606.)

type will have the same relationship to disease in all populations, the IL-1 genotype may be found less frequently in some populations than in Caucasians. It is also possible that other genetic factors may play a role in other ethnic groups. At present, it has been reported that IL-1 genotype positivity is found in approximately 30% of Caucasians[1] and Hispanics.[45] It has been reported that genotype positivity is much less common in the Chinese population.[46] Studies are in progress to determine the prevalence of the IL-1 genotype in other populations.

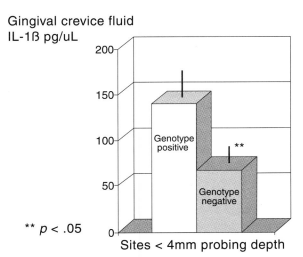

Figure 4–3. IL-1 is higher in the periodontal tissues of PST® positives. (Data from Engebretsson SP, Lamster IB, et al. The influence of interleukin-1 (IL-1) gene polymorphisms on expression of IL-1β, and tumor necrosis factor alpha (TNFα) in periodontal tissue and gingival crevicular fluid. J Periodontol 1999;70:567–73.)

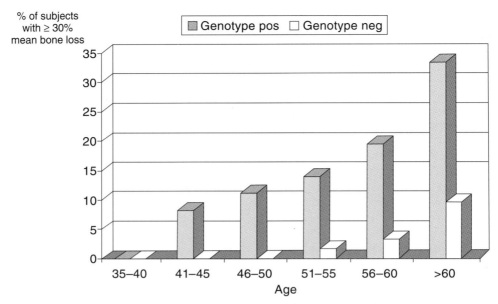

Figure 4–4. The periodontitis genotype defines a different disease susceptibility in adults. Age 35–60; odds ratio: 18.9; p < .001. The cumulative frequency distribution of non-smokers with ≥ 30% mean bone loss (severe) at different ages. The bars represent the cumulative percentage of subjects who had severe disease by the indicated age. Genotype positive (N=63). Reprinted with permission from J Clin Periodontol 1997;24:72–7.

The association between the IL-1 genotype and disease severity was unclear when heavy smokers were included in the data analysis. What does this mean? It is well documented that smoking, by itself, is a strong risk factor for more severe periodontitis. It is therefore reasonable to expect that some IL-1

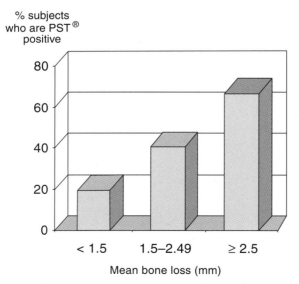

Figure 4–5. Most nonsmoker patients with severe bone loss were PST® positive. (Data from McDevitt M, Wang H-Y, Knobelman C, et al. IL-1 genetic association with periodonitits in clinical practice. J Periodontol 1999. [in press])

genotype-negative patients who are heavy smokers will be susceptible to more severe periodontitis. This will certainly confuse the data analysis of research studies unless this factor is taken into account in the analysis. One study that involves periodontal treatment shows a synergistic risk when a patient is both a smoker and is IL-1 genotype positive.[43] At present, it seems reasonable to expect that, as with risk factors for cardiovascular disease, multiple factors such as IL-1 genotype and smoking convey increased risk of more severe disease. It is likely that larger studies will help to define the magnitude of interactions between smoking and the IL-1 genotype as well as other risk factors.

Genetic Variations in IL-1 Genotype and Response to Treatment

It seems reasonable to assume that if the IL-1 genotype is associated with more severe disease, the genotype may also influence response to therapy. New data from McGuire and Nunn validate that assumption.[43] Over several years, McGuire and Nunn conducted studies to determine the effectiveness of clinical parameters in developing an accurate prognosis.[47,48] In their first study, the authors evaluated 100 treated periodontal patients under maintenance care for 5 years to determine the relationship between assigned prognoses and the clinical criteria commonly used in developing a prognosis.[47] Using multiple logistic regression models, it was shown that improvement or worsening in prognoses was strongly associated with initial tooth malposition, probing depth, furcation involvement, and smoking, when adjusted for initial prognosis. It was found that initial mobility decreased the probability of improvement in prognosis whereas good oral hygiene increased the probability of improvement in prognosis; however, neither of these factors was shown to be significant in worsening the prognosis. On the other hand, smoking doubled the probability of worsening of prognosis at 5 years and decreased the probability of improvement by 60%. According to the authors, the results of this study suggest that some clinical factors used in the assignment of prognoses are clearly associated with changes in a patient's clinical condition over time.

In their second study, McGuire and Nunn evaluated tooth loss in 100 treated periodontal patients under maintenance care to determine the effectiveness of commonly taught clinical parameters used in assigning an accurate prognosis for tooth survival.[48] Using a Cox proportional hazards regression model, it was found that initial furcation involvement, probing depth, percent bone loss, mobility, and smoking were associated with an increased risk of tooth loss. Data from the study showed a relationship between the assigned prognosis and tooth loss. The worst survival rate occurred in teeth with the worst prognosis but the commonly taught clinical parameters used in the traditional way for assigning prognosis do not adequately explain this relationship. In addition, the initial prognosis did not adequately predict survival of the tooth or explain the condition of the tooth. The results of this study indicate that when assigning prognosis, some clinical parameters should be weighted more heavily than other clinical parameters.

The latest study by McGuire and Nunn (Figure 4–6) determined that the significant predictors of tooth loss in periodontal patients who were monitored for 14 years after active therapy were heavy smoking (increased risk for tooth loss of 2.88; meaning that heavy smokers had a 288% increased risk of losing teeth after therapy as compared to non-smokers or light smokers) and the IL-1 genotype (increased risk for tooth loss of 2.66).[43] If patients were both heavy smokers and IL-1 genotype positive they were 7.7 times more likely to lose teeth after periodontal therapy than all other patients. It should be noted that even in IL-1 geno-

type-positive patients, conventional periodontal therapy and good maintenance care allowed the successful retention of most teeth.

Studies so far have shown evidence that IL-1 polymorphism analysis can provide valuable insight into an individual patient's likely response to various interventions. However, additional studies are necessary to provide greater insight into the relationships between genetic factors and periodontal and restorative therapy. This genetic marker is not diagnostic; it is a prognostic test that is used to identify individuals who have a much higher susceptibility to adverse reactions to plaque.[49]

The finding of the association between the IL-1 polymorphism and an increase in IL-1β production and more severe periodontal disease is consistent with the current model of how genetic factors influence common chronic diseases. If this model is applied to periodontitis, it would involve a disease-initiating factor, which would most certainly be a specific bacterium (ie, *P. gingivalis, Bacteroides forsythus,* and *A. actinomycetemcomitans*), and modifiers of disease mechanisms that explain the clinical severity, including certain systemic diseases, smoking, psychosocial stress, and the IL-1 genotype.[6]

Clinical Application

Despite the general overall improvement in periodontal health, periodontitis is still the number one

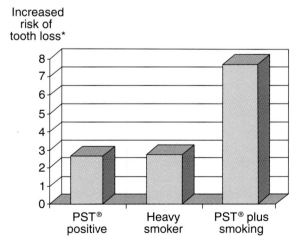

Figure 4–6. IL-1 genotype and heavy smoking were the primary predictors of tooth loss after periodontal therapy. *An increased risk of 2 indicates that the patient is two times more likely to lose teeth than patients without that risk factor. (Data from McGuire MK, Nunn ME. Prognosis versus actual outcome. IV. The effectiveness of clinical parameters and PST genotype in accurately predicting prognosis and tooth survival. J Periodontol 1999;70:49–56.

cause of tooth loss in adults. In the United States alone, over 50 million people have the disease. The cost to society in both human and economic terms is great. The indirect expenses of replacing teeth lost due to periodontitis are much higher than the direct periodontal expenditures. Patients, insurance payers, and clinicians are seeking accurate treatment and better preventive approaches. The genetic aspects of the disease have been understood and accepted with increased enthusiasm because of the tremendous strides made in molecular biology. These new insights are beginning to find their way into practical translation and use by clinicians.

This section will briefly describe how to integrate information on the genetic basis of periodontitis into the overall framework of the patient's diagnosis and treatment plan. Certain characteristics of genetic information make it different from almost any other kind of patient specific data the dental professional deals with. These include scientific, ethical, inheritance, and practical considerations unique to information about heredity. However, although different, genetic information may be viewed as (just) another type of medical information about patients and their relatives.

Use of Genetic Information in Clinical Practice

The literature in the past 5 years has had increasing amounts of space devoted to presentations of data postulating an important role for genetics in the pathogenesis of adult periodontitis. Although much of this information has been well accepted, its translation into clinically useful practice has been very slow, primarily because there have been no commercially available methods that could be used by dentists wanting to know if their patient had a specific periodontitis-implicated genotype.

Most professional organizations have developed comprehensive guidelines for diagnosis, risk assessment, and prevention of periodontitis through measures aimed at reducing the risks of disease initiation or disease progression. Dentists, dental hygienists, and their patients would like to have as much useful information as possible in order to guide decision making for periodontal treatment planning. Faced with the challenge of ascertaining all relevant risk factors and then trying to put the information together with patient preferences, the clinician manages, organizes, and synthesizes all the data to produce the best possible treatment plan. The goal is to personalize the plan and make it as accurate and predictive as possible.

Although scientific evidence and clinical experience have improved the accuracy and power of traditional methods, the ability to predict the prognosis and outcome for individual patients and individual sites has been limited.

To best appreciate how genetic information fits into the current concepts of disease, it is important to describe the scientific and clinical model of periodontitis etiology and pathogenesis that is currently accepted by the vast majority of clinicians. Importantly, the new genetic features of the disease do not replace existing elements of the paradigm and, in fact, provide clarification for many of its uncertainties.

Paradigm for Microbiologic Periodontal Disease

The main conceptual framework for the etiology of periodontitis is based on the belief that periodontitis is an infection caused by plaque (Figure 4–7). The assumptions of the model are:

1. Periodontitis begins as gingivitis.
2. In a large portion of the adult population (35%), gingivitis converts to periodontitis.
3. Approximately 10% of affected individuals will develop severe forms of the disease. If left untreated, periodontitis may progress to become more severe.
4. Plaque must be present for disease progression but the presence or the identification of specific bacteria is not predictive of periodontitis severity on an individual-site basis.
5. Intrinsic factors (genetics) and extrinsic factors (such as oral hygiene) account for the clinical variability of disease manifestation.
6. Adult periodontitis is a common, multifactorial, chronic disease.

Since there are important differences in the combination of factors causing disease, it follows that the treatment for different groups of patients with periodontitis should *not* be the same. Otherwise, there is the possibility that some patients will get too much treatment while some others do not get what they need. If 10% of patients with periodontitis will develop severe disease, then the other 90% will have only mild to moderate disease. How can patients be identified as to their risk for future severity of their disease? Are there tests or any other information that will help the clinician improve the accuracy of the predictions about the patient's future status? These are critical questions that interest all

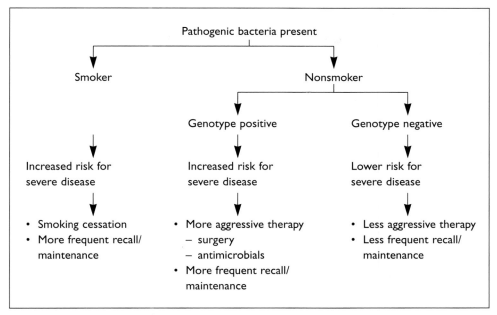

Figure 4–7. Clinical utility of genetic testing.

parties involved. Patients want the best treatment, clinicians want to provide efficient therapy, and insurance payers want to focus resources. Genetic susceptibility to the resident periodontal flora is one of the factors that determine the actual clinical presentation of disease. Assessment of other risk factors, such as smoking and systemic health, are always included in the development of a comprehensive treatment plan but practical methods available to the clinician to determine the types of bacteria at an individual periodontal site are limited.

Clinical Perspective

The practical use of genetic information offers the potential to change periodontitis treatment. Genetic predisposition to the onset of periodontitis means that some patients can be identified even before disease begins. This improves the chances of successful prevention. Genetic heterogeneity associated with disease also extends to treatment responsiveness. Distinguishing patients who are of good responders from those who are poor responders will allow more precise chemotherapeutic interventions because drug targets will be more precise. For example, there may be different response patterns to a specific anti-inflammatory drug, depending on the nature of the individual patient's cell receptors compared with those of another patient. Pharmaceutical companies are devoting vast resources to this endeavor that has been referred to as pharmacogenomics.

Available techniques, tests, diagnostic procedures, and guides to treatment have either been weakly applicable on a patient-by-patient basis, or, they have been impractical in terms of cost-effectiveness, and time management.

The main barrier to widespread use of current technology is its poor record in predicting the patient's future periodontal status. Clinical and biologic evaluations can tell the clinician about the current status of the patient's periodontium but these signs, symptoms, and clinical judgments have relatively weak prognostic value. By focusing attention on both the etiology and modifiers of periodontitis, rather than on "fixing" the results of disease, practitioners can anticipate, manage, and prevent disease much more effectively. For example, smoking, diabetes, family history, and other factors known to increase the risk and susceptibility to periodontitis are important to consider because they can influence the patient's response to therapy. Patients with more risk usually need more care. Optimum treatment implies managing the multiplicity of issues, etiologies, preferences, and physical, emotional, and inherited risk and susceptibility factors.

Ethical Considerations

The sensitivity of genetic information underscores the importance of understanding the often discussed and highly debated issues dealing with genetic information. For most dental personnel, genetic information is distinguished from other patient information because it is potentially predictive, permanent, and associated with blood relatives. Many of the most important issues are summarized in Table 4–2.

Genetic Counseling

There are two factors involved in disease risk: numerical risk and the burden or severity of the disease. Well-defined mathematical rules for predicting risk are not available for many multifactorial (non-Mendelian) disorders. In this instance, clinicians rely on empiric observations, epidemiologic data, and a variety of studies about recurrence risks. From nongenetic studies, approximate predictions and generalization can be inferred and direct application to the individual is limited. On the other hand, genetic prognosis is concerned with the prognosis for the affected individual and outlining disease risks for their different relatives.

During genetic counseling, the risks for a disease and the potential options for dealing with the risks are discussed with the individual and often with family members at risk. With diseases that are treatable, such as periodontitis, it has been shown that early intervention improves the outcome. For many common disorders, the process of family-based screening can be of value. After the initial genetic risks are determined, these risks can be more clearly defined by performing additional studies in patients and family members who are at risk.[15] Family linkage and association data are being generated for many of the genetic markers associated with periodontitis. These data will assist the counselor in describing the level of risk to the patient and family members.

For common diseases, the physician and dentist will have responsibility for counseling patients about the implications of genetic susceptibility. Genetic counselors may also be involved in this process, especially in the setting of large medical institutions.

TABLE 4–2. Summary of Genetic Information Issues for the Clinician*

Representative Issues	*Discussion*
No distinctions between genetic information and other forms of medical/dental information	1. For all diseases, whether or not there are reasonable treatments or preventive options, presymptomatic, predictive genetic testing can introduce sensitive medical/genetic information. The feature of this category of information that makes it sensitive is that it is subject to misinterpretation by patients, providers, insurers, and employers. In essence, this type of medical information is no different from other types of confidential medical facts about an individual, for example, whether or not a patient is HIV positive or negative. 2. In cases such as presymptomatic testing, the clinician must realize that the actual information about a patient's genetic make-up will, itself, impact the lives/mental health of otherwise healthy people. 3. Genetic information is not limited to the individual tested; the information is about the individual's germline/family and thus may have consequences beyond treatment planning decisions for the tested patient.
Clinical utility	1. There is a general consensus that genetic testing *should not* be withheld until enough data have been compiled to know exactly what a genetic test result means for all individuals in the general population, ie, it is not necessary to know the exact relationship between genotype and phenotype for the target marker(s). Effective treatments (therapeutics and even gene therapies) may be developed before all the complexities of interactions among genes/gene sequences and genetic and environmental variables are known. 2. Genetic testing should be introduced when • there is sufficient *analytical validity* (in essence, the test reliably determines the presence of the target marker(s) in the laboratory); • there is sufficient clinical utility (there is a clinical benefit for patients, which also is a prerequisite for reimbursement); and • patient safeguards (to ensure only informed, voluntary testing) are adhered to.

*Adapted from: M. Malinowsky, 1999.

Periodontal Disease-Specific Issues and Comments

1. Genetic tests for common diseases are *not* usually considered to be classic "diagnostic tests," and they do not eliminate the need for an accurate diagnosis and treatment plan.

   Comment: Risk assessment, including the use of genetic susceptibility testing, is an additional step, but not a substitute for a full diagnostic evaluation.

2. Common diseases are multifactorial, and because of this, genetic test results provide one piece of information needed to form a diagnosis, prognosis, and treatment plan.

   Comment: Most often, the diagnosis of a common disease is based on the identification of signs and symptoms associated with well-established criteria. Signs of periodontitis include plaque, changes in gingival color, initial attachment loss, probing depth, bleeding on probing, and suppuration. Negative genetic susceptibility test results by themselves do not rule out future occurrence of disease or disease activity because one of the other contributing factors may contribute to the observed pathology. Similarly, positive test results do not mean that disease is inevitable.

3. Another important facet of genetic test results specific to periodontitis has to do with the implications to people biologically related to the tested individual.

   Comment: Depending on the nature of the genetic association, offspring, siblings, parents, and others may carry genes that could put these people at increased disease risk. In the case of adult periodontitis, this information may be helpful in establishing treatment recommendations and preventive approaches. The decision to be tested for periodontitis susceptibility should be made by the individual patient.

4. Essential scientific characteristics of genetic susceptibility tests must meet the highest level of validity, as well as addressing ethical considerations.

   Comment: Before deciding to use genetic testing as part of patient assessment and treatment planning, the clinician must ensure that the test itself embodies certain attributes discussed in previous sections and summarized in Table 4–3. All five characteristics and considerations must be checked before the test is used.

Genetic Testing in Dentistry

Genetic testing for the IL-1 genotypes in dentistry was begun in 1997 with the introduction of the PST test (PST®, Interleukin Genetics, Inc., San Antonio, TX). Its primary use is to provide additional information about a patient's susceptibility to adult periodontitis. Since it measures the absence or presence of specific markers of the patient's inflammatory response to plaque, one of the key components of the pathogenesis of periodontitis, its clinical utility is very high. Control of inflammation is a key component of many of the treatment goals in esthetic, restorative, and reconstructive dentistry. The currently available genetic susceptibility test meets the five characteristics and conditions listed in Table 4–3.

The primary use for information about a patient's risk for disease initiation or progression is the modification and individualization of therapeutic interventions. Both the nature and the timing of therapy may be altered as a result of knowing a patient's risk for future disease. What the benefits of knowing a patient's risks for disease, including their genetic susceptibility to periodontitis, are and who should be tested are two common questions often asked by practitioners and patients. The section below discusses some essential factors about risk assessment. Knowing about these factors will provide a context for determining how the genetic susceptibility risk factor fits in the overall approach to treating and preventing periodontal disease and its relevance to restorative dentistry.

TABLE 4–3. Required Characteristics for Genetic Susceptibility Tests Associated with Common Diseases

1. The genotype must be associated with disease occurrence and, if possible, the mechanism known to be an integral part of the pathogenesis of the disease.
2. Analytical sensitivity and specificity must be determined, ie, how accurate the laboratory test and methods are in their ability to detect the genetic marker, if it is truly present.
3. Appropriate clinical validity must be ascertained: eg, odds ratio, for disease with and without the genetic marker.
4. The benefits and risks from test results must be known.
5. Treatment initiation or change as a result of the information derived from the test must be available.

Risk Factor Determination

The term "risk" is generally used to imply the probability that an unfavorable or unwanted outcome may occur in the future. Many studies have been conducted to identify the factors that increase an individual's risk for developing periodontal disease.[50,51] The findings from these studies have identified the following as risk factors for periodontitis: smoking, diabetes mellitus, advancing age, poor oral hygiene status, microbial deposits, inheritance, bleeding on probing, specific pathogenic bacteria in the subgingival flora, and previous disease experience and severity. Some risks are strongly linked to disease causation (ie, pathogenic bacteria in the subgingival flora), others may be background factors that enhance susceptibility (ie, advancing age), and some may suggest increased risk for future disease (ie, bleeding on probing). Patient decisions about treatment must be based on accurate information, including individual preferences, estimates of the patient's prognosis, expected side effects and benefits, and efficiency of the proposed treatment alternatives.[38] Although the data regarding risk factors are very good, the degree of patient variability and treatment responsiveness demonstrates the need for more research.

Patient Selection and Potential Benefit(s) of Genetic Susceptibility Testing

The list below describes some potential types of patients and the benefits that may be derived from the decision to determine the patient's genotype.

1. *Patients with early signs of periodontal disease.* Testing can be done to better determine the appropriate level of therapy and maintenance and to potentially minimize further disease progression and tooth loss.
2. *Periodontal maintenance patients.* Individuals with continuing signs of disease will potentially benefit from understanding their risk for future disease. This information should be combined with other risk factors (eg, smoking and diabetes) to determine who might benefit from more or less aggressive treatment. The information may also help to determine the level of periodontal and inflammatory risk prior to restorative or implant therapy.
3. *Patients who are resistant to accepting treatment recommendations.* If a patient is found to be genetically positive, the information may motivate him or her to reduce as many of the controllable risks as possible. This may be accomplished through better home care, more frequent dental visits, smoking cessation, pocket reduction, or any other recommended therapy. For patients who are found to be genetically negative, the information can still be used to motivate them to control other risk factors (such as smoking) and increase their chances of staying healthy.
4. *New periodontal patients* as part of an initial examination and objective measure of their risk for disease progression and patients who have a familial history of periodontitis or who have relatives who are genotype positive. Some patients may be tested after initial therapy, especially if they are not responding well.
5. *Biologic family members* of genotype-positive patients or patients with severe periodontal disease for prevention or early intervention.
6. *Patients with advanced periodontal disease* to provide information that, when combined with other risk factors, can be used to optimize therapy and determine who needs aggressive treatment and/or maintenance to minimize further disease progression and tooth loss.
7. *Patients who are candidates for complex restorative procedures* to enhance the success and maintainability of the case by considering the overall risk profile of the patient in the treatment, maintenance, and follow-up plan. Marginal inflammation and bleeding are risk factors associated with gingival recession. Patients who are "inflammation prone" due to their genetically variable response to plaque can use this information to motivate them to improve their oral hygiene.
8. *Adult orthodontic patients* as part of an initial screening for periodontal health status and risk assessment. If a patient is seen to be at risk for developing severe periodontal disease on the basis of genetic test results and/or other risk factors or already has periodontal disease, he or she may benefit from more frequent periodontal maintenance during orthodontic treatment.

CONCLUSION

With the discovery of a specific genetic factor that places individuals at a greater risk for the development of periodontitis or more severe forms of the disease, clinicians can tailor treatment for individual patients, resulting in more effective therapy. In addition, by identifying genotype-positive patients before disease initiation, clinicians may be able to prevent the development of periodontitis in some patients with the use of standard preventive measures.

There is little doubt that on the basis of risk and susceptibility factors, the practice of periodontics, will require a change of approach for dentistry and for the patients and public it serves. Risk and predisposition assessment will be used more often as first priority decision-making guides in diagnostic and therapeutic algorithms. Because clinicians can now identify and monitor periodontal risk considerably earlier than before, there is an opportunity for maximizing benefit/cost ratios. Early detection enhances appropriate treatment planning, whether it is prophylactic, medical, or surgical.

Acknowledgement

The excellent drafting and editorial assistance of Kathy Barnes and Elaine Robertson were very much appreciated in the preparation of this chapter.

REFERENCES

1. Kornman KS, Crane A, Wang H-Y, et al. The interleukin-1 genotype as a severity factor in adult periodontal disease. J Clin Periodontol 1997; 24:72–7.

2. Roberts FA, Hockett RD Jr, Bucy RP, Michalek SM. Quantitative assessment of inflammatory cytokine gene expression in chronic adult periodontitis. Oral Microbiol Immunol 1997;12(6): 336–44.

3. Haffajee AD, Socransky SS. Microbial etiological agents of destructive periodontal diseases. Periodontology 2000 1994;5:78–111.

4. Tanner AC, Kent R, Maiden MFJ, Taubman MA. Clinical, microbiological and immunological profile of health, gingivitis and putative active periodontal subjects. J Periodontal Res 1996;31: 195–204.

5. Zambon JJ. Periodontal diseases: microbial factors. Ann Periodontol 1996;1:879–925.

6. Kornman KS, di Giovine FS. Genetic variations in cytokine expression: a risk factor for severity of adult periodontitis. Ann Periodontol 1998;3(1): 327–38.

7. Hart TC, Kornman KS. Genetic factors in the pathogenesis of periodontitis. Periodontology 2000 1997;14:202–15.

8. Offenbacher S. Periodontal diseases: pathogenesis. Ann Periodontol 1996;1:821–78.

9. Hassell TM, Harris EL. Genetic influences in caries and periodontal diseases. Crit Rev Oral Biol Med 1995;6(4):319–42.

10. Hart TC. Genetic risk factors for early-onset periodontitis. J Periodontol 1996;67:355–66.

11. Alaluusua S, Asikainen S, Lai C. Intrafamilial transmission of *Actinobacillus actinomycetemcomitans*. J Periodontol 1991;62:207–10.

12. Michalowicz BS, Aeppli D, Virag JG, et al. Periodontal findings in adult twins. J Periodontol 1991;62(5):293–9.

13. Michalowicz BS, Aeppli DP, Kuba RK, et al. A twin study of genetic variation in proportional radiographic alveolar bone height. J Dent Res 1991;70(11):1431–5.

14. Corey LA, Nance WE, Hofstede P, Schenkein HA. Self-reported periodontal disease in a Virginia twin population. J Periodontol 1993;64:1205–8.

15. King RA, Rotter JI, Motulsky AG. The approach to genetic bases of common diseases. In: King RA, Rotter JI, Motulsky AG, editors. The genetic basis of common diseases. New York: Oxford University Press Inc.; 1992.

16. National Institutes of Health. Genetic architecture of complex phenotypes. Released on the Internet, June 8, 1998.

17. Newman M. Genetic, environmental, and behavioral influences on periodontal infections. Compend Contin Educ Dent 1998;19(1):25–31.

18. Dean M, Carrington M, Winkler C, et al. Genetic restriction of HIV-1 infection and progression to AIDS by a deletion allele of the CKR5 structural gene. Hemophilia Growth and Development Study, Multicenter AIDS Cohort Study, Multicenter Hemophilia Cohort Study, San Francisco City Cohort, ALIVE Study. Science 1996;273(5283):1856–62.

19. Huang Y, Paxton WA, Wolinsky SM, et al. The role of a mutant CCR5 allele in HIV-1 transmission and disease progression. Nat Med 1996;2(11): 1240–3.

20. Wilson ME, Bronson PM, Hamilton RG. Immunoglobulin G2 antibodies promote neutrophil killing of *Actinobacillus actinomycetemcomitans*. Infect Immun 1995;63(3):1070–5.

21. Kobayashi T, Westerdaal NA, Miyazak A, et al. Relevance of immunoglobulin G Fc receptor polymorphism to recurrence of adult periodontitis in Japanese patients. Infect Immun 1997; 65(9):3556–60.

22. Löe H, Anerud A, Boysen H, Morrison E. Natural history of periodontal disease in man. Rapid, moderate and no loss of attachment in Sri Lankan laborers 14 to 46 years of age. J Clin Periodontol 1986;13(5):431–45.

23. Michalowicz BS. Genetic and heritable risk factors in periodontal disease. J Periodontol 1994;65(5 Suppl):479–88.

24. Socransky SS, Haffajee AD, Cugini MA, et al. Microbial complexes in subgingival plaque. J Periodontol 1998;25:346–53.

25. di Giovine FS, Duff GW. Interleukin-1—the first interleukin. Immunol Today 1990;1:13–20.

26. Beutler B, Cerami A. The biology of cachectin/TNF-α primary mediator of the host response. Ann Rev Immunol 1989;7:625–55.

27. Probert L, Plows D, Kontogeorgos G, Kollias G. The type-i interleukin-1 receptor acts in series with tumor-necrosis-factor (TNF) to induce arthritis in TNF-transgenic mice. Eur J Immunol 1995;25:1794–7.

28. Jacob CO. Tumor-necrosis-factor-alpha in autoimmunity—pretty girl or old witch. Immunol Today 1992;13:122–5.

29. Vassalli P. The pathophysiology of tumor necrosis factors. Ann Rev Immunol 1992;10:411–52.

30. Lee HJ, Kang IK, Chung CP, Choi SM. The subgingival microflora and gingival crevicular fluid cytokines in refractory periodontitis. J Clin Periodontol 1995;22:885–90.

31. Liu C-M, Hou L-T, Wong M-Y, Rossomando EF. Relationships between clinical parameters, interleukin-1B and histopathologic findings of gingival tissue in periodontitis patients. Cytokine 1996;8:161–7.

32. Preiss DS, Meyle J. Interleukin-1 beta concentration of gingival crevicular fluid. J Periodontol 1994;65:423–8.

33. Stashenko P, Fujiyoshi P, Obernesser MS, et al. Levels of interleukin-1b in tissue from sites of active periodontal disease. J Clin Periodontol 1991;18:548–54.

34. Yavuzyilmaz E, Yamalik N, Bulut S, et al. The gingival crevicular fluid interleukin-1 beta and tumour necrosis factor-alpha levels in patients with rapidly progressive periodontitis. Aust Dent J 1995;40:46–9.

35. Cavanaugh PF Jr., Meredith MP, Buchanon W, et al. Coordinate production of PGE_2 and IL-1β in the gingival fluid of adults with periodontitis: its relationship to alveolar bone loss and disruption by twice daily treatment with ketorolac tromethamine oral rinse. J Periodontal Res 1998;33(2):75–82.

36. Pociot F, Molvig J, Wogensen L, et al. A Taq[1] polymorphism in the human interleukin-1 beta (IL-1β) gene correlates with secretion in vitro. Eur J Clin Invest 1992;22:396–402.

37. Cox A, Duff GW. Cytokines as genetic modifying factors in immune and inflammatory diseases. J Pediatr Endocrinol Metab 1996;9:129–32.

38. Newman MG, Korman KS, Holtzman S. Association of clinical risk factors with treatment outcomes. J Periodontol 1994;65:489–97.

39. di Giovine FS, Cork MJ, Crane A, et al. Novel genetic association of an IL-1β gene variation a +3953 with IL-1β protein production and psoriasis [abstract]. Cytokine 1995;7:606.

40. Engebretsson SP, Lamster IB, Herrera-Abreu M, et al. The influence of interleukin-1β gene polymorphism on expression of IL-1β, and tumor necrosis factor alpha in periodontal tissue and gingival crevicular fluid. J Periodontol 1999;70:567–73

41. Jotwani R, Avila R, Kim BO, Cutler CW. The effects of an antiseptic mouthrinse on subclinical gingivitis in IL-1 genotype-positive and -negative humans [abstract]. J Dent Res 1998; 77(B):921.

42. McDevitt M, Wang H-Y, Knobelman C, et al. IL-1 genetic association with periodontitis in clinical practice. J Periodontol 1999. [In Press]

43. McGuire MK, Nunn ME. Prognosis versus actual outcome. IV. The effectiveness of clinical parameters and PST genotype in accurately predicting prognosis and tooth survival. J Periodontol 1999;70:49–56.

44. Gore EA, Sanders JJ, Pandey JP, et al. Interleukin-1B +3953 allele 2. Association with disease status in adult periodontitis. J Clin Periodontol 1998;25:781–5.

45. Caffesse RG, R de La Rosa M, G de La Rosa M. PST genotypes in a periodontally healthy population treated for mucogingival surgery [abstract]. J Dent Res 1998;77(B):872..

46. Wu Y, Wang H-Y, di Giovine FS, Armitage GC. Low prevalence of IL-1A and IL-1B polymorphisms in a Chinese population [abstract]. J Dent Res 1998;77(B):738.

47. McGuire MK, Nunn ME. Prognosis versus actual outcome. II. The effectiveness of clinical parameters in developing an accurate prognosis. J Periodontol 1996;67(7):658–65.

48. McGuire MK, Nunn ME. Prognosis versus actual outcome. III. The effectiveness of clinical parameters in accurately predicting tooth survival. J Periodontol 1996;67(7):666–74.

49. Newman MG. Genetic risk for severe periodontal disease. Compend Contin Educ Dent 1997;18(9):881–4.

50. Genco RJ. Assessment of risk of periodontal disease. Compend Contin Educ Dent 1994;18 (Suppl):S678–83.

51. Page RC, Beck JD. Risk assessment for periodontal diseases. Int Dent J 1997;47:61–87.

CHAPTER 5

CARDIOVASCULAR DISEASES AND ORAL INFECTIONS

Robert J. Genco, DDS, PhD, Steven Offenbacher, DDS, James Beck, PhD, Terry Rees, DDS, MSD

The relationship between oral infections and cardiovascular disease is well known, particularly with respect to orally derived bacteremias as a source of organisms that infect damaged heart valves causing bacterial endocarditis. Recently, evidence has emerged relating periodontal infections to coronary artery disease and stroke.

This chapter will discuss how oral infections are related to bacterial endocarditis, coronary artery disease, and stroke. Etiologic associations, case-control studies, mechanisms, and intervention studies, where appropriate, as well as management of periodontal patients at risk for infective endocarditis and arteriosclerosis will be presented. The main goal of this chapter, therefore, is to provide a basis of knowledge relating oral infections, especially periodontal disease, to cardiovascular diseases, with clinical management guidelines outlined, where appropriate.

THE PERIODONTAL PATIENT AT RISK FOR INFECTIVE ENDOCARDITIS

Cardiovascular diseases affect over 43 million individuals in the United States, with a marked increase among the geriatric population.[1–3] Since this population group is increasing in number and since more elderly individuals are dentate than in the past, there is also an increased incidence of periodontal disease in this patient group. This, coupled with recent evidence linking severe, generalized periodontitis with coronary artery disease, suggests that the periodontist must be prepared to provide safe yet effective therapy to patients with various types of heart conditions.[4,5] Patient management requires a thorough medical history and physical examination, evaluation of vital signs, and medical consultation, when indicated.[6–12] In most instances, guidelines for periodontal management of patients with cardiovascular diseases are well established. One area, however, remains strongly controversial, with many experts voicing markedly different opinions; that is dental management of individuals with valvar heart disease.[13–17]

Infective endocarditis (IE) is a microbial infection of a native or prosthetic cardiac valve or surrounding cardiac tissue. It may be caused by a variety of microorganisms, including bacteria, fungi, rickettsiae, or chlamydia. The clinical course of IE may be classified as acute (duration of less than 6 weeks) or subacute (duration of more than 6 weeks). The two most common microorganisms associated with community-acquired IE are *Streptococcus viridans* and *Staphylococcus aureus*, either of which may, on occasion, be normal commensals in the oral cavity.[18] The biologic load of these organisms may be markedly increased in the presence of oral infection such as chronic periodontitis.[14,19,20] Other causative microorganisms for IE include enterococci, which are occasionally found in the oral cavity, or gram-negative HACEK microorganisms (*Haemophilus* species, *Actinobacillus actinomycetemcomitans*, *Cardiobacterium hominis*, *Eikenella*, and *Kingella*), some of which, especially *A. actinomycetemcomitans* and *Eikenella corrodens*, are putative periodontal pathogens. Other periodontal pathogens which have been occasionally associated with IE include *Capnocytophaga* and *Lactobacillus* species. Nosocomial IE is most commonly caused by antibiotic-resistant *S. aureus* infection.[15,21–23]

The increased use of heroin or other intravenously injected illicit drugs has further expanded the spectrum of causative organisms to include *Candida albicans* and other common skin-related microorganisms such as *S. aureus*.[22–24] Additionally, an increasing number of patients receive intravenous shunts or fistulas during hospitalization or have them permanently placed; either of these may serve as a source for systemic sepsis caused by a variety of microorganisms. For example, sepsis may be a special problem for individuals receiving renal hemodialysis or for those with diabetes mellitus that use indwelling devices for administration of insulin. A growing number of patients suffer from acquired immunodeficiency syndrome or other immunosuppressant disorders, and many individuals are prescribed drugs that induce immunosuppression.[25] Most IE occurs in individuals with no known valvar lesions although the majority of patients in this group usually have predisposing factors such as coronary artery disease, alcoholism, intravenous drug abuse, or long-term hemodialysis.[25]

Individuals with cardiac valve prostheses are especially susceptible to IE although those with native valvar damage and even those with undamaged heart valves may develop endocarditis. Infective endocarditis may occur spontaneously or as a result of focal sites of infection. Blood-borne pathogenic microorganisms may lodge directly on heart valves or on the endocardium near anatomic cardiac defects.

The incidence of IE has remained constant for several years although the epidemiology has changed. In the past, the most common cause of IE in young individuals was rheumatic fever (RF). In contrast, RF and IE are now more common among older individuals, especially those over 60 years of age with chronic heart disease or mitral valve prolapse due to calcifications of one or more of the valves or associated tissues.[22,23,25,26]

Acute IE may result from bacteremias associated with virulent strains of microorganisms. Signs and symptoms may include abrupt onset of fever, cutaneous and oral petechiae, and focal dermal gangrene. These features may be accompanied by intravascular coagulation, which markedly increases the risk for emboli and metastatic infection of any body organ.[23]

Subacute IE may begin insidiously and persist for months. Affected individuals complain of fever, night sweats, myalgias, arthralgias, malaise, anorexia, and easy fatigability.[1] In the past, clubbing of the last digits of the fingers or the presence of Osler's nodes on the hands were frequent signs of the presence of the disease. Today, however, earlier diagnosis has resulted in diminished occurrence of these signs. Patients with subacute IE are also at risk for emboli and abnormalities in the function of many organs, including the spleen and kidney. Cerebral emboli may induce stroke or seizures, altered levels of consciousness, or other neurologic manifestations. Cardiac changes are consistent with underlying valvar or congenital heart defects and may lead to congestive heart failure.[22,23]

Diagnosis of endocarditis is based on the presence of classic symptoms: a persistent bacteremia or fungemia and the presence of a heart murmur associated with valvar dysfunction. Transthoracic and transesophageal echocardiography are very accurate in the identification of anatomic heart changes associated with endocarditis. Differential diagnosis may include acute rheumatic fever and altered heart function associated with dysfunction of organs other than the heart.[23]

Infective endocarditis has a high morbidity and mortality, and therefore prevention is highly desirable. Preventive regimens include measures to reduce the potential for significant bacteremia from the oral cavity, the skin, the upper respiratory tract, and the gastrointestinal or urinary tract.[14–16,27] The following section will discuss dental management of individuals at risk for IE, particularly bacterial endocarditis (BE) related to oral infection and/or therapeutic manipulation of mouth tissues.[14–16,23,27]

VALVAR HEART DISEASE

Valvar heart disease is a significant cause of cardiac morbidity in individuals of all ages despite a significant decline in the incidence of rheumatic disease in the developed countries. The patient with valvar disease may be especially susceptible to IE. The most common valvar anomalies include mitral regurgitation, often associated with mitral valve prolapse; aortic stenosis resulting from congenital deformity of the aortic or bicuspid valve; or senile valvar calcification. Aortic regurgitation may be associated with dilatation of the aorta as well as a defective aortic valve. Thus, valvar heart disease may result from diverse pathologic processes.[8,22,28,29] Valvar calcification may be associated with congenitally acquired heart defects, mitral valve regurgitation due to mitral valve prolapse, aortic or bicuspid valve stenosis, or senility. These calcifications of the valvar leaflets or their associated chordae tendineue cordis or papillary muscles can lead to turbidity and back-flow of blood, placing the patient at risk for heart failure and/or IE. Valvar disease tends to be progressive over time because degenerative changes may be superimposed on an initial abnormality.[22,23]

Several conditions are commonly associated with valvar stenosis or regurgitation. Rheumatic fever results from streptococcal sepsis, and it occasionally induces an autoimmune phenomenon, in which antibodies against the streptococcal antigen cross-react with valvar tissue. The initial lesion of rheumatic heart disease is edema of valvar tissues. However, progressive fibrosis, calcification, and scarring may subsequently lead to valvar stenosis or incompetence.[22] Previous episodes of endocarditis may also predispose the affected individual to further valvar damage and a recurrence of IE. Despite increased use of antibiotics, RF continues to be the most common cause of mitral valve stenosis worldwide but its importance is diminishing in the developed countries due, in part, to early diagnosis and treatment.[22]

The incidence of valvar disease has increased in the geriatric population due to RF, valvar calcifications with regurgitation, mitral valve prolapse, or valvar stenosis.[22,30] As discussed earlier, an increasing number of elderly individuals are dentate yet experience a general reduction in immune response.[22,23,25,26]

Heart transplantation or ischemic heart disease may induce degenerative calcification, rupture, or scarring of perivalvar tissue, any one of which may be associated with valvar regurgitation and an increased risk for IE.[31] Degenerative calcification is a common cause of aortic stenosis in the elderly or in individuals with chronic renal dysfunction while calcification of the mitral annulus in the elderly (especially women) can also induce mitral regurgitation or stenosis.[22,31–34] Other causes of valvar stenosis include radiation therapy, the use of serotonin agonists such as methysergide, or previous use of fenfluramine and phentermine in combination.[22]

Kawasaki disease is an acute febrile disease complex of unknown etiology. It features conjunctival congestion, dryness of lips, skin, and the oral cavity, cervical lymphadenopathy, and cardiovascular changes, including coronary thromboarteritis, mitral valve insufficiency, and myocardial ischemia.[35,36]

Congenital heart anomalies may induce cardiac blood turbulence and permanent valvar damage even after surgical repair. Therefore, patients with certain congenital defects should be considered at lifetime risk for IE although the risk may be low (Tables 5–1 and 5–2).[14, 22]

TABLE 5–1. Cardiac Conditions Requiring Prophylaxis for Dental Treatment

High Risk
- Prosthetic cardiac valves, including bioprosthetic and homograft valves
- Previous infective endocarditis
- Complex congenital cardiac malformations
- Systemic pulmonary shunts (surgically constructed)

Moderate Risk
- Rheumatic heart disease, Kawasaki disease, connective tissue disorders and, other conditions associated with valvar dysfunction, even after valvar surgery
- Hypertrophic cardiomyopathy
  - Mitral valve prolapse with valvar regurgitation
  - Most other congenital cardiac malformations, except as listed below in Table 5–2

Modified from Dajani AS, Taubert KA, Wilson W, et al. Prevention of bacterial endocarditis. Recommendations by the American Heart Association. Circulation 1997;96:358–66.

Mitral valve prolapse (floppy valve syndrome) is characterized by idiopathic loss of the fibrous and elastic tissue of the mitral valve leaflets or the chordae tendineae cordis. It is found in several heritable connective tissue disorders, especially Down syndrome, Ehlers-Danlos syndrome, and Marfan syndrome.[35] It is also common in the general population, especially in young women, the elderly (especially men), and those affected by psychiatric conditions such as panic disorder, severe depression, or anorexia nervosa.[22,25,37–40] Therefore, any such history suggests a possible need for medical consultation and requires a

Table 5–2. Cardiac Conditions not Requiring Endocarditis Prophylaxis

- Isolated secundum atrial septal defect
- Surgical repair of secundum atrial septal defects, ventricular septal defects, or patent ductus arteriosus after 6 months and without residua
- Previous coronary artery bypass graft
- Mitral valve prolapse without valvar regurgitation
- Physiologic, functional, or innocent heart murmurs
- Previous rheumatic fever, Kawasaki disease or connective tissue disorders without valvar dysfunction
- Cardiac pacemakers and implanted defibrillators

Modified from Dajani AS, Taubert KA, Wilson W, et al. Prevention of bacterial endocarditis. Recommendations by the American Heart Association. Circulation 1997;96:358–66.

thorough understanding of the patient's condition and its possible ramifications.[32,33]

Systemic lupus erythematosus (SLE) may place affected individuals at risk for valvar disease and subsequent IE. Lupus erythematosus may affect virtually any body organ. Recent evidence suggests that the cardiovascular system is frequently involved. Mitral valve insufficiency may occur because SLE occasionally induces nonbacterial vegetations or thickening of the valves, sometimes leading to regurgitation; however, IE is relatively rare. Liebman Sacks verrucae associated with SLE may induce mitral valve prolapse if the valve leaflets or the chordae tendineae cordis are affected. The antiphospholipid syndrome occasionally associated with SLE or other collagen-vascular disorders may lead to myxomatous mitral valve tissue changes and prolapse, with regurgitation in approximately one-third of patients with myxomatous disease.[23] Patients with SLE often receive immunosuppressant drugs on a long-term basis which may increase susceptibility to IE.[11,22,29]

Echocardiographic examination will usually detect the presence of SLE-induced heart lesions.[22,23] Medical consultation is indicated in patients with SLE to determine any need for prophylactic antibiotic coverage during periodontal therapy. Patients with SLE that have not been medically evaluated for cardiac changes should receive only emergency dental therapy with prophylactic antibiotic coverage until medical clearance is obtained.[11,29]

Mitral regurgitation may be managed by surgical correction or by prosthetic replacement of the involved valves. Whenever possible, repair of native valves is the treatment of choice. It is most likely to be successful in the presence of myxoma-tous disease and least successful in rheumatic heart disease or endocarditis.[22,23]

Native valves may be surgically treated with commissurotomy or percutaneous balloon valvuloplasty. These therapies are often only palliative, and mitral valve prosthetic replacement may ultimately be necessary, especially if the valves are heavily scarred or calcified to such a degree that severe valve regurgitation is present. Prosthetic replacement, however, has a higher mortality and morbidity.[22]

Valvar prostheses may be either mechanical or biologic, with each type presenting certain advantages and disadvantages. Currently, more than 40 types of mechanical valve prostheses are available (Figure 5–1). They are often indicated for young or middle-aged individuals because they are generally quite durable. The greatest structural risk is fracture of the strut that holds the ball or disk in place. This, however, rarely occurs. The disadvantage of the mechanical prosthesis is that it predisposes the recipient patient to thromboembolism, necessitating the long-term use of anticoagulant medications.[22]

Bioprosthetic valves may be xenographic (usually porcine) or allographic (Figure 5–2). On occasion, an autographic valve is transplanted from one site to another following placement of a prosthesis in the donor site. Bioprostheses are more likely to deteriorate over time but durability increases in patients over age 60 years and continues to improve with the increasing age of the recipient. Xenographs offer the advantage of a lower risk for thromboembolism, and long-term anticoagulant therapy is usually not necessary.[22]

Failure of mechanical valves is rare but can have catastrophic effects (Figure 5–3). In contrast, failure of bioprosthetic valves is an expected consequence, and young recipients of these devices

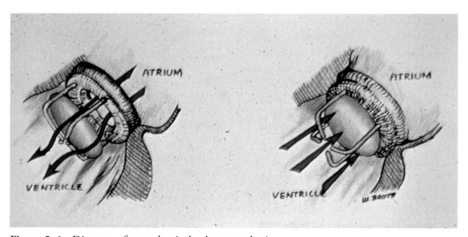

Figure 5–1. Diagram of a mechanical valvar prosthesis.

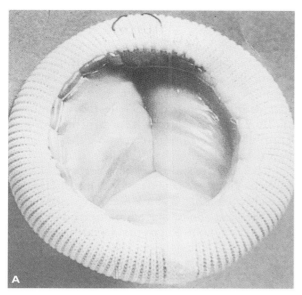 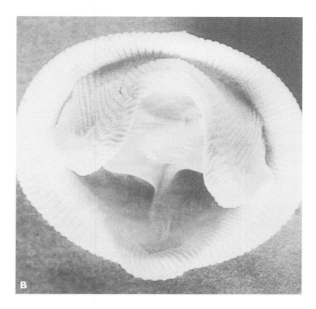

Figure 5–2. Porcine bioprosthesis: *A*, Closed. *B*, Open

should anticipate future prophylactic replacement. Fortunately, the degenerative process is slow and may take many years to manifest significant hemodynamic symptoms.[22]

DENTAL CONSIDERATIONS

The patient with valvar heart disease faces the risk of congestive heart failure, hemodynamically significant arrhythmias, and IE. Although dentists may provide dental care for patients with any of these disorders, most often they are called upon to manage patients at risk of IE.[35] Dental procedures that involve manipulation of soft tissue and result in bleeding can produce transient bacteremias. For example, 43% of patients with periodontitis experienced transient bacteremia following routine periodontal probing.[41] Administration of local intraligamental analgesia may be more likely to induce odontogenic bacteremia than tooth extraction.[42] However, available evidence clearly indicates that transient odontogenic bacteremias may be associated with routine body functions such as chewing food and brushing teeth and many authorities have challenged the benefits of prophylactic antibiotic coverage for dental treatment procedures.[14–17,25] Not all bacteremias are significant in that they may be extremely transient (2 to 3 minutes) and may not involve microorganisms likely to lodge in damaged heart tissue.[43] The incidence and severity of odontogenic bacteremias increase markedly in the presence of periodontitis

or focal oral infections, with or without manipulation of oral tissues.[14,15,25,34,44] It is generally not possible to predict which patient will develop IE or which particular procedure will be responsible.[14,45] Recently, Lamas demonstrated an absence of bacteremias among patients receiving oral mucosal biopsies except when periodontal tissues were included in the specimen.[43]

Transient bacteremias may be induced by some surgical or nonsurgical periodontal treatment procedures. However, these bacteremias rarely persist longer than 15 minutes and the majority dissipate within 3 to 5 minutes.[14,15,43] The risk of IE derived from transient bacteremias associated with manipulation of dental tissues must be weighed against the cost and risk of complications associated with administration of systemic antibiotics. Use

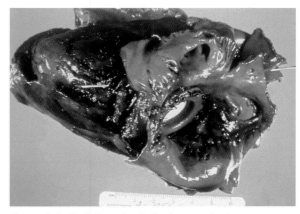

Figure 5–3. Failed mechanical valve prosthesis.

of prophylactic antibiotics may well induce a higher morbidity and mortality rate than do transient bacteremias, and several authorities have recommended more conservative use of antibiotic prophylaxis during dental treatment.[7,14,15,17,43]

In 1997, the American Heart Association (AHA) updated its recommendations for dental management of patients at risk for IE induced by odontogenic bacteremias.[14] These guidelines are applicable for prevention of endocarditis induced by oral *S. viridans* (alpha hemolytic *Streptococcus*). Dental procedures likely to induce significant bacteremia are listed in Table 5–3, and procedures at low risk of bacteremias are identified in Table 5–4.

There is some evidence that oral irrigation or use of air-abrasive polishing devices may induce bacteremia when used inappropriately or in patients with poor periodontal health, and these devices are not recommended.[14,46–49] Rinsing with antimicrobial agents containing chlorhexidine gluconate or povidone iodine prior to manipulation of dental tissues may reduce the overall bacterial bioload. This may be especially important in high-risk patients and in those with poor oral hygiene. There is, however, no conclusive evidence to confirm that prerinsing reduces the risk of oral bacteremias or IE.[50–53] Frequent home use of antiseptic rinses is not recommended due to the potential for developing resistant microorganisms.[14]

Certain cardiac conditions are more often associated with endocarditis than are others (see Tables 5–1 and 5–2). In patients at risk, antibiotic prophylaxis is recommended for *all* dental procedures likely to induce significant bleeding of hard or soft oral tissues to include surgical or nonsurgical periodontal therapy. If a series of dental procedures is required, it may be prudent to observe an interval of 9 to14 days between procedures to minimize the risk of the emergence of resistant strains of organisms.[14,54–57] In the event unanticipated bleeding occurs during low-risk dental procedures, the administration of antibiotics within 2 hours may be effective in preventing IE. There is no prophylactic benefit, however, if antibiotics are administered more than 4 hours after the incident.[14]

The AHA recommendations for specific prophylactic antibiotic regimens for dental procedures are widely published and will not be repeated in this text. For most adults, oral administration of 2 g of amoxicillin 1 hour before the dental procedure is recommended. Clindamycin (600 mg 1 hour before the dental procedure), cephalexin/cefadroxil or azithromycin/clarithromycin are recommended as alternatives in patients that are allergic to penicillin. Intramuscular or intravascular antibiotic regimens are prescribed for patients that cannot take oral medications. The recommendations are considered adequate for patients that are at high risk from IE, including those with cardiac valve prostheses.[14]

Individuals that take penicillin for secondary prevention of rheumatic fever or for other purposes may harbor oral microorganisms that are relatively resistant to penicillin, amoxicillin, or ampicillin. In such cases, the dentist should select clindamycin or another of the alternative regimens for endocarditis prophylaxis. Cephalosporins should not be used due to the potential for microbial cross-resistance between cephalosporin and penicillin derivatives.

TABLE 5–3. Dental Procedures Creating Bacteremia Risk

- Dental extractions
- Implant placement and tooth reimplantation
- Surgical and nonsurgical periodontal procedures
- Endodontic instrumentation beyond the root apex or endodontic surgery
- Initial placement of orthodontic bands
- Intraligamentary injection
- Prophylaxis when bleeding is expected
- Subgingival placement of antibiotic fibers or strips

Modified from Dajani AS, Taubert KA, Wilson W, et al. Prevention of bacterial endocarditis. Recommendations by the American Heart Association. Circulation 1997;96:358–66.

TABLE 5–4. Dental Procedures with Low Bacteremia Risk

- Restorative procedures with or without retraction cord
- Local anesthetic injections
- Placement of rubber dams
- Suture removal
- Placement or adjustment of orthodontic or removable prosthodontic appliances
- Oral impressions
- Fluoride treatments
- Oral radiographs
- Shedding of primary teeth

Modified from Dajani AS, Taubert KA, Wilson W, et al. Prevention of bacterial endocarditis. Recommendations by the American Heart Association. Circulation 1997;96:358–66.

Professional judgment may have to be used for patients that do not fit established guidelines set forth by the AHA. Tetracyclines are not recommended for prophylactic cardiovascular antibiotic coverage.[14] It has been suggested, however, that patients with periodontal diseases associated with tetracycline-sensitive organisms may be best treated by administration of tetracyclines for 2 to 3 weeks prior to periodontal treatment followed by a 1-week delay and then performance of periodontal therapy using AHA-recommended prophylactic regimens.[58] When possible, multiple dental procedures should be performed on the day of prophylactic antibiotic coverage and further treatment delayed for 9 to 14 days before the same antibiotic is used. Medical consultation should be obtained as indicated for patients that require multiple, prolonged, or unusual regimens of prophylactic antibiotic coverage. The relationship between IE and periodontal treatment procedures incorporating local delivery of antibiotics or antimicrobials into gingival pockets is not known at present although the AHA recommends systemic prophylaxis when antibiotic fibers or strips are inserted, presumably because of the potential for traumatic injury and bleeding during these procedures.[14] Antibiotic prophylaxis minimizes the risk of infective endocarditis but does not preclude its occurrence, and the clinician must remain alert for persistent fever or other symptoms associated with the condition.[14,59–61]

PROSTHETIC VALVE ENDOCARDITIS

Individuals with prosthetic heart valves have high morbidity and mortality in the event IE occurs. Therefore, these individuals may require especially diligent dental care before and after open heart surgery. Potential oral foci of infection should be eliminated before the surgery.[11,16,27] Questionable teeth should not be retained, and the patient's motivation and ability to maintain effective oral hygiene procedures should be assessed (Figure 5–4). Prior to cardiac surgery, dental procedures associated with a high risk of significant bacteremia should be accompanied by appropriate prophylactic antibiotic support. When possible, dental extractions should be accomplished at least 2 weeks prior to the heart surgery to allow adequate wound healing (Figure 5–5).

Following placement of a prosthetic heart valve, close medical-dental cooperation is essential. Periodontal therapy is usually not appropriate within 6 months of valve placement, and periodontal health

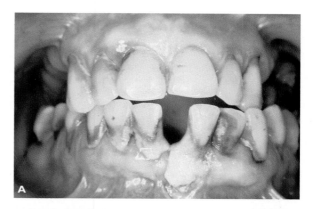
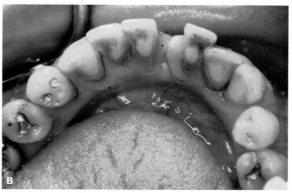
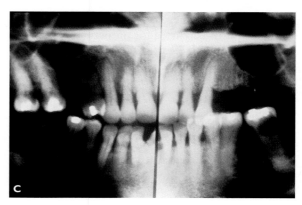

Figure 5–4. A 47-year-old Caucasian female with a history of rheumatic heart disease. The patient is scheduled for valve replacement open heart surgery in 1 month. *A*, Facial view. *B*, Mandibular anterior lingual view. *C*, Panoramic radiograph.

must be sustained, if possible, for the patient's lifetime (Figures 5–6 and 5–7). For obvious reasons, antibiotic prophylaxis is indicated for all high-risk dental treatment procedures. Some periodontal treatment procedures may be contraindicated. For example, surgical procedures that create an open wound surface (gingivectomy, free gingival grafts) should probably be avoided due to the prolonged wound healing time. These procedures also may be contraindicated in patients receiving concomitant

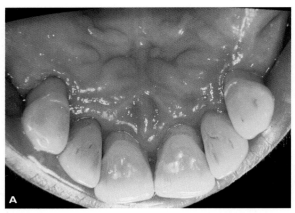 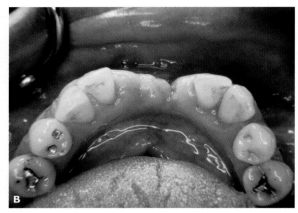

Figure 5–5. Same patient as Figure 5–4 one day before heart surgery. *A*, Maxillary anterior palatal view. Dental and periodontal infections have been eliminated. *B*, Mandibular anterior lingual view.

anticoagulant therapy to minimize the potential for postoperative hemorrhage.[27]

ANTICOAGULATED PATIENTS

Patients with prosthetic valves, thromboembolic phenomena, or other blood flow disturbances often receive anticoagulant medication immediately following heart surgery or for their lifetime. Coumarin is usually used for outpatient anticoagulation. It exerts its effect through the competitive inhibition of vitamin K, with subsequent depletion of coagulation factors dependent on that substance for their synthesis (II, VII, IX, and X). Coumarin has a delayed onset and a prolonged effect. Its effectiveness is monitored via the corrected prothrombin time known as the international normalized ratio (INR). In the past, prothrombin times (PT) varied between laboratories, potentially leading to

misleading information regarding the patient's state of coagulability. To standardize PT measurements, the World Health Organization developed an international reference thromboplastin, using human brain thromboplastin as the universal standard for comparison purposes. Each laboratory performing prothrombin tests must now compare their prothrombin against the standard. This results in a corrected normal prothrombin time for all medical laboratories.[15,34,36] Under most circumstances, the INR for patients with a normal PT is approximately 1.0. Patients requiring anticoagulant therapy are usually maintained at an INR ranging from 1.2 to 4.5. So far as is known today, patients within this range can receive all types of periodontal therapy, provided local hemostatic measures are taken. These include atraumatic surgery, adequate wound closure using sutures, application of postsurgical pressure, and the use of topical clotting agents such as thrombin, foamed gelatin, oxidized regenerated cellulose, or synthetic collagen. Oral rinses containing tranexamic acid have markedly reduced the risk of excessive hemorrhage without alteration of the INR level.[15,34,62] Tetracyclines are contraindicated in patients on anticoagulant drugs since they interfere with prothrombin formation.[54]

When contemplating procedures likely to cause bleeding, it is appropriate to communicate with the patient's physician.[63] On occasion, pharmacologic manipulation becomes necessary for the anticoagulated patient. If the patient can tolerate a wait of several hours or more, vitamin K administration will reverse the effect of coumarin. More urgent situations may require blood transfusion or infusion of fresh-frozen plasma or packed platelets.[1,15,23]

Aspirin is often used as an antithrombotic agent because of its inhibition of platelet aggregation.

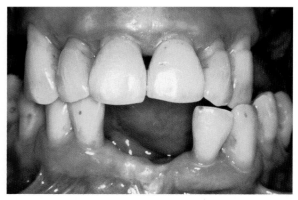

Figure 5–6. Same patient as Figure 5–4 6 months after successful placement of valvar prosthesis. *A*, Anterior view. *B*, Maxillary anterior palatal view.

Most cardiologists prescribe very small daily dosages (80 to 325 mg). At these dose levels, the medication will not significantly alter bleeding time.[15,62] On occasion, however, patients on higher aspirin levels are at a slight risk for prolonged postoperative hemorrhage following periodontal therapy. For these individuals, the medication should be discontinued for 4 to 7 days prior to the scheduled procedure with the concurrence of the cardiologist.[4,34]

Summary

The patient with valvar heart disease is frequently encountered in dental practice. Safe and effective management of such patients requires close medical and dental cooperation. Periodontal health and absence of oral foci of infection are essential, and on some occasions, prophylactic antibiotic coverage is required for dental treatment procedures. The dental practitioner must remain knowledgeable regarding current concepts in the management of such patients.

ORAL INFECTIONS AS A RISK FACTOR FOR ATHEROSCLEROSIS, CORONARY ARTERY DISEASE, AND ISCHEMIC STROKE

The role of infections in atherosclerosis has been discussed for many years. Recently, evidence has accumulated that certain common oral infections play a significant in role in atherosclerosis. Atherosclerosis lesions can occur in large- and medium-sized elastic and muscular arteries. They can lead to ischemic lesions of the brain, heart, or extremities and can result in thrombosis and infarction of affected vessels, leading to death. Cardiovascular disease, mostly associated with atherosclerosis,

remains one of the primary causes of death in the United States, Europe, and much of Asia.[64,65]

The process, supported by a considerable body of evidence, is that atherosclerosis is an inflammatory disease.[66] This concept, also termed the Ross response-to-injury hypothesis of atherosclerosis, proposes that the initial lesion results from injury to the endothelium and leads to a chronic inflammatory process in the artery. This results in the migration of monocytes through the endothelium into the underlying tissue and the proliferation of smooth muscle cells. Activation of the monocytes (macrophages) in the blood vessel leads to the release of hydrolytic enzymes, cytokines, chemokines, and growth factors, which induces further damage, leading to focal necrosis. Accumulation of lipids is a key feature of this process, and in later stages, the atheromatous plaque can be covered with a fibrous cap over the focal necrotic area. At some point, the fibrous cap may become eroded and rupture, which leads to thrombus formation and occlusion of the artery, resulting in an infarction.

The initial event in the development of an atheroma appears to be endothelial injury that results in the activation of the endothelial cells. This results in the upregulation of surface adhesin molecules and chemokines, both of which result in monocyte recruitment from the bloodstream (Figure 5–8). The monocytes then pass through the endothelium into the blood vessel and become macrophages. The macrophages in the atheroma are activated and produce growth factors, which induce smooth muscle proliferation as well as production of cytokines and other mediators that further activate the endothelium. Macrophages also accumulate lipids, especially low-density lipoproteins (LDL) in the oxidized or modified form. Modified LDL can be a major cause of injury of both the endothelium and the underlying smooth muscle. When the LDL

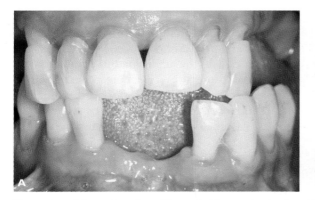
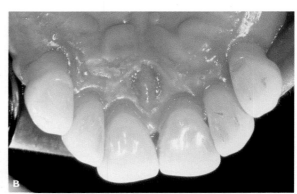

Figure 5–7. The patient from Figure 5–4 has maintained oral health for 7 years after heart surgery.

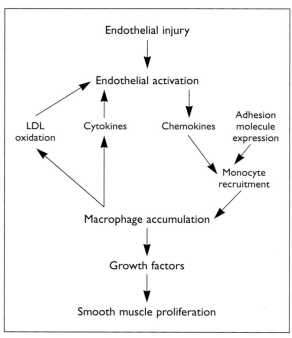

Figure 5–8. Illustration of mechanisms of atherosclerosis resulting from endothelial injury.

particles are trapped in the artery, they can undergo progressive oxidation and be internalized by macrophages, with formation of lipid peroxidases and accumulation of cholesterol esters. This results in the production of foam cells. Modified LDL is chemotactic for other monocytes and can induce the production of factors from macrophages that expand the inflammatory response.

Antioxidants can increase the resistance of LDL to oxidation, and this may explain why antioxidants, such as vitamin E, can reduce the size of fatty streaks and atherosclerotic lesions and pos-

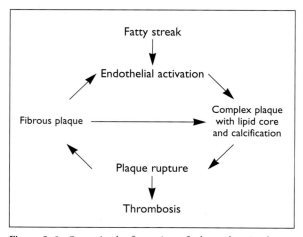

Figure 5–9. Stages in the formation of atherosclerotic plaque.

sibly protect against atheroma formation. Diabetes, through hyperglycemia and glycation of LDL and other proteins, as well as the dyslipidemia associated with diabetes, cigarette smoking, through toxic factors in smoke, and hypertension and hyperhomocystinemia are also factors that can lead to endothelial injury and the subsequent cascade of events leading to atherosclerotic lesions.

Other stages in the formation of atherosclerotic plaque are depicted in Figure 5–9. A fatty streak can become a fibrous plaque, which becomes complex with a lipid core, calcification, and deposition of extracellular matrix protein. Activated T cells may stimulate metalloproteinase production by macrophages, which remodel the fibrotic plaque. Eventually, a uniformly dense fibrous cap can cover the atheroma resulting from deposition and remodeling of the extracellular matrix in the plaque. Through remodeling of the extracellular matrix, the fibrous cap may become thin and rupture, leading to activation of the clotting system with thrombosis. It is thought that thrombosis and subsequent occlusion of the artery may be responsible for as many as one-half of the cases of acute myocardial infarction.[67]

Figure 5–10 depicts the intersecting protease cascade that connects the blood clotting system with extracellular matrix deposition and degradation. The extracellular matrix is produced by smooth muscle cells and endothelium and remodeled through degradation with endopeptidases, the matrix metalloproteinases. From Figure 5–10 it can be seen that plasminogen is converted to plasmin in the presence of tissue plasmin activator (TPA). Plasmin then activates the latent matrix metalloproteinases, which results in matrix degradation. Tissue inhibitors of matrix metalloproteinases (TIMPs) can inhibit matrix degradation whereas alpha-$_1$-antitrypsin can inhibit plasmin-mediated degradation of the extracellular matrix. Plasmin can also result in the production of fibrin from fibrinogen, which then undergoes fibrinolysis. It is likely that inflammatory mediators, such as cytokines and proteases produced by macrophages, and other cells in the atheromatous plaque, as well as bacterial proteases, contribute to extracellular matrix remodeling of fibrofatty atheromatous plaques through activation at various stages in the protease cascade depicted in Figure 5–10.

Role of Infections in Endothelial Injury

There is accumulating evidence of an association between some common infections of man and ath-

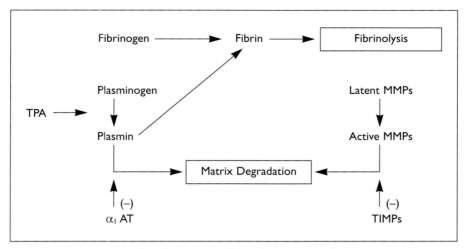

Figure 5–10. Proteases in the atheromatous plaque. TPA = tissue plasmin activator; MMP = matrix metalloproteinases; TIMPs = tissue inhibitors of matrix metalloproteinases; α1AT = α1 antitrypsin.

erosclerosis. One possible mechanism is through endothelial injury by infectious agents, triggering, in part, the inflammatory response seen in atherosclerosis. The role of infections has been recently reviewed by Danesh and colleagues,[68] and there is mounting evidence that infection with *Chlamydia pneumoniae, Helicobacter pylori,* periodontal bacteria, and cytomegalovirus are associated with heart disease (Table 5–5).

Studies Relating Oral Infections to Coronary Artery Disease

Several studies relate oral infections, including periodontal disease, to coronary artery disease. In Table 5–6, case-control and cross-sectional studies of the association between periodontal disease as well as other oral conditions and coronary artery disease are presented. In the study by Mattila and colleagues,[69] 102 controls were compared with 100 patients that had a myocardial infarction (MI). They measured oral status, using the total dental index (TDI), which is a measure of caries, periodontitis, periapical lesions, and pericoronitis, and the pantomographic index, which is a measure of periapical lesions, vertical bony defects, and furcation lesions. They found that dental health was worse in MI patients than in controls, after adjustment for age, social class, smoking, serum lipids, and diabetes. In a large cross-sectional study of 1,384 men, 45 to 64 years of age, Paunio and colleagues[70] found that a history of missing teeth was related to ischemic heart disease, after adjusting for age, hypertension, geographic area, education, and

smoking. Mattila and colleagues[71] studied 100 patients with angiographic measurements of the degree of coronary artery occlusion and previous MI. They used the dental pantomography index, which assessed periapical lesions, vertical bony defects, and furcations lesions in bone, and found that dental infections were associated with coronary atheromatosis ($p = .003$). These results were statistically significant after adjusting for age, serum lipids, body mass index, social class, and hypertension. Arbes and colleagues studied the association between the extent of periodontal attachment loss and self-reported history of heart attack from the National Health and Nutrition Examination Survey (NHANES) III data.[72] They found that when the percent of periodontal sites per person with attachment loss of ≥ 3 mm were categorized as 0%, > 0 to 33%, > 33 to 67%, and > 67%, the adjusted odds ratio with each higher category of attachment loss as relative to the 0% category was 1.4 (0.8 to 2.5), 2.3 (1.2 to 4.4), and 3.8 (1.5 to 9.7), respectively. Adjustments were made for age, sex, race, socioeconomic status, smoking, diabetes, high blood pressure, body mass

TABLE 5–5. Infections and Atherosclerosis Injury

- *Chlamydia pneumoniae*
- *Helicobacter pylori*
- Periodontal bacteria (*Porphyromonas gingivalis, Bacteroides forsythus,* and *Campylobacter rectus*)
- Cytomegalovirus

index, and serum cholesterol. This study supports findings from previous cross-sectional studies of an association between periodontal disease and coronary artery disease (CAD). These cross-sectional and case-control studies support the hypothesis that oral infections, including periodontal disease, are associated with CAD.

Perhaps more convincing evidence for the association of periodontal disease and CAD comes from a series of longitudinal and prospective studies, which are tabulated in Table 5–7. One of the first longitudinal studies to address the association between periodontal disease and coronary artery disease was published by DeStefano and colleagues in 1993.[73] They looked at 9,760 individuals in the NHANES I, who were evaluated between 1971 and 1974. These individuals were assessed at baseline for periodontal disease using the Russell periodontal index, and for decayed and missing teeth, and these individuals were followed up for 14 years for development of CAD. Subjects with periodontitis at baseline had a 25% increased risk of having CAD in the follow-up period. In males under 50 years of age, the relative risk was 1.72 after adjusting for age, blood pressure, and diabetes. Unfortunately, baseline data on smoking was available for only about one-quarter of the subjects, hence these data are only partially adjusted for smoking. Therefore, lifestyle issues, such as smoking and oral hygiene,

remain unresolved by this study. Mattila and colleagues[74] conducted a 7-year follow-up study of 214 subjects (182 men, 32 females) that had fatal and nonfatal CAD and measured the TDI as the oral condition. They found that the TDI was a statistically significant predictor of coronary artery disease after adjustment for smoking, diabetes, hypertension, socioeconomic status, previous MI, body mass index, and serum lipids.

In 1996, Beck and colleagues[75] published a study of 1,147 males enrolled in a normative aging study. Fatal and nonfatal coronary heart disease and stroke were assessed over 18 years. Baseline radiographic measurements of alveolar crestal heights were made, and the mean alveolar bone loss was dichotomized into high or low. Those individuals with high levels of mean whole mouth alveolar bone loss at baseline had a greater relative risk of total coronary heart disease (1.5; 95% CI 1.04 to 2.14) than those with low bone loss at baseline. These results remained statistically significant, after adjusting for age, body mass index, systolic blood pressure, and cholesterol. High and low alveolar bone loss at baseline was also found to be associated with fatal coronary heart disease, that is, those with high levels of alveolar bone loss had a greater chance of developing fatal heart disease with a relative risk of 1.9 (95% CI 1.10 to 3.43), after adjusting for age, smoking, systolic blood

TABLE 5–6. Summary of Case-Control and Cross-sectional Studies of the Association between Periodontal Disease and Other Oral Conditions and Coronary Artery Disease

Study	Study Design/ Subjects	Systemic Outcome	Oral Condition	Findings
Mattila et al, 1989[69]	100 myocardial infarction (MI); 102 controls	MI	Total dental index score and a "pantomographic" index of periapical lesions, vertical bony defects, and furcation lesions	Dental health worse in MI patients, after adjustments for age, social class, smoking, serum lipids, and diabetes
Paunio et al, 1993[70]	1,384 men, 45 to 64 years of age	History of angina or previous MI	Missing teeth	Number of missing teeth statistically associated (p = .0374) with ischemic heart disease, along with age, hypertension, geographic area, education, and smoking
Mattila et al, 1993[71]	100 angiography patients	Degree of coronary artery occlusion, previous MI	Dental pantomographic index	Dental infections associated with coronary atheromatosis (p = .003), after adjusting for age, serum lipids, body mass index, socio economic status class, and hypertension

TABLE 5–7. Summary of Longitudinal Studies of the Association between Periodontal Disease and Other Oral Conditions and Coronary Artery Disease

Study	Study Design/ Subjects	Systemic Outcome	Oral Condition	Findings
DeStefano et al, 1993[73]	9,760 in the National Health and Nutrition Examination Survey I	Coronary artery disease (CAD)	Russell periodontal index, number of decayed and missing teeth	Subjects with periodontitis had 25% increased risk of CAD. In males under 50 years of age, the relative risk was 1.72. Results were adjusted for age, blood pressure, diabetes, and partially adjusted for smoking
Mattila et al, 1995[74]	214 subjects (182 males, 32 females) at 7-year follow-up	Fatal and nonfatal CAD	Total dental index	The total dental index was a statistically significant predictor of CAD. Adjustments made for smoking, diabetes, hypertension, socioeconomic status, previous MI, body mass index (BMI), and serum lipids
Beck et al, 1996[75]	1,147 males	Coronary heart disease (CHD) and stroke	Radiographic interproximal alveolar crestal heights	Dichotomized mean whole mouth bone loss hi-lo at baseline associated with total CHD with relative risk of 1.5 (1.04, 2.14), after adjusting for age, BMI, systolic blood pressure, and cholesterol. Hi-lo alveolar bone loss at baseline associated with fatal CHD with relative risk of 1.9 (1.10, 3.43), after adjusting for age, smoking, systolic blood pressure, and diabetes. Cumulative incidence of CHD increased with greater levels of age-adjusted alveolar bone loss at baseline
Joshipura et al, 1996[76]	44,119 male health professionals followed up over 6 years	Coronary artery disease	Self-reported periodontal disease and self-reported number of teeth	Those who reported periodontal disease and less than 10 teeth at baseline had a relative risk of CAD of 1.67. Adjustment was made for smoking, physical activity, hypertension, cholesterol, family history of CAD, dietary and alcohol intake
Genco et al, 1997[77]	1,372 Native Americans followed up for 10 years; population has a low level of smoking	Electrocardio-graphic evidence of cardiovascular disease (CVD)	Alveolar bone level and tooth loss	Baseline periodontal disease showed that for those ≤ 60 years of age, periodontal disease was a predictor for subsequent CVD, with a relative risk of 2.68 (1.30, 5.5) after adjusting for diabetes, age, gender, cholesterol, BMI, smoking, and hypertension

pressure, and diabetes. From these studies assessing total coronary heart disease and fatal heart disease, it appears that the analyses were adjusted for many of the important risk factors that are relevant to both periodontal disease and heart disease. It is of considerable interest that Beck and colleagues[75] also found that the cumulative incidence of coronary heart disease increases with greater levels of age-adjusted alveolar bone at baseline, suggesting a dose response, that is, the more periodontal disease at baseline, the greater is the cumulative incidence of coronary heart disease over time.

Joshipura and colleagues[76] studied 44,119 male health professionals for a period of 6 years. Seven-hundred and fifty cases of CAD, including fatal and nonfatal MI, were documented. Periodontal status and number of teeth were self-reported. It was found that among those men that reported peri-odontal disease and fewer than 10 teeth at baseline, there was an increased risk of cardiovascular disease as compared with men that had 25 or more teeth at baseline (1.67 relative risk). In those that reported no previous periodontal disease, no relationship to coronary heart disease was found (1.11 relative risk). This study mainly shows an association between tooth loss (in those that reported peri-odontal disease) and coronary heart disease. It is likely that the reported tooth loss was associated with periodontal disease. Self-reported periodontal disease is fraught with inaccuracies and misclassifi-cations; however, the authors point out that when combined with assessment of tooth loss, which may be more accurately self-reported, this study does point to a possible association between heart disease and periodontal disease. The relative risk of 1.67 remained after adjustment for smoking, physical activity, hypertension, cholesterol, family history of CAD, and dietary and alcohol intake.

Genco and colleagues[77] reported a longitudi-nal study of 1,372 Native Americans, who were assessed for periodontal disease at baseline, and fol-lowed up for 10 years for electrocardiographic evi-dence of cardiovascular disease, using the Pooling criteria. Periodontal status was measured by alveo-lar bone levels. It was found that baseline peri-odontal disease for those under age 60 years was a predictor of subsequent cardiovascular disease, with a relative risk of 2.68 (95% CI 1.30 to 5.50). These results were significant, after adjusting for diabetes, age, gender, cholesterol, body mass index, smoking, and hypertension. It should be noted that in this population, the level of smoking is very low, and, in fact, smoking per se was not a risk fac-tor for either cardiovascular disease or periodontal disease. Hence, this study was carried out in a pop-ulation which minimized or eliminated smoking as a co–risk factor, which may confound the relation-ship between periodontal disease and heart disease in other studies.

All these data support the association of increased CAD, especially in men under age 60 to 65 years. The relationship, however, is weaker for men over age 60 to 65 years in most of these stud-ies. The reason for the weak association in older individuals is not yet clear but the stronger relation-ship in men under the age of 60 to 65 years remains

confirmed in all the studies reported to date. In con-clusion, there is considerable cross-sectional, case-control, and longitudinal/epidemiologic evidence of an association between periodontal infection and CAD. Other oral infections also may contribute, but the evidence suggests that caries, per se, is not related to CAD. Good evidence is not yet available to determine if there is an association of periapical lesions, pericoronal lesions, or other oral infections with heart disease. Also, little evidence is available for women, Hispanic, Black, or Asian populations with respect to the relationship between periodontal infections and heart disease.

Studies Relating Oral Infections to Stroke

There are several studies which provide suggestive evidence for an association between atherosclerosis-related ischemic stroke and oral infections (Table 5–8). One of the first studies to report this associa-tion was conducted by Syrjänen and colleagues.[78] In a case-control study, they compared 40 patients with ischemic cerebral infarction with 40 randomly selected community-based controls that were matched for age and gender. The systemic outcome was ischemic cerebral infarction, and oral condi-tions were assessed by the TDI. These investigators found a statistically significant poorer level of oral health in patients with ischemic cerebral infarction as compared to controls. However, this is a small case-control study that did not control for other co–risk or confounding factors, such as smoking, hypertriglyceridemia, hypertension, and febrile infections, which were also found to be at statisti-cally significantly higher prevalence in the patient group. Therefore, the extent to which these other confounding variables were related to the associa-tion between dental health and ischemic cerebral infarction is not clear. However, this study suggests that infections, per se, are related to ischemic cere-bral infarction, and it is not unreasonable that oral infections would also contribute.

Grau and colleagues[79] also presented a case-control study of 66 cases and 66 controls. The patients suffered from acute cerebral ischemia evi-denced by computed tomography (CT) or magnet-ic resonance imaging (MRI), or from transient cere-bral ischemia. These investigators also used the TDI, with orthopantomography as part of the index. They found that poor dental status with a TDI of > 6 was associated with cerebral ischemia (2.51, 95% CI 1.20 to 5.20). Grau and colleagues[79] also analyzed the components of the TDI and found that there was no association with the dental

TABLE 5–8. Summary of Studies of the Association between Periodontal Disease and Other Oral Conditions and Stroke

Study	Study Design/ Subjects	Systemic Outcome	Oral Condition	Findings
Syrjänen et al, 1989[78]	Case-control; 40 patients with ischemic cerebral infarction, and 40 randomly selected community controls matched for age and gender	Ischemic cerebral infarction	Total dental index (TDI) (caries, periodontitis, periapical lesions, and pericoronitis included)	A statistically significantly poorer level of oral health was found among patients as compared with controls. However, smoking, hypertriglyceridemia, hypertension, and febrile infections also greater in patients than in controls
Grau et al, 1997[79]	Case-control; 66 cases, 66 controls	Acute cerebral ischemia evidenced by CT or MRI; or transient cerebral ischemia	TDI with orthopantomography	Poor dental health (TDI >6) was associated with cerebral ischemia with an odds ratio of 2.51 (1.20, 5.2) after adjusting for current smoking, diabetes, socioeconomic status, and pre-existing vascular disease
Beck et al. 1996[75]	Longitudinal follow-up of 1,147 men	40 stroke cases, including 29 with coronary heart disease	Mean alveolar bone height, hi-lo dichotomous	High alveolar bone loss was predictive of subsequent stroke with a relative risk of 2.8 (1.45, 5.48) after adjusting for age, smoking, diabetes, diastolic blood pressure, family history, and education
Wu et al, 1999[80]	Longitudinal, NHANES I; 9,962 adults followed up for 18 years	Cerebrovascular disease, nonhemorrhagic and hemorrhagic stroke, and transient cerebral ischemia	Subjects classified as suffering from periodontitis, gingivitis, no periodontal disease, and edentulous based on Russell index	Periodontitis was associated with nonhemorrhagic stroke with a relative risk of 2.11 (1.30, 3.42). Increased risk for nonhemorrhagic stroke seen in men, women, African Americans and Caucasian Americans. The population-attributable risk for nonhemorrhagic stroke was 19% based on baseline periodontal disease.

caries component. These results were obtained after adjusting for current smoking, diabetes, socioeconomic status, and pre-existing vascular disease.

Beck and colleagues[75] provided the first longitudinal data relating stroke to oral infections. They followed up 1,147 men over 18 years of age and identified 40 stroke cases, including 29 that also had coronary heart disease. Periodontal status was measured using the mean alveolar bone height, and dichotomized into high and low groups. They found that high mean alveolar bone loss was predictive of subsequent stroke with a relative risk of

2.8 (95% CI 1.45 to 5.48). These results were obtained after adjusting for age, smoking, diabetes, diastolic blood pressure, family history, and educational level.

The largest study relating stroke to periodontal disease comes from Wu and colleagues.[80] They studied the NHANES I database on 9,962 adults followed up for 18 years. The systemic outcome was cerebrovascular disease, including nonhemorrhagic and hemorrhagic strokes and transient cerebral ischemia. Subjects were classified as suffering from periodontitis, gingivitis, or as exhibiting a healthy periodontium on the basis of the Russell periodontal index. They found that periodontitis at baseline was associated with nonhemorrhagic (ischemic) stroke, with a relative risk of 2.1 (95% CI 1.3 to 3.4). Of considerable importance was the finding that in this same population, there was no association of periodontitis with hemorrhagic stroke. Hence the association of periodontal disease with ischemic stroke, which is largely due to atherosclerotic lesions, and not with hemorrhagic stroke, which is associated with bleeding vessels, provides further evidence for the role of infections in atherosclerotic processes. The increased risk for nonhemorrhagic stroke was seen in men, women, African Americans, and Caucasians. Baseline periodontal disease accounted for 19% of the population-attributable risk for nonhemorrhagic stroke in this study, suggesting that periodontal disease is of significant public health importance in relation to stroke. This study is of interest because there was an internal control, that is, there was no relationship between periodontal disease in the same population and hemorrhagic stroke, which is not associated with atherosclerosis but rather with bleeding.

In general, the relationship of oral infections, especially periodontal disease, to fatal and nonfatal CAD as well as to nonhemorrhagic stroke, much of which is ischemic atherosclerotic stroke, strongly points to a relationship between periodontal infection and atherosclerosis and related sequelae such as coronary artery and cerebral artery disease.

MECHANISMS BY WHICH INFECTIONS MAY CONTRIBUTE TO ATHEROSCLEROSIS

Several possible mechanisms may operate independently or in concert to explain the association between infections in general and periodontal infections specifically and atherosclerosis, myocardial infarction, and stroke. For purposes of discussion, we will consider four main mechanisms: (1) direct effects of infectious agents in atheroma formation; (2) indirect or host-mediated effects triggered by infection; (3) common genetic predisposition for periodontal disease and atherosclerosis; and (4) common risk factors, such as lifestyle.

Direct Effects of Infectious Agents in Atheroma Formation

There are three lines of evidence suggesting that periodontal bacteria may have direct effects on atheroma formation. The first comes from studies finding *Porphyromonas gingivalis* in carotid and coronary atheromas.[81,82] The second comes from the findings of Deshpande and colleagues[83] showing in vitro that *P. gingivalis* can invade and may proliferate in the endothelial cells. The third line of evidence comes from studies by Herzberg and Meyer[84] showing that *P. gingivalis* is able to induce aggregation of platelets, which is thought to be associated with thrombus formation. Other possible mechanisms include protease production by *P. gingivalis* and other periodontal pathogens, which may contribute to remodeling of the extracellular matrix in atheromatous plaques. Evidence for any of these mechanisms is, at this point, in vitro or preliminary. However, it is not unreasonable to expect that organisms that infect atheromatous plaques may contribute to their formation or to the thrombotic events associated with myocardial infarction.

Indirect or Host-Mediated Effects Triggered by Infection

One possible mechanism that has garnered considerable support is that periodontitis induces an inflammatory response that is manifested, in part, by the production of acute-phase proteins, such as C-reactive protein and fibrinogen, by the liver. C-reactive protein and fibrinogen are independent risk factors for coronary artery disease, hence if they are induced, in part at least, by periodontal infection, this may help explain the link between periodontal disease and heart disease. A recent study by Wu and colleagues[85] using the NHANES III database, found that C-reactive protein and plasma fibrinogen were related to poor periodontal health, which provides support for this hypothesis.

Another indirect effect of periodontal infection that may explain the association between periodontal disease and heart disease is that periodontal organisms contain proteins which cross-react with the heart. In fact, the heat-shock protein-60, which is produced by *Bacteroides forsythus* and *P. gingivalis,* has about 60% homology with the mammalian heat-shock protein. It is known that antibodies to the heat-shock protein are found in patients with periodontal disease. It is conceivable then that these antibodies to heat-shock proteins of periodontal bacteria are cross-reactive with the heat-shock protein that is exposed in an injured endothelium or atheromatous plaque. This could set in motion autoimmune phenomena and contribute to atheroma formation.

Common Genetic Predisposition for Periodontal Disease and Atherosclerosis

There may be common genetic mechanisms which provide the link between periodontal disease and cardiovascular disease. Beck and colleagues[75] have provided a model proposing that there is a genetically determined hyperinflammatory macrophage phenotype in periodontal disease, which contributes to the susceptibility for atherosclerosis.

Common Risk Factors Affecting Both Periodontal Disease and Heart Disease

DeStefano and colleagues[73] found that periodontal disease and poor oral hygiene are stronger indicators of risk of total mortality and of coronary heart disease. They suggest that oral hygiene may be an indicator or a surrogate for lifestyle affecting personal hygiene and health care and might explain the relationship between periodontal disease and heart disease. Multiple studies showing the relationship between periodontal disease and heart disease, after adjusting for many factors associated with lifestyle, such as smoking and weight, suggest that the relationship is not simply explained by lifestyle (see Tables 5–6, 5–7, and 5–8). Also, the finding that the graded exposure of periodontal disease leads to an increased cumulative index of coronary heart disease argues against lifestyle as a simple explanation for this association.[75]

The association between periodontal disease and cardiovascular disease or stroke could be due to residual confounders or incomplete control of confounders. As with most studies that adjust for possible confounders, the adjustments may not be complete, so associations of this magnitude may be due to residual confounders. Perhaps new studies with more detailed adjustments for confounders will clarify this issue. In fact, there are two studies in progress, supported by the National Institutes of Health (NIH), which may help resolve this issue.

Further research will be needed to determine which, and to what extent, factors act singly or in concert to contribute to the formation of atheromatous plaques. It is important to know the mechanisms, however, since they add evidence to support the association between periodontal infection and atherosclerosis. In addition, knowing the mechanisms may well lead to simple, cost-effective interventions that would moderate, in part, the contribution of infection to atherosclerosis.

Management of Periodontal Disease in Patients at High Risk for Atherosclerosis

Since there is mounting evidence relating periodontal infections to atherosclerosis, it is reasonable that patients with periodontal disease that are at risk for atherosclerotic disease should be managed in the following manner:

1. Patients at high risk for atherosclerotic disease should be subjected to a complete periodontal examination.
2. Patients that have periodontal disease should have a thorough medical history evaluating systemic conditions, medications, and risk factors for atherosclerosis and related conditions such as heart disease and stroke.
3. Treatment of patients with periodontal disease and pre-existing atherosclerotic disease, such as stroke, nonfatal myocardial infarction, and atherosclerosis in general, should be coordinated among health professionals to ensure that patients are adequately managed taking into account medical as well as dental considerations and complications.
4. Aggressive prevention of periodontal disease should be undertaken in patients at high risk for atherosclerotic disease. If periodontal disease exists in these high-risk patients, comprehensive treatment should be instituted to eradicate, as much as possible, the periodontal infection and prevent its recurrence.
5. Patients should be made completely aware of the possible relationship between heart disease, stroke, and periodontal disease, without unduly alarming them, so that they may participate in the modification of risk factors for both artherosclerosis and periodontal disease, such as smoking.

REFERENCES

1. Redding S, Montgomery M. Dentistry in systemic disease: In: Diagnostic and therapeutic approach to patient management. Portland: JBK Publishing, Inc; 1990. P. 169–213.
2. Rose LF, Kaye D. Cardiovascular disorders. In: Internal medicine for dentistry. 2nd ed. Mosby Publishing Co; 1990. p. 505–14.
3. University of Washington. Medically compromised patient *with* cardiovascular disorders: a self-instructional series in rehabilitation dentistry. Seattle, WA; Module IV, Unit A.; 1986.

4. Mealey BL. Influence of periodontal infections on systemic health. Periodontol 2000 1999. [In press]

5. Mulligan R. Preventive care for the geriatric dental patient. Cal Dent Assoc J 1984;12:21–32.

6. Aragon SB, Buckley SB, Tilson HB. Oral surgery management of the geriatric patient. Spec Care Dent 1984;4:124–9.

7. Little JW, Falace, DA. Therapeutic considerations in special patients. Dent Clin North Am 1984; 28:455–69.

8. Little JW, Falace DA. Dental management of the medically compromised patient. 3rd ed. St. Louis: Mosby Publishing Co.; 1988. p. 83–195.

9. Matsuura H. Systemic complications and their management during dental treatment. Int Dent J 1989;39:113–21.

10. McCarthy FM, Pallasch TJ, Gates, R. Documenting safe treatment of the medical-risk patient. J Am Dent Assoc 1989;119:383–9.

11. Mulligan R. Pretreatment for the cardiovascularly compromised geriatric dental patient. Spec Care Dent 1985;5:116–23.

12. Thornton JB, Wright JT. Special and medically compromised patients in dentistry. St. Louis: Mosby Year-Book Publishers; 1989. p. 149–68.

13. Cash J, Raab RW, Coke JM. Understanding your patient with cardiac disease. J Colorado Dent Assoc 1990;68:16–9.

14. Dajani AS, Taubert KA, Wilson W, et al. Prevention of bacterial endocarditis. Recommendations by the American Heart Association. JAMA 1997;277:1794–801. Circulation 1997;96: 358–66.

15. Mealey BL. Periodontal implications: medically compromised patients. Ann Periodontol 1996; 1:256–321.

16. Rees TD. Adjunctive therapy. Discussion section X. In: Nevins M, Becker W, Kornman K, editors. Proceedings of the world workshop in clinical periodontics. Chicago, IL: The American Academy of Periodontology; 1989.

17. Strom BL, Abrutyn E, Berlin JA, et al. Dental and cardiac risk factors for infective endocarditis. A population-based, case-control study. Ann Intern Med 1998;129:761–9.

18. Younessi OJ, Walker DM, Ellis P, Dwyer DF. Fatal *Staphylococcus aureus* infective endocarditis: dental implications. Oral Surg Oral Med Oral Pathol Oral Radiol Endod 1998;85:168–72.

19. Burne RA. Concise review. Oral streptococci, products of their environment. J Dent Res 1998; 77:445–52.

20. Slots J. Causal or casual relationship between peri-odontal infection and non-oral disease [guest editorial]. J Dent Res 1998;77:1764–5.

21. Atkinson BA, Abu-Al-Jaibat A, LeBlanc DJ. Antibiotic resistance among enterococci isolated from clinical specimens between 1953 and 1954. Antimicrobial Agents Chemother 1997; 41:1598–600.

22. Griffin BP. Valvular heart disease. In: Dale DC, Federman DD, editors. Scientific American Medicine. New York, NY: Scientific American Inc.; 1998.

23. Karchmer AW. Infective endocarditis. In: Dale DC, Federman DD, editors. Scientific American Medicine. New York, NY: Scientific American, Inc.; 1999.

24. Sanabria TJ, Alpert JS, Goldberg R, et al. Increasing frequency of staphylococcal infective endocarditis. Experience at a university hospital, 1981 through 1988. Arch Intern Med 1990; 150:1305–9.

25. Cowper TR. Pharmacologic management of the patient with disorders of the cardiovascular system. Infective endocarditis. Dent Clin North Am 1996;40:611–47.

26. Kupferwasser HD, Muller AM, Morh-Kahaly S, et al. Clinical and morphological characteristics in *Streptococcus bovis* endocarditis: a comparison with other causative microorganisms in 177 cases. Heart 1998;80:276–80.

27. Rees TD. Dental management of the medically compromised patient. In: McDonald RE, Hurt WC, Gilmore HW, Middleton, RA, editors. Current therapy in dentistry. 7th ed. St. Louis: C.V. Mosby Co.; 1980. p. 1–30.

28. McKinsey DS, Ratts TE, Bisno AL. Underlying cardiac lesions in adults with infective endocarditis. Am J Med 1987;82:681–8.

29. Zysset MK, Montgomery MT, Redding SW, Dell' Italia LJ. Systemic lupus erythematosus: a consideration for antimicrobial prophylaxis. Oral Surg Oral Med Oral Pathol Oral Radiol Endod 1987;64:30–4.

30. Friedlander AH, Yoshikaua TT. Pathogenesis, management, and prevention of infective endocarditis in the elderly dental patient. Oral Surg Oral Med Oral Pathol Oral Radiol Endod 1990; 69:177–81.

31. Friedlander AH. Risk assessment of the older dental patient: a review of the pathophysiology of the cardiovascular system. Spec Care Dent 1987; 7:41–2.

32. Bayer AS, Lam K, Ginzton L, et al. *Staphylococcus aureus* bacteremia. Arch Intern Med 1987;147: 457–62.

33. Devereux RB, Kramer-Fox R, Kligfield P. Mitral valve prolapse: causes, clinical manifestations, and management. Ann Intern Med 1989;111: 305–17.

34. Rees TD. Periodontal considerations in patients with bone marrow or solid organ transplants. 1999. In: Periodontal Medicine *etc.*

35. Rees, TD, Rose LF. Periodontal management of patients with cardiovascular diseases [position paper, American Academy of Periodontology]. J Periodontol 1996;67:627–35.

36. Taylor MH, Peterson DS. Kawasaki's disease. J Am Dent Assoc 1982;104:44–7.

37. Barnett ML, Friedman D, Kastner, T. The prevalence of mitral valve prolapse in patients with Down's syndrome: implications for dental management. Oral Surg Oral Med Oral Pathol 1988;66:445–7.

38. Clemens JD, Ransohoff DF. A quantitative assessment of pre-dental antibiotic prophylaxis for patients with mitral-valve prolapse. J Chron Dis 1984;37:531–41.

39. Friedlander AH, Gorelick DA. Panic disorder: its association with mitral valve prolapse and appropriate dental management. Oral Surg Oral Med Oral Pathol Oral Radiol Endod 1987; 63:309–12.

40. Meyers DG, Starke H, Pearson PH, Wilken MK. Mitral valve prolapse in anorexia nervosa. Ann Intern Med 1986;105:384–6.

41. Daly C, Mitchell D, Grossberg D, et al. Bacteraemia caused by periodontal probing. Aust Dent J 1997;42:77–80.

42. Roberts GJ, Simmons NB, Longhurst P. Odontogenic bacteraemia and intraligamental analgesia. Br Dent J 1992;173:195.

43. Lamas WP. A study of transient bacteremia following an intraoral soft tissue biopsy [thesis]. Dallas, TX: Baylor College of Dentistry-TAMUS; 1998.

44. Francis JL. Significance of bacteremias of dental origin. J Am Dent Assoc 1986;112:306–8.

45. Pallasch TJ. Antibiotic prophylaxis: theory and reality. Calif. Dent Assoc J 1989;17:27–39.

46. Berger SA, Weitzman S, Edberg SC, Coreg JI. Bacteremia after the use of an oral irrigating device. Ann Intern Med 1974;80:510–1.

47. Felix JE, Rosen S, App GR. Detection of bacteremia after the use of an oral irrigation device on subjects with periodontitis. J Periodontol 1971;42:785–7.

48. Hunter KM, Holborow DW, Kardos TB, et al. Bacteremia and tissue damage resulting from air polishing. Br Dent J 1989;167:275–7.

49. Romans AR, App GR. Bacteremia, a result from oral irrigation in subjects with gingivitis. J Periodontol 1971;42:757–60.

50. Barco CT. Prevention of infective endocarditis: a review of the medical and dental literature. J Periodontol 1991;62:510–23.

51. Bender IB, Naidorf IJ, Garvey GJ. Bacterial endocarditis: a consideration for physician and dentist. J Am Dent Assoc 1984;109:415–20.

52. MacFarlane TW, Ferguson MM, Mulgrew CJ. Post-extraction bacteremia: role of antiseptics and antibiotics. Br Dent J 1984;156:179–81.

53. Tzukert AA, Leviner E, Sela M. Prevention of infective endocarditis: not by antibiotics alone. Oral Surg Oral Med Oral Pathol Oral Radiol Endod 1986;62:385–8.

54. Fay JT, O'Neal RB. Dental responsibility for the medically compromised patient IV. J Oral Med 1984;39:218–25.

55. Kilmartin C, Munroe C. The dental management of the cardiac patient requiring antibiotic prophylaxis. J Can Dent Assoc 1986;52:77–82.

56. Kilmartin C, Munroe CO. Cardiovascular diseases and the dental patient. J Can Dent Assoc 1986; 52:513–8.

57. Leviner E, Tzukert AA, Berioliol R, et al. Development of resistant oral viridans streptococci after administration of prophylactic antibiotics: time management in the dental treatment of patients susceptible to infective endocarditis. Oral Surg Oral Med Oral Pathol Oral Radiol Endod 1987;64:417–20.

58. Slots J, Rosling BG, Genco RJ. Suppression of penicillin-resistant oral *Actinobacillus actinomycetemcomitans* with tetracycline: considerations in endocarditis prophylaxis. J Periodontol 1983; 54:193–6.

59. American Dental Association. Patients with cardiovascular disease. Oral Health Care Guidelines 1989; September:1–13.

60. Baltch AL, Pressman HL, Schaffer C, et al. Bacteremia in patients undergoing oral procedures. Arch Intern Med 1988;148:1084–8.

61. Steinberg BJ, Brown S. Dental treatment of the health compromised. Medical and psychological considerations. Alpha Omegan 1986;79:34–41.

62. Glasser S. The problems of patients with cardiovascular disease undergoing dental treatment. J Am Dent Assoc 1977;94:1158–62.

63. Mulligan R, Weitzel KG. Pretreatment management of the patient receiving anticoagulant drugs J Am Dent Assoc 1988;117:479–83.

64. Breslow JL. Cardiovascular disease burden increases, NIH funding decreases. Nat Med 1997;3:600–1.

65. Braunwald E. Shattuck Lecture—cardiovascular medicine at the turn of the millennium: triumphs, concerns, and opportunities. N Engl J Med 1997;337:1360–9.

66. Ross R. Atherosclerosis—an inflammatory disease. N Engl J Med 1999;340:115–26.

67. Falk E, Shah PK, Fuster V. Pathogenesis of plaque disruption. In: Fuster V, Ross R, Topol EJ, editors. Atherosclerosis and coronary artery disease. Vol 2. Philadelphia: Lippincott-Raven; 1996. p. 492–510.

68. Danesh J, Collins R, Peto R. Chronic infections and coronary heart disease: is there a link? Lancet 1997;350:430–6.

69. Mattila K, Nieminen M, Valtonen V, et al. Association between dental health and acute myocardial infarction. BMJ 1989;298:779–82.

70. Paunio K, Impivaara O, Tiekso J, Maki J. Missing teeth and ischaemic heart disease in men aged 45-64 years. Eur Heart J 1993;14Suppl:54–6.

71. Mattila KJ, Valle M, Nieminen MS, et al. Dental infections and coronary atherosclerosis. Atherosclerosis 1993;103:205–11.

72. Arbes S, Slade GD, Beck JD. Association between extent of periodontal attachment loss and self-reported history of heart attack: an analysis of NHANES III data. J Dent Res 1999. [In press]

73. DeStefano F, Anda RF, Kahn HS, et al. Dental disease and risk of coronary heart disease. BMJ 1993;306:688–91.

74. Mattila KJ, Valtonen VV, Nieminen M, Huttunen JK. Dental infection and the risk of new coronary events: prospective study of patients with documented coronary artery disease. Clin Infect Dis 1995;20:588–92.

75. Beck J, Garcia J, Heiss G, et al. Periodontal disease and cardiovascular disease. J Periodontol 1996; 67:1123–37.

76. Joshipura KJ, Rimm EB, Douglass CW, et al. Poor oral health and coronary heart disease. J Dent Res 1996;75:1631–6.

77. Genco RJ, Chadda S, Grossi S, et al. Periodontal disease is a predictor of cardiovascular disease in a Native American population [abstract]. J Dent Res 1997;76(Special Issue):3158.

78. Syrjänen J, Peltola J, Valtonen V, et al. Dental infections in association with cerebral infarction in young and middle-aged men. J Intern Med 1989;255:179–84.

79. Grau AJ, Buggle F, Ziegler C, et al. Association between acute cerebrovascular ischemia and chronic and recurrent infection. Stroke 1997; 28:1724–9.

80. Wu T, Trevisan M, Genco RJ, et al. Periodontal disease and risk of cerebrovascular disease: the first National Health and Nutrition Examination Survey and its follow-up study. JAMA 1999. [In press]

81. Haraszthy VI, Zambon JJ, Trevisan M, et al. Identification of pathogens in atheromatous plaques [abstract]. J Dent Res 1998;77(Special Issue): 273.

82. Chiu B, Viira E, Evans RT, Genco RJ. Detection of an odontopathogen: *Porphyromonas gingivalis* in atherosclerotic plaques: an immunohistochemical and in situ hybridization study. Appl Immunohistochem Molec Morphol 1999. [In press]

83. Deshpande RG, Kahn MB, Genco CA. Invasion of aortic and heart endothelial cells by *Porphyromonas gingivalis*. Infect Immun 1998;66:5337–43.

84. Herzberg MC, Meyer MW. Effects of oral flora on platelets: possible consequences in cardiovascular disease. J Periodontol 1996;67:1138–42.

85. Wu T, Trevisan M, Genco RJ, et al. An examination of the relation between periodontal health status and cardiovascular risk factors: serum total and HDL cholesterol, C-reactive protein, and plasma fibrinogen. Am J Epidemiol 1999. [In press]

CHAPTER 6

Relationships between Periodontal and Respiratory Diseases

Frank A. Scannapieco, DMD, PhD

Respiratory diseases are responsible for a significant number of deaths and considerable suffering in humans. These diseases are widely prevalent. For example, lower respiratory infections were the third commonest cause of mortality worldwide in 1990 (causing 4.3 million deaths), and chronic obstructive pulmonary disease (COPD) was the sixth leading cause of mortality (2.2 million deaths);[1] it was the fourth leading cause of death in the United States in 1996,[2] claiming 100,000 lives while pneumonia and influenza together caused almost 84,000 deaths.

Accumulating evidence suggests that oral disorders, particularly periodontal disease, may influence the course of respiratory infection. This chapter will describe the major respiratory diseases caused or influenced by bacteria, the epidemiologic evidence that supports a role for oral bacteria in the process of respiratory infection, and possible mechanisms that may explain the role of oral bacteria in the process of respiratory infection.

RESPIRATORY DISEASES

Bacterial Pneumonia

Pneumonia is a group of related diseases caused by a wide variety of infectious agents, including bacteria, mycoplasma, fungi, parasites, and viruses, resulting in infection of the pulmonary parenchyma (Figure 6–1). Pneumonia can be a life-threatening infection, especially in the elderly and immunocompromised patient,[3,4] and it is a significant cause of morbidity and mortality in patients of all ages. Bacterial pneumonia, a common form of the disease, can arise de novo or as a superinfection of an underlying viral pneumonia. Up until the early part of this century, bacterial pneumonia was a common, severe, and often fatal infection.[5] With the advent of the widespread use of antibiotics, many of these infections became treatable. However, the continuing emergence of antibiotic-resistant bacteria (eg, penicillin-resistant pneumococci) suggests that the number of cases of bacterial pneumonia caused by resistant organisms will increase in the years to come.[6] Thus, knowledge of the pathogenesis of and the risk factors for bacterial pneumonia is critical to the development of strategies for the treatment and prevention of these infections.

Pneumonia can be classified as community acquired or hospital acquired (nosocomial). These types of pneumonia differ with respect to their causative agents (Table 6–1). Community-acquired bacterial pneumonia is usually associated with *Streptococcus pneumoniae* and *Haemophilus influenzae,* with other species such as *Mycoplasma pneumoniae, Chlamydia pneumoniae, Legionella pneumophila,* and a variety of anaerobic species also involved.[7,8] The spectrum of organisms responsible for nosocomial pneumonia is quite different, with gram-negative bacilli (including enterics such as *Escherichia coli, Klebsiella pneumoniae, Serratia* spp., and *Enterobacter* spp. as well as *Pseudomonas aeruginosa*) and *Staphylococcus aureus* being the most prevalent.[4,8–10] The spectrum of organisms prevalent in nursing homes is even broader, with pathogens common to both community- and hospital-acquired pneumonias involved.[4]

Infections are of particular concern in the hospital environment. Greater than 5% of all hospitalized patients develop an infection following their admission to the hospital, and pneumonia typically accounts for 10 to 20% of these.[10–13] Hospital-acquired pneumonia often prolongs hospital stay, increases patient care costs, and causes significant morbidity and mortality.[14] There are more than 300,000 nosocomial respiratory infections each year,[11] leading to about 20,000 deaths,[13] and such infection adds 7 to 9 days to the average length of stay in the hospital.[13] The annual direct cost of diagnosing and treating nosocomial pneumonia may exceed $2 billion.[15] While also contributing to a significant number of deaths by acting as a complicating or secondary factor, pneumonia is of special significance in the elderly population, accounting for the majority of admissions to hospitals from nursing homes.[4,16]

Chronic Obstructive Pulmonary Disease

Another severe respiratory disease affecting a significant segment of the population is COPD. This condition is characterized by chronic obstruction to airflow, with excess production of sputum resulting from chronic bronchitis (CB) and/or emphysema.[17] Chronic bronchitis is the result of irritation to the bronchial airway, which causes an expansion of the proportion of mucus-secreting cells within the airway epithelium (Figure 6–2). These cells secrete excessive tracheobronchial mucus sufficient to cause cough with expectoration for at least 3 months of the year over two consecutive years.[18] Emphysema is defined as the distention of the air spaces distal to the terminal bronchiole with destruction of the alveolar septa.

Chronic bronchitis is quite prevalent, with 20 to 30% of all adults over 45 years reporting a history of asthma or chronic bronchitis.[19] Chronic bronchitis is more prevalent in men than in woman, with about 20% of all adult males displaying some evidence of it.[17] The prevalence of the disease in women is on the rise since more women are smok-

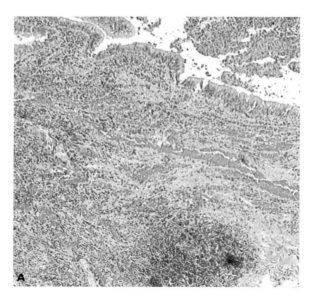

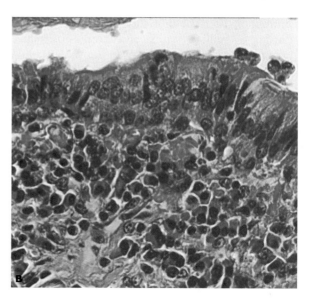

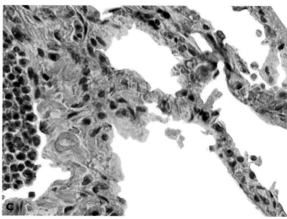

Figure 6–1. Histopathology of bronchopneumonia. *A,* Low power of a bronchiole showing the presence of an inflammatory exudate in its lumen. A patchy inflammatory cell infiltrate is observed in the subephithelial region. (Hematoxylin-eosin stain, original magnification × 20) *B,* Higher power view illustrates the simple columnar ciliated epithelium that lines the bronchiole. The lamina propria and lumen of the bronchiole contain numerous inflammatory cells. (Hematoxylin-eosin stain, original magnification × 400) *C,* High power view of pulmonary alveoli shows early red hepatization characterized by capillary congestion in the septae. In addition, an extensive neutrophilic exudation in the alveoli is also observed. (Hematoxylin-eosin stain, original magnification × 400)

TABLE 6–1. Etiology of Bacterial Pneumonia

Community-Acquired Pneumonia	*Nosocomial Pneumonia*
• *Streptococcus pneumoniae* • *Haemophilus influenzae* • *Mycoplasma pneumoniae* • *Chlamydia pneumoniae* • *Legionella pneumophila* • *Staphylococcus aureus* • *Candida albicans* • Anaerobic species	• Gram-negative bacilli (including enterics such as *Escherichia coli*, *Klebsiella pneumoniae*, *Serratia* spp, *Enterobacter* spp, *Pseudomonas aeruginosa*) • *Staphylococcus aureus*

ing than ever before. The incidence of emphysema is less well known since the main tool for noninvasive diagnosis (computed tomographic [CT] scanning) cannot be applied to population studies. It is interesting that it is rare to find lungs completely free of emphysema post mortem. However, the vast majority of individuals, while showing well-defined histologic evidence of emphysema, will not have clinical symptoms of the disease.

The major risk factor for COPD is a history of prolonged cigarette smoking, with chronic exposure to toxic atmospheric pollutants (eg, second-hand smoke) also being a contributory factor. Genetic conditions, such as the presence of a defective alpha$_1$-antitrypsin gene, variant alpha$_1$-antichymotrypsin, alpha$_2$-macroglobulin, vitamin D–binding protein, and blood group antigen genes, may also predispose subjects to this disease.[20]

One of the major complications of COPD is the occurrence of "exacerbations," or episodes in which there are objective signs that the disease has worsened such as increased sputum production showing a change in color and/or consistency, cough, dyspnea, chest tightness, and fatigue. The factors responsible for the initiation of exacerbation are not completely known although they are thought to be provoked, in part, by bacterial infection.[21,22] The organisms most closely associated with exacerbations are nontypeable *H. influenzae*, *S. pneumoniae*, and *Moraxella catarrhalis*. It should be pointed out that the frequency of exacerbations in COPD patients varies from individual to individual. The frequency of exacerbations is not related to the severity of lung disease. Although viral infections, fluid overload, and allergy have been suggested to enhance the risk for exacerbation, no studies have yet proven the role of these factors in the disease process.[17]

Pathogenesis and Risk Factors for Lung Infection

The lung is composed of numerous units formed by the progressive branching of the airways. The airway of each terminal respiratory unit (bronchiole, alveolar duct, alveolar sac, and alveoli) is lined by epithelial cells in close proximity on their basal aspect to the capillaries, which permits the efficient exchange of gases. In normal healthy individuals, the lower airways are normally sterile, in spite of the fact that the secretions of the upper airways are heavily contaminated with microorganisms seeded from the oral and nasal surfaces.[23,24] Sterility of the lower airway is maintained by intact cough reflexes, the action of the tracheobronchial secretions, mucociliary trans-

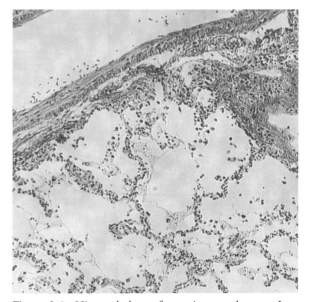

Figure 6–2. Histopathology of panacinar emphysema. Low power view shows distended alveoli, destruction of the alveolar walls, and fibrosis. (Hematoxylin-eosin stain, original magnification × 20)

port of inhaled microorganisms and particulate material from the lower respiratory tract to the oropharynx, and immune and nonimmune defense factors (cell-mediated immunity, humoral immunity, and polymorphonuclear leukocytes).[5,25] Other defense factors contained within the secretions that coat the pulmonary epithelium include surfactant, other proteins such as fibronectin, complement, and immunoglobulins. The lung also contains a rich system of phagocytic cells, which remove microorganisms and particulate debris.

Microorganisms can contaminate the lower airways by four possible routes: aspiration of oropharyngeal contents,[26] inhalation of infectious aerosols,[11] spread of infection from contiguous sites,[27] and hematogenous spread from extrapulmonary sites of infection (eg, translocation from the gastrointestinal tract).[27] Aspiration of the oropharyngeal contents is the commonest route of infection. While claims have been made supporting the stomach as a primary source of nosocomial respiratory pathogens,[28] especially in patients treated with H$_2$-blockers and other antiulcer medications, it is more likely that most pathogens first colonize the surfaces of the oral cavity or pharyngeal mucosa before aspiration.[29] These pathogens can colonize from an exogenous source or can emerge following overgrowth of the normal oral flora after antibiotic treatment. Common respiratory pathogens such as *S. pneumoniae, Streptococcus pyogenes, M. pneumonia,* and *H. influenzae* can colonize the oropharynx and be aspirated into the lower airways. As will be discussed below, other species thought to comprise the normal oral flora, including *Actinobacillus actinomycetemcomitans,* and anaerobes such as *Porphyromonas gingivalis* and *Fusobacterium* spp., can also be aspirated into the lower airways to cause pneumonia. Indeed, studies using careful sampling and strict anaerobic culture conditions have found that a considerable proportion of community-acquired and nosocomial pneumonia may involve anaerobic agents.[26,30] Pneumonia can be the result of a mixed infection, with anaerobes combining with facultative agents such as oral viridans streptococci or enteric rods.[31,32]

Aspiration of oropharyngeal secretions is not uncommon, even in healthy subjects. Studies have demonstrated that 50% of normal adults aspirate oropharyngeal contents during sleep. However, aspiration occurs more frequently in individuals with impaired consciousness, such as alcoholics, drug abusers, and epileptics, and those with chronic swallowing disorders or mechanical interventions such as nasogastric or endotracheal tubes.[26,33]

All these patient groups tend to have a greater incidence of bacterial pneumonia than the population as a whole.[34]

Generally accepted risk factors that predispose to nosocomial pneumonia include the presence of underlying diseases such as chronic lung disease, congestive heart failure, or diabetes mellitus, age > 70 years; mechanical ventilation or intubation, a history of smoking, previous antibiotic treatment, immunosuppression, a long preoperative stay, and/or prolonged surgical procedures.[10–12,28] Other commonly accepted risk factors in mechanically ventilated patients include placement of intracranial pressure monitors, anti–stress ulcer therapy, hospitalization in the fall or winter seasons, and changes of ventilatory circuits every 24 hours.[12,28] In nursing home residents, risk factors for pneumonia include difficulty with oropharyngeal secretions, deteriorating health status, and occurrence of unusual events (confusion, agitation, falls, or wandering).[35]

It is possible that oral disorders such as periodontal disease may also predispose subjects to nosocomial pneumonia. For example, hospitalized patients, especially those admitted to an intensive care unit, are likely to pay less attention to personal hygiene than less ill patients. One important dimension of this personal neglect may be diminished attention to oral hygiene. A lapse in oral hygiene may optimize conditions that contribute to the initiation of pneumonia.

DENTAL CONSIDERATIONS

Oral Bacteria as Etiologic Agents of Respiratory Infection

It is possible that the teeth can serve as a reservoir for respiratory infection. Indeed, the notion that the oral cavity may influence the bacterial flora of the lower bronchi is not new. For example, Potter and colleagues noted in 1968 that infected teeth were present in 25% of 80 patients with potential respiratory pathogens in the bronchi, as against only 7.5% of 80 patients free of pathogens in the bronchi.[36] Oral bacteria can be released from the dental plaque into the salivary secretions, which are then aspirated into the lower respiratory tract to cause pneumonia (Figure 6–3). It has long been known that severe anaerobic lung infections can occur following aspiration of salivary secretions, especially in patients with periodontal disease.[5,25,34,37] Estimates have been made that 30 to 40% of all cases of aspiration pneumonia, necrotizing pneumonia, or lung abscess involve anaerobic bacteria.[38] A variety of oral anaerobes and facultative species have been cultured from infected lung fluids, including *P. gingivalis, Bacteroides gracilus, Bacteroides oralis, Bacteroides buccae, Eikenella corrodens, Fusobacterium nucleatum, Fusobacterium necrophorum, A. actinomycetemcomitans, Peptostreptococcus, Clostridium,* and *Actinomyces.*[38–47] Most, if not all, of these organisms have been implicated as etiologic agents in the pathogenesis of periodontal disease.[48,49] It is also possible that viridans streptococci, thought to be exclusively benign members of the oral flora, may participate in the initiation and/or progression of pneumonia.[32,43,50–52]

Oral bacteria may also have a role in the exacerbations of COPD. For example, oral bacteria can be cultured from a significant proportion of the lung fluids obtained from transtracheal aspiration, a technique that avoids contamination with oropharyngeal secretions. Thus, anaerobic bacteria (presumably from the oral cavity) were cultured from 17% of transtracheal aspirates from patients with COPD.[53] The distal airway of COPD subjects frequently shows bacterial colonization by presumably nonpathogenic oral bacteria, including oral streptococci (Table 6–2).[24] Indeed, *Streptococcus viridans* was found to be the cause of pneumonia in 4% of COPD patients.[54]

Laboratory studies suggest that oral anaerobes such as *P. gingivalis* can cause marked inflammation when instilled into the lungs of laboratory animals.[55] A relationship between the systemic humoral response to *Prevotella* species (bacteria associated with periodontal disease) and ventilator-associated pneumonia in hospitalized patients has also been described. Thus, colonization of patients by *Prevotella* species may be associated with an infectious process leading to ventilator-associated pneumonia and a systemic humoral response.[56]

Dental Plaque as a Reservoir of Respiratory Pathogens

Ill persons probably do not pay close attention to oral hygiene. Several studies have documented that hospitalized individuals tend to have poorer oral hygiene than matched ambulatory, community-dwelling controls.[57–62] Lack of attention to oral hygiene results in an increase in the mass and complexity of dental plaque, which may foster bacterial interactions between indigenous plaque bacteria and acknowledged respiratory pathogens such as *P. aeruginosa* and enteric bacilli.[63] These interactions may result in colonization of the dental plaque by

respiratory pathogens. Dental plaque may therefore provide a reservoir for colonization of respiratory pathogens that can be shed into saliva. Contamination of the distal portions of the respiratory tree by saliva containing such organisms may result in pulmonary infections. It should also be pointed out that respiratory pathogens that establish in dental plaque may be difficult to eradicate. It is well known that bacteria in biofilms are much more resistant to antibiotics than planktonic bacteria.[64]

Previous studies have documented that patients admitted to medical intensive care units (ICU) have poorer oral hygiene than nonhospitalized patients and have a higher prevalence of respiratory pathogen colonization on the teeth and oral mucosa than do age- and gender-matched outpa-

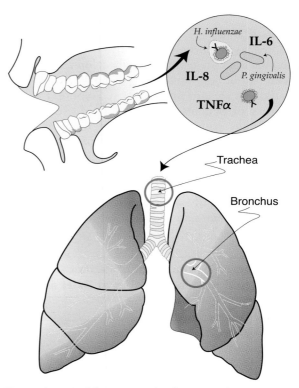

Figure 6–3. Oral bacteria, oral infection, and pneumonia. Bacteria that colonize the supra- or subgingival dental plaque are shed into the saliva. These pathogenic bacteria can be either those associated with periodontal disease (*P. gingivalis, Fusobacterium nucleatum*) or respiratory pathogens (*P. aeruginosa, Klebsiella pneumonia*). The saliva is aspirated into the lower respiratory tract (bronchus), where an infection can ensue. Cytokines from diseased periodontal tissues can enter the saliva from the gingival crevice fluid and also be aspirated to stimulate local inflammatory processes that contribute to the initiation and/or progression of infection in the lung. With permission from Scannapieco FA. Role of oral bacteria in respiratory infection. J Periodontol 1998;70:793–802.

TABLE 6–2. Bacterial Colonization of the Lower Airway Determined by Bronchoscopic Protected Specimen Brush

Subjects	Number of Patients	Percent Colonized	Flora
Healthy	15	12	Viridans streptococci, group D streptococci, S. aureus
Bronchogenic carcinoma	33	39	Viridans streptococci, Neisseria, Staphylococcus, H. influenzae, S. pneumoniae
COPD	18	83	Viridans streptococci, Neisseria, Staphylococcus, Corynebacterium, Candida, Haemophilus, S. pneumoniae, S. aureus
Bronchiectasis	17	82	Viridans streptococci, group D streptococci, Staphylococcus
Long-term tracheostomy	32	38	Viridans streptococci, Corynebacterium, M. catarrhalis, S. aureus

COPD= chronic obstructive pulmonary disease.
With permission from Cabello H, Torres A, Celis R, et al. Bacterial colonization of distal airways in healthy subjects and chronic lung disease: a bronchoscopic study. Eur Resp J 1997;10:1137–44.

tients (Table 6–3).[59,65] In some cases, respiratory pathogens comprise up to 100% of the cultivable aerobic flora. In general, heavily colonized patients tend to be on antibiotic therapy. Respiratory pathogens are also more likely to colonize the oral cavities of patients with teeth or dentures than edentulous patients not wearing dentures. This finding suggests that respiratory pathogen colonization is favored by the presence of nonshedding surfaces and/or the conditioning of mucosal surfaces by dental plaque.

More recently, a prospective study of 57 consecutive patients admitted to medical ICU during a 3-month period assessed the colonization of dental plaque by respiratory pathogens.[61] The amount of dental plaque on the teeth of inpatients increased over time, as did the proportion of respiratory pathogens in their dental plaque. A high concordance was found between respiratory colonization of dental plaque by pathogens and the presence of the same pathogens in tracheal aspirate cultures and between salivary and dental plaque cultures. Clinically, 21 patients developed a nosocomial infection in the ICU. Dental plaque colonization on days 0 and 5 was significantly associated with the occurrence of nosocomial pneumonia and bacteremia. In

TABLE 6–3. Comparison of Patient Characteristics between the Preventive Dentistry Clinic (PDC) and the Medical ICUs at BGH and VAMC

	PDC	BGH	VAMC
Mean age (years)	62.4	63.6	63.8
Gender (male/total numer patients studied)	23/25	12/19	32/34
Mean APACHE II score*	Not done	14.8	17.1
Oral hygiene (mean plaque score)[†]	1.4	1.7	1.9
% positive oral cultures[‡]	16 (4/25)	58 (11/19)[§]	65 (22/34)[§]

BGH = Buffalo General Hospital; VAMC = Veterans Administration Medical Center; ICU = intensive care unit;
APACHE = Acute Physiology, Age, Chronic Health Evaluation; PDC = Preventive Dental Clinic
*APACHE II score was used to semiquantitate the physiologic status of each patient at the time of admission to the medical ICU.[65a] This system evaluates a variety of parameters, including physiologic information (temperature, mean arterial pressure, heart rate, respiratory rate, oxygenation, arterial pH, serum levels of Na, K, and creatinine, hematocrit, white blood count), the patient's age, chronic health status, and cardiovascular, renal, respiratory, and immune status. The higher the score, the more severely ill is the patient.
[†]Plaque score performed as described by Silness and Löe.[65a]
[‡]% of patients having colonization of buccal mucosa and/or dental plaque with a target respiratory pathogen (enteric rod, P. aeruginosa, S. aureus).
[§]The differences observed were found to be significantly different from PDC patients by contingency table analysis.[59,65b]

six cases of nosocomial infection, the pathogen was first isolated from the dental plaque.

Taken together, these results strongly suggest that patients admitted to medical ICUs have a significant risk for oral colonization by respiratory pathogens. Thus, the oral cavity may serve as important nidus of infection for respiratory disease in high-risk subjects, such as hospitalized or COPD patients.

It has been suggested that high-risk patients in nursing home settings are also at risk for lower respiratory tract infection. The possibility therefore exists that, like the hospital intensive care environment, poor oral health may predispose nursing home residents to oral colonization by respiratory pathogens.[66,67] Recently, the prevalence and distribution patterns of suspected respiratory pathogens in the dental plaque of older individuals living in a long-term care facility were studied.[62] Findings from this group were compared with those from a similar number of age-, race-, and gender-matched community-dwelling subjects. Briefly, no differences were noted in the prevalence of colonization by respiratory pathogens between the long-term care facility subjects and dental outpatient subjects; 25% (7 of 28) of long-term care facility subjects were colonized with respiratory pathogens versus 27% (8 of 30) of dental clinic outpatients. However, when only those subjects that were positively colonized were considered (with the respiratory pathogen comprising ≥ 0.1% of the total cultivable flora), there was a statistically significant difference between the prevalence of subjects that were colonized in each group (14% [4 of 28] of the long-term care facility subjects versus 0% [0 of 30] of the dental clinic outpatients). Nursing home subjects harbored more dental plaque than did the dental outpatients (Figure 6–4). Colonized long-term care facility subjects tended to be colonized to a much greater degree than did those dental clinic outpatient subjects (42.88 ± 53.4 versus 0.02 ± 0.04).

In summary, these results suggest that nursing home subjects (who are at greater risk for lower respiratory infection) have a greater tendency for their dental plaque to be colonized by respiratory pathogens. This finding is substantiated by the report of Mojon and colleagues,[68] who found that poor oral hygiene may be a major risk factor for respiratory tract infection in elderly institutionalized individuals.

Oral Status and Chronic Obstructive Pulmonary Disease

To evaluate the relationship between COPD and oral health status, a study was performed and data from the National Health and Nutrition Examination Survey I (HANES I) was analyzed.[69] Of 23,808 individuals, 386 reported a suspected respiratory condition that was further assessed by a physician. These subjects were categorized as having a confirmed chronic respiratory disease (chronic bronchitis or emphysema), acute respiratory disease (influenza, pneumonia, acute bronchitis), or not to have a respiratory disease.

Significant differences were noted between subjects having no disease and those having a chronic respiratory disease confirmed by a physician. Individuals with a confirmed chronic respiratory disease had a significantly greater oral hygiene index (OHI) than had subjects without a respiratory disease. Logistic regression analysis was performed to simultaneously control for multiple variables including gender, age, race, OHI, and smok-

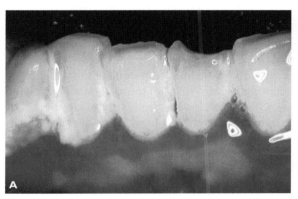 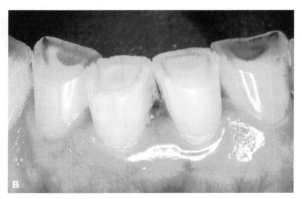

Figure 6–4. Comparison of dental plaque status of community-dwelling and nursing home residents. *A*, Facial aspect of mandibular anterior teeth of a typical community-dwelling elder. *B*, Facial aspect of mandibular anterior teeth of a typical nursing home resident elder (Courtesy of Dr. Stephanie Russell, New York University School of Dentistry).

ing status. The final model included OHI and smoking status alone. The results of this analysis suggest that for patients having the highest OHI values, the odds ratio for chronic respiratory disease was 4.5. These data are supported by the recent study of Hayes and colleagues,[70] who found that periodontal disease, measured as alveolar bone loss from periapical radiographs, was an independent risk factor for COPD in adult males enrolled in the Veterans Administration Normative Aging study.

Potential Mechanisms of Action of Oral Bacteria in the Pathogenesis of Respiratory Infection

Several mechanisms can be envisioned to help explain how oral bacteria can participate in the pathogenesis of respiratory infection: (1) oral pathogens (such as *P. gingivalis, A. actinomycetemcomitans*) may be aspirated into the lung to cause infection; (2) periodontal disease–associated enzymes in saliva may modify mucosal surfaces to promote adhesion and colonization by respiratory pathogens; (3) periodontal disease–associated enzymes may destroy salivary pellicles on pathogenic bacteria; and (4) cytokines originating from periodontal tissues may alter respiratory epithelium to promote infection by respiratory pathogens.

Periodontal Disease–Associated Enzymes in Saliva Modifying Mucosal Surfaces

Previous studies have shown that respiratory pathogens such as *P. aeruginosa* may adhere better to oral epithelial cells obtained from patients colonized by respiratory pathogens than to cells harvested from noncolonized patients.[71,72] Trypsin treatment of epithelial cells from noncolonized patients in vitro resulted in increased adhesion by respiratory pathogens. These data suggest that a mucosal alteration promoted enhanced bacterial adhesion by these bacteria, perhaps the loss of fibronectin from the epithelial cell surface.[73] Buccal epithelial cells from critically ill patients, all colonized by *P. aeruginosa,* interacted with greater numbers of bacterial cells in vitro and possessed lesser amounts of surface fibronectin as determined by immunofluorescence. The removal of fibronectin (by exposure to proteases) may unmask mucosal surface receptors for respiratory pathogen adhesins. Other investigators have also pointed out an inverse relationship between the amount of mucosal epithelial cell fibronectin and gram-negative bacilli binding to these cells.[74]

Saliva contains many hydrolytic enzymes, and the amount of enzyme activity in saliva is related to the periodontal and oral hygiene status of the subjects tested.[75–77] For example, a direct relationship has been found between the ability of saliva to degrade fibronectin and oral hygiene status.[77] Subjects practicing meticulous oral hygiene (dental hygiene students) have very low levels of salivary fibronectin degrading enzymes. In contrast, saliva samples collected from laboratory workers having less than ideal oral hygiene had higher amounts of enzyme activity, and saliva collected on awakening in the latter group had even higher levels. The source of these enzymes has been attributed to bacteria[75,76,78–80] or polymorphonuclear leukocytes, which enter the saliva from the gingival sulcus.[81] It is conceivable that in subjects with periodontal disease that harbor dental plaque with elevated levels of bacteria such as *P. gingivalis* and spirochetes (bacteria known to be prolific producers of proteases), protease activity may alter the mucosal epithelium in such a way as to increase the adhesion and colonization by respiratory pathogens (Figure 6–5A). Such bacteria may also produce other enzymes such as mannosidase, fucosidase, hexosaminidase, and sialidase, known to be elevated in the saliva of such patients.[82,83] Exposure of the epithelium and glycoproteins to such enzymes may increase the adhesion of gram-negative bacteria to the mucosal surface by exposing the "buried" adhesin receptors on the mucosal epithelium,[84] which may foster increased adhesion and colonization by respiratory pathogens.

Destruction of Protective Salivary Pellicles by Oral Bacteria

Recent evidence suggests that the respiratory pathogen *H. influenzae* binds to mucins contained within the mucosal secretions.[85–87] This binding may involve sialic acid residues.[85,88] In the context of COPD, it is possible that subjects with poor oral hygiene may have elevated levels of hydrolytic enzymes (eg, sialidase) in their saliva. These enzymes may process mucins to reduce their ability to bind to and clear pathogens such as *H. influenzae* (Figure 6–5B). Conversely, the enzymes may process the respiratory epithelium to modulate the adhesion of such pathogens to the mucosal surface (Figure 6–5C). Indeed, several studies have suggested that certain oral bacteria can break down a variety of salivary components.[89,90] Thus, poor oral hygiene results in increased dental plaque load and salivary hydrolytic enzyme levels. These enzymes may then destroy the protective domains of the host secretory components (eg, mucins), thus diminishing nonspecific host defense against respiratory pathogens in high-risk subjects.

Cytokines That May Alter Respiratory Epithelium

Periodontal disease (periodontitis) is a localized chronic inflammatory disease caused by bacterial infection of the periodontal tissues by bacteria in dental plaque, resulting in the destruction of the supporting bone and connective tissues. In untreated periodontal disease, oral pathogens continuously stimulate the cells of the periodontium (epithelial cells, endothelial cells, fibroblasts, macrophages, white cells) to release a wide variety of cytokines and other biologically active molecules.[91,92] Cytokines produced by epithelial and connective tissue cells in response to these bacteria including interleukin (IL)-1α, IL-1β, IL-6, IL-8, and TNF-α.[92] Oral bacteria can also stimulate the peripheral mononuclear cells to release cytokines (IL-1α and TNF-α). In fact, oral streptococci (for example, *Streptococcus sanguis*), which are abundant in dental plaque, stimulate the release of high levels of these cytokines from such cells.[93] Epithelial cells are also known to alter the expression of the adhesion molecules on the surface of various cells in response to cytokine stimulation. Variation in the expression of such adhesion molecules may alter the interaction of the bacterial pathogens with the mucosal surface.[94]

One mechanism proposed for the gross airway epithelial damage observed in COPD involves release of proinflammatory cytokines (ie, IL-8) from the respiratory epithelium, resulting in the recruitment and infiltration of neutrophils and the subsequent release of proteolytic enzymes and toxic oxygen radicals from the neutrophils.[95,96]. The mechanism of release of cytokines from the respiratory epithelium may be the result of the binding of respiratory pathogens (eg, *H. influenzae*) or their products to the respiratory epithelial cells, followed by stimulation of the respiratory epithelial cells to produce a variety of cytokines. This mechanism has been demonstrated for medical pathogens such as *S. pneumoniae* and *H. influenzae*, which are also known to attach to mucosal receptors and to stimulate cytokine production by the underlying cells.[97] It is also conceivable that the oral bacteria in secretions come in contact with the respiratory epithelial surfaces and may adhere to the mucosal surface. Oral bacteria are routinely cultivated, for example, from

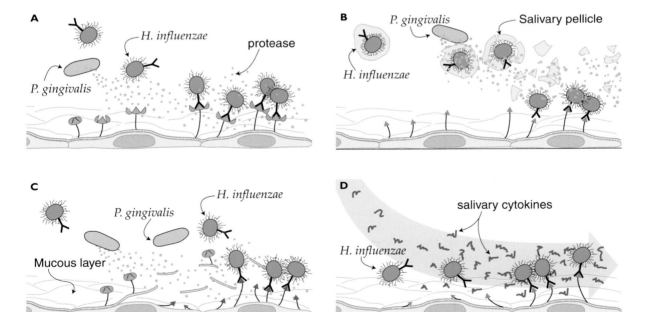

Figure 6–5. *A,* Dental pathogens such as *P. gingivalis* produce enzymes (such as proteases) that alter mucosal surface adhesion receptors for respiratory pathogens such as *H. influenzae*, which adhere, colonize, and can subsequently be aspirated into the lung to cause infection. *B,* Oral bacteria such as *P. gingivalis* produce enzymes that degrade the salivary molecules that normally form a pellicle on the pathogens, which prevents the pathogens from adhering to mucosal surfaces. *C,* Oral bacteria produce enzymes that degrade the salivary pellicle on the mucosal surface, thereby exposing adhesion receptors for respiratory pathogens. *D,* Cytokines from the saliva, from inflamed periodontal tissues, upregulate the expression of adhesion receptors on the mucosal surfaces to promote respiratory pathogen colonization. With permission from Scannapieco FA. Role of oral bacteria in respiratory infection. J Periodontol 1998;70:793–802.

tonsillar epithelium.[98] These bound oral bacteria may stimulate cytokine production by mucosal epithelium. It is also possible that cytokines originating from the oral tissues (for example, from the gingival crevicular fluids[99–101]), which exit the gingival sulcus to be mixed with whole saliva, may contaminate the distal respiratory epithelium to stimulate the respiratory epithelial cells. These stimulated respiratory cells may then release other cytokines that recruit inflammatory cells (eg, neutrophils) to the site. These inflammatory cells may release hydrolytic enzymes and other modifying molecules, resulting in damaged epithelium that may be more susceptible to colonization by respiratory pathogens.

Oral bacteria may influence the expression and effects of cytokines in more novel ways. Darveau and colleagues[102] have shown that IL-8 is secreted by gingival epithelial cells in response to components of the normal oral flora. In contrast, *P. gingivalis* strongly inhibits IL-8 accumulation from the gingival epithelial cells. Inhibition was shown to be associated with a decrease in mRNA for IL-8. Antagonism of IL-8 accumulation did not occur in KB cells, an epithelial cell line that does not support high levels of intracellular invasion by *P. gingivalis*. Furthermore, a noninvasive mutant of *P. gingivalis* was unable to antagonize IL-8 accumulation. They concluded that invasion-dependent destruction of the gingival IL-8 chemokine gradient at sites of *P. gingivalis* colonization may impair mucosal defense. It is not yet known if *P. gingivalis* would have a similar effect on the respiratory epithelium. Such an effect might result in perturbation of local cytokine networks and thus promote a destructive inflammatory lesion within the lung.

Prevention of Oral Colonization by Potential Respiratory Pathogens

Few studies have evaluated the role of poor oral hygiene and/or periodontal disease in the development of pneumonia in high-risk patients (for example, those that are mechanically ventilated). Several reports have documented a strong association between periodontal disease and an increased frequency of oral infections in nursing home residents.[57,103] However, there are no studies that have identified an association between poor oral hygiene and the increased incidence of pneumonia in such subjects. A possible link between poor oral hygiene and the increased incidence of pneumonia in nursing home residents has been suggested but no supporting evidence was provided.[65] Recently, Terpenning and colleagues, in a preliminary report

of a longitudinal study of medical and dental conditions in nursing home residents, observed an association between the development of aspiration pneumonia and dental status.[104] Among 26 dentate nursing home residents followed up for 1 year, 5 (19.8%) developed pneumonia compared with 2 (7.6%) of 26 edentulous nursing home residents.

Because of the key role that oropharyngeal bacterial colonization plays in the pathogenesis of bacterial pneumonia, several methods have been proposed to reduce or eliminate colonization in susceptible patients, such as those on mechanical ventilation. We hypothesize that improved oral hygiene in the hospital setting may decrease the occurrence of oropharyngeal colonization by respiratory pathogens and thus decrease the risk of nosocomial pneumonia. Current oral hygiene measures recommended by nursing educators are probably inadequate to prevent dental plaque formation.[105] One method, called selective digestive decontamination (SDD), uses antibiotics topically applied to the surfaces of the gastrointestinal tract (including the oral cavity) to reduce the carriage of pathogenic bacteria and thus to prevent respiratory infection.[106–108] For example, the use of lozenges containing polymyxin B, tobramycin, and amphotericin B have been shown to diminish oral colonization by gram-negative bacilli.[109] The study by Pugin and colleagues[110] has particular relevance because it focused on the elimination of oropharyngeal colonization by pathogens and the subsequent development of pneumonia. These investigators used topical oropharyngeal antibiotics (versus topical placebo) in mechanically ventilated patients. Oropharyngeal colonization by aerobic gram-negative bacilli and *S. aureus* and also pneumonia rates were significantly reduced in the treated population versus the placebo group (16% versus 78%; $p < .0001$). These findings suggest that focusing specifically on factors promoting oropharyngeal bacterial colonization may be useful in developing other strategies to prevent colonization and thereby prevent bacterial pneumonia in susceptible populations. However, while diminishing the colonization rate of pathogenic bacteria in the hospital setting, SDD does not appear to have an effect on the mortality rate[111] and seems to foster the selection of antibiotic-resistant bacteria and cross-infection.[112,113] These findings have raised doubts about the widespread use of SDD. Other approaches to reduce colonization of these pathogens certainly deserve more study.

Maintenance of good oral hygiene may, by itself, reduce oropharyngeal colonization by respiratory pathogens. Methods of maintaining good oral hygiene in mechanically ventilated patients, if as effective as SDD in reducing pneumonia occurrence, may be much less expensive than SDD regimens, may lessen the risk of emergence of antibiotic resistance among bacteria indigenous to the intensive care unit, and may lessen antibiotic use. The overall effect may be a reduction in the cost of intensive care. Similarly, if providing and maintaining good oral hygiene in nursing home residents is effective in reducing pneumonia rates, significant benefits to this high-risk population would include reduced morbidity and mortality related to pneumonia occurrence, reduced medical care costs because hospital admissions will be reduced, and an enhanced sense of well being.[58]

Although antiseptics with demonstrable ability to disinfect the oral environment are available,[114,115] little research has been done concerning the efficacy of these agents to inhibit oral respiratory pathogen colonization in institutionalized patients. Chlorhexidine appears to be a reasonable choice for this as it has been shown to reduce plaque and salivary levels of bacteria by up to 85%.[116] Interestingly, chlorhexidine gluconate has been shown to reduce transfer of group B streptococci from mother to infant during parturition.[117] An analogous method used in the mouth may inhibit oral colonization by respiratory pathogens, with minimal risk. Chlorhexidine has had widespread use in dentistry to inhibit dental plaque formation,[114] gingivitis,[118] and oral mucosal ulcerations.[119] This agent also appears to inhibit the production of proteases by subgingival bacteria.[120] By inhibiting protease activity, chlorhexidine may diminish the potential of these enzymes to process oral surfaces to expose "cryptitopes" that may act as receptors for bacterial adhesins.[84]

An interesting report by DeRiso and colleagues[121] suggests that a 0.12% chlorhexidine gluconate oral rinse reduced the overall nosocomial infection rate by 65% in 353 patients admitted to a cardiovascular ICU, and the incidence of total respiratory tract infections by 69%. These investigators also noted a 43% reduction in the use of nonprophylactic antibiotics in chlorhexidine-treated patients. Finally, overall mortality was reduced to 1.16% in the chlorhexidine-treated group versus 5.56% in the placebo group.

A variety of recommendations have been made to reduce the incidence of nosocomial pneumonia.[12] Fastidious infection control remains the cornerstone of prevention. Surveillance of potential pathogens, identification of high-risk patients, staff education, hand washing, and the proper use of gloves and gowns, all have a positive impact on reducing nosocomial pneumonia. Additional attention paid to oral hygiene may even further reduce the risk of nosocomial pneumonia. Unfortunately, little information is available concerning the effect of improved oral hygiene on infection rates in the hospital or nursing home setting. It would, therefore, seem reasonable to perform appropriate studies to evaluate the effect of improved oral hygiene on respiratory pathogen colonization in high-risk subjects.

REFERENCES

1. Harvard School of Public Health B, Massachusetts, US. Mortality by cause for eight regions of the world: global burden of disease study. Lancet 1997;349:1269–76.
2. Petty TL, Weinmann GG. Building a national strategy for the prevention and management of and research in chronic obstructive pulmonary disease. JAMA 1997;277:246–53.
3. Garibaldi RA, Brodine S, Matsumiya S. Infections among patients in nursing homes: policies, prevalence and problems. N Engl J Med 1981; 305:731–5.
4. Bentley DW. Bacterial pneumonia in the elderly: clinical features, diagnosis, etiology, and treatment. Gerontologist 1984;30:297–307.
5. Donowitz GR, Mandell GL. Acute pneumonia. In: Mandell GL, Douglas RG, Bennett JE, editors. Principles and practice of infectious diseases. New York: Churchill Liningstone; 1990.
6. Levy SB. The challenge of antibiotic resistance. Sci Am 1998;278:46–53.
7. Østergaard L, Andersen PL. Etiology of community-acquired pneumonia. Evaluation by transtracheal aspiration, blood culture, or serology. Chest 1993;104:1400–7.
8. Rosenthal S, Tager IB. Prevalence of gram-negative rods in the normal pharyngeal flora. Ann Intern Med 1975;83:355–7.
9. Bartlett JG, O'Keefe P, Tally FP, et al. Bacteriology of hospital-acquired pneumonia. Arch Intern Med 1986;146:868–71.
10. Cunha BA. Hospital-acquired pneumonias, clinical diagnosis and treatment. Hosp Phys 1986;22: 12–7.
11. Toews GB. Nosocomial pneumonia. Am J Med Sci 1986;291:355–67.
12. Craven DE, Steger KE, Barber TW. Preventing nosocomial pneumonia: state of the art and perspectives for the 1990s. Am J Med 1991;91:44S–53S.

13. Wenzel RP. Epidemiology of hospital-acquired infection. In: Balows A, Hausler WJ, Herrmann KI, et al, editors. Manual of clinical microbiology. Washington, D.C.: American Society for Microbiology; 1991. p. 147–50.

14. Boyce JM, Potter-Bynoe G, Dziobek L, Solomon SL. Nosocomial pneumonia in Medicare patients. Hospital costs and reimbursement patterns under the prospective payment system. Arch Intern Med 1991;151:1109–14.

15. Wenzel RP. Hospital-acquired pneumonia: overview of the current state of the art prevention and control. Eur J Clin Microbiol Infect Dis 1989;8:56–60.

16. McDonald AM, Dietsche L, Litsche M, et al. A retrospective study of nosocomial pneumonia at a long-term care facility. Am J Infect Cont 1992; 20:234–8.

17. Ingram RH. Chronic bronchitis, emphysema, and airways obstruction. In: Isselbacher KJ, Braunwald E, Wilson JD, et al, editors. Harrison's Principles of internal medicine. New York: McGraw-Hill; 1994. p. 1197–206.

18. Society AT. Standards for the diagnosis and care of patients with chronic obstructive pulmonary disease. Am J Respir Crit Care Med 1995;152: S77–121.

19. Renwick DS, Connolly MJ. Prevalence and treatment of chronic airways obstruction in adults over the age of 45. Thorax 1996;51:164–8.

20. Sandford AJ, Weir TD, Pare PD. Genetic risk factors for chronic obstructive pulmonary disease. Eur Resp J 1997;10:1380–91.

21. Murphy TF, Sethi S. Bacterial infection in chronic obstructive pulmonary disease. Am Rev Respir Dis 1992;146:1067–83.

22. Fagon JY, Chastre J. Severe exacerbations of COPD patients: the role of pulmonary infections. Semin Respir Infect 1996;11:109–18.

23. Laurenzi GA, Potter RT, Hass EH. Bacteriologic flora of the lower respiratory tract. N Engl J Med 1961;265:1273–8.

24. Cabello H, Torres A, Celis R, et al. Bacterial colonization of distal airways in healthy subjects and chronic lung disease: a bronchoscopic study. Eur Respir J 1997;10:1137–44.

25. Levison ME. Pneumonia, including necrotizing pulmonary infections (lung abscess). In: Isselbacher KJ, Braunwald E, Wilson JD, et al, editors. Harrison's Principles of internal medicine. New York: McGraw-Hill; 1994. p. 1184–91.

26. Megran DW, Chow AW. Bacterial aspiration and anaerobic pleuropulmonary infections. In: Sande MA, Hudson LD, Root RK, editors. Respiratory infections. New York: Churchill Livingstone; 1986. p. 269–92.

27. Fiddian-Green R, Baker S. Nosocomial pneumonia in the critical ill: product of aspiration or translocation? Crit Care Med 1991;19:793–9.

28. Sinclair DG, Evans TW. Nosocomial pneumonia in the intensive care unit. Br J Hosp Med 1994; 51:177–80.

29. Bonten MJM, Gaillard CA, Tiel FHV, et al. The stomach is not a source for colonization of the upper respiratory tract and pneumonia in ICU patients. Chest 1994;105:878–84.

30. Bartlett JG, Finegold SM. Anaerobic infections of the lung and pleural space. Am Rev Respir Dis 1974;110:56–77.

31. Bartlett JG. Anaerobic bacterial infections of the lung. Chest 1987;91:901–9.

32. Shinzato T, Saito A. A mechanism of pathogenicity of "*Streptococcus milleri* group" in pulmonary infection: synergy with an anaerobe. J Med Microbiol 1994;40:118–23.

33. Elpern EH, Scott MG, Petro L, Ries MH. Pulmonary aspiration in mechanically ventilated patients with tracheostomies. Chest 1994;105: 563–6.

34. Finegold SM. Aspiration pneumonia. Rev Infect Dis 1991;13:S737–42.

35. Harkness GA, Bentley DW, Roghman KJ. Risk factors for nosocomial pneumonia in the elderly. Am J Med 1990;89:457–63.

36. Potter RT, Rotman F, Fernandez F, et al. The bacteriology of the lower respiratory tract. Bronchoscopic study of 100 clinical cases. Am Rev Respir Dis 1968;97:1051–61.

37. Schreiner A. Anaerobic pulmonary infections. Scand J Infect Dis 1979;19 Suppl:77–9.

38. Brook I, Frazier EH. Aerobic and anaerobic microbiology of empyema. A retrospective review in two military hospitals. Chest 1993;103:1502–7.

39. Goldstein EJ, Kirby BD, Finegold SM. Isolation of *Eikenella corrodens* from pulmonary infections. Am Rev Respir Dis 1979;119:55–8.

40. Suwanagool S, Rothkopf MM, Smith SM, et al. Pathogenicity of *Eikenella corrodens* in humans. Arch Intern Med 1983;143:2265–68.

41. Joshi N, O'Bryan T, Appelbaum PC. Pleuropulmonary infections caused by *Eikenella corrodens*. Rev Infect Dis 1991;13:1207–12.

42. Zijlstra EE, Swart GR, Godfroy FJM, Degener JE. Pericarditis, pneumonia and brain abscess due to a combined *Actinomyces-Actinobacillus actinomycetemcomitans* infection. J Infect 1992;25: 83–7.

43. Mahomed AG, Feldman C, Smith C, et al. Does

primary *Streptococcus viridans* pneumonia exist? S Afr Med J 1992;82:432–4.

44. Lorenz KA, Weiss PJ. Capnocytophageal pneumonia in a healthy man. West J Med 1994;160:79–80.

45. Morris JF, Sewell DL. Necrotizing pneumonia caused by mixed infection with *Actinobacillus actinomycetemcomitans* and *Actinomyces israelii*: Case report and review. Clin Infect Dis 1994;18:450–2.

46. Yuan A, Luh KT, Yang PC. *Actinobacillus actinomycetemcomitans* pneumonia with possible septic embolization [letter]. Chest 1994;105:646.

47. Chen AC, Liu CC, Yao WJ, et al. *Actinobacillus actinomycetemcomitans* pneumonia with chest wall and subphrenic abscess. Scand J Infect Dis 1995;27:289–90.

48. Moore WEC, Moore LVH. The bacteria of periodontal disease. Periodontol 2000 1994;5:66–77.

49. Slots J, Rams TE. Microbiology of periodontal disease. In: Slots J, Taubman MA, editors. Contemporary oral microbiology and immunology. St. Louis, MO: Mosby-Year Book Inc.; 1992. p. 425–43.

50. Appelbaum PC, Cameron EW, Hutton WS, et al. The bacteriology of chronic destructive pneumonia. S Afr Med J 1978;53:541–2.

51. Pratter MR, Irwin RS. Viridans streptococcal pulmonary parenchymal infections. JAMA 1980;243:2515–7.

52. Marrie TJ. Bacteremic community-acquired pneumonia due to viridans group streptococci. Clin Invest Med 1993;16:38–44.

53. Haas H, Morris JF, Samson S, et al. Bacterial flora of the respiratory tract in chronic bronchitis: comparison of transtracheal, fiberbronchoscopic, and oropharyngeal sampling methods. Am Rev Respir Dis 1977;116:41–7.

54. Torres A, Dorca J, Zalacain R, et al. Community-acquired pneumonia in chronic obstructive pulmonary disease: a Spanish multicenter study. Am J Respir Crit Care Med 1996;154:1456–61.

55. Nelson S, Laughon BE, Summer WR, et al. Characterization of the pulmonary inflammatory response to an anaerobic bacterial challenge. Am Rev Respir Dis 1986;133:212–7.

56. Grollier G, Dore P, Robert R, et al. Antibody response to *Prevotella* spp. in patients with ventilator-associated pneumonia. Clin Diag Lab Immunol 1996;3:61–5.

57. Bagramian RA, Heller RP. Dental health assessment of a population of nursing home residents. J Gerontol 1977;32:168–74.

58. Karuza J, Miller WA, Lieberman D, et al. Oral status and resident well-being in a skilled nursing facility population. Gerontologist 1992;32:104–12.

59. Scannapieco FA, Stewart EM, Mylotte JM. Colonization of dental plaque by respiratory pathogens in medical intensive care patients. Crit Care Med 1992;20:740–5.

60. Kiyak HA, Grayston MN, Crinean CL. Oral health problems and needs of nursing home residents. Comm Dent Oral Epidemiol 1993;21:49–52.

61. Fourrier F, Duvivier B, Boutigny H, et al. Colonization of dental plaque: a source of nosocomial infections in intensive care unit patients. Crit Care Med 1998;26:301–8.

62. Russell SL, Boylan RJ, Kaslick R, et al. Respiratory pathogen colonization of the dental plaque of institutionalized elders. Spec Care Dent 1999;19:1–7.

63. Komiyama K, Tynan JJ, Habbick BF, et al. *Pseudomonas aeruginosa* in the oral cavity and sputum of patients with cystic fibrosis. Oral Surg Oral Med Oral Pathol 1985;59:590–4.

64. Costerton JW, Lewandowski Z, Caldwell DE, et al. Microbial biofilms. Ann Rev Microbiol 1995;49:711–45.

65. Scannapieco FA, Mylotte JM. Relationships between periodontal disease and bacterial pneumonia. J Periodontol 1996;67:1114–22.

65a. Silness J, Löe H. Periodontal disease in pregnancy. II. Correlation between oral hygiene and periodontal condition. Acta Odontol Scand 1964;24:747–59.

65b. Knaus WA, Draper EA, Wagner DP, Zimmerman JE. APACHE II: a severity of disease classification system. Crit Care Med 1985;13:818–29.

66. Limeback H. The relationship between oral health and systemic infections among elderly residents of chronic care facilities: a review. Gerodontologist 1988;7:131–7.

67. Limeback H. Implications of oral infections on systemic diseases in the institutionalized elderly with a special focus on pneumonia. Ann Periodontol 1998;3:262–75.

68. Mojon P, Budtz-Jørgensen E, Michel JP, Limeback H. Oral health and history of respiratory tract infection in frail institutionalised elders. Gerodontologist 1997;14:9–16.

69. Scannapieco FA, Papandonatos GD, Dunford RG. Associations between oral conditions and respiratory disease in a national sample survey population. Ann Periodontol 1998;3:251–6.

70. Hayes C, Sparrow D, Cohen M, et al. Periodontal

disease and pulmonary function: the VA longitudinal study. Ann Periodontol 1998; 257–61.

71. Johanson WG, Pierce AK, Sanford AK, Thomas JP. Nosocomial respiratory infections with gram-negative bacilli: the significance of colonization of the respiratory tract. Ann Intern Med 1972; 77:701–6.

72. Johanson WG, Higuchi JH, Chaudhuri TR, Woods DE. Bacterial adherence to epithelial cells in bacillary colonization of the respiratory tract. Am Rev Respir Dis 1980;121:55–63.

73. Woods DE, Straus DC, Johanson WG, Bass JA. Role of fibronectin in the prevention of adherence of *Pseudomonas aeruginosa* to buccal cells. J Infect Dis 1981;143:784–90.

74. Abraham SN, Beachey EH, Simpson WA. Adherence of *Streptococcus pyogenes*, *Escherichia coli* and *Pseudomonas aeruginosa* to fibronectin-coated and uncoated epithelial cells. Infect Immun 1983;41:1261–8.

75. Nakamura M, Slots J. Salivary enzymes. Origin and relationship to periodontal disease. J Periodontal Res 1983;18:559–69.

76. Zambon JJ, Nakamura M, Slots J. Effect of periodontal therapy on salivary enzyme activity. J Periodontal Res 1985;20:652–9.

77. Gibbons RJ, Etherden I. Fibronectin-degrading enzymes in saliva and their relation to oral cleanliness. J Periodontal Res 1986;21:386–95.

78. Loesche WJ, Syed SA, Stoll J. Trypsin-like activity in subgingival plaque. A diagnostic marker for spirochetes and periodontal disease. J Periodontol 1987;58:266–73.

79. Wikstrom M, Linde A. Ability of oral bacteria to degrade fibronectin. Infect Immun 1986;51:707–11.

80. Frandsen EG, Reinholdt J, Kilian M. Enzymatic and antigenic characterization of immunoglobulin A1 proteases from *Bacteroides* and *Capnocytophaga* spp. Infect Immun 1987;55:631–8.

81. Cimasoni G, Ishikawa I, Jacccard F. Enzyme activity in the gingival crevice. In: Lehner T, editor. Borderland between caries and periodontal disease. London: Academic Press; 1977. p. 13–41.

82. Quinn MO, Miller VE, Dal Nogare AR. Increased salivary exoglycosidase activity during critical illness. Am J Respir Crit Care Med 1994;150:179–83.

83. Weinmeister KD, Dal Nogare AR. Buccal cell carbohydrates are altered during critical illness. Am J Respir Crit Care Med 1994;150:131–4.

84. Gibbons RJ, Hay DI, Childs WC, Davis G. Role of cryptic receptors (cryptitopes) in bacterial adhesion to oral surfaces. Arch Oral Biol 1990;35:107S–114S.

85. Reddy MS, Murphy TF, Faden HS, Bernstein JM. Middle ear mucin glycoprotein: purification and interaction with nontypable *Haemophilus influenzae* and *Moraxella catarrhalis*. Otolaryngol Head Neck Surg 1997;116:175–80.

86. Davies J, Carlstedt I, Nilsson AK, et al. Binding of *Haemophilus influenzae* to purified mucins from the human respiratory tract. Infect Immun 1995;63:2485–92.

87. Barsum W, Wilson R, Read RC, et al. Interaction of fimbriated and nonfimbriated strains of unencapsulated *Haemophilus influenzae* with human respiratory tract mucus in vitro. Eur Respir J 1995;8:709–14.

88. Fakih MG, Murphy TF, Pattoli MA, Berenson CS. Specific binding of *Haemophilus influenzae* to minor gangliosides of human respiratory epithelial cells. Infect Immun 1997;65:1695–700.

89. van der Hoeven JS, van den Kieboom CW, Camp PJM. Utilization of mucin by oral *Streptococcus* species. Antonie van Leeuwenhoek 1990;57:165–72.

90. Scannapieco FA. Saliva-bacterium interactions in oral microbial ecology. Crit Rev Oral Biol Med 1994;5:203–48.

91. Reddi K, Wilson M, Nair S, et al. Comparison of the pro-inflammatory cytokine-stimulating activity of the surface-associated proteins of periodontopathic bacteria. J Periodontal Res 1996;31:120–30.

92. Wilson M, Reddi K, Henderson B. Cytokine-inducing components of periodontopathogenic bacteria. J Periodontal Res 1996; 31:393–407.

93. Kjeldsen M, Holmstrup P, Lindemann RA, Bendtzen K. Bacterial-stimulated cytokine production of peripheral mononuclear cells from patients of various periodontitis categories. J Periodontol 1995;66:139–44.

94. Svanborg C, Hedlund M, Connell H, et al. Bacterial adherence and mucosal cytokine responses. Receptors and transmembrane signaling. Ann N Y Acad Sci 1996;797:177–90.

95. Khair OA, Davies RJ, Devalia JL. Bacterial-induced release of inflammatory mediators by bronchial epithelial cells. Eur Respir J 1996;9:1913–22.

96. Durum SK, Oppenheim J. Proinflammatory cytokines and immunity. In: Paul WE, editor. Fundamental immunology. New York, NY: Raven Press Ltd.; 1993.

97. Håkansson A, Carlstedt I, Davies J, et al. Aspects on the interactions of *Streptococcus pneumoniae* and *Haemophilus influenzae* with human respiratory tract mucosa. Am J Respir Crit Care Med 1996;154:S187–91.

98. Brook I, Yocum P, Foote PAJ. Changes in the core tonsillar bacteriology of recurrent tonsillitis: 1977–1993. Clin Infect Dis 1995;21:171–6.

99. Rossomando EF, White L. A novel method for the detection of TNF-alpha in gingival crevicular fluid. J Periodontol 1993;64:445–9.

100. Tatakis DN. Interleukin-1 and bone metabolism: a review. J Periodontol 1993;64:416–31.

101. Birkedal-Hansen H. Role of cytokines and inflammatory mediators in tissue destruction. J Periodontal Res 1993;28:500–10.

102. Darveau RP, Belton CM, Reife RA, Lamont RJ. Local chemokine paralysis, a novel pathogenic mechanism for *Porphyromonas gingivalis*. Infect Immun 1998;66:1660–5.

103. Viglid M. Oral hygiene and periodontal conditions among 201 dentate institutionalized elderly. Gerodontologist. 1988;4:140–5.

104. Terpenning M, Bretz W, Lopatin D, et al. Bacterial colonization of saliva and plaque in the elderly. Clin Infect Dis 1993;16 Suppl:314–6.

105. Luckman J, Sorensen KC. Medical-surgical nursing. Philadelphia, PA: W.B. Saunders Co.; 1987.

106. Kerver AJH, Rommes JH, Mevissen-Verhage EAE, et al. Prevention of colonization and infection in critically ill patients: a prospective randomized study. Crit Care Med 1988;16:1087–93.

107. Nord CE, Heindahl A. Impact of orally administered antimicrobial agents on human oropharyngeal and colonic microflora. J Antimicrob Ther 1986;18 Suppl C:159–64.

108. Stoutenbeek CP, Hendrik HKF, Miranda DR, et al. The effect of oropharyngeal decontamination using topical nonabsorbable antibiotics on the incidence of nosocomial respiratory tract infections in multiple trauma patients. J Trauma 1987;27:357–64.

109. Spijkervet FKL, Saene HKFV, Saene JJMV, et al. Effect of selective elimination of the oral flora on mucositis in irradiated head and neck cancer patients. J Surg Oncol 1991;46:167–73.

110. Pugin J, Auckenthaler R, Lew DP, Suter PM. Oropharyngeal decontamination decreases incidence of ventilator-associated pneumonia. A randomized, placebo-controlled, double-blind clinical trial. JAMA 1991;265:2704–10.

111. Gastinne H, Wolff M, Delatour F, et al. A controlled trial in intensive care units of selective decontamination of the digestive tract with nonabsorbable antibiotics. N Engl J Med 1992;326:594–9.

112. Johanson WG, Seidenfeld JJ, de los Santos R, et al. Prevention of nosocomial pneumonia using topical and parenteral antimicrobial agents. Am Rev Respir Dis 1988;137:265–72.

113. Hurley JC. Prophylaxis with enteral antibiotics in ventilated patients: selective decontamination or selective cross-infection? Antimicrob Agents Chemother 1995;39:941–7.

114. Tonelli PM, Hume WR, Kenney EB. Chlorhexidine: a review of the literature. J West Soc Periodontol 1983;31:5–30.

115. Exner M, Gregori G, Pau HW, Vogel F. In vivo studies on the microbicidal activity of antiseptics on the flora of the oropharyngeal cavity. J Hosp Infect 1985;6 Suppl:185–8.

116. Balbuena L, Stambaugh KI, Ramirez SG, Yeager C. Effects of topical oral antiseptic rinses on bacterial counts of saliva in healthy human subjects. Otolaryngol Head Neck Surg 1998;118:625–9.

117. Nilsson G, Larsson L, Christensen K, et al. Chlorhexidine for prevention of neonatal colonization with group B streptococci. V. Chlorhexidine concentrations in blood following vaginal washing during delivery. Eur J Obstet Gynec Reprod Biol 1989;31:221–6.

118. Lang NP, Brecx MC. Chlorhexidine gluconate—an agent for chemical plaque control and prevention of gingival inflammation. J Periodontal Res 1986;21 Suppl 16:74–89.

119. Ferretti GA, Ash RC, Brown AT, et al. Control of oral mucositis and candidiasis in marrow transplantation: a prospective double blind trial of chlorhexidine. Bone Marrow Transplant 1988;3:483–94.

120. Radford JR, Homer KA, Naylor MN, Beighton D. Inhibition of human subgingival plaque protease activity by chlorhexidine. Arch Oral Biol 1992;37:245–8.

121. DeRiso AJN, Ladowski JS, Dillon TA, et al. Chlorhexidine gluconate 0.12% oral rinse reduces the incidence of total nosocomial respiratory infection and nonprophylactic systemic antibiotic use in patients undergoing heart surgery. Chest 1996;109:1556–61.

CHAPTER 7

TOBACCO USE AND INTERVENTION

Robert E. Mecklenburg, DDS, MPH
Sara G. Grossi, DDS, MS

The good news is that three-quarters of the adult population in the United States do not use tobacco. Smoking decreased in the general population from 42% in 1965 to 25% by 1995.[1] Among adults aged 18 to 24 years, tobacco use was approximately half as high in 1991 (23%) as in 1965 (46%).[2] Among high school seniors, the prevalence of daily smoking decreased from 29% in 1976 to 17% in 1992.[3] Public awareness of the risks associated with tobacco use is increasing, and some public policy ground has been gained, such as the enactment of several community, state, and federal clean-air laws.

The bad news is that trends in tobacco use reversed during the 1990s.[3] Large, protracted tobacco industry advertising and promotion campaigns influenced the susceptible adolescent population. Youth use of tobacco increased year by year after 1991 to 43% of U.S. high school students using cigarettes, smokeless tobacco, or cigars in 1997, which is a 32% increase. By 1997, this trend led to a new increase in tobacco use among adults aged 18 to 24 years.[3a] Some cigarette smokers switched to or started using smokeless/spit tobacco and/or cigars, and some never-smokers began using smokeless/spit tobacco and/or cigars only. A common mistaken belief is that a reduced risk is equivalent to a negligible risk.[3b,3c] Also, few youths appreciate the addictive properties of nicotine inherent in the use of any tobacco product, non adults perceive the extent of their tobacco-related health risks.[3]

Cigarette smoking is the single most important and modifiable factor responsible for cases of lung cancer, hypertension, and cardiovascular diseases in the western world. Malignant and premalignant oral lesions alike have been associated with cigarette smoking.[4,5] Generally speaking, soft tissue conditions, dental caries, and delayed wound healing are exceedingly more prevalent in smokers compared with nonsmokers. Periodontal disease has been added to the ever-increasing list of health consequences (oral and systemic) of tobacco smoking.[6-12] Chronic exposure to many substances in tobacco and tobacco byproducts significantly affects the prevalence and progression of periodontal diseases.[8,9,12,13] So profound is the negative effect of cigarette smoking on the periodontium that exposure to second-hand smoke accounts for 30% of periodontal disease in nonsmokers.[14] In addition, tobacco use complicates periodontal therapy and substantially reduces the possibility of favorable treatment outcomes.[15–17] Integrating tobacco intervention services within clinical practice is a prudent clinical step and professional obligation. From a broader perspective, providing such services is a civic duty. All scientifically sound clinical intervention services available to the health professional should be applied to help dental patients overcome this life-endangering behavior.

COST OF USING TOBACCO

Most adults and adolescents are aware that tobacco use jeopardizes their health but may not realize how great the risk is compared with other behaviors that are considered risky.[1] Cigarette smoking is the most important preventable cause of morbidity and mortality in the United States. It is responsible for more than 400,000 deaths each year (1998 estimate, 430,700).[18] Indeed, nearly one of every five American deaths can be attributed to cigarette smoking. Each year, more than 140,000 women die as a result of smoking-related diseases. Among women, cardiovascular disease is the most common cause of smoking-related death.[19] Lung cancer, the second most common cause, has been rising rapidly since the early 1960s and, in 1989, exceeded breast cancer as the most common form of cancer death among women.[20] The lung cancer mortality rate among men has stabilized but remains the leading cause of cancer in all male age groups ages 15 and older.[21–23]

Tobacco use produces massive economic costs to society. The direct annual cost of treating smoking related illness is greater than the gross sales of tobacco products.[24,25] When the indirect costs of smoking during pregnancy, lost workdays, lost output from early death or retirement and the external costs, such as fires caused by smoking, are added to medical costs, the burden to the U.S. economy in 1998 approaches $130 billion per year, more than two and a half times the gross sales of tobacco products.[25,26] Intangible costs add to the burden, such as tobacco-related suffering, disability, and worsening in the quality of life. Cigar and pipe smoking and the use of smokeless/spit tobacco significantly elevate health risks and are not safe alternatives to cigarette smoking.[3c,27,28] Their relatively low proportion of use and recent increase in popularity do not provide as solid an evidence base for adverse economic consequences as does the overwhelming evidence attributed to cigarette smoking.

On a global perspective tobacco use is responsible for about 4 million deaths each year. That figure represents more deaths than are caused by HIV, tuberculosis, maternal mortality, motor vehicle accidents, suicides, and homicides combined. By 2030, the World Health Organization projects that tobacco will be the leading cause of death and disability, killing more than 10 million people annually. [28a,28b] These statistics are even more alarming when one considers that all smoking-related deaths are essentially preventable. The decline in cigarette smoking in the United States over the last 25 years has not been equal across all populations. The number of adults currently remains high, and adult prevalence has changed little from 1993 to 1997.[1] Increased trends in tobacco use by youths in the United States portends a worsening state of tobacco-related diseases.

Cost to the Periodontium: Risk Factors

Cigarette smoking accounts for approximately half the cases of periodontitis diagnosed in young adults (< 35 years).[29] A meta-analysis from six cross-sectional and case-control studies reported an odds ratio of 2.82 (95% CI 2.36 to 3.39) for "severe" periodontal disease (Figure 7–1).[30] Smokers are, therefore, almost three times more likely to show severe periodontal disease compared with non-

smokers. Since smokers with slight or moderate periodontitis were either excluded from this analysis or included as controls, this figure may represent an underestimation of the real magnitude of the association. Current smokers were also 3.3 times more likely to attend a periodontal practice office compared with nonsmokers.[31] The effect of smoking on periodontal tissues is cumulative and dose dependent (Figures 7–2 and 7–3). Evidence for this biologic gradient is demonstrated in the Erie County Study, where 80% of individuals smoking at least 20 pack-years exhibited moderate to severe periodontal disease, measured by either clinical attachment loss (see Figure 7–2)[8] or alveolar bone loss (see Figure 7–3).[9] Clinically, smoking-associated periodontal disease presents with thick inflamed marginal gingiva and generalized recession. The buccal marginal gingiva of both upper and lower anterior teeth often present with the characteristic stain of smoker melanosis (Figure 7–4). The degree of alveolar bone destruction far exceeds the periodontal destruction evident clinically (Figures 7–5 and 7–6). If these figures do not speak for themselves, 30% of the incidence of periodontal disease in nonsmokers is accounted for by exposure to environmental (household) second-hand smoke.[14] Thus, cigarette smoking is the single, modifiable environmental factor responsible for the excess prevalence of periodontal disease in the population. Cases of periodontal disease attributed solely to smoking are by far greater than the ones owed to other important factors such as diabetes mellitus.[7] Accordingly, cigarette smoking has been demonstrated to fit all of the nine "Bradford Hill criteria" for causation and, as such, is proposed as a causal factor in severe periodontal disease.[32]

Mechanisms of Tobacco Toxicity to the Periodontium

There is an established biologic rationale for the negative effect of cigarette smoking on periodontal tissues. First and foremost, smoking has an immunosuppressive effect on the host, adversely affecting host-parasite interactions. Peripheral blood polymorphonuclear leukocyte motility, chemotaxis, and phagocytosis are significantly impaired,[33-36] thus, compromising this very important first line of defense against subgingival bacteria. In addition, smokers have decreased antibody production, especially IgG$_2$,[37] the subclass most important in the opsonization of periodontal bacteria, and decreased immunoregulatory T-cell subset ratios.[38] The net result is that periodontal organisms in current ciga-

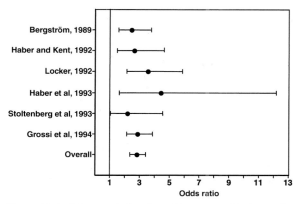

Figure 7–1. Meta-analysis of smoking as a risk factor for periodontal diseases. Bars indicate the 95% confidence limits for the depicted odds ratios. Adapted from Papapanou, PN. Periodontal diseases: epidemiology. Ann Periodontol 1996;1:1–36.

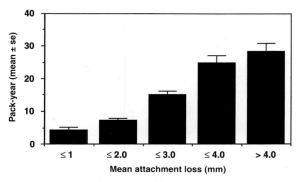

Figure 7–2. Dose-dependent effect of cigarette smoking and severity of attachment loss. For every 10 pack-years increment, there is 1 mm increase in mean attachment loss. Adapted from Grossi et al. J Periodontol 1994;65:260–7.

rette smokers escape specific and nonspecific immune clearance mechanisms allowing them to establish as subgingival inhabitants. Alteration in the physical subgingival environment, such as decreased oxygen tension, would allow the overgrowth of an essentially anaerobic flora.[39,40] In additon, cigarette smoking also increases bacterial adhesion to epithelial cells.[41] Indeed, current smokers are significantly more likely to be infected with *Bacteroides forsythus* and *Porphyromonas gingivalis* compared with nonsmokers.[42]

Several studies have demonstrated the absorption of nicotine in periodontal tissues. Nicotine has been detected on root surfaces in smokers with periodontal disease.[43] Cotinine, the major metabolite of nicotine, is found in the serum, saliva, and gingival crevicular fluid of smokers.[44] Fibroblasts exposed to nicotine have shown reduced proliferation,[45] migration, and attachment to root surfaces.[46] In addition, fibroblasts have been shown to nonspecifically bind and internalize nicotine,[47] which could, in turn, result in an alteration of the cell metabolism, including collagen synthesis and protein secretion. In summary, cigarette smoking appears to trigger a cycle of impaired immune response, anaerobic subgingival infection, and connective tissue cytotoxicity, leading to greater severity of periodontal disease and impaired wound healing.

Tobacco Use and Response to Periodontal Therapy

Nonsurgical Therapy
Scientific evidence shows that smoking impairs wound healing throughout the body, including the

oral cavity. Periodontal intervention studies consistently demonstrate that smokers do not heal as well as nonsmokers after periodontal therapy. The clinical outcomes of periodontal therapy, that is reduction in pocket depth and gain in probing attachment level, are significantly reduced in current smokers compared with former and nonsmokers (Figure 7–7)[15,17,48,49] The reduced clinical response to mechanical therapy seen in current smokers is paralleled by a persistence of subgingival *B. forsythus* and *P. gingivalis* compared with nonsmokers or former smokers (Figure 7–8).[16] This reduced clinical response is directly related to active smoking. Former smokers, on the other hand, respond to periodontal therapy in a manner similar to never-smokers.[16] Although no studies have specifically addressed the effect of smoking cessation on periodontal therapy, indirect data from intervention studies that have included former smokers indicate that smoking cessation restores the host's

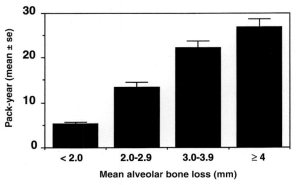

Figure 7–3. Severity of alveolar bone loss is directly proportional to the overall lifetime exposure to tobacco smoke, measured as pack-years. Adapted from Grossi et al. J Periodontol 1995;66:23–9.

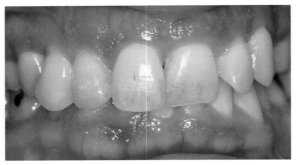

Figure 7–4. Female heavy smoker (more than 20 pack-years). Attached gingiva is thick, chronically inflamed, and fibrotic. Smoker melanosis is evident as well.

healing capacity to levels comparable with those who never smoked.

Surgical, Regenerative, and Implant Therapy

Current cigarette smoking impairs wound healing following surgical periodontal therapy to a greater extent than following nonsurgical therapy. Smokers that underwent periodontal surgery with either modified Widman flap or mucoperiosteal flap had significantly less reduction in pocket depth and gain in probing attachment levels compared with nonsmokers.[50] Cigarette smoking has also been associated with a reduced healing response after guided tissue-regeneration therapy in the deep intrabony defects[51,52] and with an 80% failure rate in the treatment of furcation defects.[53] Current smoking also decreases the percentage of root coverage that takes place after tissue grafting.[54] Eighty percent of current smokers undergoing intraoral bone grafting and simultaneous implant placement showed impaired wound healing, defined as loss of bone or implant, compared with only 10% of non-

smokers.[55] In a 15-year prospective study of mandibular implant prostheses, current smoking was more closely associated with marginal bone loss around implants than was poor oral hygiene.[56] In summary, current smoking is by far the most significant factor responsible for impaired periodontal wound healing and poor clinical outcome following flap and regenerative surgery and implant failure.[51,52,54–57]

Supportive Periodontal Therapy and Need for Re-treatment

Two independent studies on the long-term effects of supportive periodontal therapy (SPT) consistently agreed that smokers have a less favorable response to SPT compared with nonsmokers.[17,50] This reduced response is dose dependent in that heavy smokers, that is, > 20 cigarettes per day, respond less favorably than light smokers (< 19 cigarettes/day) to long-term SPT.[17] Both studies report the encouraging finding that former smokers respond to STP in a manner similar to those that never smoked. A similar benefit of smoking cessation has been reported for dental implant survival.[58] Ninety percent of patients diagnosed with refractory periodontitis are current smokers.[36] Thus, not only does smoking result in reduced response to all modalities of periodontal treatment and less favorable outcome, susceptibility to recurrence and need for re-treatment are increased as well.

Cost to Patient and Provider to Treat Tobacco-Related Periodontal Conditions

When one considers the simple fact that severe periodontal disease will result in more clinic visits, longer clinic appointments, and more complex treatment procedures than will less severe forms of disease, the

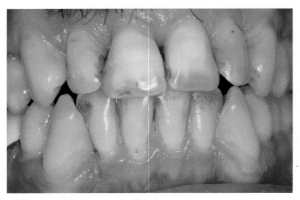

Figure 7–5. Male heavy smoker (more than 20 pack-years) with severe periodontal disease. Gingival tissue is thick, fibrotic, and with receded margins.

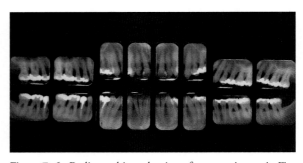

Figure 7–6. Radiographic evaluation of same patient as in Figure 7–5. Generalized severe alveolar bone loss is evident, involving 50% of the root length or more. Furcation involvement (class III) in all molars is evident. Degree of alveolar bone destruction in this patient exceeds the clinical involvement.

increased cost of treating smoking-related periodontal disease to both patient and provider becomes evident. If one then considers that 80% of moderate to severe periodontal disease is associated with heavy smoking, the figures are rather staggering. If the costs of periodontal treatment are calculated, smoking is second only to number of remaining teeth and age. Following the same trend seen for disease severity and response to periodontal therapy, smoking, measured as number of cigarettes per day, has a significant effect both on the treatment cost per patient and per individual tooth.[59] Thus, in addition to causing and exacerbating oral diseases and conditions, tobacco use adversely affects oral health care. Occasionally, patients that exhibit tobacco-related diseases may require special planning, premedication, consultation, or unanticipated medical care during their oral health care. Conversely, tobacco intervention services for the prevention and treatment of oral diseases also benefit the general health and well-being of the patient and reduce collateral risks to clinical practice and society.[60]

UNDERLYING DISEASE

Understanding of the nature of nicotine dependency is essential to applying substantive, efficient means to treat this debilitating condition. Providing periodontal therapy or several other clinical services to tobacco users without treating their tobacco dependency is analogous to painting a rusty surface—a major underlying cause and/or major contributor to the problem is not addressed, thus predisposing to recurrence.

Nicotine dependency is a progressive, chronic, relapsing disease; it is a brain disease imbedded in a social context. That is, nicotine governs tobacco-using behavior, but many psychologic and social cues reinforce the process. Nicotine is considered as addictive as other commonly used substances of abuse; however, more tobacco experimenters become dependent and, once dependent, have greater difficulty while quitting and lower success rates.[61] This is partly because of the low cost and easy availability of tobacco and partly because use is socially acceptable in some environments.[62]

At the molecular-cellular level, nicotine is a tertiary amine that is highly psychoactive. In the brain, chronic exposure to nicotine stimulates release of dopamine and other neurotransmitter monoamines into the CNS neuronal cleft and other sites. In the presence of repeated exposure, nicotinic acetylcholine receptors proliferate on the

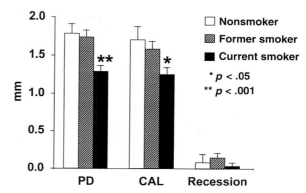

Figure 7–7. Clinical response to mechanical periodontal therapy in smokers and nonsmokers at 3 months after therapy, in deep sites (pocket depth ≥ 5 mm). Current smokers had significantly less ($p < .001$) reduction in pocket depth and gain in clinical attachment ($p < .05$) in deep pockets compared with former and nonsmokers. The clinical response to mechanical therapy in former smokers was comparable with that in nonsmokers, suggesting the benefit of smoking cessation in response to periodontal therapy. PD = pocket depth; CAL = clinical attachment loss.

postsynaptic neurons. Intraneuronal changes occur that alter gene expression. With repeated exposure, central nervous system (CNS) stimulation by nicotine gradually wanes, and more nicotine becomes necessary to ward off withdrawal symptoms. Brain metabolism initially increases and then stabilizes in the presence of nicotine. Thus, continued periodic dosing with nicotine becomes a necessity for individuals to function normally as they would had

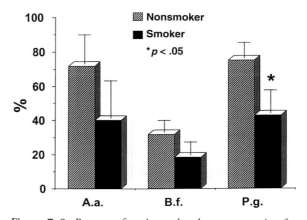

Figure 7–8. Percent of patients that became negative for *A. actinomycetemcomitans*, *B. forsythus*, and *P. gingivalis* at 3 months following mechanical periodontal therapy. Half as many smokers continued to become negative for any of these periodontal organisms after treatment compared with nonsmokers, suggesting that the reduced clinical response to periodontal treatment seen in smokers is due to persistence of periodontal infection of these patients.

they never been exposed. A pack-a-day smoker, drawing ten puffs, self-administers about 200 "hits" each day. This frequently repeated behavior becomes part of the dependency.

The presence of low levels of nicotine in the body over time produces many other effects. For example, in the cardiovascular system, nicotine increases circulating catecholamines, modulates heart A-V node conduction, contracts collateral arteries, promotes platelet aggregation, increases low density lipoproteins, decreases high density lipoproteins, and promotes formation of atherosclerotic plaques. In the respiratory tract, it decreases cilia motility, increases airway resistance, and decreases lung tissue elasticity.

Physical dependency on nicotine is recognized by a cluster of specific patterns of behavior. Dependent individuals typically construct their daily activities around the self-administration of nicotine.

The American Psychiatric Association diagnostic criteria for substance dependency, which includes nicotine addiction are given below:

DMS-IV Diagnostic Criteria for Substance Dependence

A maladaptive pattern of substance use, leading to clinically significant impairment or distress, as manifested by three or more of the following, occurring at any time in the same 12-month period:

Tolerance, as defined by
- a need for markedly increased amounts of the substance to achieve the desired effect, or
- markedly diminished effect with continued use of the same amount of the substance.

Withdrawal, as manifested by
- the characteristic withdrawal syndrome for the substance;
- the substance is taken to relieve or avoid withdrawal symptoms; or
- the substance is often taken in larger amounts or over longer periods than was intended.

There is persistent desire or unsuccessful effort to cut down substance use
- A great deal of time is spent in activities necessary to abstain from the substance, use the substance, or recover from its effects.
- Important social, occupational, or recreational activities are given up or reduced because of substance use. The substance use is continued despite knowledge of having a persistent or recurrent physical or psychological problem that

is likely to have been caused or exacerbated by the substance.

A nicotine-dependent individual uses the drug for avoidance of withdrawal symptoms as much as or more than for perceived benefits such as calming, stimulation, or suppression of hunger. A major component of the "pleasure" of smoking or chewing is relief from the building withdrawal symptoms produced by nicotine depletion.

With permission from Henningfield JE, Cohen C, Pickworth WB. Psychopharmacology of nicotine. In: Orleans CT, Slade J, editors. Nicotine addiction: principles and management. New York, NY: Oxford University Press; 1993.

DMS-IV Criteria for Nicotine Withdrawal
A. Daily use of nicotine for at least several weeks.

B. Abrupt cessation of nicotine use, or reduction in the amount of nicotine used, followed within 24 hours by four (or more) of the following signs:
1. dysphoric or depressed mood
2. insomnia
3. irritability, frustration or, anger
4. anxiety
5. difficulty concentrating
6. restlessness
7. decreased heart rate
8. increased appetite or weight gain

C. The symptoms in criterion B cause clinically significant distress or impairment in social, occupational, or other important areas of functioning.

D. The symptoms are not due to a general medical condition and are not better accounted for by another mental disorder.

With permission from Hughes JR. Nicotine withdrawal, dependence, and abuse. In: Widiger TA, Frances AJ, Pincus HA, editors. DMS-IV sourcebook. Washington, D.C.: American Psychiatric Association; 1994. p.109–16.[63]

EPIDEMIOLOGY OF TOBACCO USE

Physical dependency upon nicotine is not, of course, a factor when an individual is first exposed. Initially, a very small level of exposure can produce symptoms of nicotine intoxication such as dizziness, nausea, and confusion. Establishing patterns of tobacco use occur gradually over months to years and occur for a variety of psychologic and social reasons.[64–66] Desire for tobacco products in adolescents is cultivated by tobacco industry advertising and promotions. A wide variety of communication channels are used. Also, the tobacco industry actively attempts to circumvent and abolish barriers to youth access, recognizing that adolescents, although comprising less than 10% of the market, are vital to the industry's long-term profitability.

Nearly 90% of users begin as children and adolescents, long before they become old enough to legally purchase tobacco products. It is estimated that of the more than 5,000 young people each day that try smoking for the first time, more than 3,000 become regular smokers, many for decades and some for life.[67] Few adolescents smoke daily. However, long before a daily pattern is established, nicotine dependency has begun. An individual that has smoked as few as 100 cigarettes is at high risk of becoming a long-term, dependent smoker. Smokeless tobacco users quickly develop high nicotine tolerance and dependency due to the steady transfer of nicotine across the oral mucosa and throughout the body.

With continued exposure, the effects of nicotine on the central nervous system gradually increase, building up to a physical dependency that dominates the pattern of use.[68] Once dependency is established, the desire for nicotine becomes the principal reason that individuals continue to use tobacco products. Indeed, nicotine is one of the most addictive substances known, and the vast majority of people that quit smoking relapse within days.[69,70] Thus, each year, only 2 to 3% of smokers become nonsmokers without help.[71]

About 70% of adults that smoke would like to stop, and about 34% attempt to quit each year.[72] More women than men would like to stop, but women have greater difficulty in doing so. Adolescent patterns are similar, with 50 to 74% of 12- to 18-year-olds wanting to stop and 40 to 49% percent making an attempt to quit. One survey showed that among adolescents that smoked at some time within the past month but are not smoking daily, over 30% found they could not quit.[73]

NICOTINE DEPENDENCY RISK FACTORS

Smoking prevalence has consistently been in inverse relation to education and income. In 1993, the prevalence of current smoking among adults was 37% for persons that had completed 9 to 11 years of education, 29% among high school graduates, and less than 2% for individuals that had at least 4 years of college education.[72] As defined by the Social Security Administration, 22% of individuals above the poverty level smoked and 28% of those below the poverty level. In addition to poverty, other sociodemographic factors associated with higher prevalence of smoking are being a blue collar worker, separated or divorced, and in active military service.[72]

The prevalence of cigarette smoking is highest among American Indians and Alaska Natives (39%), intermediate in African Americans (26%) and European Americans (25%), and lowest in Hispanics (20%) and Asian Americans and Pacific Islanders (18%).[74] Smokeless tobacco use is also highest among American Indians and Alaska Natives of both genders, followed by European Americans (12%), Hispanics (5%), and African Americans (2%). Cultural and socioeconomic factors may influence initiation, but genetic factors may contribute to some races being more susceptible than others once exposed to nicotine.[75,76] Within any race, genetic factors in some individuals predispose them to nicotine dependency when exposed.[77]

No single factor determines patterns of tobacco use among racial/ethnic minority groups. These patterns are the result of complex interactions of multiple factors, such as socioeconomic status, cultural characteristics, acculturation, stress, biologic elements, targeted advertising, price of tobacco products, and varying capacities of communities to mount effective tobacco control initiatives.[78]

Certain effects of nicotine, such as its ability to suppress appetite, may selectively increase the risk of nicotine dependency in women. Evidence indicates that people with depression are especially vulnerable to nicotine dependency, and since the prevalence of depression is twice as high in women as in men, this relationship may be particularly important for women.[79]

It is alarming that by 1997, tobacco use in high school students was 43%. This exceedingly high smoking prevalence in adolescents suggests a commensurate rise in the number of adults that will want to quit, as well as an increase in the incidence of tobacco-related morbidity and mortality.

WHO QUITS?

In recent years, tobacco use among men has declined more rapidly than among women so that rates are similar (27 versus 24%), and differences may become smaller in the future. Men are somewhat less interested than women in quitting (67 versus 73%), but a greater number of men than women have quit (51 versus 47%).[72]

Surveys of gender differences in the ratios of cigarette smoking cessation suggest that men have an easier time of it (49 versus 40%). When the ratios are adjusted for the use of other tobacco products (cigars, pipes, smokeless tobacco), however, the ratios are quite similar (42 versus 40%). More men than women merely switch from cigarettes to other forms of tobacco to sustain their nicotine dependency rather than truly quit. Long-term abstinence rates for those that quit show virtually no difference by gender.[80] Thus, men and women may have different reasons for initiation, continuing to use, wanting to quit, quitting, and staying abstinent, but the net behavior outcome is not very significant. Nevertheless, helping patients during the quitting process requires an appreciation of gender differences; physiologic factors, such as differential sensitivity and tolerance to nicotine, more intense withdrawal symptoms by women, timing of quit attempts in relation to the menstrual cycle; and behavioral and psychologic factors, such as women's fear of weight gain, greater need for social support, and their lower confidence in their ability to quit.[81]

DENTAL PROFESSION'S ROLE IN TREATING NICOTINE ADDICTION

In recent years, dentists have been acquiring clinical tobacco intervention skills. A quarter of dentists (24%) routinely identify their patients' status of tobacco-use and accordingly advise them to quit.[82] More than half the dentists that do not provide such services state that they desire training that would enable them to do so.[83,84] The reasons for providing clinical tobacco intervention services are compelling.

Of course, helping patients quit and stay abstinent is an ethical obligation. Overwhelming evidence indicates that tobacco is harmful to oral health and that smoking status is an important factor in the prognoses of several dental therapies, including periodontal therapy, oral surgery, implant dentistry, and cosmetic dentistry. Second, clinical tobacco intervention services have a moral basis as well. It is a regular act of citizenship to attempt to preserve life and prevent injury and death. Smoking kills half the regular users, and half of these will die prematurely, losing, on average, two decades of life.[28b] Third, clinical tobacco intervention services

are cost effective. Long-term tobacco users develop chronic conditions that often become time-consuming patient management problems. Smokers are ill more often than are nonsmokers, which frequently leads to problems with appointments, medical considerations, and emergencies during treatment. Many patients are prematurely lost to practice when tobacco-related disabilities severely restrict their mobility and resources.

Many professional organizations have developed support systems that help clinicians integrate cessation services into their practices. For example, several dental organizations have adopted tobacco-related clinical policies. The American Dental Association (ADA) now has published and distributed a guide to therapeutics titled "Tobacco counseling for the control and prevention of oral disease," established a service code (01320) and included tobacco use status and interest in quitting questions in the ADA Health History Form. Educational guidelines have been developed for educational institutions. Such infrastructure developments help ease the integration of clinical tobacco intervention services into practice.[85]

TREATING NICOTINE DEPENDENCY

Nicotine dependency is not merely a "risk factor" for other disease, but it is a disease requiring treatment in its own right.[86] There are numerous methods for helping nicotine-dependent patients. Unfortunately, most are not supported by scientific evidence, even though some seem attractive or are popular. Until recently, empirical approaches, primarily combinations of methods, have been used. Any method will yield its success stories. When studied, using scientifically sound methods, and critically analyzed, success rates for most methods do not compare favorably with not using the method. Often individual successes can be explained by other factors.

Systematic studies of smoking cessation began in earnest during the early 1980s.[87] Randomized controlled trials demonstrated that physicians, using minimum clinical intervention methods, could be effective in increasing patient cessation rates.[88–92] Dentists and other clinicians subsequently were also shown to be as effective.[93–96] Currently, there is overwhelming evidence that medical and dental practices are an essential part of helping the public avoid and discontinue tobacco use.[97]

Within the scientific community, "success" is considered long-term abstinence, with "long-term" defined as being tobacco-free for 6 months or longer. Studies that do not include follow-up for at least 5 months are generally not seriously considered when assessing effectiveness. "Abstinence" is defined as being tobacco free, not nicotine free. Food and Drug Administration (FDA)-approved nicotine replacement products are routinely used to help individuals quit using tobacco. Some products are available without prescription.

In 1981, a 2-mg nicotine gum was approved by the FDA to supplement behavioral interventions. During the 1990s, a variety of nicotine replacement products and one non-nicotine tablet were approved. Other pharmaceutical agents are under investigation. Research on nicotine addiction and CNS function promises to provide more effective treatments in the future. There is no "silver bullet" method or pharmaceutical agent. Although a selected combination of clinical methods combined with an FDA-approved pharmaceutical agent can significantly increase cessation rates, none sustain long-term abstinence for as many as half the number of the individuals that make a cessation attempt.[97a]

Since 1996, Clinical Practice Guideline Number 18: Smoking Cessation of the Agency for Health Care Policy and Research (AHCPR) has become the international gold standard for clinical tobacco intervention services.[98] This guideline and its subsequent revisions (one scheduled for early 2000) can help focus valuable clinician time on services that are evidence based and return the highest success rates for the time invested. The following statements and recommendations are based on or taken from the guideline, except where supplemental references are shown.

Although the long-duration, intensive treatments are more effective than the brief treatments, such interventions can be reserved for smoking cessation specialists and other specialists in the management of patients who experience multiple relapses, have multiple drug dependencies, are mentally challenged, or have severe psychiatric disorders. Guidelines are available for such clinicians.[99,100] However, most patients can be approached by and benefit from brief, practical interventions by even the busiest clinician of any health discipline.

RECOMMENDED MINIMUM CLINICAL INTERVENTION METHODS

A practical routine should be integrated into every clinical practice. Basic steps are known as the "4 A's,"

Ask, Advise, Assist, and Arrange (Table 7–1).[101,102] First proposed by Marc Manley and Thomas Glynn of the National Cancer Institute, the steps have remained the core of successful clinical programs, even when other names are applied. The basic steps are as follows:

Ask

Identify the tobacco use status of every patient. "Do you use tobacco?" This information should be considered a vital sign.[103,104] Inquiry can be integrated within existing patient questionnaire systems. It is essential that each patient record show the current tobacco use status so that all clinic staff are aware of it.[105] As nicotine dependency is chronic and relapsing, it is important to ask this question at every encounter. Of course, since most patients do not use tobacco, the answer under most circumstances is a brief "no." Tobacco users must be asked about the duration and intensity of their use, past experience with quitting, and especially about their desire to stop. "How interested are you in quitting now?"

Advise

This step focuses on building the patient's motivation to be tobacco free. Although brief and simple, building motivation is one of three basic clinical intervention services. Commend never-users and former users on the wisdom of their behavior. This is an especially important message to children and adolescents to help prevent and postpone initiation and to former users, who are vulnerable to relapse.

1. Advise all tobacco users in clear language that you think they should quit. Patients place great weight on such advice by clinicians.

TABLE 7–1. Basic Steps of Successful Smoking Cessation Program

"4 A's"	
• Ask	Identify the tobacco use status of every patient
• Advise	Increase the tobacco user's interest in quitting
• Assist	Help those who are ready with their problem solving skills and with pharmacotherapy
• Arrange	Arrange follow-up support throughout the quitting process

2. Associate use with existing patient health conditions. When possible, show the patient his or her own tobacco-related conditions. Patients also should understand other health risks and tobacco risks to planned health services and prognoses, but not only that.

3. Ask each patient for his or her own reasons for wanting to quit. Most will have a reason, perhaps several. Expressing those reasons helps strengthen them, even though many have little to do with health. The patient's reasons provide clues to which the clinician can add motivating ideas and perspectives that help dispel unwarranted hesitancy. The clinician should be as upbeat as possible. Emphasize the benefits of quitting in terms that are specific to each patient's interests, circumstances, and culture.

Many patients will not be interested in quitting at the moment, but the "Advice" step strengthens the decision-making process that individuals must progress through to initiate a behavior change. The discussion clarifies in the patient's mind the opinion of a respected individual. It introduces to contented users ideas that will begin to offset their reasons for continuing. Discussion helps individuals that are generally interested in quitting to begin thinking more seriously about what they are doing to themselves and about their prospects for living tobacco free. Discussion identifies highly motivated patients, that is, those that previously attempted to quit or have an intention to quit in the foreseeable future. A clinician's advice to quit can trigger the decision to act.

The patient's desire for clinical therapy to be successful and enduring can influence his or her desire to quit. Other personal benefits become bonus advantages in this situation. The ever-present goal of doing everything possible to save each patient's life may remain a silent imperative in the clinician's mind.

Patients that are not interested in quitting at the moment should be offered assistance in the future, "When (not if) you are ready, I'll be glad to help." In addition, patients should be given motivational literature that is appropriate to their interests, circumstances, and, if possible, culture.

Assist

While "Ask" and "Advise" are routine steps for all patients, the "Assist" step is used with a subset of patients that are ready to quit. This step focuses on helping patients cope with the quitting process.

The clinician acts as a caring, skilled facilitator because, of course, the primary responsibility remains with the individual that must quit. Three specific components are essential: establishing a plan for (1) preparing to quit, (2) coping with psychologic and social cues during the quitting process, and (3) managing the physical challenges of nicotine withdrawal.

Preparing to Quit

Ask the patient to choose a quit date. The date ideally should be within 2 weeks, but not so soon that there is no time for mental preparation. Give the patient a reminder of the date, perhaps on a prescription form, that can be posted at home.

Suggest that the patient inform family, friends, and co-workers and solicit their support. One's spouse can be an especially important ally. The patient should arrange to have others that use tobacco not use it in their presence during the quitting process.

The final use of tobacco should be during the day before the selected quit date. Advise the patient to remove all tobacco products and the materials that they use from home, car, work place, and any other readily accessible site.

Advise that other forms of tobacco also contain nicotine and their use will work against the goal of quitting for good.

Coping with Psychologic and Social Cues

Ask the patient what is most likely to lead to a relapse and how he or she would plan to manage that. Encourage the patient to solve the problem. Then offer specific suggestions and answer patient concerns.

Advise that even a single puff is dangerous and often leads to relapse.

Caution that alcohol and other drug use impairs judgment and can lead to relapse.

Stress and weight gain are two common concerns. The quit date selected should be at a time of least possible stress; however, the management of stress should be discussed, and the patient should be advised that the transition period is often accompanied by a period of anxiety, restlessness, insomnia, and reduced ability to concentrate while the brain adjusts to the absence of nicotine. Help the patient with stress management strategies that are alternatives to using tobacco.

Although dieting should be postponed during the first few weeks, alternatives to adding calories and approaches to burning calories should be addressed. Advise the patient that weight gain is a minor risk compared with continuing to use tobacco. Tell the patient to tackle one problem at a time; first be confident that they have quit using tobacco for good before working on weight gain. The use of nicotine gum may delay weight gain.

If the patient has previously attempted to quit and relapsed, address how to deal with that specific situation. Determine if the precipitating event was due to nicotine withdrawal, psychologic, or a social situation.

Provide literature on the quitting process. This saves clinician time and can be referred to as often as wanted. The AHCPR's booklet "You can quit," available in eight languages, the National Cancer Institute's "Clearing the air," and other organization pamphlets provide reinforcement to motivation and offer suggestions for preparing to quit and managing the effects of quitting, such as nicotine withdrawal and weight gain. Such booklets describe coping strategies not commonly shown in the flyers aimed at motivating various segments of the public.

As with other substances of abuse, individuals that successfully quit must appreciate that permanent CNS neuron changes have occurred. They must be alert to the possibility that even a single exposure can rapidly lead to complete relapse, even years after quitting.

Certain psychologic states, such as acute stress, depression, or encountering a previously learned social cue, can trigger a relapse.

Managing the Physical Dynamics of Nicotine Withdrawal

1. Prescribe or recommend an FDA-approved nicotine replacement for use, beginning on the quit date. The intent is to reduce the intensity and duration of nicotine withdrawal symptoms while the patient is learning to cope with the psychologic challenges and social cues that had become part of the addiction. It extends the use of the one drug that drives tobacco use behavior, but places its administration under supervision and in amounts that do not produce the "hits" or peaks of nicotine in the brain. Also, the patient learns how to live without possessing tobacco products and going through the rituals of using tobacco-associated paraphernalia.

   Nicotine transdermal patches approximately double long-term abstinence compared with abstinence using behavioral intervention alone.[106] Patches are often the preferred route for clinical use because there are few compli-

ance problems, and little clinician time and effort are required to train patients in their effective use. A patch is applied to a different skin area each day to minimize irritation. Three brands of patch are available in three strengths, according to patch size, and are used either for 16 or 24 hours each (Table 7–2). The largest patch is used for the initial 4 weeks and the next smaller sizes for two 2-week, stepped withdrawal periods. The midsize patch should be used initially by patients that are light smokers (less than 10 cigarettes daily) or are of small stature (weight less than 100 pounds). One patch is used for 16 hours only and patches are used for 6 weeks, after which use is discontinued entirely. If the particular patch is not effective for a patient, another brand may help.

TABLE 7–2. Recommended Agents to Manage Nicotine Withdrawal

Nicotine Replacement Agents
  Patch
  • Habitrol® (*Novartis*)
      Nicotine
      21 mg
      14 mg
      7 mg
  • Prostep® (*Lederle Labs*)
      22 mg/24 h
      11 mg/24 h
  • Nicotrol® (*McNeil Consumer*)
      15 mg/16 h
  • Nicoderm® CQ® (*SmithKline Beecham Consumer*)
      – Step I   21 mg/24 h
      – Step II   14 mg/24 h
      – Step III   7 mg/24 h
  Gum
  • Nicorette® (*SmithKline Beecham Consumer*)
      2 mg or 4 mg
  Nasal spray
  • Nicotrol® NS (*McNeil Consumer*)
      Nicotine
      0.5 mg
  Inhaler
  • Nicotrol® Inhaler (*McNeil Consumer*)
      2 mg
      4 mg
Non-nicotine agents
  Bupropion HCL
  • Zyban® (*Glaxo Wellcome*)
      150 mg

The 4-mg nicotine gum (nicotine polacrilex) is usually preferred when a skin disease or adhesive allergy rules out use of a patch, when a patient has not been successful with using a patch, as a supplement to a patch, or when gum is preferred by the patient for any reason.[107] One piece should be used every 1 to 2 hours for 6 weeks, then every 2 to 4 hours for 3 weeks, and 4 to 8 hours for 3 weeks. Patients must be instructed to chew each piece until a peppery taste is noticeable, and then to park the gum as nicotine absorption occurs. The "chew and park" routine is followed for about 30 minutes per piece. The patient must be instructed to stop using acidic liquids such as coffee, soft drinks, and fruit juices, at least 15 minutes before using the gum since the nicotine is not absorbed in an acidic environment. Light smokers may use a 2-mg gum. Long-term quit rates are about 40 to 60% higher in using nicotine gum than in using behavioral intervention alone.

The nicotine nasal spray is an option that simulates the rapid delivery effect of cigarette smoking.[108,109] The recommended dosage is one spray into each nostril 8 to 16 times daily. Long-term quit rates reported are from 18 to 27%. The nicotine oral inhaler is another option.[110,111] Its ritual and sensory aspects resemble smoking. The recommended dosage is up to 16 cartridges per day. Long-term quit rates are reported to range from 13 to 28%. Use of any of the products are recommended for an 8- to 10-week period.[112]

Contraindications for all nicotine replacements are similar. They are not recommended for patients in an immediate postmyocardial infarction period, those that have severe arrhythmias, or those that have a severe or worsening angina pectoris. Specific contraindications include skin disorders for patches, asthma or chronic nasal disorders for nasal spray and inhalation systems, and temporomandibular joint disorders or dentures for nicotine gum.

Because of the serious risks of smoking to both mother and fetus, pregnant smokers should be offered intensive counseling. Nicotine replacement should be used during pregnancy only if the increased likelihood of smoking cessation, with its potential benefits, outweigh the risk of nicotine replacement and potential concomitant smoking.

Nicotine replacement should be considered for adolescents, only when there is clear evidence of nicotine dependency and a clear desire to quit using tobacco.

Many individuals that are not successful in becoming nicotine free are able to become tobacco free by using a nicotine replacement for several months or indefinitely.[113,114] Although continued use of a nicotine replacement beyond a 10- to 12-week period is not recommended, it is infinitely better than returning to tobacco use. Nicotine is harmful, but not as much as many other tobacco constituents. Of the at least 2,550 known compounds in tobacco and over 4,000 compounds in tobacco smoke, primary tobacco biohazards include at least 43 carcinogens, such as the nicotine nitrosamines, and alpha-emitting radionuclides, such as Polonium 210. Tobacco smoke contains carbon monoxide, thiocyanate, herbicide, fungicide, and pesticide residues, tars, and many other substances that promote disease and impair body functions. Tobacco is a highly polluting nicotine delivery system.

2. Bupropion HCl (Zyban) is a nicotine replacement alternative. Bupropion is used in tobacco use cessation treatment as a centrally acting non-nicotine agent. The long-term abstinence rate through its use is equivalent to that through using a nicotine patch.[115] Patients that are strongly dependent upon nicotine may use bupropion in combination with a nicotine replacement.

The patient's medical history, current medical status, and patterns of behavior must be carefully evaluated before recommending bupropion. It interacts with many drugs, including alcohol, antipsychotic agents, hepatic enzyme inducers and inhibitors, levodopa, and monoamine (MAO) inhibitors. This is of concern because many of these potentiate the risk of seizures. The use of bupropion is contraindicated in patients being treated with Wellbutrin (which is also bupropion HCl), antipsychotics, antidepressants, theophylline, or systemic steroids and in patients that abruptly discontinue use of a benzodiazepine or another agent that lowers seizure threshold. Bupropion is contraindicated in patients with anorexia nervosa or bulimia, bipolar disorders, CNS tumor, a history of head trauma or drug abuse, hepatic or renal impairment, recent history of myocardial infarct, unstable heart disease, psychosis, or seizure disorders.[116]

The use of bupropion differs from nicotine replacement in that bupropion treatment should begin 7 to 10 days before the patient-selected quit date, whereas the pharmaceutical nicotine substitution should begin on the quit date.

A recent review of randomized clinical trials and of meta-analyses of smoking intervention studies concludes that pharmacotherapy for smoking cessation should be made available to all smokers.[117] All currently available therapies appear equally efficacious, approximately doubling the quit rate compared with placebo. In addition, combined therapies are more successful in obtaining long-term success. Thus, combining patch with gum or patch with bupropion may increase the quit rate compared with any single treatment.[117]

3. Consult package inserts, the *Physician's Desk Reference*, the *ADA Guide to Accepted Dental Therapeutics*, and comparable resources for dosage and management information on specific FDA-approved pharmaceutical agents for tobacco use cessation.

4. Other pharmaceutical agents have been studied. There is little scientific evidence for the use of clonidine, either as a primary or as an adjunctive pharmacologic treatment for tobacco use cessation. There is no scientific evidence demonstrating the effectiveness of any antidepressant other than bupropion. The use of anxiolytics, benzodiazepines, lobeline, silver acetate, cotinine, beta blockers, glucose, sodium bicarbonate, and stimulants have not been shown to be effective. The use of mecamylamine, buspirone, phenylpropanolamine, and various other drugs, independently and in combination with approved agents, are under investigation but not recommended for use outside the research protocols.

Other behavioral intervention methods and nonpharmacologic agents have been assessed. Of the self-help methods, hotline/helpline support is effective, but providing video and audiotapes, lists of community programs, and pamphlets and booklets is not. Group counseling is beneficial for selected individuals but is no more effective than the basic clinical interventions described above. Evidence does not support methods based on motivation, weight/diet/nutrition counseling, exercise/fitness, contingency contracting, relaxation/breathing, or nicotine fading. Aversive smoking increases cessation rates and may be used, with caution, with smokers that desire such treatment or have been unsuccessful using other interventions. There is insufficient evidence to assess the effectiveness of hypnosis or acupuncture. There is no evidence supporting the use of herbal products and foods for tobacco intervention.

It is recommended that those few practical (brief) methods that are supported by substantial scientific evidence be mastered and routinely used. They can become the basis for developing one's art and practice, as the science of clinical tobacco intervention services evolves. Clinical interventions against an addictive behavior must be considered incremental. Indeed, most patients relapse, but this should not be a deterrent. Other adverse health conditions also have recurrences. As with other chronic diseases and conditions, cures for smoking cessation are unusual, but the absence of a high success rate from single intervention attempts are never a reason to withhold treatment, especially when continued tobacco use is clearly a high risk to a multitude of diseases and life itself.

Arrange

Establish a schedule for follow-up contacts, either in person or by telephone. Although some increase in patient quit rates can be anticipated from a single encounter, long-term abstinence is dramatically improved, three to four-fold, when there is timely follow-up.

Schedule a first contact by clinic staff for a day or two before the patient-selected quit date. This serves as a quit date reminder, as an expression of support and encouragement, and as an opportunity to solicit questions and concerns related to preparations.

The recommended post–quit-date follow-up contact schedule is four to seven contacts over a 3-month period. The first follow-up contact should be within 2 weeks of the quit date, preferably within the first week. The second, third, and fourth contacts should be near the end of the first, second, and third months. Studies suggest that fewer than four and more than seven contacts yield lower results than this follow-up interval and frequency.

During each follow-up contact, the clinician should applaud success. If a lapse occurred, the patient should be asked for a recommitment to total abstinence. Remind the patient that a lapse can be used as a learning experience, and review the circumstances that caused it. Ask the patient how he or she could better manage that situation next time. Suggest alternative behaviors.

Even if the patient remains abstinent, identify problems encountered and anticipate challenges in the immediate future. Review the benefits, including potential health benefits, to be derived from cessation. Discuss specific problems such as weight gain, negative mood/depression, prolonged nicotine withdrawal, and lack of support for cessation from others. Discussion helps the patient to clarify and cope with such problems.

All treatment strategies apply to individuals that are of any age, gender, or ethnic origin, generally healthy or ill, or inpatient or outpatient. All treatment strategies apply to adolescents who want to quit using tobacco. Clinicians should be firm but nonjudgmental and should personalize the encounter to the individual situation.

One primary finding has been that all types of clinicians are about equally effective, that is, regardless of discipline. Providing a brief intervention can yield about a 50% increase in patient quit rates compared with not helping. It is significant that interventions by multiple providers reinforce and nearly quadruple patient quit rates. Success may be partially due to previous efforts by colleagues; lack of immediate success with a patient actually serves as an important preparation for a subsequent clinician contact that becomes persuasive. Thus, each clinician is part of a broad, not necessarily known-by-name, professional tobacco intervention network.

As little as 3 minutes' cessation helps produce a significant increase in long-term abstinence from tobacco. However, even less than 3 minutes' cessation yields a measurable benefit over self-help methods. If 3 or more minutes are not available, even the briefest help should be employed, given the ever increasing life-threatening risk when the individual continues to use tobacco and the importance of reinforcement by multiple providers, to achieve a commitment to quitting and long-term abstinence. More intense interventions, that is more time-per-patient contact, increase long-term abstinence rates.

In general, actual cessation rates vary widely by demographic factors, such as income and educational level. The practical clinical intervention methods recommended above compare the relative increase in long-term abstinence compared to withholding clinician intervention and are not absolute values. Also, any quit attempt is useful as preparation for long-term abstinence. It is estimated that unsuccessful cigarette smokers, on average, make three to four attempts before achieving long-term abstinence.[118]

Tobacco users with psychiatric comorbidity should be offered the same treatments recommended to other individuals. Although it is not necessary to assess psychiatric comorbidity prior to initiating an intervention, such an assessment may be helpful in that it allows the clinician to prepare for an increased likelihood of relapse or for exacerbation of the comorbid condition as a result of nicotine withdrawal. Individuals that experience depressive and anxiety symptoms are at higher risk for smoking initiation.[119] Individuals experiencing psychiatric disorders are at high risk of initiation and may smoke as a form of self-treatment.[120] Individuals with a history of clinical depression are more likely to experience a recurrence during the quitting process.[121]

TREATMENT ENVIRONMENT

Providing clinical intervention services requires a team approach. Clinic personnel, the office environment, and the management system need a few simple adjustments for services to be provided efficiently, effectively, and pleasantly. First, one individual, usually not the primary-care provider, needs to be responsible for the service operation. All members of the clinic team need to understand the objectives and methods employed. The "ASK" step is usually managed by the reception/receiving staff, as well as the recording of the patient's tobacco use status. This is verified when other vital signs are taken and initial work-up begun. Diagnosis and treatment planning must include the "Advice" step. "Assist" is often begun by the primary clinician or other provider. Other staff may provide more detailed help for the patient that commits to a quit date and ensure that the "Arrange" step is done so that follow-up will occur.

Clinic staff that use tobacco present a special consideration. Patients should not be able to determine that staff do so, for mixed messages are sent about the clinic being a responsible health unit. Offers to help patients quit may lack credibility if smelly hands, hair, or clothes are detected. Every effort must be made to encourage tobacco-using staff to quit. Intense help may be needed. Employee unions, personnel offices, and facility directors may need to be involved.

The clinic's physical environment should convey a positive tobacco-free message. A "Thank you for not Smoking" sign establishes the authority of the office in a manner that invites cooperation. The absence of ash trays and presence of posters and a display of motivational literature enhances the message. Magazines available for patients should not carry tobacco advertizing. The back covers are especially important since they may be seen by several patients at once.

Patient records should have an identifying mark so that all clinic staff can easily recognize the tobacco use status of each patient. Records of patients who are tobacco-free also need an identifying mark so that patients whose tobacco use status has not been determined will be easily recognized. Basic information required is patient status and interest in quitting. More complete information includes details about duration, intensity, and type of tobacco used, the level of patient dependency on nicotine, factors that would enhance or hinder a quit attempt, and the history of previous quit attempts. Such information, when completed by patients saves clinic staff time. The record should include progress notes on cessation attempts. Also, the recall system should be able to trigger a contact with patients who are making a quit attempt. The contacts should be scheduled for a day or two before the quit date, during the first few days post quit date, and at least once a month through the quitting period.

The clinic system should trigger an inquiry about all patients of any age. Of course, prenatal visits focus on the importance of both mother and fetus being tobacco free until term. The caregivers of infants and children less than age 5 years need the "4 As." Ask about tobacco use in the home and other tobacco smoke exposure. Advise that steps be taken to protect the infants and children from exposure. In addition to discussion with caregivers, children aged 5 to 11 years should be asked directly, commended for not using tobacco, and be given other reinforcing messages to help counter the allure already being transmitted by the tobacco industry and to prevent initiation. Adolescents need to be encouraged to quit as well as given proved messages to avoid tobacco and exposure to tobacco smoke.

Beyond individual patient contact, clinicians have unlimited opportunity to prevent adolescent interest in tobacco, prevent initiation, prevent nicotine addiction, and promote cessation. Health professionals are respected opinion leaders in professional affairs, religious and other community organizations, hobby and other personal interests, and with patients that are involved in the development of public policy, worksite policies, administrative affairs, and public education. Educated views about tobacco, born of one's experience with patients and organized initiatives, carry weight. It is from such discussions that community norms evolve. Each health professional has a continuing stream of unique opportunities to counter the influence of the tobacco industry by helping prevent nicotine addiction among youths and increasing the determination of adult tobacco users who are trying to break free.

Studies supported by the National Cancer Institute during the 1980s and statewide demonstration projects in the 1990s demonstrated that tobacco use among adults can decline at twice the rate of secular trends when media, community, business, policy, and professional tobacco education and public health promotion efforts are made concurrently. Messages via these channels reinforce each other, helping the public conclude that avoiding tobacco use is in their own best interests and those of their loved ones and communities.

During the 1990s, concurrent with media coverage of the struggle between public health and the tobacco industry, the FDA approved several pharmacologic agents to aid smoking cessation. Advertising and promotion by pharmaceutical companies contributed to public awareness that smoking cessation is possible and desirable and that certain drugs could help. Nicotine replacement products were determined to be sufficiently safe, delivering substantially lower peak doses than self-administered tobacco products. Two brands of nicotine patch and two strengths of nicotine gum were approved for over-the-counter sales.

The public is better informed about risks in tobacco use, including nicotine dependency, than ever before. There is a willingness, indeed an expectation, that health professionals are informed and interested in helping patients quit. National Center for Health Statistics surveys consistently show that each year about 70% of smokers want to quit and about a third make a quit attempt. Yet, only slightly over 60% of U.S. physicians report that they identify patient smoking status, and slightly over a fifth report counseling their patients that are smokers. It is even less encouraging when it is noted that most counseling is selective, primarily restricted to patients already exhibiting clinical symptoms of smoking-related diseases. Few smoking patients that do not exhibit a smoking-related disease are counseled.[122]

Primary barriers to counseling have been a belief that intervention is not effective, not knowing which methods are effective, lack of compensation for the service, and perceived time available to provide help. The AHCPR *Clinical Practice Guideline* responds to such concerns. Many methods are examined, and those most effective are recommended. Recommendations are targeted at clinicians that have little time, specialists, researchers, educators, administrators, and health policy makers. Studies show that the health-care system must support tobacco cessation services. Managed-care programs are taking note that tobacco cessation has been found to be more cost effective than any other preventive medical service.[123] Standards for facility accreditation are being upgraded to include clinical tobacco intervention services. Having the *Clinical Practice Guideline* as an evidence-based model, several health professions are integrating tobacco topics appropriately into educational curricula and continuing education programs. As the 1990s draw to a close, the health professions are developing the necessary infrastructure.

SUMMARY AND CONCLUSION

The late 1980s and 1990s have brought an overwhelming body of evidence to substantiate unequivocally that tobacco use has a profound negative effect on periodontal disease severity, prevalence, incidence, and progression. Tobacco use has also a profound negative effect on the health and well being of users, society, and clinical practice. The public is increasingly aware of this fact. Tobacco use is preventable. Most nicotine dependent individuals want to quit and can quit, when guided by proper support.

Advances in the art and science of addiction medicine, and especially nicotine addiction medicine, are being increasingly published in the professional literature and presented in scientific forums. Some convergence is occurring in the understanding and treatment of all substances of abuse, binding stronger relations between the behavioral and bench sciences. In recent years, several pharmacologic agents for smoking cessation have been approved by the FDA. Additional pharmacologic agents and refined behavioral intervention methods should be expected.

Adoption of scientifically sound clinical tobacco cessation services is a professional obligation, a moral imperative, and a practical matter. Three to five minutes of cessation assistance integrated into other clinical services is a life-saving service that benefits patients, community, and practice. Periodontal health and prognoses for periodontal therapy substantially improve when patients quit smoking.

The AHCPR's *Clinical Practice Guideline Number 18: Smoking Cessation* provides the information needed to develop the art and skill neces-

sary to make cessation services a routine practice. The experience of a few successful cases provides satisfaction and ensures commitment to bringing hope of successful cessation to people whose tobacco use places them at high risk of developing major life-threatening illnesses.

Clinicians also have expanding opportunities to help patients in a collective manner. Professional opinion and guidance are important to the public's development of self-directed health behaviors.

AREAS OF FUTURE RESEARCH

Tobacco-related research questions abound. Major conferences, government agencies, and public advocacy organizations frequently update information on tobacco and behavior, tobacco as a risk factor, tobacco dependency, tobacco and adolescents, tobacco cessation, tobacco economics, and tobacco intervention policy research agenda. On the one hand, fruits of such areas of research benefit individuals engaged in the tobacco-related aspects of oral health care, research, education, program management, and policy making. On the other, experts in oral health affairs provide insights into related general health and human behavior research questions, professional education system content, health-care policies and practices, and monitoring and assessment systems.

Some areas of research need leadership by oral health investigators. Their focus is on how each of the many forms of tobacco and tobacco use practices impact on oral health and oral health care. Research is needed on the public response to the dental profession as a resource for tobacco cessation assistance and how the profession regards its ability to help the public through its clinical and extraclinical endeavors. More research is needed on how to provide effective intervention when available smoking cessation therapies are ineffective; the impact of tobacco use on the oral and craniofacial development of the growing fetus, infants, children, adolescents; and the direct and contributing influence of tobacco on oral diseases and conditions and on prognoses, recovery, and recurrence. Tobacco-related oral health research is needed within subpopulations, on the basis of race/ ethnicity, gender, age, lifestyle, codependencies, and environmental factors.

Assessment of the expanding scientific base for tobacco intervention services is a professional imperative for researchers, educators, and clinicians. Such monitoring ensures that professional education and practice are evidence-based, that health service resources expended are in the best interests of both patient and public, and that the dental profession is a viable member of a broad community of professional, public, and private sectors committed to creating a tobacco-free society.

REFERENCES

1. U.S. Department of Health and Human Services. Cigarette smoking among adults—United States, 1995. MMWR 1997;46:1217–20.

2. U.S. Department of Health and Human Services. Surveillance for selected tobacco-use behaviors —United States, 1900–1994. MMWR 1994;43 (SS-3):34.

3. U.S. Department of Health and Human Services. Tobacco use among high school students— United States, 1997. MMWR 1998;47:229–33.

3a. Wechester H, Riggot NA, Gledhill-Hoyt J, Lee H. Increasing levels of cigarette use among college students: a cause for national concern. JAMA 1998;280:1673–8.

3b. Krall EA, Garvey AJ, Garcia RI. Alveolar bone loss and tooth loss in male cigar and pipe smokers. J Am Dental Assoc 1999;130:57–64.

3c. Iribarren C, Tekawa IS, Sidney S, Friedman GD. Effects of cigar smoking on the risk of cardiovascular disease, chronic obstructive pulmonary disease, and cancer in men. NEJM 1999;340: 1773–80.

3d. Ayaian JZ, Cleary PD. Perceived risks of heart disease and cancer among cigarette smokers. JAMA 1999;281:1019–21.

4. Research, Science and Therapy Committee. Tobacco use and the periodontal patient. J Periodontol 1996;67:51–6.

5. Mecklenburg RE, Greenspan D, Manley MW, et al. Tobacco effects in the mouth. Bethesda, MD: NIH publication No. 93–3330;1991.p 5–13.

6. Burgan SW. The role of tobacco use in periodontal diseases: a literature review. Gen Dent 1997;45: 449–60.

7. Haber J, Wattles J, Crowley M, et al. Evidence for cigarette smoking as a major risk factor for periodontitis. J Periodontol 1993;64:16–23.

8. Grossi SG, Zambon JJ, Ho AW, et al. Assessment of risk for periodontal disease. I. Risk indicators for attachment loss. J Periodontol 1994;65:260–7.

9. Grossi SG, Genco RJ, Machtei EE, et al. Assessment of risk for periodontal disease. II. Risk indicators for alveolar bone loss. J Periodontol 1995;66:23–9.

10. Mandel I. Smoke signals: an alert for oral disease. J Am Dent Assoc 1994;125:872–8.

11. Genco RJ. Risk factors for periodontal diseases. J Periodontol 1996;67:1041–9.

12. Bergstrom J. Cigarette smoking as risk factor in chronic periodontal disease. Dent Oral Epidemiol 1989;17:245–7.

13. Machtei EE, Dunford R, Hausmann E, et al. Longitudinal study of prognostic factors in established periodontitis patients. J Clin Periodontol 1997;24(2):102–9.

14. Ho AW, Grossi SG, Genco RJ. Assessment of passive smoking and risk for periodontal disease [abstract]. J Dent Res 1999;78:542.

15. Kinane DF, Rafvar M. The effects of smoking on mechanical and antimicrobial periodontal therapy. J Periodontol 1997;68:467–72.

16. Grossi SG, Zambon J, Machtei EE, et al. Effects of smoking and smoking cessation on healing after mechanical periodontal therapy. J Am Dent Assoc 1997;128:599–607.

17. Kaldahl WB, Johnson GK, Patil KD, Kalkwarf KL. Levels of cigarette consumption and response to periodontal therapy. J Periodontol 1996;67: 675–81.

18. U.S. Department of Health and Human Services. Reducing the health consequences of smoking: 25 years of progress: a report of the Surgeon General. U.S. Department of Health and Human Services, Public Health Service, Centers for Disease Control, Center for Chronic Disease Prevention and Health Promotion, Office on Smoking and Health, DHHS Publication No. (CDC) 89–8411;1989. p. 204–17.

19. McGinnis JM, Foege WH. Actual causes of death in the United States. JAMA 1993;270:2207–12.

20. U.S. Department of Health and Human Services. Mortality trends for selected smoking-related cancers and breast cancer—United States 1950– 1990. MMWR 1993;42:857,863–6.

21. U.S. Department of Health and Human Services. Cigarette smoking-attributable mortality and years of potential life lost—United States, 1990. MMWR 1993;42:645–9.

22. Wingo PA, Tong T, Bolden S. Cancer statistics, 1995. Cancer 1995;45:8–30.

23. Landis SH, Murray T, Bolden S, Wingo PA. Cancer statistics, 1998. Cancer 1998;48:6–29.

24. U.S. Department of Agriculture. Tobacco outlook and situation report. April 1996;TBS-234: tables 1,33,34.

25. U.S. Department of Health and Human Services. Medical-care expenditures attributed to cigarette smoking—United States, 1993. MMWR 1994;43:469–72.

26. Summers LH. The economic case for comprehensive tobacco legislation. Department of the Treasury remarks at the George Washington School of Health; March 25, 1998. Table 1.

27. National Cancer Institute. Cigars: health effects and trends. Smoking and tobacco control, monograph 9. National Cancer Institute; 1998. NIH Publication No. 98–1302.

28. National Cancer Institute. Smokeless tobacco or health: an international perspective. Smoking and tobacco control, monograph 2. National Cancer Institute; 1992. NIH Publication No. 93–3461.

28a. Hurt RD. Treat tobacco dependence and "bend to treat." Bull World Health Org 1999;77:367.

28b. Peto R, Lopez AD, Boreham J, Thun M, Health C Jr. Mortality from tobacco in developed countries: indirect estimations from national vital statistics. Lancet 1992;339:1268–78.

29. Linden GJ, Mullally BH. Cigarette smoking and periodontal destruction in young adults. J Periodontol 1994;65:718–23.

30. Papapanou PN. Periodontal diseases: epidemiology. Ann Periodontol 1996;1:1–36.

31. Haber J, Kent RL. Cigarette smoking in a periodontal practice. J Periodontol 1992;63:100–6.

32. Gelskey SC. Cigarette smoking and periodontitis: methodology to assess the strength of evidence in support of a casual association. Comm Dent Oral Epidemiol 1999;27:16–24.

33. Kenney EB, Kraal JH, Saxe SR, Jones J. The effect of cigarette smoke on human oral polymorphonuclear leukocytes. J Periodontal Res 1977;12:223–34.

34. Noble R, Penny B. Comparison of leukocyte count and function in smoking and nonsmoking young men. Infect Immun 1975;12:550–5.

35. Corberand J, Laharraghe P, Nguyen F, et al. In vitro effect of tobacco smoke components on the function of normal human polymorphonuclear leukocytes. Infect Immun. 1980;30:649–55.

36. MacFarlane GD, Herzberg MC, Wolff LF, Hardie NA. Refractory periodontitis associated with abnormal polymorphonuclear leukocyte phagocytosis and cigarette smoking. J Periodontol 1992;63:908–13.

37. Tew JG, Zhang J-B, Quinn S, et al. Antibody of the IgG$_2$ subclass, Actinobacillus actinomycetemeomitans and early-onset periodontitis. J Periodontol 1996;67(Suppl):317–22.

38. Costabel U, Bross KJ, Reuter C, et al. Alterations in immunoregulatory T-cell subsets in cigarette smokers: a phenotypic analysis of brochoalveolar and blood lymphocytes. Chest 1986;90:39–44.

39. Loeshe WJ, Gusberti F, Mettraux G, et al. Relationship between oxygen tension and subgingival bacterial flora in untreated human periodontal pockets. Infect Immun 1983;42:659–67.

40. Mettraux G, Gusberti F, Graf H. Oxygen tension (pO2) in untreated human periodontal pockets. J Periodontol 1984;55:516–21.

41. Venditto MA. Therapeutic considerations: lower respiratory tract infections in smokers. J Am Osteopath Assoc 1992;92:897–900.

42. Zambon JJ, Grossi SG, Machtei EE, et al. Cigarette smoking and subgingival infection. J Periodontol 1996;67:1050–5.

43. Cuff MJ, McQuade MJ, Scheidt MJ, et al. The presence of nicotine on root surfaces of periodontally diseased teeth in smokers. J Periodontol 1989; 60(10):564–9.

44. McGuire JR, McQuade MJ, Rossman JA, et al. Cotinine in saliva and gingival crevicular fluid of smokers with periodontal disease. J Periodontol 1989;60(4):176–81.

45. Silverstein P. Smoking and wound healing. Am J Med 1992;93(1A):22s–24s.

46. Raulin LA, McPherson JC III, McQuade MJ, Hanson BS. The effect of nicotine on the attachment of human fibroblasts to glass and human root surfaces in vitro. J Periodontol 1988;59(5):318–25.

47. Hanes PJ, Schuster GS, Lubas S. Binding, uptake and release of nicotine by human gingival fibroblasts. J Periodontol 1991;62(2):142–7.

48. Preber H, Begström J. The effect of non-surgical treatment on periodontal pockets in smokers and nonsmokers. J Clin Periodontol 1986; 13(4):319–23.

49. Grossi SG, Skrepcinski FB, DeCaro T, et al. Response to periodontal therapy in diabetics and smokers. J Periodontol 1996;67:1094–102.

50. Ah MK, Johnson GK, Kaldahl WB, et al. The effect of smoking on the response to periodontal therapy. J Clin Periodontol 1994;21(2):91–7.

51. Tonetti MS, Pini-Prato G, Cortellini P. Effect of cigarette smoking on periodontal healing following GTR in infrabony defects: a preliminary retrospective study. J Clin Periodontol 1995; 22(3):229–34.

52. Rosen PS, Marks MH, Reynolds MA. Influence of smoking on long-term clinical results of intrabony defects treated with regenerative therapy. J Periodontol 1996;67:1159–63.

53. Rosenberg ES, Cutler SA. The effect of cigarette smoking on the long-term success of guided tissue regeneration: a preliminary study. Ann R Austral Coll Dent Surg 1994;12(4):89–93.

54. Miller PD Jr. Root coverage with the free gingival

graft: factors associated with incomplete coverage. J Periodontol 1987;58(10):674–81.

55. Jones JK, Triplett RG. The relationship of cigarete smoking to impaired intraoral wound healing: a review of evidence and implications for patient care. J Oral Maxillofac Surg 1992;50(3):237–40.

56. Lindquist LW, Carlsson GE, Jemt T. A prospective 15-year follow-up study of mandibular fixed prosthesis supported by osseointegrated implants. Clin Oral Implant Res 1996;7:329–36.

57. Bain CA, Moy PK. The association between the failure of dental implants and cigarette smoking. Int J Oral Maxillofac Implants 1993;8:609–615.

58. Bain CA. Smoking and implant failure—benefits of a smoking cessation protocol. J Oral Maxillofac Implants 1996;11:756–759.

59. Sintonen H, Tuominen R. Exploring the determinants of periodontal treatment costs: a special focus on cigarette smoking. Soc Sci Med 1989; 29:835–44.

60. U.S. Department of Health and Human Services. The health benefits of smoking cessation: a report of the Surgeon General. Rockville, MD:U.S. Department of Health and Human Services, Centers for Disease Control and Prevention, Center for Chronic Disease Prevention and Health Education, Office on Smoking and Health; 1990. DHHS Publication No. (CDC) 90–8416, vii-viii.

61. Henningfield JE, Cohen C, Pickworth WB. Psychopharmacology of nicotine. In: Orleans CT, Slade J, editors Nicotine addiction: principles and management. New York, NY: Oxford University Press; 1993.

62. Hughes JR. Smoking as a drug dependence, a reply to Robinson and Pritchard. Psychopharmacology 1993;113:282–3.

63. Hughes JR. Nicotine withdrawal, dependence, and abuse. In Widiger TA, Frances AJ, Pincus HA, et al, editors. DMS-IV sourcebook. Washington, D.C.: American Psychiatric Association; 1994. p. 109–16.

64. U.S. Department of Health and Human Services. Preventing tobacco use among young people: a report of the Surgeon General. Washington, D.C.: U.S. Department of Health and Human Services, Public Health Service, Centers for Disease Control and Prevention, Center for Chronic Disease Prevention and Health Promotion, Office on Smoking and Health; 1994.

65. Institute of Medicine. Lynch BS, Bonnie RJ, editors. Growing up tobacco free: preventing nicotine addiction in children and youths. Washington, D.C.: National Academy Press; 1994.

66. U.S. Department of Health and Human Services. Preventing tobacco use among young people: a report of the Surgeon General. Washington, D.C.: U.S. Department of Health and Human Services, Public Health Service, Centers for Disease Control and Prevention, Center for Chronic Disease Prevention and Health Promotion, Office on Smoking and Health; 1994. p. 125–46.

67. Pierce JP, Fiore MC, Novotny TE, et al. Trends in cigarette smoking in the United States. JAMA 1989;261:61–5.

68. U.S. Department of Health and Human Services. The health consequences of smoking: nicotine addiction: a report of the Surgeon General. Rockville, MD: U.S. Department of Health and Human Services, Public Health Service, Centers for Disease Control, Center for Health Promotion and Education, Office on Smoking and Health; 1988.

69. Henningfield JE, Cohen C, Slade JD. Is nicotine more addictive than cocaine? Br J Addict 1991; 86:565–9.

70. Hughes JR, Gulliver SB, Fenwick JW. Smoking cessation among self-quitters. Health Psychol 1992;11:331–4.

71. Fiore MC. Trends in cigarette smoking in the United States: the epidemiology of tobacco use. Med Clin North Am 1992;76:289–303.

72. U.S. Department of Health and Human Services. Cigarette smoking among adults: United States, 1993. MMWR 1994;43:925–30.

73. U.S. Department of Health and Human Services. Preventing tobacco use among young people: a report of the Surgeon General. Washington, D.C.: U.S. Department of Health and Human Services, Centers for Disease Control and Prevention, Center for Chronic Disease Prevention and Health Promotion, Office on Smoking and Health; 1994.

74. Giovino GA, Henningfield JE, Tomar SL, et al. Epidemiology of tobacco use and dependence. Epidemiol Rev 1995;17:48–65.

75. Caraballo RS, Giovino GA, Pechacek TF, et al. Racial and ethnic differences in serum cotinine levels of cigarette smokers. JAMA 1998;280:135–9.

76. Perez-Stable EJ, Herrera B, Jacob P III, Benowitz NL. Nicotine metabolism and intake in black and white smokers. JAMA 1998;280:152–6.

77. Spitz MR, Shi H, Yang F, et al. Case-control study of D2 dopamine receptor gene and smoking status in lung cancer patients. J Natl Cancer Inst 1998;90:358–63.

78. U.S. Department of Health and Human Services. Tobacco use among U.S. racial/ethnic minority

groups—African Americans, American Indians and Alaska Natives, Asian Americans and Pacific Islanders, and Hispanics: a report of the Surgeon General. Atlanta, GA: U.S. Department of Health and Human Services, Centers for Disease Control and Prevention, National Center for Chronic Disease Prevention and Health Promotion, Office on Smoking and Health; 1998.

79. Fant RV, Everson D, Dayton G, et al. Nicotine dependence in women. J Am Med Wom Assoc 1996;51:19–20,22–3.

80. U.S. Department of Health and Human Services. The health benefits of smoking cessation: a report of the Surgeon General. Washington, D.C.: U.S. Government Printing Office; 1990 DHHS Publication No. (CDC) 90–8416.

81. Gritz ER, Nielsen IR, Brooks LA. Smoking cessation and gender: the influence of physiological, psychological, and behavioral factors. J Am Med Wom Assoc 1996;51:35–42.

82. Tomar SL, Husten CG, Manley MW. Do dentists and physicians advise tobacco users to quit? J Am Dent Assoc 1996;127:259–65.

83. Dolan TA, McGorray SP, Grinstead-Skigen CL, Mecklenburg RE. Tobacco control activities in U.S. dental practices. J Am Dent Assoc 1997; 128:1669–79.

84. Hayes C, Kressin N, Garcia R, et al. Tobacco control practices: how do Massachusetts dentists compare with dentists nationwide? J Massachusetts Dent Soc 1997;46:9–12,14.

85. Mecklenburg RE. Tobacco: addiction, oral health, and cessation. Quint Int 1998;29:250–2.

86. Orleans CT. In: Orleans CT, Slade J, editors: Nicotine addiction: principles and management. New York, NY: Oxford University Press; 1993. P. ix.

87. National Cancer Institute. Smoking, tobacco, and cancer program: 1985–1989 status report. Bethesda, MD: U.S. Department of Health and Human Services, Public Health Service, National Institutes of Health, National Cancer Institute; 1990. NIH Publication No. 90–3107.

88. Ockene JK, Kristellar J, Goldberg R. Increasing the efficacy of physician-delivered smoking interventions: a randomized clinical trial. J Gen Intern Med 1991;6:1–8.

89. Cohen SJ, Stookey GK, Katz BP, et al. Encouraging primary care physicians to help smokers quit: a randomized, controlled trial. Ann Intern Med 1989;110:648–52.

90. Cummings SR, Coates TJ, Richard RJ, et al. Training physicians in counseling about smoking cessation: a randomized trial of the "Quit for Life"

program. Ann Intern Med 1989;110:640–7.

91. Wilson DMC, Taylor DW, Gilbert JR, et al. A randomized trial of a family physician intervention for smoking cessation. JAMA 1988;260:1570–4.

92. Kottke TE, Brekkle MI, Solberg LI, Hughes JR. A randomized trial to increase smoking intervention by physicians: doctors helping smokers, round I. JAMA 1989;261:2101–6.

93. Cohen SJ, Stookey GK, Katz BP, et al. Helping smokers quit: a randomized controlled trial with private practice dentists. J Am Dent Assoc 1989;118:41–5.

94. Hollis JF, Lichtenstein E, Vogt TM, et al. Nurse-assisted counseling for smokers in primary care. Ann Intern Med 1993;118:521–5.

95. Dix SM, McGhan WF, Lauger G. Pharmacist counseling and outcomes of smoking cessation. Am Pharm 1995;NS35:20–32.

96. Wewers ME, Bowen JM, Stanislaw AE, Desimone VB. A nurse-delivered smoking cessation intervention among hospitalized postoperative patients—influence of a smoking-related diagnosis: a pilot study. Heart Lung 1994;23:151–6.

97. National Cancer Institute. Tobacco and the clinician: interventions for medical and dental practitioners. U.S. Department of Health and Human Services, Public Health Service, National Institutes of Health, 1994. NIH Publication No. 94–3693.

97a. Cincirpini PM, McClure JB. Smoking cessation: recent developments in behavioral and pharmacologic interventions. Table 2. Oncology 1998; 12:249–259.

98. Fiore MC, Bailey WC, Cohen SJ, et al. Clinic practice guideline number 18: smoking cessation. U.S. Department of Health and Human Services, Public Health Service, Agency for Health Care Policy and Research, Centers for Disease Control and Prevention; 1996. AHCPR Publication No. 96–0692.

99. Fiore MC, Bailey WC, Cohen SJ, et al. Smoking cessation: information for specialists. U.S. Department of Health and Human Services, Public Health Service, Agency for Health Care Policy and Research, Centers for Disease Control and Prevention; 1996. AHCPR Publication No. 96–0694.

100. Hughes JR, Fiester S, Goldstein MG, et al. Practice guidelines for the treatment of patients with nicotine dependence. Am J Psychiatry 1996; 153:S1–31.

101. Glynn TJ, Manley MW. How to help your patients stop smoking: a National Cancer Institute manual for physicians. U.S. Department of Health

and Human Services, Public Health Service, National Institutes of Health; 1989. NIH Publication No. 90–3064.

102. Husten CG, Manley MW. How to help your patients stop smoking. Am Fam Phys 1990;42: 1017–26.

103. Fiore MC. The new vital sign. JAMA 1991;266: 3183–4.

104. Fiore MC, Jorenby DE, Schensky AE, et al. Smoking status as the new vital sign: effect on assessment and intervention in patients who smoke. Mayo Clin Proc 1995;70:209–13.

105. Cohen SJ, Christen AG, Katz BP, et al. Counseling medical and dental patients about cigarette smoking: the impact of nicotine gum and chart reminders. Am J Public Health 1987;77:313–6.

106. Fiore MC, Jorenby DE, Baker TB, Kenford SL. Tobacco dependence and the nicotine patch: clinical guidelines for effective use. JAMA 1992;268:2687–94.

107. Henningfield JE. Nicotine medications for smoking cessation. N Eng J Med 1995;333:1196–203.

108. Hjalmarson A, Franzon M, Westin A, Wiklund O. Effect of nicotine nasal spray on smoking cessation. A randomized, placebo-controlled, double-blind study. Arch Intern Med 1994;154: 2567–72.

109. Benowitz NL, Zevin S, Jacob P III. Sources of variability in nicotine and cotinine levels with use of nicotine nasal spray, transdermal nicotine, and cigarette smoking. Br J Clin Pharmacol 1997; 43:259–67.

110. Leischow SJ, Nilsson F, Franzon M, et al. Efficacy of the nicotine inhaler as an adjunct to smoking cessation. Am J Health Behav 1996;20:364–71.

111. Schneider NG, Olmstead R, Nilsson F, et al. Efficacy of a nicotine inhaler in smoking cessation: a double-blind, placebo-controlled trial. Addiction 1996;91:1293–306.

112. Ostrowski DJ, DeNelsky GY. Pharmacologic management of patients using smoking cessation aids. Dent Clin North Am 1996;40:779–801.

113. Fagerstrom KO, Tejding R, Westin A, Lunell E. Aiding reduction of smoking with nicotine replacement medications: hope for the recalcitrant smoker? Tobacco Cont 1997;6:311–6.

114. Warner KE, Slade J, Sweanor DT. The emerging market for long-term nicotine maintenance. JAMA 1997;278:1087–92.

115. Hurt RD, Sachs DPL, Glover ED, et al. A comparison of sustained-release bupropion and placebo for smoking cessation. N Engl J Med 1997;337:1195–202.

116. Somerman M, Mecklenburg RE. Cessation of tobacco use. In Ciancio SG, editors. ADA guide to dental therapeutics. Chicago, IL: ADA Publishing Company; 1998. p. 505–16.

117. Hughes JR, Goldstein MG, Hurt RD, Shiffman S. Recent advances in the pharmacotherapy of smoking. JAMA 1999;281:72–6.

118. Prochaska J, DeClemente C, Norcross J. In search of how people change: applications to addiction behaviors. Am Psychol 1992;47:1102–14.

119. Patton GC, Carlin JB, Coffey C, et al. Depression, anxiety, and smoking initiation: a prospective study over 3 years. Am J Public Health 1998;88: 1518–22.

120. Nisell M, Nomikos GG, Svenson TH. Nicotine dependence, midbrain dopamine systems and psychiatric disorders. J Pharmacol 1995;76: 157–62.

121. Glassman AH, Helzer JE, Covey LS, et al. Smoking, smoking cessation, and major depression. JAMA 1990;264:1546–9.

122. Thorndyke AN, Rigotti NA, Stafford RS, Singer DE. National patterns in the treatment of smokers by physicians. JAMA 1998;279:604–8.

123. Cromwell J, Bartosch WJ, Fiore MC, et al. Cost-effectiveness of the clinical recommendations in the AHCPR guideline for smoking cessation. JAMA 1997;278:1759–66.

CHAPTER 8

DIABETES MELLITUS

Brian Mealey, DDS, MS

Diabetes mellitus is a disease of metabolic dysregulation, primarily of carbohydrate metabolism, characterized by hyperglycemia (elevated blood glucose) that results from defects in insulin secretion, impaired insulin action, or both. Alterations in lipid and protein metabolism are also seen. Chronic elevation in blood glucose is associated with long-term dysfunction and damage to numerous organs, especially the eyes, kidneys, heart, nerves, and blood vessels.

Approximately 16 million Americans (6 to 7% of the population) have diabetes, but about half these individuals are unaware that they have the disease.[1] More than 600,000 new cases are diagnosed each year, and the worldwide prevalence of diabetes is projected to double between 1994 and 2010, to 240 million.[2,3] The number of cases in the United States continues to rise due to increasing population and life expectancy, combined with an increased prevalence of obesity, which is strongly associated with the most common form of diabetes. The total direct and indirect costs of diabetes constitute almost 12% of all annual health care costs in the United States, exceeding $90 billion.[4] Given the high prevalence of this disease, it is likely that every practicing dentist will encounter patients with diabetes. In a dental practice with 2,000 patients and an average prevalence of 6 to 7%, approximately 120 to 140 patients would have diabetes. Again, only half these people would be aware of their diabetic condition.

CLASSIFICATION AND PATHOPHYSIOLOGY OF DIABETES

Over the past three decades, the diagnosis and classification of diabetes has undergone numerous changes. In 1997, the American Diabetes Association provided the current classification.[5] The two most common forms are type 1 diabetes, formerly called insulin-dependent diabetes, and type 2 diabetes, previously known as non–insulin-dependent diabetes (Table 8–1). Because insulin injection is frequently used in the treatment of both forms of diabetes, the terms "insulin-dependent" and "non–insulin-dependent" were often confusing. The new classification is based on the underlying pathophysiology of the disease types, rather than on treatment approaches.

Gestational diabetes is another form of the disease that occurs during pregnancy and generally resolves after parturition. Other, less common forms of diabetes may be related to genetic defects in insulin-secreting cells in the pancreas, genetic defects in insulin action, pancreatic diseases or injuries, drug- or chemical-induced changes in metabolism, other endocrine disorders, infections, and genetic syndromes of which diabetes is one component.[5]

TABLE 8–1. Classification of Diabetes Mellitus

- Type 1 diabetes (formerly, insulin-dependent diabetes)
- Type 2 diabetes (formerly, non–insulin-dependent diabetes)
- Gestational diabetes
- Other types of diabetes
  - Genetic defects in β cell function
  - Genetic defects in insulin action
  - Pancreatic diseases or injuries
    Pancreatitis, neoplasia, cystic fibrosis, trauma, pancreatectomy
  - Infections
    Cytomegalovirus, congenital rubella
  - Drug-induced or chemical-induced diabetes
    Glucocorticoids, thyroid hormone
  - Endocrinopathies
    Acromegaly, pheochromocytoma, glucagonoma, hyperthyroidism, Cushing's syndrome
  - Other genetic syndromes with associated diabetes

During digestion, most foods are broken down into glucose, which then enters the circulatory system and is subsequently used by tissue cells for energy and growth (Figure 8–1). Most cells, excluding those in the brain and central nervous system, require the presence of insulin to allow glucose entry. Insulin binds to specific cellular receptors to exert its effects. Insulin is produced by the β cells of the pancreas, and increased insulin secretion occurs in response to increased blood glucose concentrations. With the secretion of insulin from the pancreas into the circulatory system and its subsequent binding to its cellular receptors, glucose is able to exit the bloodstream and enter the tissues, resulting in its utilization by the cells and thus decreased blood glucose concentrations. Decreased insulin production or diminished insulin action will alter glucose metabolism and result in hyperglycemia. Conversely, increased insulin levels may cause hypoglycemia (low blood glucose).

The excess glucose that is not required by the body for current activity is stored in the liver in the form of glycogen. In the fasting state, or when glucose demand exceeds glucose available from recent food consumption, the liver breaks down glycogen and releases glucose into the bloodstream through the process of glycogenolysis. The liver also produces glucose through the process of gluconeogenesis—the production of glucose from noncarbohydrate sources such as amino acids and fatty acids.

Insulin is the primary hormone that reduces blood glucose levels. A group of counter-regulato-ry hormones serve to balance glycemia (Table 8–2). While these hormones have a wide variety of functions, they all result in elevation of blood glucose. If insulin function is normal, as in the nondiabetic patient, elevated blood glucose levels resulting from secretion of counter-regulatory hormones are quickly normalized through compensatory secretion of endogenous insulin. If, however, insulin secretion is impaired, as in the diabetic patient, elevated blood glucose levels in response to counter-regulatory hormone release will remain elevated. For example, if an individual with type 1 diabetes is placed under significant stress, epinephrine and cortisol are released. This causes an increase in blood glucose levels. Since the patient is unable to secrete insulin, hyperglycemia results.

Type 1 Diabetes

Type 1 diabetes is caused by cell-mediated autoimmune destruction of the insulin-producing β cells in the pancreas. This results in absolute insulin deficiency; the individual no longer produces insulin. The rate of β-cell destruction is variable. Some individuals, especially children and adolescents, quickly develop signs and symptoms of type 1 diabetes following rapid destruction of β cells. Others retain some insulin-producing capacity as the β cells are slowly destroyed. Numerous markers are available for assessing risk and aiding diagnosis of type 1 diabetes, including autoantibodies to pancreatic islet cells, insulin, glutamic acid decarboxylase, and tyrosine phosphatases.[5] One or more of these markers can be detected in 90% of type 1 diabetic patients at the time of initial diagnosis.

Type 1 diabetes has multiple genetic predispositions but is also strongly related to various environmental factors. Monozygous (identical) twins have a concordance rate for type 1 diabetes of approximately 30 to 50%. Thus, less than half the monozygous siblings of patients with type 1 diabetes will be diagnosed with the disease. This suggests that envi-

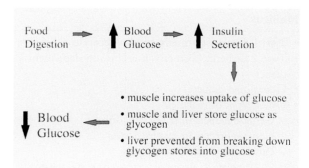

Figure 8–1. Insulin control of blood glucose. Hormonal control of blood glucose by insulin. Ingestion of food results in increased blood glucose levels. The pancreas is stimulated to increase insulin secretion. Insulin then allows glucose to enter cells, especially muscle. Insulin also stimulates storage of excess glucose by muscle and the liver in the form of glycogen. Insulin prevents the breakdown of stored glycogen into glucose by the liver. The net result is a decrease in blood glucose levels. Glycogen stores are used during periods of fasting or increased tissue glucose demand.

TABLE 8–2. Hormonal Control of Glycemia

Hormones that raise blood glucose
- Glucagon
- Catecholamines (epinephrine)
- Growth hormone
- Thyroid hormone
- Glucocorticoids (cortisol)

Hormone that lowers blood glucose
- Insulin

TABLE 8–3. Characteristics of Type 1 and Type 2 Diabetes

	Type 1 Diabetes	Type 2 Diabetes
Age at onset	Generally <30 years	Generally in adulthood
Most common body type	Thin or normal stature	Obese
Race most commonly affected (in the United States)	White	African American, Hispanic, American Indian, Pacific Islanders
Family history	Common	More common
Rapidity of clinical onset	Abrupt	Slow
Pathogenesis	Autoimmune β cell destruction	Insulin resistance, impaired insulin secretion, increased liver glucose production
Endogenous insulin production	None	Decreased, normal, or elevated
Susceptibility to ketoacidosis	High	Low
Treatment may include	Diet, exercise, insulin	Diet, exercise, oral agents, insulin

ronmental influences are superimposed on the genetic components. Susceptibility to type 1 diabetes is linked to the presence of certain genetically determined antigens found on the cell surface of lymphocytes (human leukocyte antigens [HLA]). These HLA associations are linked primarily to DQ and DR genes. Some HLA loci, such as DR3 and DR4, are associated with increased risk for developing type 1 diabetes while other loci may be protective. Alterations in these major histocompatibility complex (MHC) antigens on cell surfaces may explain why individuals become intolerant of self-antigens, resulting in T-cell-mediated destruction of pancreatic β cells. The complex genetic susceptibility of type 1 diabetes is not clearly understood.

Onset of β–cell destruction in people with a genetic susceptibility to type 1 diabetes may be initiated by an environmental event. Viral infections have long been targeted as possible triggering events although evidence is not conclusive. Of particular interest are coxsackie virus, cytomegalovirus, and rubella infections. A working model of type 1 diabetes suggests that an environmental event may cause focal damage to pancreatic β cells.[3] The autoantigens that are then released from the damaged β cells are taken up by antigen-presenting cells such as macrophages. The autoantigens are then processed and presented to host T helper cells, which respond via increased cytokine production. These cytokines cause influx into the pancreatic islets of both nonspecific and antigen-specific mononuclear inflammatory cells. These cells release cytokines that eventually result in the death of β cells and loss of insulin production.

The onset of type 1 diabetes occurs most often before the age of 30 years; in fact, type 1 diabetes was once known as "juvenile" diabetes (Table 8–3). However, it may be diagnosed at any age. Onset of clinical symptoms is usually abrupt. Most people with type 1 diabetes are of normal weight or are thin in stature. The lack of endogenous insulin production makes the type 1 individual dependent on exogenous insulin injections for survival.

People with type 1 diabetes are highly susceptible to ketoacidosis.[2] In the absence of adequate insulin levels, glucose cannot be used by the tissue and remains in the bloodstream, leading to cellular starvation. Body fat stores are then broken down for energy through the process of lipolysis. The glycerol portion of triglyceride is converted to glucose, and free fatty acids are released. With prolonged insulin deficiency, lipolysis continues and fatty acids are converted to ketones. Increased ketone levels in body fluids lead to excretion of ketones in the urine. Large amounts of water are excreted along with ketones, resulting in dehydration. Diabetic ketoacidosis results from accumulation of ketones in body fluids, increased loss of electrolytes in the urine, and alterations in the bicarbonate buffer system (Table 8–4). If not treated properly, severe acidosis can lead to coma or death.

Severe diabetic ketoacidosis usually occurs when the signs and symptoms of undiagnosed type 1 diabetes are not recognized or when the known diabetic patient's glycemia is poorly controlled. For many individuals, a diagnosis of type 1 diabetes is not made until they are hospitalized for treatment of acute ketoacidosis. In the patient with previously diagnosed type 1 diabetes, ketoacidosis may be precipitated by systemic infection or stress. Elevated levels of cortisol, epinephrine, or glucagon as a result of stress promote increased

TABLE 8–4. Signs, Symptoms, and Laboratory Findings in Diabetic Ketoacidosis

Nausea and vomiting
Abdominal pain
Dehydration
  • Dry mucous membranes
  • Tachycardia
  • Hypotension
  • Abnormal skin turgor
Kussmaul's respiration
Altered mental state
Possible coma
Hyperglycemia
Increased blood urea nitrogen (BUN) and serum
  creatinine
Decreased serum potassium and phosphorus
Acidosis (arterial pH <7.3)

hepatic glucose production and ketogenesis. Ketoacidosis is often seen when the type 1 diabetic person remains hyperglycemic for several days or longer due to inadequate amounts of exogenous insulin or excessive amounts of glucose intake. Many people with type 1 diabetes suffer multiple episodes of diabetic ketoacidosis as a result of poor daily glycemic control.

Type 2 Diabetes

Type 2 diabetes is much more common than type 1, constituting 90% of all diabetic cases. While type 1 diabetes is most common in Caucasian Americans, the prevalence of type 2 is higher in African Americans, Hispanics, American Indians, and Pacific Islanders.[5] The highest prevalence and incidence of type 2 diabetes in the United States is found in the Pima Indian population of Arizona, in which almost 50% of those between 30 and 65 years of age have the disease. Type 2 diabetes commonly leads not only to hyperglycemia but also to hypertension, dyslipidemia (elevated triglycerides and/or decreased high-density lipoprotein), central obesity (abdominal), and atherosclerosis. This group of disorders is often called "the insulin resistance syndrome," or "syndrome X."[5,6]

The pathophysiology of type 2 diabetes is different from that of type 1. While the specific etiologies are not known, autoimmune destruction of β cells does not occur. Type 2 diabetes is characterized by three major abnormalities: (1) peripheral resistance to insulin, particularly in muscle; (2) impaired pancreatic insulin secretion; and (3) increased glucose production by the liver. The clinical effect of these disorders is the same as in type 1 diabetes, namely, hyperglycemia. Evidence strongly suggests that the initial defect in the pathogenesis of type 2 diabetes is insulin resistance, which is eventually followed by impaired insulin secretion.[7]

Even though the pancreas still produces insulin, the presence of insulin resistance prevents transport of glucose into tissue cells, causing hyperglycemia. Relative to nondiabetic individuals, pancreatic insulin secretion may also be decreased, worsening hyperglycemia. Paradoxically, in many type 2 diabetic patients, there is actually an increase in insulin production. This is a direct result of insulin resistance and the subsequent decrease in glucose utilization. The pancreas may respond to poor glucose utilization and hyperglycemia by a compensatory increase in insulin production, resulting in hyperinsulinemia. There may also be differences in pathophysiology within the type 2 diabetic population. The majority of people with type 2 diabetes are obese, and these individuals tend to exhibit significant insulin resistance accompanied by hyperinsulinemia. Obesity itself can result in insulin resistance, even in the absence of diabetes.[8] Conversely, thin individuals with type 2 diabetes primarily suffer from impaired insulin secretion, with insulin resistance being less severe than in obese people.[5]

Type 2 diabetes has a stronger genetic component than type 1, with a concordance rate of up to 90% in identical twins.[9] Unfortunately, while over 250 genes have been tested for possible relationships with type 2 diabetes, none has shown consistent associations in multiple study populations.[10] It is possible that no single genetic defect is responsible for type 2 diabetes. Besides obesity, acquired risk factors for type 2 diabetes include advancing age and a sedentary lifestyle.

Unlike the sudden onset of clinical symptoms in type 1 diabetes, type 2 diabetes may remain undiagnosed for years. Thus, it is estimated that about half of all patients with type 2 diabetes are unaware of their condition. Because they still produce endogenous insulin, people with type 2 diabetes are not generally dependent on exogenous insulin administration for survival. However, a large number of these individuals take insulin injections as a part of their treatment regimen. Type 2 diabetic patients are also resistant to ketosis since their pancreatic insulin production is usually sufficient to suppress ketone formation. Under conditions of extreme physiologic stress, type 2 patients may develop ketoacidosis. With prolonged hyperglycemia, individuals with type 2 diabetes may develop hyperosmolar nonketotic acidosis. Excretion of large amounts of glucose in the urine is accompanied by significant water loss. Failure to replace lost fluids may lead to electrolyte imbalance and acidosis in the absence of ketones. Another similar entity called hyperosmolar nonacidotic diabetes is characterized by severe hyperglycemia (plasma glucose >600 mg/dL), hyperosmolarity, and dehydration. This disorder is associated with severe fluid depletion and renal impairment, with a high mortality rate.

Impaired Glucose Tolerance/Impaired Fasting Glucose

Impaired glucose tolerance (IGT) and impaired fasting glucose (IFG) imply a metabolic state between normal glycemia and diabetes. Many people with IGT have normal blood glucose levels most of the time, often manifesting hyperglycemia only after challenge with a large glucose load.[4] Those with IFG have elevated fasting glucose levels but may be normal in a fed state. Both IGT and IFG are not considered to be clinical entities in themselves. Rather, they are primarily risk factors for future development of diabetes.[11] In fact, they can be seen as intermediate stages in all types of diabetes. Both IGT and IFG are strongly associated with insulin resistance and with syndrome X.[6] Endogenous insulin production is normal and remains so in the majority of IGT/IFG patients. However, about 30 to 40% of patients with IGT/IFG will develop type 2 diabetes within 10 years after initial diagnosis. During the transition to type 2 diabetes, several changes occur.[5] Insulin resistance increases and insulin secretion is impaired as β-cell function diminishes. Hepatic glucose production also increases. Eventually, the patient manifests overt clinical and laboratory signs of diabetes.

Patients with IGT/IFG are not at increased risk for microvascular complications such as those seen in diabetic individuals. However, they are at greater risk for cardiovascular disease than are people with normal glucose tolerance. The reasons why IGT and IFG increase the risk of cardiovascular disease are not well understood. Both IGT and IFG are frequently associated with hypertension, hypertriglyceridemia, and low levels of high-density lipoproteins (HDL), all well-known risk factors for cardiovascular disease. Thus, IGT/IFG may not be directly involved in the pathogenesis of cardio-

vascular disease but may be risk factors in conjunction with other components of syndrome X.

Gestational Diabetes

Gestational diabetes usually develops during the third trimester of pregnancy but can occur earlier. About 4% of all pregnancies in the United States are complicated by gestational diabetes.[12] An increased prevalence of gestational diabetes is seen in women who are overweight, older than 25 years of age, have a family history of diabetes, and are members of ethnic groups with higher prevalence rates for type 2 diabetes (African American, Hispanic, American Indian).[13,14] The disorder appears to have a similar pathophysiology to IGT/IFG and type 2 diabetes, ie, it is strongly associated with insulin resistance.

Gestational diabetes significantly increases perinatal morbidity and mortality as well as increasing the rate of cesarean delivery.[15] Diagnosis of gestational diabetes is important because proper management significantly improves pregnancy outcomes.[16] About 6 weeks or more after parturition, women with gestational diabetes are reclassified as having either diabetes, IGT, IFG, or normoglycemia. Most patients who develop gestational diabetes return to normal after delivery. Others will be diagnosed at some time postpartum with IGT, IFG, type 1 or type 2 diabetes. It is estimated that 30 to 50% of women with a history of gestational diabetes will develop type 2 diabetes within 10 years of the initial diagnosis.

CLASSIC COMPLICATIONS OF DIABETES

In addition to dysregulation in carbohydrate, lipid and protein metabolism, type 1 and type 2 diabetes are associated with a classic group of microvascular and macrovascular complications (Table 8–5). While the microvascular complications of retinopathy, nephropathy, and neuropathy are specifically associated with diabetes, macrovascular diseases occur in the nondiabetic population as well. However, the risk of macrovascular disease is greatly increased in diabetic patients.

These complications are the major cause of the high morbidity and mortality of diabetes. The diabetic patient has a dramatically increased risk for visual impairment or blindness, kidney failure, limb amputation, stroke, and myocardial infarction. Sustained hyperglycemia plays a central role

TABLE 8–5. Classic Complications of Diabetes Mellitus

Retinopathy
- Blindness

Nephropathy
- Renal failure

Neuropathy
- Sensory
- Autonomic

Macrovascular disease (accelerated atherosclerosis)
- Peripheral
- Cardiovascular (coronary artery disease)
- Cerebrovascular (stroke)

Altered wound healing

in the onset and progression of diabetic complications. The duration of diabetes is an important risk factor as the prevalence of these complications increases with longer duration of disease. Hypertension and dyslipidemia are also risk factors for both microvascular and macrovascular complications. There are also genetic influences affecting the propensity to develop these complications.

Vascular complications of diabetes result from microangiopathy and atherosclerosis.[17–19] Changes in the blood vessels include endothelial proliferation and thickening of the basement membrane, thickening of the walls of larger vessels, and increased lipid deposition and atheroma formation. These changes occur throughout the body and are primarily responsible for the majority of diabetic complications.

Diabetic retinopathy consists of both proliferative and nonproliferative changes in the retina. Development of retinopathy increases as the duration of diabetes increases and is more common in type 1 diabetes.[19] After 15 years' duration of type 1 diabetes, about 95% of individuals have some degree of retinopathy, with about 50% having the more advanced form of proliferative retinopathy. The earliest retinal changes are nonproliferative and include dilation, occlusion, and increased permeability of retinal blood vessels. The basement membrane of retinal capillaries thickens, and microaneurysms develop. Extravasation of blood from the capillaries results in soft and hard exudate formation on the retina. Microaneurysms tend to occur near the macula, the region of the retina responsible for visual acuity and central vision. Macular edema may result from hemorrhages and deposit formation, leading to loss of central vision and acuity. Capillary occlusion causes retinal ischemia, which may then lead to proliferation of abnormal blood vessels and fibrous tissue from the surface of the retina out into the vitreous, a process known as proliferative retinopathy. These new blood vessels are fragile and may bleed into the vitreous. As that blood is reabsorbed from the vitreous, scarring occurs. Over time, macular edema and proliferative retinopathy may lead to severe vision loss or blindness.[2,19]

Renal failure is the leading cause of death in the type 1 diabetic population. Approximately 35 to 45% of type 1 patients develop nephropathy, compared with about 20% of type 2 individuals. The mesangium, the membrane supporting the capillary loops in the renal glomeruli, expands due to increased production of mesangial matrix proteins.[18] As the mesangium expands, the surface area for glomerular capillary filtration decreases, and the glomerular filtration rate (GFR) declines. The basement membrane in glomerular capillaries also thickens, further decreasing glomerular filtration. Clinically, the earliest sign of diabetic nephropathy is the excretion of small amounts of albumin in the urine (microalbuminuria). With progressive disease and reduction in glomerular filtration capacity, macroalbuminuria may develop, with large amounts of protein excreted in the urine (proteinuria). Increased renal blood pressure may also occur. The expanding mesangium, thickening of capillary basement membranes, renal hypertension, and declining GFR may then progress to end-stage renal disease. Patients with end-stage renal disease are treated with hemodialysis, peritoneal dialysis, or kidney transplantation, each of which has its own host of potential complications and adverse sequelae.

Diabetic neuropathy occurs in up to 50% of diabetic patients, its prevalence increasing with the duration of diabetes.[20] Neuropathy may affect the sensory, motor, and autonomic nerves. Peripheral sensorimotor neuropathy is the most common variety, frequently manifesting as numbness or tingling of the toes or feet. This may be accompanied by muscle weakness or cramping, alterations in gait, and burning pain. As neuropathy worsens, the paresthesia or dysesthesia may disappear and be replaced by hypoesthesia or even anesthesia. This reduction in sensory ability makes the affected areas highly prone to injury since the patient is unable to perceive painful stimuli. Diabetic foot ulcers resulting from repetitive injury to an insensate foot are a major cause of hospitalization and amputation. The patient is unable to perceive pain in the limb, leading to repeated trauma. When combined with alterations in wound healing capacity and changes in the peripheral vasculature, this otherwise relatively minor injury may lead to gangrene and amputation of the affected area (Figures 8–2).

Diabetic neuropathy may also affect the autonomic nervous system. Cardiovascular autonomic neuropathy can lead to dysrhythmias and alterations in blood pressure. Genitourinary neuropathy may cause incontinence due to hypotonia or atonia of the bladder. Sensory and autonomic genitourinary neuropathy often leads to impotence in diabetic men. Diabetic gastroparesis results from gastrointestinal neuropathy and manifests as delayed gastric emptying, sensation of fullness, nausea and vomiting. Diabetic diarrhea may present as nocturnal diarrhea or incontinence, alternating with periods of constipation. The mechanisms involved in diabetic neuropathy are not completely understood. Sustained hyperglycemia is certainly involved and alterations in specific glucose-linked biochemical processes may lead to progressive structural and functional nerve changes.[2,20]

The most common cause of death in type 2 diabetes is myocardial infarction, underlining the importance of macrovascular complications in these individuals.[17] Similarly, macrovascular complications are very common in type 1 diabetes. Atherosclerosis affects the cardiac, cerebral, and peripheral vasculature. Atherosclerosis and coronary artery disease are not unique to the diabetic population, but the risk and incidence of these changes are significantly increased in diabetes. Hyperglycemia plays an important role in macrovascular disease. Increased intimal thickness and atheroma formation are related to hyperglycemia-induced tissue alterations. Increased thickness of vessel walls leads to partial obstruction and reduced blood flow. Atheroma formation further narrows the vessels, diminishing the flow of blood. Decreased blood flow in peripheral vessels leads to alteration in tissue homeostasis and wound healing. In central vessels, reduction in blood flow places major organs such as the heart and brain at risk for altered function.[17]

Poorly controlled or previously undiagnosed diabetic patients have major modifications in their lipoprotein metabolism.[21,22] Triglyceride levels are often dramatically elevated while HDL levels are decreased. Low-density lipoprotein (LDL) levels may be normal, but there are often changes in LDL composition. In some cases, LDL levels are also markedly elevated. Improved glycemic control generally improves lipoprotein metabolism.

Hyperglycemia increases the oxidation of LDL, and oxidized LDL is much more atherogenic than the native form. Thrombus formation is also greatly enhanced in the diabetic patient. Increased fibrin deposition along the vessel wall and increased platelet aggregation lead to formation of intravascular microthrombi.[22] These alterations can cause intermittent hypercoagulation. Increased formation of atheromas and microthrombi in the diabetic patient results in increased risk for thromboembolic events such as stroke and myocardial infarction. Peripheral thromboemboli place end-terminal organs at risk for poor oxygenation and exchange of metabolic waste products. Risk factors commonly associated with atherosclerosis, coronary artery disease, and stroke in the nondiabetic population—smoking, hypertension, obesity, and dyslipidemia—also apply to diabetes patients. The presence of diabetes, however, warrants more aggressive management and alteration of these risk factors.

The underlying pathophysiology of diabetes complications is complex and diverse. Hyperglycemia is, in large part, responsible for both the macrovascular and microvascular complications. Hyperglycemia alters cell function and produces a cascade of events leading to the structural changes seen in affected tissues. Current research has focused on alterations in lipoprotein metabolism and on nonenzymatic glycosylation of proteins as possible common links between these various complications.

Because the physical and chemical properties of membranes are determined, in part, by the fatty

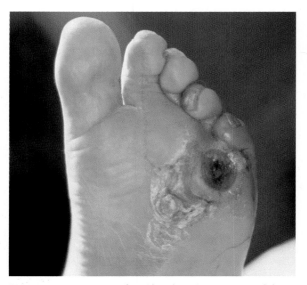

Figure 8–2. Gangrenous foot (dorsal view) in patient with long-standing diabetes mellitus. Foot was amputated due to extensive tissue necrosis (Photograph courtesy of Dr. Kathyrn Cripps).

acids within the phospholipid bilayer, alterations in lipid metabolism may have wide-ranging effects on cellular function.[21] Oxidization of LDL in the hyperglycemic patient may increase oxidant stress, inducing chemotaxis of monocytes/macrophages in affected tissues such as vessel walls. Once resident within the affected tissue site, oxidized LDL may induce alterations in cellular adhesion as well as increased production of chemotactic factors, cytokines, and growth factors.[23] This may then lead to increased vessel wall thickness and formation of atheromas and microthrombi in the large vessels and alterations in endothelial cell function and vascular permeability in the microvasculature.

Another common link between the complications of diabetes is the glycosylation of proteins, lipids, and nucleic acids.[24,25] In many diabetic patients, the small blood vessels of the retina, glomerulus, and endoneurial region and the walls of the large blood vessels accumulate deposits of carbohydrate-containing plasma proteins. In addition, expansion of the extracellular matrix is seen in all these sites. Increased basement membrane thickness is noted in the retina and around the nerves, the mesangial matrix is thickened in the glomerulus, and accumulation of collagen is seen in the diabetic arteries. The cumulative effect is a progressive narrowing of the vessel lumen and decreased perfusion of affected organs.

The carbohydrate-containing proteins which accumulate in patients with sustained hyperglycemia are known as advanced glycosylation end-products (AGEs).[24-26] Formation of AGEs begins with the attachment of glucose to the amino groups on proteins to form an unstable Schiff base adduct (Figure 8–3). Through a slow chemical rearrange-ment, these are converted to a more stable but still reversible glucose-protein adduct known as an Amadori product. Normalization of glycemia at this stage results in reversal of the Amadori product. Thus, while these early glycosylation products increase when blood glucose levels are elevated, a return to normal glycemia results in their reversal, and they do not accumulate in tissues. If hyperglycemia is sustained, the Amadori products become highly stable and form AGEs. Because AGEs are irreversible, once formed, they remain attached to proteins for the lifetime of those proteins. Thus, even if hyperglycemia is corrected, the level of AGEs in the affected tissues does not return to normal.

Formation of AGEs varies among individuals; AGEs form in everyone, not only in people with diabetes. The accumulation of AGEs also increases with age and may be the basis for many age-related physiologic changes. However, AGE accumulation is greatly increased in many diabetic patients.[24,25] There is significant heterogeneity in AGE formation within the diabetic population. It is thought that this heterogeneity may provide a partial explanation for the variation in the incidence of complications seen in diabetes. While hyperglycemia is distinctly linked to the onset and progression of diabetic complications, there are many poorly controlled diabetic individuals who do not develop significant complications. Conversely, some patients with well-controlled diabetes still develop complications. It is postulated that the differences between individuals in AGE accumulation may explain some of this variance in complications within the diabetic population.

Advanced glycosylation end-products form on collagen, a major component of the extracellular matrix. Once formed, AGEs cause increased collagen cross-linking, resulting in the formation of highly stable collagen macromolecules that are resistant to normal enzymatic degradation and tissue turnover.[24-26] This causes the accumulation of protein at the affected site. In the blood vessel wall, AGE-modified collagen accumulates, thickening the vessel wall and narrowing the lumen. In addition, circulating LDL in the vessel lumen is immobilized in the presence of AGE-modified arterial collagen.[21,24,25] The amount of LDL that covalently cross-links to collagen increases as levels of AGE increase. Therefore, hyperglycemia contributes to formation of increasing levels of AGE-modified collagen in the vessel wall. Circulating LDL becomes cross-linked to this AGE-modified collagen and contributes to atheroma formation in the diabetic macrovasculature.

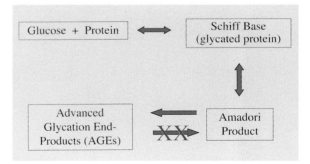

Figure 8–3. Advanced glycosylation end-product formation. Glucose attaches to the amino-terminal end of proteins to form unstable Schiff-base adduct. Over a period of weeks, this product stabilizes to form a reversible Amadori product. With sustained hyperglycemia, the Amadori product rearranges to form irreversible advanced glycosylation end-product.

The formation of AGEs occurs in both the central and peripheral diabetic arteries and is thought to contribute greatly to macrovascular complications of diabetes. The modification of collagen by AGEs also occurs in the basement membrane of small blood vessels. Again, AGE-modified collagen accumulates and increases basement membrane thickness, altering normal homeostatic transport across the membrane.

At the cellular level, AGEs have significant effects. Accumulation of AGEs not only affects extracellular matrix components but can affect matrix-to-matrix interactions and cell-to-matrix interactions. A receptor for AGEs known as RAGE (receptor for AGE) has been identified on the surface of smooth muscle cells, endothelial cells, neurons, and monocytes/macrophages.[27–29] Hyperglycemia results in increased RAGE expression and AGE-RAGE interaction. The effect on the endothelial cells is an increase in vascular permeability and thrombus formation.[30] The AGE-RAGE interaction on smooth muscle cells results in cellular proliferation within the arterial wall. As AGEs are chemotactic for monocytes, AGE-RAGE interaction induces increased cellular oxidant stress and activates the transcription factor Nf-κB on monocytes. This then alters the phenotype of the monocyte/macrophage and results in increased production of proinflammatory cytokines and growth factors such as interleukin-1 (IL-1), tumor necrosis factor (TNF), platelet-derived growth factor (PDGF), and insulin-like growth factor (IGF).[27,28,31,32] All these cytokines and growth factors have been shown to contribute to the chronic inflammatory process in the formation of atheromatous lesions. Interestingly, oxidized LDL, elevated in many diabetic patients, also activates NF-κB, and may result in similar processes. Thus, alterations in lipid and protein metabolism induced by the sustained hyperglycemia characteristic of diabetes may play a major role and provide a common link between all the classic complications of this disease.

CLINICAL PRESENTATION AND DIAGNOSIS OF DIABETES

The onset of type 1 diabetes is usually quite sudden while type 2 diabetes may be present for years before the patient develops symptoms. The classic signs and symptoms of undiagnosed diabetes are polydipsia (excessive thirst), polyuria (excessive urination), unexplained weight loss, and polyphagia (excessive hunger). Patients may also suffer from weakness, malaise, irritability, blurriness or other changes in vision, nausea, and dry mouth. The type 1 patient who does not seek medical evaluation quickly may develop diabetic ketoacidosis.

The diagnosis of diabetes is established through recognition of its signs and symptoms and by laboratory evaluation. Urinalysis was once a primary diagnostic tool, but is no longer used in this manner. Hyperglycemia may lead to excretion of glucose in the urine. Urinary glucose can be detected by use of a urine dip-stick test. However, many diabetic patients do not excrete large amounts of glucose, even at relatively high blood glucose levels. Conversely, finding glucose in the urine is not diagnostic for diabetes as glucose may be excreted from the kidneys in nondiabetic conditions.

The primary methods used to diagnose diabetes mellitus and monitor blood glucose levels have been the fasting blood glucose, a combination of fasting blood glucose plus a 2-hour test after glucose loading (2-hour postprandial), and oral glucose tolerance tests. In 1997, the American Diabetes Association provided the most current laboratory diagnostic parameters for diabetes[33] (Table 8–6). The new diagnostic guidelines allow use of a casual (nonfasting) plasma glucose for diagnosis and restrict routine use of the oral glucose tolerance test. These diagnostic tests clearly demonstrate the individual's capacity to regulate plasma glucose levels.

The fasting and casual plasma glucose tests and the oral glucose tolerance test allow determination of glycemia at the moment in time when the blood sample is drawn. They do not allow evaluation of glycemic control over a more extended time period. The primary test used for this purpose is the glycosylated hemoglobin assay (also called the glycohemoglobin test). This test measures the amount of glucose bound to the hemoglobin molecule on red blood cells. Glucose binds irreversibly to hemoglobin to form glycosylated hemoglobin and will remain bound for the lifespan of the red blood cell, ranging from about 30 to 90 days. This process is an example of AGE formation. The higher the blood glucose levels over time, the greater is the percentage of glycosylated hemoglobin. The glycosylated hemoglobin value is proportional to the blood glucose levels; thus, this test gives a measure of the blood glucose status over the preceding 30 to 90 days.

Two different glycosylated hemoglobin tests are available: the hemoglobin A1 (HbA1) test and the hemoglobin A1c (HbA1c) test. Each has a dif-

Table 8–6. Laboratory Diagnostic Criteria for Diabetes

Laboratory Methods*
1. Symptoms of diabetes plus casual (nonfasting) plasma glucose ≥ 200 mg/dL. Casual glucose may be drawn at any time of day without regard to time since the last meal. Classic symptoms of diabetes include polyuria, polydipsia, and unexplained weight loss.
2. Fasting plasma glucose ≥126 mg/dL. Fasting is defined as no caloric intake for at least 8 hours.
3. Two-hour postprandial glucose ≥200 mg/dL during an oral glucose tolerance test. The test should be performed using a glucose load containing the equivalent of 75 g of anhydrous glucose dissolved in water.†

Categories of fasting plasma glucose (FPG)
1. FPG <110 mg/dL = normal fasting glucose
2. FPG ≥110 mg/dL and <126 mg/dL = Impaired fasting glucose (IFG)
3. FPG ≥126 mg/dL = provisional diagnosis of diabetes (must be confirmed on subsequent day as described below)

Categories of 2-hour postprandial glucose (2hPG)
1. 2hPG <140 mg/dL = normal glucose tolerance
2. 2hPG ≥140 mg/dL and <200 mg/dL = impaired glucose tolerance (IGT)
3. 2hPG ≥200 mg/dL = provisional diagnosis of diabetes (must be confirmed on subsequent day as described below)

*Whatever method is used, it must be confirmed on a subsequent day by using any one of the three methods.
†The third method is not recommended for routine clinical use.

ferent range of normal values, with the normal HbA1 being less than about 8% and the normal HbA1c less than 6 to 6.5%.[34,35] Because different laboratories use different forms of the assay, glycosylated hemoglobin values must be interpreted in the context of the range of normal values for the individual medical laboratory performing the service. The American Diabetes Association recommends that diabetic patients try to achieve a target HbA1c of <7%.[36] An HbA1c >8% suggests that alteration in patient management is needed to improve glycemic control.

More recently, glycosylated albumin and fructosamine tests have been developed as monitoring tools although they are not used as commonly as the glycosylated hemoglobin assay. Fructosamine levels provide assessment of glycemic control over the past 4 to 6 weeks.[37] The normal range for fructosamine is 2 to 2.80 mmol/L.

While the above laboratory tests are available for professional diagnosis of diabetes and determination of glycemic control, the advent of self-blood glucose monitoring (SBGM) has allowed the individual diabetic patient to rapidly assess his or her own blood glucose levels almost instantaneously. Almost all diabetic patients using insulin and many on oral agents have a glucometer for SBGM. A small sterile lancet is used to create a puncture on the finger. A drop of capillary blood is drawn from the puncture site (Figure 8–4) and placed on

a strip which is inserted in the glucometer (Figure 8–5). A reading of capillary whole blood glucose is given in 1 to 2 minutes. The person can then adjust their medication, food consumption, or activity level on the basis of the test results.

There are numerous glucometers on the market, each with slightly different user instructions. The frequency with which the diabetic patient uses SBGM depends on the patient's individual treatment regimen. In some cases, the blood glucose may be checked once a day, or even less often. In other patients, especially those using insulin, the blood glucose may be checked many times daily. In general, the more intensively a diabetes patient is managed, the more frequently he or she will use SBGM.

ORAL DISEASES AND DIABETES

Oral complications of diabetes may include alterations in salivary flow and constituents, increased incidence of infection, burning mouth, altered wound healing, and increased prevalence and severity of periodontal disease. Xerostomia and parotid gland enlargement may occur in the diabetic individual.[38,39] These complications may be related to the degree of glycemic control.[40] Diabetes patients may complain of burning mouth syndrome associated with decreased salivary flow. Dry mucosal surfaces are easily irritated and often

TABLE 8–7. Oral Agents for Treatment of Diabetes

Sulfonylureas
- First generation
  - Chlorpropamide
  - Tolazamide
  - Tolbutamide
- Second generation
  - Glyburide
  - Glipizide
  - Glimepiride

Nonsulfonylurea insulin secretogogues
- Repaglinide

Biguanides
- Metformin

Thiazolidinediones
- Troglitazone

α-glucosidase inhibitors
- Acarbose

provide a favorable substrate for the growth of fungal organisms. The incidence of candidiasis may be increased in patients with diabetes[41] although not all studies support this relationship.[42]

Dental caries rates may also be altered in diabetes. While some studies have shown an increased caries incidence in diabetes,[43] others have demonstrated similar or lower rates than in nondiabetic individuals.[44,45] An increased caries rate may be associated with decreased salivation or with increased glucose concentrations in the saliva and gingival crevicular fluid (GCF). Conversely, most diabetic patients restrict fermentable carbohydrate intake as part of their disease management diet. This less cariogenic diet may be associated with decreased caries rates. In addition to medica-

tions used to manage blood glucose levels, many diabetic patients also take other drugs for treatment of related complications or unrelated disorders. These drugs can have xerostomic effects. Therefore, xerostomia may result not from the diabetic condition itself but from medications taken by the patient. Autonomic neuropathy may also cause disturbances in the regulation of saliva secretion.[46] Salivary flow is controlled by sympathetic and parasympathetic pathways. Diabetic neuropathy may disturb these pathways, leading to decreased salivation.

In recent studies of type 2 diabetic subjects and nondiabetic controls, no significant differences in salivary flow rates were seen.[46] There were also no differences between groups in the organic constituents of saliva. However, the effect of xerostomic medications on salivary flow rates was greater in diabetic individuals than in control patients. No differences were seen in the prevalence of coronal caries or root caries.[47] The salivary counts of acidogenic bacteria (*Streptococcus mutans* and lactobacilli) were similar between the diabetic

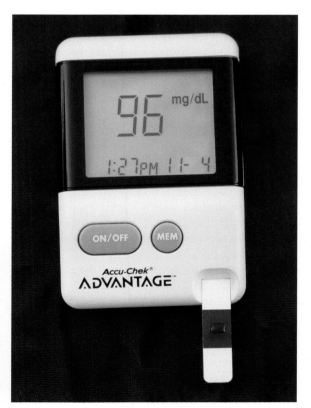

Figure 8–5. Test strip in glucometer with glucose reading. Blood is placed on a specific area of the glucometer strip. After an appropriate period of time, blood glucose reading is given by the glucometer.

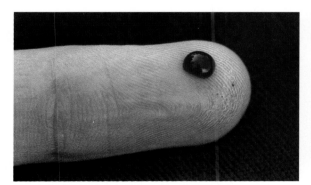

Figure 8–4. Obtaining drop of blood for glucometer testing. Finger lancet used to "prick" finger and drop of blood "milked" from puncture site.

and nondiabetic subjects. Likewise, carriage of salivary yeasts was similar between groups.

Diabetes and Periodontal Disease

The influence of diabetes on the periodontium has been thoroughly studied. It is difficult to make definitive conclusions from many of these studies owing to the heterogeneity of study designs, differences in the populations studied, changes in the classification of periodontal diseases and diabetes over the years, changes in the methods for diagnosing diabetes and evaluating glycemic control, inadequacy of study controls, and differences in periodontal parameters or outcome variables measured. Some research with relatively small numbers of subjects suggests that diabetes has little influence on the prevalence and severity of periodontal diseases. However, modern epidemiologic methods used in large populations have clearly established that diabetes is a risk factor for periodontal disease.

Diabetes is often associated with increased gingival inflammation in response to bacterial plaque.[48–50] This response may be related to the level of glycemic control, with subjects with well-controlled diabetes having a similar degree of gingivitis as nondiabetic individuals and poorly controlled diabetic subjects having significantly increased inflammation.[51,52] Increased gingival inflammation may be seen in diabetic subjects even though plaque levels are similar to nondiabetic controls.

The prevalence of periodontitis in diabetic adolescents and young adults is significantly greater than similar-aged nondiabetic individuals.[49] While some young diabetic people develop periodontitis, especially those with poor metabolic control, periodontal disease is much more common in adults. In a thorough analysis of the literature, Papapanou demonstrated that the majority of studies show a more severe periodontal condition in adult patients with diabetes than in nondiabetic adults.[53]

In large populations, type 2 diabetes has been shown to be a significant risk factor for periodontitis. The Pima Indian population of Arizona, with the highest prevalence of type 2 diabetes in the world, has been extensively studied.[54,55] The prevalence of attachment loss and bone loss was greater among diabetic subjects than among nondiabetic control subjects in all age groups. The differences in disease prevalence were most pronounced in the younger age groups. In addition, periodontal destruction was more severe in diabetic patients, with greater mean bone loss and attachment loss. Again, the differences in disease severity were greatest in the younger age groups. For example, diabetic subjects from 15 to 34 years of age had mean attachment loss and bone loss scores approximately twice as high as similar-aged nondiabetic subjects. In a multivariate risk analysis, it was determined that diabetic subjects had a risk of periodontitis 2.8 to 3.4 times higher than nondiabetic subjects after adjusting for the effects of confounding variables such as age, sex, and oral hygiene measures.

A recent meta-analysis of data from several studies of type 2 diabetes and periodontal disease was performed.[53] These studies included a total of 3,524 adults over 18 years of age and clearly demonstrated a significant association between periodontitis and diabetes mellitus. Diabetes may influence not only the prevalence and severity of periodontitis but also the progression of disease. Taylor and colleagues demonstrated that type 2 diabetes significantly increased the rate of alveolar bone loss progression over a 2-year period when compared to nondiabetic subjects.[56] The risk for progressive bone loss was 4.2 times greater in diabetic subjects, with the greatest increase in risk occurring in patients under the age of 34 years.

The relationship between metabolic control of diabetes and periodontal disease is not clear.[57] Some diabetic patients with poor glycemic control develop extensive periodontal destruction while others do not. Conversely, many patients with well-controlled diabetes have excellent periodontal health, but others develop periodontitis. In this way, periodontal disease is similar to the classic complications of diabetes. Poor glycemic control is clearly associated with increased risk for complications, but not all patients with poorly controlled diabetes develop these complications. While there is no unequivocal dose-response relationship between glycemia and periodontitis, many studies support the clinical observation that patients with poorly controlled diabetes of long duration tend to develop more advanced periodontal destruction than diabetic patients with good metabolic control. Over 2 to 3 years, Seppala and colleagues demonstrated that subjects with poorly controlled diabetes had significantly greater longitudinal attachment loss and bone loss than did subjects with well controlled diabetes.[58] Tervonen and Oliver showed that subjects with poor metabolic control over the preceding 2 to 5 years had a significantly greater prevalence of deep probing depths and advanced attachment loss than did subjects with good glycemic control.[59] Longitudinally, Taylor and colleagues found that poor glycemic control was associated with significantly increased risk of progressive bone loss compared with better metabolic control.[56] Thus, metabolic control of diabetes may be an important variable in the onset and progression of periodontal disease. Patients with well-controlled diabetes may be similar to nondiabetic individuals. It is important to remember that periodontal disease prevalence and severity varies greatly within the nondiabetic population. Presence of periodontal disease in a diabetic individual may therefore have more to do with other risk factors for periodontitis such as poor oral hygiene and smoking than it does with the mere presence of a diabetic state.

An important question for the dental practitioner is, Will diabetic patients with periodontal disease respond favorably to periodontal treatment In a study of patients with predominantly well-controlled diabetes and moderate to advanced periodontal disease, Christgau and colleagues found similar responses to nonsurgical scaling and root planing when compared with nondiabetic subjects 4 months after treatment.[60] Conversely, patients with poorly controlled diabetes often have a less favorable response to treatment than those with well-controlled diabetes.[61] Westfelt and colleagues performed a longitudinal assessment of diabetic subjects and nondiabetic controls with moderate to advanced periodontitis.[62] Patients received scaling and root planing, modified Widman flap surgery and supportive periodontal therapy every 3 months. Five years after the study began, there was a similar percentage of sites gaining or losing attachment, and a similar percentage of sites with stable attachment levels when comparing diabetic and nondiabetic subject groups. Most of the diabetic patients in this study had well-controlled or moderately well-controlled glycemia.

Diabetic patients must be examined individually to assess their potential response to periodontal therapy. The mere presence of diabetes does not condemn the person to a less favorable periodontal outcome. A diabetic patient with good glycemic control can be expected to respond in a fashion similar to the nondiabetic subject. The presence of poor glycemic control may place the patient at risk of a less favorable response. In addition, other factors such as smoking or poor plaque control may adversely affect the response to periodontal therapy in diabetic individuals, just as they may in a nondiabetic person.

Mechanisms of Diabetic Influence on Periodontium

A number of possible mechanisms have been proposed by which diabetes may affect the periodontium. These are primarily related to changes in the subgingival microbiota, GCF glucose levels, periodontal vasculature, host response, and collagen metabolism.[57] While early studies showed possible differences in subgingival bacterial colonization between diabetic and nondiabetic patients with periodontitis, more recent research has demonstrated few differences. Periodontally diseased sites in diabetic patients harbor similar species as comparable sites in nondiabetic individuals.[60,63,64] This lack of significant differences between diabetic and nondiabetic individuals in the primary bacterial etiologic agents of periodontal disease suggests that the increased prevalence and severity of periodontitis in diabetes may be due to differences in host response factors.

Increased blood glucose levels in diabetes are reflected in increased levels of GCF glucose.[65,66] In vitro studies show decreased chemotaxis of periodontal ligament fibroblasts to PDGF when placed in a hyperglycemic environment compared with normoglycemic conditions.[67] Thus, elevated GCF glucose levels in diabetes may adversely affect periodontal wound healing events and the local host response to microbial challenge.

Changes affecting the renal, retinal, and perineural vasculature in diabetes also occur in the periodontium. Increased thickness of gingival capillary endothelial cell basement membranes and the walls of small blood vessels may be seen in diabetic individuals.[68–70] This thickening may impair oxygen diffusion and nutrient provision across basement membranes. Increased thickness of small vessel walls results in narrowing of the lumen, altering normal periodontal tissue homeostasis.

The formation of AGEs occurs in the periodontium as it does in other tissue sites. Schmidt and colleagues have demonstrated a two fold increase in AGE accumulation in diabetic gingiva compared with gingiva from nondiabetic subjects. Increased oxidant stress was also noted in diabetic tissues.[71] Enhanced oxidant stress has been targeted as the underlying mechanism responsible for the widespread vascular injury associated with diabetes. The formation of AGEs stimulates arterial smooth muscle cell proliferation, increasing thickness of vessel walls. In the capillaries, enhanced cross-linking of AGE-modified collagen in the basement membrane inhibits the normal degradation of these proteins, increasing the thickness of the basement membrane. Elevated LDL levels, especially common in type 2 diabetes, may cause changes in the gingival vasculature.[21] The AGE-modified arterial collagen in gingival blood vessel walls can bind circulating LDL, resulting in atheroma formation and further narrowing of the vessel lumen. All these events may play a role in altering the tissue response to periodontopathic bacteria, resulting in increased severity and progression of periodontitis.

Altered host defenses have long been considered important in the pathogenesis of periodontitis associated with diabetes. Defects in polymorphonuclear leukocyte (PMN) adherence, chemotaxis, and phagocytosis have been observed in some individuals with diabetes.[57,72,73] Many of these PMN abnormalities can be corrected with improved glycemic control. Defects affecting this first line of defense against subgingival microbial agents may result in significantly increased tissue destruction. In many diabetic patients, PMN function is normal. Oliver and colleagues have even suggested hyper-responsiveness or increased numbers of PMNs within the gingival crevice of poorly controlled diabetic patients as indicated by elevated levels of the PMN-derived enzyme β-glucuronidase.[74]

The monocyte/macrophage cell line is critical to cell-mediated host defense in periodontal diseases. Studies suggest that many diabetic patients possess a hyper-responsive monocyte/macrophage phenotype in which stimulation by bacterial antigens such as lipopolysaccharide (LPS) results in dramatically increased proinflammatory cytokine production.[75] Salvi and colleagues have demonstrated significantly increased production of proinflammatory cytokines by monocytes derived from patients with diabetes compared with nondiabetic subjects.[76] In response to LPS from the periodontal pathogen *P. gingivalis*, diabetic monocytes produced 24 to 32 times the level of TNFα compared with nondiabetic monocytes. Also, there was a four fold increase LPS-stimulated monocyte production of PGE_2 and IL-1β in diabetic subjects than in nondiabetic subjects.[77] The gingival crevicular fluid levels of PGE_2 and IL-1β were significantly higher in diabetic patients with periodontitis than in nondiabetic subjects with a similar degree of periodontal destruction.

It is likely that there is a genetic component to the development of a hyper-responsive monocyte/macrophage phenotype in some diabetic patients. Not all individuals with diabetes have this phenotype. The formation of AGEs also plays an important role in the upregulation of the monocyte/macrophage cell line. Accumulation of AGEs in the periodontium stimulates influx of monocytes. Once in the tissue, AGEs interact with the receptor RAGE on monocyte cell surfaces. This halts the migration of the monocytes, fixing them at the local site. The AGE-RAGE interaction then induces a change in monocyte phenotype, upregulating the cell and significantly increasing proinflammatory cytokine production. This provides another explanation for increased GCF production of TNFα, PGE_2 and IL-1β noted in diabetic patients with periodontitis.[28,32]

As previously discussed, there is a great deal of heterogeneity in AGE formation within the diabetic population. Thus, these AGE-associated changes may be present in some patients but absent in others. Those individuals at greatest risk for increased AGE accumulation and its adverse effects are those with poor glycemic control, who may accumulate large deposits of AGEs within target tissues. Similarly, the patient with poorly controlled diabetes is most likely to suffer more rapid and advanced periodontal destruction. However, just as some individuals with poorly controlled diabetes do not develop classic vascular complications of the disease, some such patients have little, if any, significant periodontal disease. The variability in AGE formation may provide some explanation for the variance in risk of periodontal complications of diabetes.

Collagen is the primary constituent of gingival connective tissue and the organic matrix of alveolar bone. Changes in collagen metabolism contribute to alterations in wound healing and to periodontal disease initiation and progression. Proteinases are enzymes involved in matrix degradation. In the periodontium, these matrix metalloproteinases (MMPs) include collagenases, gelatinases, and elastases.[78,79] There are at least 12 distinct members of the MMP family, and these enzymes are responsible for the breakdown of bone and connective tissue during periodontal disease. Matrix metalloproteinases are produced by all of the major cell types in the periodontium when activated by various cytokines and growth factors, including PMNs, fibroblasts, macrophages, endothelial cells, osteoblasts, and osteoclasts.[78]

Increased collagen breakdown through stimulation of collagenase activity has been observed in the periodontium of diabetic patients.[80] Collagenases primarily degrade more newly formed and, therefore, more soluble collagen macromolecules. Sustained hyperglycemia results in AGE modification of existing collagen, with increased cross-linking. The net effect of these alterations in collagen metabolism is a rapid degradation of recently synthesized collagen by host collagenase and a predominance of older, highly cross-linked, AGE-modified collagen. Since collagen production and degradation exist as a highly balanced homeostatic mechanism, changes in collagen metabolism result in altered wound healing in response to physical or microbial wounding of the periodontium. Impaired wound healing is a well-recognized complication of diabetes and may affect any tissue site, including the periodontium.

Reduction in host collagenase production can be achieved by tetracycline therapy.[78,81,82] This is accomplished via mechanisms which are independent of the antimicrobial properties of these agents. Low-dose tetracyclines and chemically modified tetracyclines (CMTs), which have no antimicrobial effect, have been shown to significantly decrease collagenase production and collagen degradation.[83–85] Although CMTs are not yet available for routine use, tetracyclines such as doxycycline, minocycline, and tetracycline HCl have been used for many years. Low-dose doxycycline is now available as well[86] although its use in diabetic patients has not yet been reported. Due to their anticollagenolytic effect, tetracyclines and CMTs have potential benefits in inhibiting the onset and progression of periodontitis, arthritis, and osteoporosis, among other conditions.[85] In a disease such as diabetes, where collagenase production is significantly increased, these agents may have even greater beneficial effects by normalizing collagen metabolism and wound healing events.

EFFECTS OF PERIODONTAL INFECTION ON GLYCEMIC CONTROL OF DIABETES

While diabetes significantly impacts the periodontium, evidence also suggests the potential for periodontal infection to adversely influence glycemic control in diabetes. Taylor and colleagues examined subjects with type 2 diabetes to determine whether severe periodontitis increased the risk for poor glycemic control.[87] The subjects, some of whom had severe periodontitis and others who did not, all had relatively well-controlled glycemia at baseline, as indicated by glycosylated hemoglobin (HbA1) levels of less than 9%. At re-examination 2 years later, a greater proportion of subjects with severe periodontitis had poor glycemic control (HbA1 >9%) than did subjects without severe periodontitis. Severe periodontitis at baseline was associated with a six fold increased risk of poor glycemic control at follow-up.

In a case-control study of diabetic adults having gingivitis or mild periodontitis compared with patients with severe periodontitis, those with severe periodontal disease had a significantly greater prevalence of cardiovascular and kidney complications during the 1- to 11-year follow-up period than did patients with minimal periodontal disease.[88] This was true despite the fact that HbA1c levels were similar in both groups, indicating a similar level of long-term glycemic control. Thus, the classic complications of diabetes may be closely associated with periodontal disease in these individuals, lending further credence to the concept that periodontal disease may be the "sixth complication of diabetes."[89]

If periodontal infection adversely affects glycemic control in diabetes, then the question arises, Can periodontal treatment directed at elimination of pathogenic organisms and reduction of inflammation have a positive impact on glycemic control? In case studies of patients with poorly controlled diabetes and periodontitis, improvement in metabolic control has been noted coincident with improvement in periodontal health following treatment. In 1960, Williams and Mahan performed extractions and periodontal surgery in combination with systemic antibiotic therapy on 9 diabetic patients with severe periodontitis to eliminate periodontal infection.[90] The metabolic parameters, including daily insulin dose and periodic blood glucose readings, were crude by today's standard but were routinely used at the time. With improved periodontal health, 7 of the 9 patients had decreased daily insulin requirements, some by over 50%. Miller and colleagues evaluated the effect of scaling and root planing combined with 14 days of systemic doxycycline on glycemia in 9 poorly controlled type 1 diabetic patients with periodontitis.[91] At post-treatment examinations 4 and 8 weeks after therapy, 5 of 9 patients had significant improvement in bleeding on probing. These same 5 subjects also had improvement in metabolic control, indicated by significant reductions in HbA1c values. The 4 patients who had no improvement in bleeding on probing also had no improvement in glycemic control. This noncontrolled case study suggests that improved periodontal health may be accompanied by a parallel improvement in metabolic control of diabetes, and indicates the potential systemic benefits of periodontal treatment in patients with poorly controlled diabetes and periodontitis.

In the first long-term placebo-controlled study of its kind, Grossi and colleagues examined a large group of poorly controlled type 2 diabetic patients with severe periodontitis following non-surgical débridement combined with either systemic doxy-cycline (100 mg/day) or placebo for 14 days.[92,93] All patient groups had significant reductions in gingival bleeding and probing depths, with gains in clinical attachment. Doxycycline-treated patients had a greater reduction in prevalence of *P. gingivalis* at 3 and 6 months. The doxycycline-treated patients also demonstrated significant reductions in HbA1c at 3 months, which gradually reverted to baseline levels by 6 months. Placebo-treated subjects had no significant change in HbA1c levels at any time point. Consequently, the combination of subgingival débridement and systemic doxycycline resulted in significant short-term improvement in the parameters of metabolic control.

Conversely, subjects with well-controlled or moderately controlled diabetes and periodontitis who receive scaling and root planing without adjunctive systemic antibiotic therapy may demonstrate no significant changes in glycemic control despite improvement in their periodontal parameters.[60,94] The mechanisms by which adjunctive antibiotics may induce positive changes in glycemic control when combined with thorough mechanical débridement are unknown at this time. It is possible that improved glycemia is associated with the more complete elimination of pathogenic organisms in antibiotic-treated patients. Tetracyclines and CMTs are also known to suppress glycosylation of proteins, AGE formation, and MMP activity.[78]

Acute bacterial and viral infections have been shown to increase insulin resistance and aggravate glycemic control.[95,96] This occurs in both diabetic and nondiabetic individuals. Insulin resistance persists for an extended period of time after clinical recovery from infection, often for weeks or months. In the type 2 diabetes patient, who already has significant insulin resistance, further resistance induced by infection may considerably exacerbate poor glycemic control. In type 1 patients, prescribed doses of injected insulin may be insufficient to maintain good glycemic control in the presence of infection-induced tissue resistance. It is possible that chronic gram-negative periodontal infections may also result in increased insulin resistance and poor glycemic control.[97] Periodontal treatment designed to decrease the bacterial challenge and reduce inflammation might restore insulin sensitivity over time, resulting in improved metabolic control. The improved glycemic control seen in studies of combined mechanical and antibiotic periodontal therapy would support such a hypothesis.

DIABETES AND DENTAL IMPLANT THERAPY

There is little scientific evidence regarding the success or failure of dental implant therapy in diabetic individuals. Diabetes is often considered a relative contraindication to implant placement, but in well-controlled diabetes there is no reason to avoid implant therapy. Patients with poorly controlled diabetes may not respond well to any surgical treatment, including implant placement, due to impaired wound healing. In animal models, diabetes has been associated with decreased bone-to-implant contact and decreased bone density in the peri-implant region.[98,99] It is not known if this occurs in humans. The effect of diabetes on long-term clinical implant stability is also unknown at this time.

MEDICAL MANAGEMENT OF DIABETES

Treatment of diabetes aims to achieve blood glucose levels as close to normal as possible and to prevent diabetic complications. The American Diabetes Association has standards of care to guide treatment, with a goal of achieving HbA1c levels <7%.[37] This goal is difficult to attain for most diabetic patients, and the majority of these individuals have less than ideal metabolic control.[2,5,100] Specific goals of therapy include maintaining normal growth and development, attaining normal body weight, avoiding sustained hyperglycemia or symptomatic hypoglycemia, preventing diabetic ketoacidosis and nonketotic acidosis, and immediately detecting and treating long-term diabetic complications. Treatment options for type 2 diabetes may include diet, exercise, weight control, oral medications, and insulin injections. Generally, a combination of these therapeutic approaches is used. While treatment for type 1 diabetes also involves diet, exercise, and weight control, insulin injection is essential to sustain life.

Diet, exercise, and weight control are the mainstay of therapy. Proper diet allows intake of carbohydrate, protein and fat in proportions commensurate with the target weight and nutritional needs. Obesity is common in type 2 diabetes and contributes substantially to insulin resistance. Exercise and weight reduction significantly improve tissue sensitivity to insulin and utilization of glucose by target tissues. Even small reductions in body weight can have dramatic effects on insulin sensitivity. Many patients with type 2 diabetes take oral medications which either increase pancreatic insulin production, decrease production of glucose by the liver, improve tissue sensitivity to insulin, or alter absorption of carbohydrate from the gut. All type 1 diabetic patients and many type 2 patients inject exogenous insulin to allow glucose utilization by the tissues. Self-blood glucose monitoring through use of a glucometer is recommended for all type 1 and most type 2 diabetic individuals as it provides vital feedback to the patient regarding blood glucose levels and allows tailoring and adjustment of individual treatment regimens on the basis of knowledge of glucose levels at different times of the day.

In the course of a typical day, blood glucose levels rise after meals, resulting in increased pancreatic insulin secretion (see Figure 8–1). Insulin allows glucose to be removed from the bloodstream for tissue utilization and storage; thus, blood glucose levels fall. A feedback mechanism then results in decreased insulin secretion until the next meal when the cycle is repeated (Figure 8–6). In healthy subjects, blood glucose fluctuations are held within a relatively tight range throughout the day, rarely falling below 60 mg/dL or rising above 150 mg/dL. In diabetes mellitus, wide ranges in glycemic fluctuation are common even with treatment. Deficiencies in plasma insulin levels result in hyperglycemia while excess levels of insulin cause hypoglycemia. The ideal treatment of the diabetic individual would establish glycemic patterns similar to those of nondiabetic persons.

In 1985, a prospective, randomized, controlled, multicenter clinical trial known as the Diabetes Control and Complications Trial (DCCT) was begun to determine the relationship between glycemic control and diabetic complications.[100] This landmark study compared the effects of intensive insulin therapy directed at near normalization of glycemia with the effects of conventional insulin therapy on the initiation and progression of microvascular complications in type 1 diabetes.

In the DCCT, 1,441 type 1 diabetic subjects were followed for 3 to 9 years after being randomly assigned to one of two groups. The first was a conventional insulin therapy group, who took 1 or 2 insulin injections each day. The second was an intensive insulin therapy group, who took 3 or 4 daily injections or used an external subcutaneous insulin infusion pump. The study was designed to determine whether intensive insulin therapy, used to maintain blood glucose values within the normal range over a long period of time, could prevent

the initial development of retinopathy, nephropathy, and neuropathy in subjects who entered the study free of these complications. The study also determined the effect of intensive insulin therapy on the progression of these complications in patients who began the study with pre-existing early complications.

The results of the DCCT provided strong evidence that improved glycemic control, achieved through intensified insulin regimens, inhibited the onset and delayed the progression of diabetic complications.[101,102] The risk of developing retinopathy was reduced by 76% in intensively treated patients compared with those on conventional insulin regimens. The progression of existing retinopathy decreased by 54% in the intensively treated group. Albuminuria, a sign of nephropathy, and clinical neuropathy were reduced by 54% and 60%, respectively. Thus, change from conventional insulin regimens, which rarely achieve normoglycemia, to intensive regimens resulted in improved glycemic control and dramatic reductions in the risk of microvascular complications. Improvement in glycemic control was also associated with a reduction in macrovascular complications.[103] The potential reduction in morbidity and mortality related to diabetic complications seen in the DCCT led the American Diabetes Association to issue a position statement declaring that a primary goal in treating type 1 diabetes is to attain blood glucose control "at least equal to that achieved in the intensively treated cohort" of the DCCT.[104] Physicians have begun to intensify insulin regi-

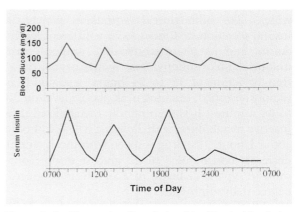

Figure 8–6. Glucose-insulin relationship. Rise in blood glucose following each meal or snack stimulates increased insulin secretion, which then allows glucose utilization and storage. Blood glucose levels decrease until the next meal, when the cycle is repeated. In healthy subjects, glycemic fluctuations are held within a tight range between approximately 60 and 150 mg/dL.

mens in response to these results, and diabetic patients who know about the DCCT are motivated to improve their glycemic control.[105,106]

Several studies have substantiated the conclusions of the DCCT for individuals with type 2 diabetes as well.[107,108] In one study with a similar design, the patient group that maintained near-normal blood glucose values over a 6-year study period had a 69% reduction in the risk of retinopathy compared with the group with poorly controlled diabetes.[107] The risk of neuropathy and nephropathy decreased by 57% and 70%, respectively. The risk of cardiac, cerebral, and peripheral macrovascular complications was reduced by 54%. Thus, it is likely that dental professionals will encounter increasing numbers of type 1 and type 2 diabetic patients using intensified treatment regimens.

Oral Agents Used in Diabetes

A number of oral agents are used to treat type 2 diabetes[5,34,109] (Table 8–7). Sulfonylureas stimulate the β cells of the pancreas to increase insulin secretion. First-generation sulfonylureas are used infrequently today. Second-generation agents (glipizide, glyburide, and glimepiride) are more potent, produce less significant side effects, and have fewer drug interactions than first-generation sulfonylureas. However, the major complication of sulfonylurea therapy is hypoglycemia, which may be more frequent with second-generation agents. As pancreatic insulin secretion increases in response to sulfonylureas, food intake must be adequate to avoid low blood glucose levels.

Repaglinide is a new antidiabetic agent, which, like sulfonylureas, stimulates pancreatic insulin secretion.[110] It does so via a different mechanism, and its pharmacodynamic properties are unique. Unlike sulfonylureas which have a duration of action of 12 to 24 hours, repaglinide is rapidly absorbed, reaching peak plasma levels in 30 to 60 minutes. It is then rapidly metabolized into inactive metabolites, with a plasma half-life of only about 1 hour. The drug is taken with meals, and it decreases postprandial blood glucose peaks, common in type 2 diabetes, to a significantly greater degree than sulfonylureas.

Metformin lowers blood glucose primarily by preventing glycogenolysis in the liver. It also increases tissue uptake and utilization of glucose, counteracting the insulin resistance characteristic of type 2 diabetes. Unlike sulfonylureas, metformin rarely causes hypoglycemia. Troglitazone, a relatively new thiazolidinedione agent, increases tissue sensitivity to insulin, thereby stimulating glucose utilization in muscle. It also reduces blood glucose levels by suppressing gluconeogenesis in the liver. Like metformin, troglitazone generally does not cause hypoglycemia.

The α-glucosidase inhibitor acarbose works in a manner different from other oral agents. Taken with meals, acarbose slows the digestion and uptake of carbohydrates from the gut, thus lowering postprandial peaks in blood glucose. Since acarbose is not absorbed, few systemic effects are seen although gastrointestinal side effects are not uncommon. Acarbose may be used by both type 1 and type 2 diabetic patients. While acarbose itself does not cause hypoglycemia, when taken by a patient who also uses insulin or sulfonylureas, the delay in glucose absorption from the gut into the bloodstream can lead to relative insulin excess and hypoglycemia.

Insulin Therapy

Insulin is used by all patients with type 1 diabetes and many patients with type 2 diabetes. Insulin is administered by subcutaneous injection, usually with a syringe. Insulin pumps provide an insulin infusion through a subcutaneous catheter. The amount of insulin taken each day and the exact regimen for insulin delivery vary with each patient.[111]

Insulins vary in their onset, peak, and duration of activity and are classified as rapid-, short-, intermediate-, or long-acting (Table 8–8). While human insulin is currently the most used, beef and pork insulins are also still encountered. An ideal insulin profile obtained by insulin injection would closely mimic daily insulin fluctuations in nondiabetic individuals (see Figure 8–6), a very difficult goal to achieve. Lispro and regular insulin are generally taken close to meal time in an attempt to match the peak absorption of glucose from the gut into the bloodstream with the peak activity of the injected insulin. Ultralente insulin is taken to simulate the basal metabolic rate of insulin secreted from a normally functioning pancreas. Ultralente is often called "peakless" insulin due to its very slow onset, minimal peak activity and long duration of action. Intermediate-acting insulins such as NPH and lente have a slower onset and peak activity than rapid- or short-acting insulins. Thus, NPH or Lente insulin injected at 7:00 AM will usually reach its peak activity sometime around noon or shortly thereafter.

While many regimens exist, some conventional daily insulin injection regimens include (1) a

TABLE 8–8. Types of Insulin

Insulin Type	Insulin Classification	Onset of Activity	Peak Activity	Duration of Activity
Lispro	Rapid-acting	15 min	30 to 90 min	<5 h
Regular	Short-acting	30 to 60 min	2 to 3 h	4 to 12 h
NPH	Intermediate-acting	2 to 4 h	4 to 10 h	14 to 18 h
Lente	Intermediate-acting	3 to 4 h	4 to 12 h	16 to 20 h
Ultralente	Long-acting	6 to 10 h	12 to 16 h	20 to 30 h

single morning injection of intermediate-acting insulin; (2) a single morning injection of intermediate-acting insulin mixed with regular or lispro insulin; (3) twice-daily injections of intermediate-acting insulin; or (4) twice-daily injections of intermediate-acting insulin mixed with regular or lispro insulin (Figures 8–7, 8–8, 8–9). While the insulin injection regimen in Figure 8–9 appears to closely mimic the normal pancreatic insulin secretion profile seen in Figure 8–6, even this regimen often results in relatively poor glycemic control with wide fluctuations in blood glucose levels throughout the day. This was clear in the DCCT, where glycemic control with all conventional regimens was poor compared with intensive regimens. The variability in the activity of injected insulin makes it very difficult to match peak plasma insulin levels with peak blood glucose levels following ingestion of food.

Intensive insulin regimens such as those used in the DCCT generally dictate injection of regular or lispro insulin before each meal since these insulins have less variability in absorption and activity than either intermediate- or long-acting insulins. Insulin injection is timed so that peak plasma insulin levels coincide with peak postprandial glucose levels. Intensive regimens may also include intermediate- or long-acting insulin to provide a basal metabolic level of plasma insulin (Figure 8–10, 8–11).

Insulin pumps use either regular or lispro insulin only. A continuous basal metabolic infusion rate is programmed into the pump to mimic normal pancreatic basal secretion. Then the patient programs a bolus of insulin prior to each meal. The pump is battery operated and delivers insulin from a storage syringe within the pump through tubing into a subcutaneous catheter. The catheter and infusion set are changed every 2 to 3 days. Since the results of the DCCT were published, the number of patients using intensive insulin regimens has increased significantly.[112] However, even the most intensive insulin regimens used in highly motivated patients are relatively poor substitutes for a normally functioning pancreas.

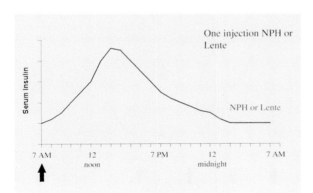

Figure 8–7. Conventional insulin injection regimen: one injection of NPH/Lente. Example of conventional insulin regimen using single injection of intermediate-acting insulin (NPH or Lente) each day. Arrow indicates time of injection. The only meal that is covered by injected insulin is lunch. Glucose absorbed from breakfast, dinner, and evening snack remains in the bloodstream due to insufficient insulin levels, resulting in hyperglycemia.

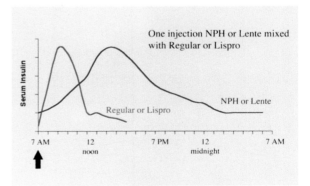

Figure 8–8. Conventional insulin injection regimen: one injection of NPH/Lente mixed with Regular/Lispro. Example of conventional insulin regimen using single injection of intermediate-acting insulin (NPH or Lente) mixed with short-acting (Regular) or rapid-acting (Lispro) insulin. Arrow indicates time of injection. Glucose absorption from breakfast and lunch is covered by injected insulin but that from dinner and evening snack is not.

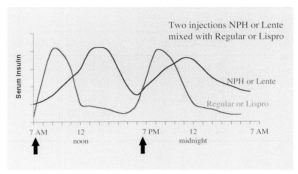

Figure 8–9. Conventional insulin injection regimen: two injections of mixed Regular/Lispro and NPH/Lente. Example of conventional insulin regimen using both morning and evening injections of intermediate-acting insulin (NPH or Lente) mixed with short-acting (Regular) or rapid-acting (Lispro) insulin. Arrows indicate time of injection. Theoretically, glucose absorption from all meals is covered.

Hypoglycemia is the most common complication of insulin therapy. Hypoglycemia can and does occur in patients using oral sulfonylurea agents; however, its incidence is higher in those taking insulin injections. While intensified treatment regimens decrease the risk of long-term diabetic complications, they increase the risk of hypoglycemia. In the DCCT, the incidence of severe hypoglycemia was three times higher in the intensive insulin group compared with the conventional therapy group.[113,114] Severe hypoglycemia was defined as hypoglycemia in which the neurologic impairment was so severe that the patient required the assistance of another person. One-third of all severe hypoglycemic episodes in the DCCT led to seizures or loss of consciousness. Perhaps even more significant,

36% of severe hypoglycemic reactions occurred without warning symptoms for the patient. In another 51% of cases, warning symptoms occurred but were not recognized as such by the patient. This suggests the seriousness with which dental practitioners should manage hypoglycemia, especially in insulin-using diabetic patients.

DENTAL MANAGEMENT OF THE DIABETIC PATIENT

Patients who present to the dental office with intraoral findings suggestive of a previously undiagnosed diabetic condition should be questioned closely. Questions should be targeted toward eliciting a clear history of polydipsia, polyuria, polyphagia, or recent unexplained weight loss. Patients should also be asked about family history of diabetes.

The patient in Figure 8–12, a 50-year-old Mexican-American male, presented with generalized moderate adult periodontitis. Heavy accumulations of plaque and calculus were noted. The patient was healthy, although obese, and was taking no medications. Following scaling and root planing, he failed to return for re-evaluation. Five years later, he presented again to the periodontist. This time, severe bone loss was noted in the incisor and molar regions (Figure 8–12B). Oral hygiene was poor, but the rapidity of bone loss was inconsistent with adult periodontitis. Upon questioning, the patient stated that it was common for him to urinate three to five times a night. The positive his-

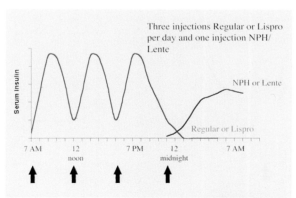

Figure 8–11. Intensive insulin regimen: three daily injections of Regular/Lispro plus one injection of NPH/Lente. Example of intensive insulin regimen using injections of Regular or Lispro insulin before breakfast, lunch, and dinner. A single injection of intermediate-acting (NPH or Lente) insulin is taken at bedtime to cover an evening snack and the increased glucose production that normally occurs before awakening in the morning.

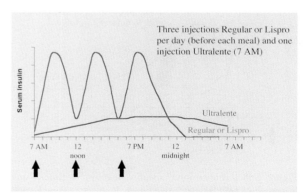

Figure 8–10. Intensive insulin regimen: three daily injections of Regular/Lispro plus one injection of Ultralente. Example of intensive insulin regimen using injections of Regular or Lispro insulin before breakfast, lunch, and dinner. A single injection of long-acting (Ultralente) insulin in the morning provides basal metabolic insulin levels during the day.

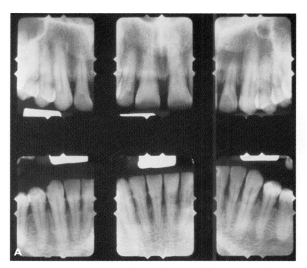 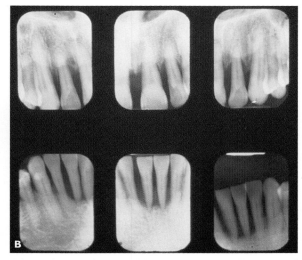

Figure 8–12. *A,* Six-radiograph set of anterior teeth (minimal bone loss). Fifty-year-old patient prior to diagnosis of diabetes. Heavy local factors with mild to moderate adult periodontitis. *B,* Six-radiograph set of anterior teeth (severe bone loss). Five years after initial presentation, patient in Figure 8–12 has severe bone loss. Patient had undiagnosed type 2 diabetes.

tory of polyuria led to appropriate laboratory evaluation and diagnosis of type 2 diabetes.

Rapid attachment loss and bone loss that are inconsistent with local factors may indicate an underlying systemic component to the patient's periodontal condition. When supported by a thorough review of the medical history, clinical examination and laboratory evaluation, a previously undiagnosed diabetic state may be revealed. Other periodontal manifestations of undiagnosed diabetes include enlarged, hemorrhagic gingival tissues and multiple periodontal abscesses (Figure 8–13). If the clinician suspects undiagnosed diabetes, laboratory evaluation and physician referral are indicated (see Table 8–6).

Previously diagnosed but poorly controlled diabetic patients may present with oral manifestations similar to the undiagnosed diabetic individual. The patient in Figures 8–13 and 8–14 had type 2 diabetes. Her glycemic control had worsened considerably over the previous 12 months as indicated by a rise in HbA1c values from 7.7 to 13.9% in 1 year. She acknowledged poor compliance with her oral antidiabetic medication regimen. In patients with suspected poorly controlled diabetes, dental treatment should be limited initially to provision of emergency care.[34] Referral to the patient's physician should include a description of intraoral findings and a brief outline of the patient's dental treatment needs. The dental practitioner should request evaluation of the patient's glycemic control and appropriate medical management prior to elective dental treatment.

In known diabetic patients, it is important to establish the level of glycemic control early in the examination process. This can be done through physician referral or review of medical records. Most patients who do SBGM record their glucose readings for future review by their diabetes management team. Having the patient bring this log to the dental office may provide the practitioner with information regarding the patient's overall glycemic control and normal blood glucose fluctuations during the day. It is helpful to determine the patient's most recent glycosylated hemoglobin values, since this test provides a measure of glycemic control over the preceding 2 to 3 months (Table 8–9). Comparison with past values provides information on the stability of glycemic control over time. Addressing the issue of glycemic control at the beginning of treatment often results in improved periodontal status, affording a more accurate assessment of actual treatment needs. Periodontal therapy, if needed, involves numerous patient visits and regularly scheduled maintenance following active treatment. Thus, the dentist and dental hygienist are in a perfect position to encourage patient compliance and control.

The patient with well-controlled diabetes with no significant complications can generally be managed in a fashion similar to the nondiabetic dental patient, with the notable exception of the need to monitor for signs and symptoms of hypoglycemia during treatment. Key considerations related to dental treatment of the diabetic patient include stress reduction, diet modification, inpatient versus

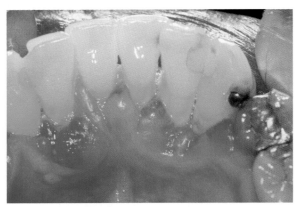

Figure 8–13. Mandibular anterior teeth from lingual view. Sixty-year-old African American female with poorly controlled type 2 diabetes. Enlarged, hemorrhagic gingival tissue at multiple sites.

outpatient care, antibiotic use, changes in medication regimens, and appointment timing.[115,116]

Stress reduction and adequate pain control are important in treating the diabetic patient. Epinephrine and cortisol secretion often increases in stressful situations. Both these hormones elevate blood glucose levels and interfere with glycemic control. Efforts to allay patient apprehension and minimize discomfort are important and may include preoperative sedation and analgesia.[116,117]

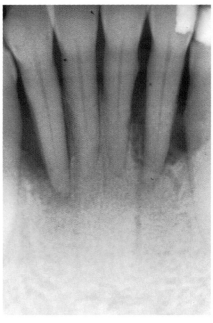

Figure 8–14. Radiograph of mandibular anterior teeth (severe incisor bone loss) from patient in Figure 8–14.

Local anesthetics used in conjunction with most dental procedures may contain varying concentrations of vasoconstrictors (eg, 1/100,000 epinephrine). Use of these agents has minimal effect on blood glucose levels, probably due to their relatively slow absorption from the local site and the low concentrations and small volumes used. Profound anesthesia with such agents minimizes endogenous epinephrine release.[34]

Periodontal therapy often requires surgical procedures that may result in mild to moderate postoperative discomfort. Modification of the diabetic patient's diet may be needed as a result of compromised chewing and swallowing that can accompany extensive dental procedures.[34,115] While many diabetic individuals are very knowledgeable about diet and medication modifications, others are not. It may be necessary to consult the patient's diabetes management team prior to the appointment for suggested liquid or semi-solid dietary alternatives.

Most diabetic patients can be easily managed in the dental office on an outpatient basis.[115,116] However, for those with very poor glycemic control, severe medical complications, and extensive treatment needs that will alter dietary and medication regimens for extended periods of time, hospitalization may be considered. Diabetic patients with severe head and neck infections should be treated in a controlled medical environment to avert possible life-threatening complications.

Antibiotics are not necessary for routine dental treatment in most diabetic patients but may be considered in the presence of overt infection.[34] Antibiotic coverage prior to surgical treatment should be considered in patients with poorly controlled diabetes.[115] Since elective procedures are generally deferred until adequate glycemic control is achieved, this most often applies to emergency situations such as periodontal and periapical abscesses or other acute odontogenic infections. Adjunctive antibiotic therapy may also be considered in the management of periodontal disease. As previously discussed, the

TABLE 8–9. Laboratory Evaluation of Diabetes Control

Glycated Hemoglobin Assay (HbA1c):	
4 to 6%	Normal
<7%	Good diabetes control
7 to 8%	Moderate diabetes control
>8%	Action suggested to improve diabetes control

use of systemic tetracycline antibiotics in conjunction with mechanical root débridement may have beneficial effects not only on the periodontium but on glycemic control as well.

At one time, a general recommendation was made for diabetic patients to have their dental appointments in the morning. This recommendation was also made for many other medically compromised patients. While morning appointments may be preferable for some diabetic patients, others may be better treated in the afternoon. Appointment timing often depends on the particular medication regimen used by each individual patient. When possible, it is best to plan dental treatment either before or after periods of peak insulin activity because hypoglycemic reactions are more likely to occur when insulin levels are high.[34,116] Type 2 diabetic patients taking sulfonylureas are at risk for hypoglycemia. In their case, it is prudent, when possible, to plan dental treatment to avoid periods of peak drug activity. Metformin and troglitazone rarely cause hypoglycemia.

If the patient takes insulin, the dentist should determine the exact type being used. Its onset of activity and time of peak activity relative to the planned dental therapy should be determined (see Table 8–8). The greatest risk of hypoglycemia is usually during the time of peak insulin activity: 30 to 90 minutes after injection of lispro insulin; 2 to 4 hours after injection of regular insulin, or approximately 6 to 8 hours after injection of NPH or Lente insulin (see Figures 8–7 to 8–11). The primary factor to consider is the peak action of the insulin taken and the amount of glucose being absorbed from the gut following the last meal. A key question to consider is, Will the amount and type of food eaten 'match' the level of insulin activity? To determine the answer, other questions must be asked. Did the patient follow his or her usual routine, eat the same amount and type of food, and take the same amount of insulin as always? Or did they skip a meal or reduce the amount of food eaten before their dental appointment? These are important questions to ask since any reduction in normal food consumption, if not accompanied by a reduction in insulin dose, may place the patient at higher risk of hypoglycemia during the dental treatment. For example, the patient who takes intermediate-acting insulin in the morning (see Figures 8–7 to 8–9) but then skips lunch before the afternoon dental appointment faces a significant risk of hypoglycemia. The NPH or Lente insulin will peak in the early afternoon, and blood glucose levels may fall precipitously since the patient has not had any food.

It may be impossible to plan dental appointments to avoid peak insulin activity. In these instances, the dentist simply needs to be aware that the patient is at risk for hypoglycemia, assess the patient's pretreatment blood glucose level with their glucometer, and have a carbohydrate source readily available. Just as patients with asthma are encouraged to bring their inhaler to the dental appointment, or patients with angina to bring their nitroglycerine, dental practitioners should recommend that diabetic patients who do SBGM bring their glucometer to the dental office for each visit. Patients can check their blood glucose levels at the beginning of the appointment. If glucose levels are at or near the lower end of normal, the patient may consume some carbohydrates before starting treatment to avoid hypoglycemia during the appointment. For example, if a long dental procedure is planned and the patient's pretreatment blood glucose is below 70 to 80mg/dL, having the patient drink 120 mL (4 oz) of fruit juice may prevent hypoglycemia during treatment. On the other hand, a markedly elevated pretreatment blood glucose (eg, greater than 300mg/dL) may suggest postponement of the procedure until metabolic control is assessed and improved.

In addition to determining pretreatment glucose levels, the dentist should determine the type of insulin the patient takes, when it was last taken, and the amount taken. Next, it is important to find out when the patient last ate, what they ate, and how the last food consumption relates to the normal intake at that time of day.[34,115,116] For example, if the patient took their usual dose of regular insulin in the morning before breakfast but then either failed to eat or ate a lighter breakfast than usual, the patient is at increased risk for hypoglycemia if the dental appointment is scheduled in the morning. Carbohydrate intake must be adequate to "match" plasma insulin levels or hypoglycemia will result. If dental treatment requires alteration in diet either before or after the appointment, the patient's medication regimen may need to be changed. Patients who are on NPO (nothing by mouth) orders before dental treatment may need to have their insulin regimen altered. Sulfonylurea doses may also need adjustment. In these cases, physician consultation may be indicated. Physicians frequently recommend reduction in the insulin dose that immediately precedes lengthy or extensive procedures. Longer-term adjustments are often made when diet modifications will occur.

Management of Diabetic Emergencies

Medical emergencies related to diabetic complications may occur in the dental office. For example, macrovascular disease can lead to myocardial infarction or a cerebrovascular accident, and nephropathy may cause renal failure. However, the most common medical emergency in diabetic patients is hypoglycemia. As seen in the DCCT, hypoglycemia is a potentially grave complication.[113,114] Frequent causes of hypoglycemia are (1) injection of excess insulin; (2) delaying or skipping meals or snacks while taking the usual dose of insulin or oral sulfonylurea; (3) increasing exercise without adjusting food intake or the dose of insulin or sulfonylurea; (4) consuming alcohol and confusing signs of hypoglycemia with those of alcohol intoxication; and, (5) stress.[34,115,116]

Symptoms of hypoglycemia include confusion, shakiness or tremors, agitation, sweating, and tachycardia (Table 8–10). If unrecognized and untreated, hypoglycemia may lead to seizures, coma, and death. If a patient has symptoms of hypoglycemia and brought a glucometer to the dental appointment, they should immediately check the blood glucose level. Symptoms of hypoglycemia are likely to occur if the blood glucose drops below 60 mg/dL but may occur in some patients at higher or lower threshold levels.

To treat hypoglycemia in a conscious patient, the dentist should give approximately 15 g of oral carbohydrate in a form that will be rapidly absorbed (Table 8–11). About 120 to 180 mL (4 to 6 oz) of fruit juice or soda is usually adequate to relieve symptoms. Alternatively, 3 or 4 teaspoons of table sugar or an appropriate amount of hard candy may be given. Tubes of cake icing are easy to store and provide a rapid source of readily absorbed carbohydrate. Oral carbohydrate in these forms will generally elevate blood glucose within 10 to 20 minutes, with relief of symptoms. Changes in blood glucose can be confirmed by glucometer. If symptoms have not resolved in a short period of time or the glucometer readings show persistent low blood glucose, another 15 g of carbohydrate should be given. If this does not elevate blood glucose, the parenteral route of treatment should be considered.[116]

In these cases, or when the patient is sedated or unable to take food or drink by mouth, 25 to 30 mL of 50% dextrose or 1 mg of glucagon can be given intravenously. In the absence of intravenous access, 1 mg of glucagon can be injected subcutaneously or intramuscularly at practically any location of the body. Glucagon injection results in glycogenolysis in the liver, releasing glucose from glycogen stores and rapidly increasing blood sugar levels. The patient should recover within 5 to 15 minutes following treatment. If not, a call for emergency medical assistance is warranted. When a patient experiences symptomatic hypoglycemia requiring emergency treatment in the dental office, they should be monitored for approximately 1 hour to ensure complete recovery. Evaluation of the blood glucose level by glucometer can confirm normoglycemia.

In some cases, hyperglycemia may present with symptoms similar to hypoglycemia. If a glucometer is not available to accurately determine blood glucose levels and the patient has symptoms

---

TABLE 8–10. Signs and Symptoms of Hypoglycemia

Confusion
Shakiness, tremors
Agitation
Anxiety
Sweating
Dizziness
Tachycardia
Feeling of "impending doom"
Seizures
Loss of consciousness

TABLE 8–11. Emergency Treatment of Hypoglycemia

Establish blood glucose level with glucometer, if possible.
In awake patient, give 15 g of carbohydrate orally; in the form of
  • 120 to 180 mL (4 to 6 oz) fruit juice or sugared soda;
  • 3 to 4 tsp table sugar;
  • hard candy; or
  • cake frosting in tube.
If patient unable to use oral route and IV is in place, administer
  • 25 to 30 mL 50% dextrose (D50) IV; or
  • 1 mg glucagon IV.
If patient unable to use oral route and IV is *not* in place, administer
  • 1 mg glucagon subcutaneously or intramuscularly.
Monitor patient for 1 hour after recovery.
Seek emergency medical assistance if patient does not respond.

suggestive of hypoglycemia, immediate carbohydrate intake or administration of glucose-elevating medication is indicated. When in doubt, the patient who is known to have diabetes and experiences shakiness, sweating, tachycardia, or agitation should be treated presumptively for hypoglycemia. If the symptoms turn out to have been caused by hyperglycemia rather than hypoglycemia, the small amount of additional carbohydrate given will generally not have a significant negative effect. Conversely, if carbohydrate or medication to elevate blood glucose levels is withheld from a patient who is actually experiencing hypoglycemia, in the mistaken belief that the symptoms are being caused by hyperglycemia, severe sequelae are possible. The best means of rapidly determining the true nature of the emergency is measurement of capillary blood glucose with a glucometer.

Hyperglycemic crisis is a far less common emergency in the dental office than is hypoglycemia. Prolonged hyperglycemia may result in diabetic ketoacidosis in people with type 1 diabetes while in type 2 diabetes it may cause hyperosmolar nonketotic acidosis or hyperosmolar nonacidotic diabetes.[116] Onset of hyperglycemic emergencies occurs more slowly than does hypoglycemia, generally after protracted elevation of blood glucose. Hyperglycemic emergencies require immediate medical evaluation and treatment. Basic life support procedures should be performed, including opening the airway, administering oxygen, evaluating circulation, and monitoring vital signs. The emergency medical system should be activated and the patient transported to a hospital as soon as possible.

The classic signs and symptoms of hypoglycemia may not be present immediately prior to a severe hypoglycemic reaction. The patient receiving conscious sedation in conjunction with dental therapy may have even more difficulty recognizing the warning symptoms. Constant verbal and visual contact and assessment of the patient's subjective symptoms is necessary. The danger of hypoglycemia may be reduced by periodic glucose monitoring during longer dental appointments.

As part of the initial medical history, diabetic patients should be questioned about their past history of hypoglycemic episodes. In the DCCT, patients with a history of previous severe hypoglycemia had a 112% higher risk of having another severe hypoglycemic reaction compared with those with no prior history.[113] The strongest predictor of severe hypoglycemia was the number of previous hypoglycemic episodes.[114] The patient's glycemic control may also relate to the risk for

hypoglycemia. In what seems at first glance to be a paradox, the risk for hypoglycemic emergencies increases as glycemic control improves and glycosylated hemoglobin values decrease.[113] Determining the patient's past glycosylated hemoglobin values prior to treatment not only provides an excellent assessment of the patient's degree of metabolic control but may also suggest their relative risk for severe hypoglycemia. For example, the patient with a recent HbA1c of 7.5% may pose a greater risk of hypoglycemia than a patient with a recent HbA1c of 11%.

With time, some diabetic patients lose their ability to recognize impending hypoglycemia, a phenomenon known as hypoglycemia unawareness.[118] Hypoglycemia unawareness may occur not only in intensively treated patients but in those on conventional insulin regimens or oral agents as well. While signs and symptoms of hypoglycemia are common when blood glucose levels fall below 60 mg/dL, patients with hypoglycemia unawareness may feel completely normal at levels of 40 mg/dL or lower. This places the patient at risk of developing severe hypoglycemia and impairs their ability to take appropriate corrective measures. Onset of emergencies in patients with hypoglycemia unawareness may be immediate and without warning. Dental practitioners should question their diabetic patients as to the frequency of hypoglycemic episodes and the most common symptoms experienced by them.

THE DIABETIC PATIENT AND THE ROAD TO ORAL HEALTH

Ensuring oral health in patients with diabetes requires an expanded scope of medical and dental knowledge. There is undoubtedly a close relationship between diabetes and periodontal disease, a relationship requiring further study and exploration. Diabetes increases the risk of periodontal destruction, especially in patients whose glycemic control is poor. These same patients are most likely to report to the dental office with significant periodontal treatment needs. All diabetic patients should have routine dental evaluation and preventive therapy. The practitioner who understands the role of diabetes in the etiology of oral diseases, the potential for oral infections to influence glycemic control, the current medical therapeutic approaches to diabetes, and the implications of diabetes on dental care provides the patient with the best chances of successful treatment outcomes.

REFERENCES

1. National Diabetes Data Group: Diabetes in America, 2 ed. Bethesda, MD: National Institutes of Health. NIH Publication No 95-1468; 1995.

2. De Sanctis RW, Dec GW. Cardiomyopathies. In: Dale DC, Federman DD, editors. Scientific American Medicine. New York: Scientific American Inc.; 1995.

3. Mandrup-Poulsen T. Recent advances—Diabetes. Br Med J 1998;316:1221–5.

4. Edelman SV. Type II diabetes mellitus. Adv Internal Med 1998; 43:449–500.

5. American Diabetes Association. Report of the Expert Committee on the Diagnosis and Classification of Diabetes Mellitus. Diabetes Care 1997;20:1183–97.

6. Reaven GM. Role of insulin resistance in human disease. Diabetes 1988;37:1595–607.

7. Eriksson J, Franssila-Kallunki A, Ekstrand A, et al. Early metabolic defects in persons at increased risk for non-insulin-dependent diabetes mellitus. N Engl J Med 1989; 321:337–43.

8. Bogardus C, Lillioja S, Mott DM, et al. Relationship between degree of obesity and in vivo insulin action in man. Am J Physiol 1985;248:E286–91.

9. Newman B, Selby JV, Slemenda C, et al. Concordance for type 2 (non-insulin-dependent) diabetes mellitus in male twins. Diabetologia 1987;30:763–8.

10. Ghosh S, Schork NJ. Genetic analysis of NIDDM. Diabetes 1996;45:1–14.

11. Charles MA, Fontboune A, Thibult N, et al. Risk factors for NIDDM in white populations: Paris Prospective Study. Diabetes 1991;40:796–9.

12. Engelgau MM, Herman WH, Smith PJ, et al. The epidemiology of diabetes and pregnancy in the U.S., 1988. Diabetes Care 1995;18:1029–33.

13. Dietrich ML, Dolnicek TF, Rayburn WR. Gestational diabetes screening in a private midwestern American population. Am J Obstet Gynecol 1987;156:1403–8.

14. Marquette GP, Klein VR, Niebyl JR. Efficacy of screening for gestational diabetes. Am J Perinatol 1985;2:7–14.

15. Magee MS, Walden CE, Benedetti TJ. Influence of diagnostic criteria on the incidence of gestational diabetes and perinatal morbidity. JAMA 1993;269:609–15.

16. Langer O, Rodriguez DA, Xenakis EMJ, et al. Intensified versus conventional management of gestational diabetes. Am J Obstet Gynecol 1994;170:1036–47.

17. Steinberg D. Diabetes and atherosclerosis. In: Porte D, Sherwin RS, editors. Diabetes mellitus. 5th ed. Stamford, CT: Appleton & Lange; 1997.

18. Steffes MW. Pathophysiology of renal complications. In: Porte D, Sherwin RS, editors. Diabetes mellitus. 5th ed. Stamford, CT: Appleton & Lange; 1997.

19. Klein R. Retinopathy and other ocular complications in diabetes. In: Porte D, Sherwin RS, editors. Diabetes mellitus. 5th ed. Stamford, CT: Appleton & Lange; 1997.

20. Greene DA, Feldman EL, Stevens MJ, et al. Diabetic neuropathy. In: Porte D, Sherwin RS, editors. Diabetes mellitus. 5th ed. Stamford, CT: Appleton & Lange; 1997.

21. Iacopino AM. Diabetic periodontitis: possible lipid-induced defect in tissue repair through alteration of macrophage phenotype and function. Oral Diseases 1995;1:214–29.

22. Colwell JA, Jokl R. Vascular thrombosis in diabetes. In: Porte D, Sherwin RS, editors. Diabetes mellitus. 5th ed. Stamford, CT: Appleton & Lange; 1997.

23. Brunzell JD, Chait A. Diabetic dyslipidemia: pathology and treatment. In: Porte D, Sherwin RS, editors. Diabetes mellitus. 5th ed. Stamford, CT: Appleton & Lange; 1997.

24. Vlassara H. Recent progress on the biologic and clinical significance of advanced glycosylation end products. J Lab Clin Med 1994;124:19–30.

25. Brownlee M. Glycosylation and diabetic complications. Diabetes 1994;43:836–41.

26. Monnier VM, Glomb M, Elgawish A, Sell DR. The mechanism of collagen cross-linking in diabetes. A puzzle nearing resolution. Diabetes 1996:45(Suppl 3):S67–72.

27. Schmidt AM, Hori O, Brett J, et al. Cellular receptors for advanced glycosylation end products. Implications for induction of oxidant stress and cellular dysfunction in the pathogenesis of vascular lesions. Atheroscler Thromb 1994;14: 1521–8.

28. Schmidt AM, Hori O, Cao R, et al. RAGE. A novel cellular receptor for advanced glycosylation end products. Diabetes 1996;45(Suppl 3):S77–80.

29. Vlassara H, Bucala R. Recent progress in advanced glycosylation and diabetic vascular disease: role of advanced glycosylation end product receptors. Diabetes 1996;45(Suppl 3):S65–6.

30. Esposito C, Gerlach H, Brett J, et al. Endothelial receptor-mediated binding of glucose-modified albumin is associated with increased monolayer permeability and modulation of cell surface coagulant properties. J Exp Med 1992;170: 1387–407.

31. Kirstein M, Aston C, Hintz R, Vlassara H. Receptor-specific induction of insulin-like growth fac-

tor I in human monocytes by advanced glycosylation end product-modified proteins. J Clin Invest 1992;90:439–46.

32. Vlassara H, Brownlee M, Monogue K, et al. Cachetin/TNF and IL-1 induced by glucose-modified proteins: role in normal tissue remodeling. Science 1988;240:1546–8.

33. American Diabetes Association Expert Committee on the Diagnosis and Classification of Diabetes Mellitus. Committee Report. Diabetes Care 1997;20:1183–97.

34. Mealey BL. Impact of advances in diabetes care on dental treatment of the diabetic patient. Compend Contin Educ Dent 1998;19:41–58.

35. Tsuji I, Nakamoto K, Hasegawa T, et al. Receiver operating characteristic analysis of fasting plasma glucose, HbA1c, and fructosamine on diabetes screening. Diabetes Care 1991;14:1075–7.

36. American Diabetes Association. Standards of medical care for patients with diabetes mellitus. Diabetes Care 1998;21(Suppl 1):S23–31.

37. American Diabetes Association. Self-monitoring of blood glucose (consensus statement). Diabetes Care 1993;16:60–5.

38. Thorstensson H, Flak H, Hugoson A, Olsson J. Some salivary factors in insulin-dependent diabetics. Acta Odontol Scand 1989;47:175–83.

39. Sreebny LM, Yu A, Green A, Valdini A. Xerostomia in diabetes mellitus. Diabetes Care 1992;15: 900–4.

40. Harrison R, Bowden WH. Flow rate and organic constituents of whole saliva in insulin-dependent diabetic children and adolescents. Pediatr Dent 1987;9:287–90.

41. Fisher BM, Lamey PJ, Samaranayake LP, et al. Carriage of *Candida* species in the oral cavity in diabetic patients: relationship to glycaemic control. J Oral Pathol 1987;16:282–4.

42. Phelan JA, Levin SM. A prevalence study of denture stomatitis in subjects with diabetes mellitus or elevated plasma glucose levels. Oral Surg Oral Med Oral Pathol 1986;62:303–5.

43. Jones RB, McCallum RM, Kay EJ, et al. Oral health and oral health behavior in a population of diabetic clinic attenders. Community Dent Oral Epidemiol 1992;20:204–7.

44. Tenovuo J, Alanen P, Larjava H, et al. Oral health of patients with insulin dependent diabetes mellitus. Scand J Dent Res 1986;94:338–46.

45. Tavares M, DePaola P, Soparkar P, Joshipura K. Prevalence of root caries in a diabetic population. J Dent Res 1991;70:979–83.

46. Meurman JH, Collin HL, Niskanen L, et al. Saliva in non-insulin-dependent diabetic patients and control subjects. The role of the autonomic nervous system. Oral Surg Oral Med Oral Pathol Oral Radiol Endod 1998;86:69–76.

47. Collin HL, Uusitupa M, Niskanen L, et al. Caries in patients with non-insulin-dependent diabetes mellitus. Oral Surg Oral Med Oral Pathol Oral Radiol Endod 1998;85:680–5.

48. Gusberti FA, Syed SA, Bacon G, et al. Puberty gingivitis in insulin-dependent diabetic children. J Periodontol 1983;54:714–20.

49. Cianciola LJ, Park BH, Bruck E, et al. Prevalence of periodontal disease in insulin-dependent diabetes mellitus (juvenile diabetes). J Am Dent Assoc 1982;104:653–60.

50. De Pommereau V, Dargent-Pare C, Robert JJ, Brion M. Periodontal status in insulin-dependent diabetic adolescents. J Clin Periodontol 1992;19:628–32.

51. Ervasti T, Knuuttila M, Pohjamo L, Haukipuro K. Relation between control of diabetes and gingival bleeding. J Periodontol 1985;56:154–7.

52. Karjalainen KM, Knuuttila MLE. The onset of diabetes and poor metabolic control increases gingival bleeding in children and adolescents with insulin-dependent diabetes mellitus. J Clin Periodontol 1996;23:1060–7.

53. Papapanou PN. 1996 World Workshop in Clinical Periodontics. Periodontal diseases: epidemiology. Ann Periodontol 1996;1:1–36.

54. Emrich LJ, Shlossman M, Genco RJ. Periodontal disease in non-insulin-dependent diabetes mellitus. J Periodontol 1991;62:123–30.

55. Shlossman M, Knowler WC, Pettitt DJ, Genco RJ. Type 2 diabetes mellitus and periodontal disease. J Am Dent Assoc 1990;121:532–6.

56. Taylor GW, Burt BA, Becker MP, et al. Non-insulin dependent diabetes mellitus and alveolar bone loss progression over 2 years. J Periodontol 1998;69:76–83.

57. Oliver RC, Tervonen T. Diabetes—a risk factor for periodontitis in adults? J Periodontol 1994;65: 530–8.

58. Seppala B, Seppala M, Ainamo J. A longitudinal study on insulin-dependent diabetes mellitus and periodontal disease. J Clin Periodontol 1993;20:161–5.

59. Tervonen T, Oliver RC. Long-term control of diabetes mellitus and periodontitis. J Clin Periodontol 1993;20:431–5.

60. Christgau M, Palitzsch KD, Schmalz G, et al. Healing response to non-surgical periodontal therapy in patients with diabetes mellitus: clinical, microbiological, and immunological results. J Clin Periodontol 1998;25:112–24.

61. Tervonen T, Karjalainen K. Periodontal disease related to diabetic status. A pilot study of the response to periodontal therapy in type 1 diabetes. J Clin Periodontol 1997;24:505–10.

62. Westfelt E, Rylander H, Blohme G, et al. The effect of periodontal therapy in diabetics. Results after 5 years. J Clin Periodontol 1996;23:92–100.

63. Zambon JJ, Reynolds H, Fisher JG, et al. Microbiological and immunological studies of adult periodontitis in patients with non-insulin dependent diabetes mellitus. J Periodontol 1988;59:23–31.

64. Sastrowijoto SH, Hillemans P, van Steenbergen TJ, et al. Periodontal condition and microbiology of healthy and diseased periodontal pockets in type 1 diabetes mellitus patients. J Clin Periodontol 1989;16:316–22

65. Kjellman O. The presence of glucose in gingival exudate and resting saliva of subjects with insulin-treated diabetes mellitus. Swed Dent J 1970;63:11–9.

66. Ficara AJ, Levin MP, Grower MF, Kramer GD. A comparison of the glucose and protein content of gingival crevicular fluid from diabetics and nondiabetics. J Periodontal Res 1975;10:171–5.

67. Nishimura F, Takahashi K, Kurihara M, et al. Periodontal disease as a complication of diabetes mellitus. Ann Periodontol 1998;3:20–9.

68. Frantzis TG, Reeve CM, Brown AL. The ultrastructure of capillary basement membranes in the attached gingiva of diabetic and non-diabetic patients with periodontal disease. J Periodontol 1971;42:406–11.

69. Listgarten MA, Ricker FH, Laster L, et al. Vascular basement membrane lamina thickness in the normal and inflamed gingiva of diabetics and nondiabetics. J Periodontol 1974;45:676–84.

70. Seppala B, Sorsa T, Ainamo J. Morphometric analysis of cellular and vascular changes in gingival connective tissue in long-term insulin-dependent diabetes. J Periodontol 1997;68:1237–45.

71. Schmidt AM, Weidman E, Lalla E, et al. Advanced glycosylation endproducts (AGEs) induce oxidant stress in the gingiva: a potential mechanism underlying accelerated periodontal disease associated with diabetes. J Periodontal Res 1996; 31:508–15.

72. Manoucher-Pour M, Spagnuolo PJ, Rodman HM, Bissada NF. Comparison of neutrophil chemotactic response in diabetic patients with mild and severe periodontal disease. J Periodontol 1981;52:410–5.

73. McMullen JA, van Dyke TE, Horoszewicz HU, Genco RJ. Neutrophil chemotaxis in individuals with advanced periodontal disease and a genetic predisposition to diabetes mellitus. J Periodontol 1981;52:167–73.

74. Oliver RC, Tervonen T, Flynn DG, Keenan KM. Enzyme activity in crevicular fluid in relation to metabolic control of diabetes and other periodontal risk factors. J Periodontol 1993;64:358–62.

75. Offenbacher S. 1996 World Workshop in Clinical Periodontics. Periodontal diseases: pathogenesis. Ann Periodontol 1996;1:821–78.

76. Salvi GE, Collins JG, Yalda B, et al. Monocytic TNF-α secretion patterns in IDDM patients with periodontal diseases. J Clin Periodontol 1997;24:8–16.

77. Salvi GE, Yalda B, Collins JG, et al. Inflammatory mediator response as a potential risk marker for periodontal diseases in insulin-dependent diabetes mellitus patients. J Periodontol 1997;68:127–35.

78. Ryan ME, Ramamurthy NS, Golub LM. Matrix metalloproteinases and their inhibition in periodontal treatment. Curr Opin Periodont 1996;3:85–96.

79. Birkedal-Hansen H. Role of matrix metalloproteinases in human periodontal disease. J Periodontol 1993;64:474–84.

80. Ramamurthy NS, Golub LM. Diabetes increases collagenase activity in extracts of rat gingiva and skin. J Periodontal Res 1983;18:23–30.

81. Golub LM, Lee HM, Lehrer G, et al. Minocycline reduces gingival collagenolytic activity during diabetes: preliminary observations and a proposed new mechanism. J Periodontal Res 1983; 18:516–26.

82. McCulloch CAG, Birek P, Overall C, et al. Randomized controlled clinical trial of doxycycline in prevention of recurrent periodontitis in high risk patients: antimicrobial activity and collagenase inhibition. J Clin Periodontol 1990;17:616–22.

83. Golub LM, Lee HM, Greenwald RA, et al. A matrix metalloproteinase inhibitor reduces bone-type collagen degradation fragments and specific collagenases in gingival crevicular fluid during adult periodontitis. Inflamm Res 1997; 46:310–9.

84. Bain S, Ramamurthy NS, Impeduglia T, et al. Tetracycline prevents cancellous bone loss and maintains near-normal rates of bone formation in streptozotocin diabetic rats. Bone 1997;21:147–53.

85. Greenwald RA, Golub LM, Ramamurthy NS, et al. In vitro sensitivity of the three mammalian col-

lagenases to tetracycline inhibition: relationship to bone and cartilage degradation. Bone 1998; 22:33–8.

86. Caton J, Ciancio S, Crout R, et al. Adjunctive use of subantimicrobial doxycycline therapy for periodontitis (Abstract). J Dent Res 1998;77:1001.

87. Taylor GW, Burt BA, Becker MP, et al. Severe periodontitis and risk for poor glycemic control in patients with non-insulin-dependent diabetes mellitus. J Periodontol 1996;67:1085–93.

88. Thorstensson H, Kuylensteirna J, Hugoson A. Medical status and complications in relation to periodontal disease experience in insulin-dependent diabetics. J Clin Periodontol 1996;23:194–202.

89. Loe H. Periodontal disease. The sixth complication of diabetes mellitus. Diabetes Care 1993;16 (Suppl 1):329–34.

90. Williams RC, Mahan CJ. Periodontal disease and diabetes in young adults. JAMA 1960;172: 776–8.

91. Miller LS, Manwell MA, Newbold D, et al. The relationship between reduction in periodontal inflammation and diabetes control: a report of 9 cases. J Periodontol 1992;63:843–8.

92. Grossi SG, Skrepcinski FB, DeCaro T, et al. Response to periodontal therapy in diabetics and smokers. J Periodontol 1996;67:1094–102.

93. Grossi SG, Skrepcinski FB, DeCaro T, et al. Treatment of periodontal disease in diabetics reduces glycosylated hemoglobin. J Periodontol 1997; 68:713–9.

94. Aldridge JP, Lester V, Watts TLP, et al. Single-blind studies of the effects of improved periodontal health on metabolic control in type 1 diabetes mellitus. J Clin Periodontol 1995;22:271–5.

95. Sammalkorpi K. Glucose intolerance in acute infections. J Intern Med 1989;225:15–9.

96. Yki-Jarvinen H, Sammalkorpi K, Koivisto VA, Nikkila EA. Severity, duration and mechanism of insulin resistance during acute infections. J Clin Endocrinol Metab 1989;69:317–23.

97. Grossi SG, Genco RJ. Periodontal disease and diabetes mellitus: a two-way relationship. Ann Periodontol 1998;3:51–61.

98. Nevins ML, Karimbux NY, Weber HP, et al. Wound healing around endosseous implants in experimental diabetes. Int J Oral Maxillofac Implants 1998;13:620–9.

99. Takeshita F, Murai K, Iyama S, et al. Uncontrolled diabetes hinders bone formation around titanium implants in rat tibiae. A light and fluorescence microscopy, and image processing study. J Periodontol 1998; 69:314–20.

100. Diabetes Control and Complications Trial Research Group. The Diabetes Control and Complications Trial (DCCT): design and methodologic considerations for the feasibility phase. Diabetes 1986;35:530–45.

101. Diabetes Control and Complications Trial Research Group. The effect of intensive treatment of diabetes on the development and progression of long-term complications in insulin-dependent diabetes mellitus. N Engl J Med 1993;329:977–86.

102. Diabetes Control and Complications Trial Research Group. Progression of retinopathy with intensive versus conventional treatment in the Diabetes Control and Complications Trial. Ophthalmology 1995;102:647–61.

103. Diabetes Control and Complications Trial Research Group. Effect of intensive diabetes management on macrovascular and microvascular events and risk factors in the Diabetes Control and Complications Trial. Am J Cardiol 1995;75:894–903.

104. American Diabetes Association Position Statement. Implications of the Diabetes Control and Complications Trial. Diabetes Spectrum 1993;6:225–7.

105. Diabetes Control and Complications Trial Research Group. Lifetime benefits and costs of intensive therapy as practiced in the Diabetes Control and Complications Trial. JAMA 1996;276:1409–15.

106. Thompson CJ, Cummings JF, Chalmers J, et al. How have patients reacted to the implications of the DCCT? Diabetes Care 1996;19:876–9.

107. Ohkubo Y, Kishikawa H, Araki E, et al. Intensive insulin therapy prevents the progression of diabetic microvascular complications in Japanese patients with non-insulin-dependent diabetes mellitus: a randomized prospective 6-year study. Diabetes Res Clin Pract 1995;28:103–17.

108. Andersson DKG, Svardsudd K. Long-term glycemic control relates to mortality in type II diabetes. Diabetes Care 1995;18:1534–43.

109. Scheen AJ, Lefebvre PJ. Oral antidiabetic agents. A guide to selection. Drugs 1998;55:225–36.

110. Wolffenbuttel BHR, Nijst L, Sels JPJE, et al. Effects of a new oral hypoglycaemic agent, repaglinide, on metabolic control in sulfonylurea-treated patients with NIDDM. Eur J Clin Pharmacol 1993;45:113–6.

111. Lebovitz HE: Oral antidiabetic agents. In: Kahn CR, Weir GC, editors. Joslin's diabetes mellitus, 13th ed. Malvern (PA): Lea & Febiger; 1994.

112. Peterson KA, Smith CK. The DCCT findings and standards of care for diabetes. Am Fam Physician 1995;2:1092–8.

113. Diabetes Control and Complications Trial Research Group. Epidemiology of severe hypoglycemia in the Diabetes Control and Complications Trial. Am J Med 1991;90:450–9.

114. Diabetes Control and Complications Trial Research Group. Hypoglycemia in the Diabetes Control and Complications Trial. Diabetes 1997;46:271–86.

115. Rees TD. The diabetic dental patient. Dent Clin North Am 1994;38:447–63.

116. Mealey BL. 1996 World Workshop in Clinical Periodontics. Periodontal implications: medically compromised patients. Ann Periodontol 1996;1:256–321.

117. Galili D, Findler M, Garfunkel AA. Oral and dental complications associated with diabetes and their treatment. Compend Contin Educ Dent 1994;15:496–509.

118. Heller SR, Herbert M, MacDonald IA, Tattersall RB. Influence of sympathetic nervous system on hypoglycemic warning symptoms. Lancet 1987;2:359–63.

CHAPTER 9

PERIODONTAL MEDICINE AND THE FEMALE PATIENT

Joan Otomo-Corgel, DDS, MPH
Barbara J. Steinberg, DDS

Women's life cycle changes present unique challenges to the oral health care profession. Hormonal influences associated with the reproductive process alter periodontal and oral-tissue responses to local factors creating diagnostic and therapeutic dilemmas. It is imperative, therefore, that the clinician recognize, customize, and vary periodontal therapy according to the individual female and the stage of her life cycle.

This chapter will deal with phases of the female life cycle during the reproductive years: puberty, menses, and pregnancy. Oral contraceptives, periodontal manifestations, systemic effects, and clinical management will also be discussed.

PUBERTY

Periodontal Manifestations

During puberty, the female experiences an increase in the production of sex hormones (estrogen and progesterone) that remains relatively constant following puberty throughout the normal female lifetime reproductive phase. There is also an increase in the prevalence of gingivitis without an increase in the amount of plaque.[1]

Gram-negative anaerobes, especially *Prevotella intermedia,* have been implicated in association with puberty gingivitis. Kornman and Loesche postulated that this anaerobic organism may use ovarian hormone as a substitute for vitamin K growth factor.[1] Delaney and Kornman suggest that levels of black-pigmented bacteroides, especially *Bacteroides intermedius,* increase with increased levels of gonadotrophic hormones in puberty. *Capnocytophaga* species also increase in incidence as well as in proportion. These organisms have been implicated in the increased bleeding tendency observed during puberty.[2] Recent studies associated with puberty gingivitis indicate proportionately elevated motile rods, spirochetes, and *Prevotella intermedia.*[3] Statistically significant increases in gingival inflammation and in the proportion of *Prevotella intermedia* and *Prevotella nigrescens* were seen in puberty gingivitis.[4]

Clinically, during puberty, there may be a nodular hyperplastic reaction of the gingiva in areas where food debris, materia alba, plaque, and calculus are deposited. The inflamed tissues are erythematous and may be lobulated and retractable (Figure 9–1). Bleeding may occur with brushing or mastication. Histologically, the appearance is consistent with inflammatory hyperplasia.

Management

Preventive care, including a vigorous program of oral hygiene, is vital. Milder gingivitis cases respond well to scaling and root planing with frequent oral hygiene instructions.[5] Severe cases of gingivitis may require microbial culturing, antimicrobial mouthwashes and local site delivery, or

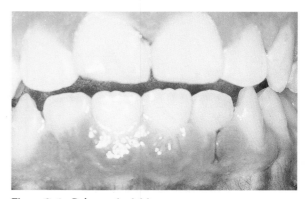

Figure 9–1. Puberty gingivitis.

antibiotic therapy. Supportive periodontal therapy visits may need increased frequency. Whenever possible, involvement of a parent or caregiver with home care procedures is recommended.

Eating Disorders

This age group also is susceptible to eating disorders, bulimia nervosa, and anorexia nervosa. The clinician should recognize the intraoral effects of chronic regurgitation of gastric contents on intraoral tissues. Perimylolysis, or smooth erosion of the enamel and dentin, typically on the lingual surfaces of maxillary anterior teeth, varies with the duration and frequency of the behavior.[6] Also, parotid gland enlargement (occasionally, sublingual glands) has been estimated at between 10 to 50 percent in the patient who binges and purges.[7] Therefore, there may also be a diminished salivary flow rate, which will increase oral mucous membrane sensitivity and gingival erythema. One should also rule out other etiologies that alter salivary flow, that is, systemic conditions or medications.

MENSES

Periodontal Manifestations

During the reproductive years, there are ongoing changes in the concentration of the gonadotrophins and ovarian hormones during the monthly menstrual cycle (Figure 9–2). Estrogen and progesterone are steroid hormones produced by the ovaries during the menstrual cycle. The gonadotrophins follicle-stimulating hormone (FSH) and luteinizing hormone (LH) influence estrogen and

progesterone to prepare the uterus for implantation of the egg. There are two phases of the monthly reproductive cycle. During the follicular phase I, estrogen causes cellular proliferation of the stroma cells, blood vessels, and glands of the endometrium. Phase II is called the luteal phase. Note that estrogen peaks to 0.2 ng/mL and progesterone to 10.0 ng/mL to complete the rebuilding of the endometrium for fertilized egg implantation. The corpus luteum involutes, ovarian hormone levels drop, and menstruation ensues.

The concept that ovarian hormones may increase inflammation in gingival tissues and exaggerate the response to local irritants has been postulated by several studies. Gingival inflammation seems to be aggravated by an imbalance and/or increase in sex hormones.[8–11]

Progesterone has been associated with increased permeability of the microvasculature, altering the rate and pattern of collagen production in the gingiva;[8] increasing folate metabolism,[9,10] and altering the immune response. During menses, progesterone increases from the second week, peaks at approximately 10 days, and dramatically drops prior to menstruation. (Note that this is based on a 28-day cycle and individual cycles are variable.) Progesterone plays a role in stimulating the production of prostaglandins that mediate the body's response to inflammation. Prostaglandin E$_2$ (PGE$_2$) is one of the major secretory products of monocytes and is higher in inflamed gingiva.[10] Miyagi and colleagues found that the chemotaxis of polymorphonuclear leukocytes (PMNs) was enhanced by progesterone, whereas it was reduced by estradiol.[11] Testosterone did not have a measurable effect on PMN chemotaxis. They suggested that the altered PMN chemotaxis associated with gingival inflammation may be due to the effects of sex hormones.

Gingival tissues have been reported to be more edematous and erythematous preceding the onset of menses in some individuals. In addition, an increase of gingival exudate has been observed during the menstrual period and is sometimes associated with a minor increase in tooth mobility.[12]

Intraoral recurrent aphthous ulcers,[13] herpes labialis lesions, and Candidae infections occur in some women as a cyclic pattern associated with the luteal phase of their cycle when progesterone is the highest. Because the esophageal sphincter is relaxed by progesterone, women may be more susceptible to gastroesophageal reflux disease (GERD) during this time of the cycle as well. Symptoms of GERD include heartburn, regurgitation, and chest pain; when reflux is severe, some people will develop

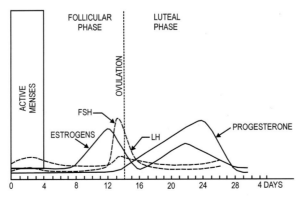

Figure 9–2. Female reproductive cycle. Note peak of progesterone and estrogen to follicle-stimulating hormone (FSH) and luteinizing hormone (LH).

unexplained coughing, hoarseness, sore throat, gingivitis, or asthma.

During the peak level of progesterone (about 7 to 10 days prior to menstruation), premenstrual syndrome (PMS) also occurs. There appears to be no significant differences in estrogen and progesterone levels between women who suffer from PMS and women who do not. Yet, women with PMS seem to have lower levels of certain neurotransmitters such as enkephalins, endorphins, γ-aminobutyric acid (GABA) and serotonin. Depression, irritability, mood swings, and difficulty with memory and concentration may be symptoms of neurotransmitter reduction.

Management

For the women who have increased gingival bleeding and tenderness associated with the menstrual cycle, adherence to 3 to 4-month supportive periodontal therapy appointments is recommended. Antimicrobial mouthrinses prior to cyclic inflammation may be indicated. Particular emphasis should be placed on oral hygiene.

During PMS, physical symptoms may include fatigue, sweet and salty food cravings, abdominal bloating, swollen hands or feet, headaches, breast tenderness, and nausea or gastrointestinal upset.[14] Gastroesophageal reflux disease may make it more uncomfortable for the patient to lay fully supine, especially within the hours immediately after consumption of a meal. Care should be taken during dental treatment to prevent stimulating the more sensitive gag reflex. The clinician should be aware that nonsteroidal anti-inflammatory medication, infection, and acidic foods exacerbate GERD. Patients taking over-the-counter antacids, H_2 receptor antagonists (cimetidine, famotidine, nizatidine, and ranitidine), prokinetic agents (cisapride and metcloplamide), and proton pump inhibitors (lansoprazole and omeprazole) may be GERD candidates.[15] The aforementioned medications have interactions with some antibiotics and antifungal medications, therefore, review of the pharmacology is necessary if they are used in periodontal therapy. Fluoride rinses and/or trays, frequent periodontal débridement, and avoidance of mouthwashes with high alcohol content may reduce the associated gingival and caries sequelae.

It is common for physicians to treat PMS by increasing the levels of deficient neurotransmitters. Alprazolam mimics GABA. Fluoxetine increases the amount of serotonin in the circulation and has a reported 70 percent response rate. It is one of the 10 most-prescribed medications in the United States in the late 1990s. The clinician should be aware that patients on fluoxetine will have increased side effects with highly protein-bound drugs (eg, aspirin) and the half-life of diazepam and other central nervous system (CNS) depressants will be increased. Other common selective serotonin reuptake inhibitors are sertraline and peroxetine.

The PMS patient may be difficult to treat due to emotional and physiologic sensitivity. Treat the gingival and oral mucosal tissues gently. Moisten gauzes or cotton rolls with a lubricant, chlorhexidine rinse, or water before placing them in the aphthous prone patient. Careful retraction of the oral mucosa, cheeks, and lips will be necessary in both the aphthous and herpetic prone patient. Since the hypoglycemic threshold is elevated, advise the patient to have a light snack prior to her appointment. Note that 70 percent of menstruating women have PMS symptoms, but only 5 percent meet the strict diagnostic criteria.

PREGNANCY

Pregnancy provides unique diagnostic and treatment challenges to the periodontal clinician. It is an opportunity to individualize care at a time when the patient may experience the most profound physiologic and psychologic changes in her life. Awareness exists regarding pregnancy and its effect on periodontal disease; however, recent evidence indicates an inverse relationship to systemic disease. Current research implies that periodontal disease may alter the systemic health of the patient as well as adversely effect the well-being of the fetus by elevating the risk of low-birth-weight, preterm infants.

Periodontal Manifestations

Periodontal Diseases
In 1877, Pinard recorded the first case of "pregnancy gingivitis."[16] Only recently has periodontal research began to focus on causative mechanisms. Pregnancy gingivitis is extremely common, occurring in approximately 30 to 75 percent of all pregnant women.[17–19] It is characterized by erythema, edema, hyperplasia, and increased bleeding. Histologically, the description is the same as gingivitis. The etiologic factors, however, are different despite clinical and histologic similarities. Cases range from mild inflammation (Figure 9–3) to severe hyperplasia, pain, and bleeding (Figure 9–4).

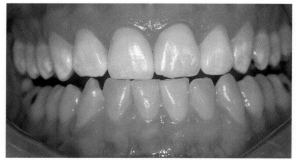 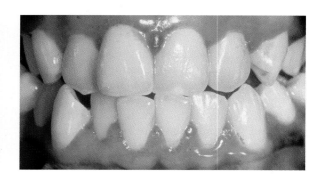

Figure 9–3. Mild to moderate pregnancy gingivitis.

Alterations in immunocompetency during pregnancy may create an exaggerated response in periodontal supporting structures (Figure 9–5). Periodontal status prior to pregnancy may influence the progression or severity as the circulating hormones fluctuate. The anterior region of the mouth is more commonly affected, and interproximal sites tend to be most involved.[20] Increased tissue edema may lead to increased pocket depths and relate to a transient tooth mobility.[21] Anterior site inflammation may be exacerbated by increased mouthbreathing, primarily in the third trimester from "pregnancy rhinitis."

Pyogenic granulomas occur during pregnancy at a prevalence of 0.2 to 9.6 percent. The "pregnancy tumor" or "pregnancy epulis" are clinically and histologically indistinguishable from pyogenic granulomas occurring in women who are not pregnant or in men. They appear most commonly during the second or third month of pregnancy. The gingiva is the most common site involved (approximately 70% of all cases), followed by tongue and lips, buccal mucosa, and palate.[22]

Clinically, pregnancy tumors appear to be tumorlike growths that generally appear on the interdental papillae of maxillary anterior teeth.

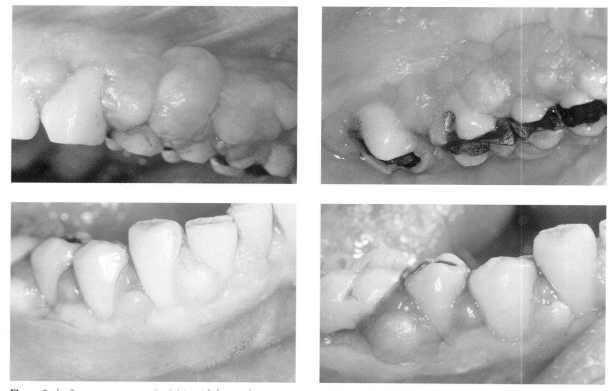

Figure 9–4. Severe pregnancy gingivitis with hyperplasia in a patient with non-insulin-dependent diabetes mellitus in poor control.

They usually grow rapidly, bleed easily, and become hyperplastic and nodular. They may be sessile or pedunculated and may be ulcerated. Color ranges from purplish red to deep blue, depending on the vascularity of the lesion and the degree of venous stasis. The lesion classically occurs in an area of gingivitis and is associated with poor oral hygiene. Often calculus is present. Osseous destruction is not usually associated with pyogenic granulomas of pregnancy.

Etiologic Factors

Despite the clinical/histologic diagnoses of gingivitis or pyogenic granuloma, a variety of other etiologic factors contribute to these periodontal conditions during pregnancy (Table 9–1). Alterations in the composition of subgingival plaque, maternal immunoresponsiveness, and sex hormone concentrations create a myriad of responses in the periodontium.

Subgingival Plaque Composition. There is an alteration in the composition of subgingival plaque during pregnancy. Kornman and Loesche found that during the second trimester there was an increase in gingivitis and gingival bleeding without an increase in plaque levels.[23] Bacterial anaerobic-to-aerobic ratios increased, as well as *Bacteroides melaninogenicus*, and *Prevotella intermedia* proportions (2.2 to 10.1%). There was also an increase in *Porphyromonas gingivalis*. These authors suggested that estradiol or progesterone can substitute for menadione (vitamin K) as an essential growth factor for *P. intermedia* but not *P. gingivalis* or *Bacteroides coherences*.

Maternal Immunoresponse. Recent studies support alteration of immunocomponents during pregnancy. These changes in maternal immunoresponsiveness suggest increased susceptibility to gingival inflammation. In one study, gingival index was higher, but percentages of T3, T4, and B cells appear to decrease in peripheral blood and gingival tissues during pregnancy as compared to a control group.[24] Other studies report decreased neutrophil chemotaxis, depression of cell-mediated immunity and phagocytosis as well as a decreased T-cell response with elevated levels of ovarian hormone, especially progesterone.[25] A decrease in in vitro responses of peripheral blood lymphocytes to several bacterial antigens has been reported[26–28] and there is evidence for a decrease in the absolute numbers of CD4-positive cells in peripheral blood during pregnancy as compared to the number of these cells post partum.[29,30] Lapp and colleagues suggest that high levels of progesterone during pregnancy affect the development of localized inflammation by down-regulation of IL-6 production, rendering the gingiva less efficient at resisting the inflammatory challenges produced by the bacteria.[31]

Also, ovarian hormone stimulates the production of prostaglandins, mediators of the inflammatory response. With the prostaglandin acting as an immunosuppressant, gingival inflammation may increase when the mediator level is high.[32,33] Kinnby and colleagues found that high progesterone during pregnancy influenced plasminogen activator inhibitor type 2 (PAI-2) and disturbed the balance of the fibrinolytic system.[34] Because PAI-2 serves as an

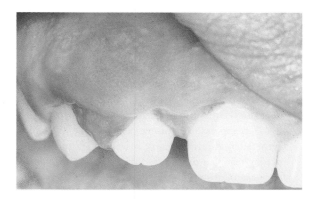

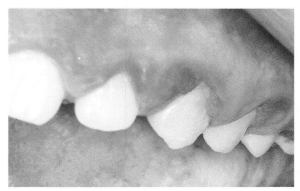

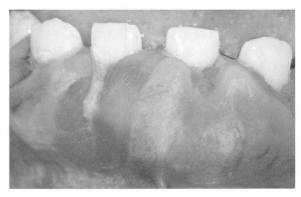

Figure 9–5. Pregnant (5½ months) patient with severe hyperplasia and acute monocytic leukemia.

important inhibitor of tissue proteolysis, the research by Kinnby and colleagues implies that components of the fibrinolytic system may be involved in the development of pregnancy gingivitis.

TABLE 9–1. Etiology of Gingival Responses to Elevated Estrogen and Progesterone during Pregnancy

Subgingival Plaque Composition
  Anaerobic-to-aerobic ratio increases
  Higher concentrations of *Prevotella intermedia* (substitutes sex hormone for vitamin K growth factor)
  Higher concentrations of *Bacteroides melaninogenicus*
  Higher concentrations of *Porphyromonas gingivalis*
Maternal Immunoresponse
  Depression of cell-mediated immunity
  Decreased neutrophil chemotaxis
  Depression of antibody and T cell responses
  Decrease in the ratio of peripheral T helper cells to T suppressor-cytotoxic cells (CD4/CD8 ratio)
  Cytotoxicity directed against macrophages and β cells may result in diminished immunoresponsiveness
  Decrease in absolute numbers of CD3-, CD4- and CD19-positive cells in peripheral blood during pregnancy versus post partum
  Stimulation of prostaglandin production
Sex Hormone Concentration
  Estrogen
    Increases cellular proliferation in blood vessels (known in the endometrium)
    Decreases keratinization while increasing epithelial glycogen
    Specific receptors are found in gingival tissues
  Progesterone
    Increases vascular dilation and thus increases permeability (results in edema and accumulation of inflammatory cells)
    Increases proliferation of newly formed capillaries in gingival tissues (increased bleeding tendency)
    Alters rate and pattern of collagen production
    Increases metabolic breakdown of folate (a deficiency can inhibit tissue repair)
    Specific receptors are found in gingival tissues
    Decreases plasminogen activator inhibitor factor type 2 and thus increases tissue proteolysis
  Estrogen and Progesterone
    Affect ground substance of connective tissue by increasing fluidity
    Concentrations increase in saliva and fluid with increased concentrations in serum

Sex Hormone Concentration. During pregnancy, progesterone reaches levels of 100 ng/mL, 10 times the peak luteal phase of menses. Estradiol in the plasma may be 30 times higher than that during the reproductive cycle. Estrogens and progesterones have different roles. Estrogen may regulate cellular proliferation, differentiation, and keratinization, while progesterone influences the permeability of the microvasculature,[35,36] alters the rate and pattern of collagen production, and increases the metabolic breakdown of folate (necessary for tissue maintenance).[37] A high concentration of sex hormones in gingival tissues, saliva, serum, and crevicular fluid may exaggerate the response as well. Vittek and colleagues have demonstrated specific estrogen and progesterone receptors in gingival tissues.[38] This is direct biochemical evidence that this tissue may function as a target organ for sex hormones. Muramatsu and Takaesu found increasing concentration of sex hormones in saliva from the first month of gestation, peaking in the ninth month along with increasing percentages of *Prevotella intermedia*. With increasing depth, the number of gingival sites with bleeding and redness increased until 1 month post partum.[39] There is also evidence of sex hormone concentration in crevicular fluid, providing a growth media for periodontal pathogens.

Periodontal Disease and Preterm Low-Birth-weight Births. Due to the pioneering research of Offenbacher and co-workers, evidence exists that untreated periodontal disease in pregnant women may be a significant risk factor for preterm (< 37 weeks) low-birth-weight (< 2,500 g) babies.[40] The relationship with genito-urinary tract infection and preterm low birth weight (PLBW) is well documented in human and animal studies. Periodontal researchers suspecting periodontal disease as another source of infection found that mothers of low-birth-weight infants, otherwise having low risk, had significantly more periodontal attachment loss than control mothers having normal-weight infants at birth. The current opinion is that PLBW occurs as a result of infection and is mediated indirectly, principally by the translocation of bacterial products such as endotoxin (lipopolysaccharide [LPS]) and by the action of maternally produced inflammatory mediators.[41] Biologically active molecules such as prostaglandin E_2 (PGE$_2$) and tumor necrosis factor (TNF), which are involved in normal parturition, are raised to artificially high levels by the infection process, which may foster premature labor.[42] Gram-negative bacteria in periodontal diseases, therefore, may permit selective overgrowth or invasion of gram-negative bacteria within the genito-urinary tract. Recently, gingival crevicular fluid levels of PGE_2 were positively associated with intra-amniotic PGE_2 levels, suggesting that gram-negative periodontal infection may present a systemic challenge sufficient to initiate the onset of premature labor as a source of LPS and/or through stimulation of secondary inflammatory mediators such as PGE_2 and interleukin-1 beta (IL-1β).[43] There is ongoing research supporting the association of periodontal disease and PLBW.[44,45] Offenbacher has recently published data suggesting a dose-response relationship for increasing gingival crevicular fluid PGE_2 as a marker of current periodontal disease activity and decreasing birth weight. Four organisms associated with mature plaque and progressing periodontitis (*Bacteroides forsythus, Porphyromonas gingivalis, Actinobacillus actinomycetemcomitans,* and *Treponema denticola*) were detected at higher levels in PLBW mothers, as compared to normal birth weight controls.[46] Further longitudinal studies and intervention trials are needed to clarify the relationship between periodontal infection and PLBW.

Other Oral Manifestations of Pregnancy

Perimylolysis or acid erosion of teeth may occur if "morning sickness" or esophageal reflux is severe and involves repeated vomiting of gastric contents. Severe reflux may cause scarring of the esophageal sphincter, and the patient may become a more likely candidate for GERD later in life.

Xerostomia is a frequent complaint among pregnant women. One study found this persistent dryness in 44 percent of pregnant participants.[47]

A rare finding in pregnancy is ptyalism, or sialorrhea. This excessive secretion of saliva usually begins at 2 to 3 weeks of gestation and may abate at the end of the first trimester. While its etiology has not been identified, ptyalism may result from the inability of nauseated gravid women to swallow normal amounts of saliva rather than from a true increase in the production of saliva.[48]

Because pregnancy places the woman in an immunocompromised state, the clinician must be aware of the total health of the patient (see Figure 9–4). Gestational diabetes, leukemia, and other medical conditions may appear during pregnancy.

Management

The periodontal evaluation of the pregnant patient begins with a thorough medical history. This history should note any complications the patient has encountered in the pregnancy and record any previous miscarriages, recent cramping, spotting, or pernicious vomiting. If possible, the next step is to contact the obstetrician to discuss the patient's medical status, dental needs, and proposed treatment plan.

The most important objectives in planning dental treatment for the pregnant patient are to establish a healthy oral environment and to obtain optimum oral hygiene levels. These are achieved by means of a good preventive dental program, consisting of nutritional counseling and rigorous plaque control measures in the dental office and at home.

Preventive program

Nutrition. The quality of the diet affects caries formation and pregnancy gingivitis. Diet is also important for the developing dentition in the fetus. Pregnant patients normally receive nutritional guidance from their obstetricians, which may be re-inforced by the dental team. It is imperative that the mother's diet supplies sufficient levels of needed nutrients, including vitamins A, C, and D, protein, calcium, and phosphorus (Table 9–2).

Patients should select nutritious snacks, but because so many foods contain sugars and starches that can contribute to caries development, it is advisable to limit the number of times they snack between meals.

Plaque Control. The pregnant patient should be provided with a comprehensive plaque control program to minimize the exaggerated inflammatory response of the gingival tissues. The heightened tendency for gingival inflammation may be clearly explained to the patient so that acceptable oral hygiene techniques may be taught, re-inforced, and monitored throughout pregnancy. Scaling, polishing, and root planing may be performed whenever necessary throughout the pregnancy. Some practitioners avoid the use of high-alcohol-content antimicrobial mouthrinses in pregnant women and prefer to use non-alcohol-based mouthrinses.

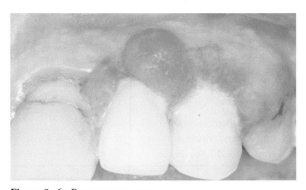

Figure 9–6. Pregnancy tumor.

Prenatal Fluoride. The prescribing of prenatal fluoride supplements has been an area of controversy for quite some time. Although two studies have claimed beneficial results,[49,50] others suggest that the clinical efficacy of prenatal fluoride supplements is uncertain and that the mechanism by which prenatal fluorides might impart cariostasis is unclear.[51]

The American Dental Association (ADA) does not recommend the use of prenatal fluoride, because its efficacy has not been demonstrated. The American Academy of Pediatric Dentistry supports this position as well. The American Academy of Pediatrics has no stated position on prescribing prenatal fluorides.

Baby-Bottle Tooth Decay. When discussing preventive oral health with the patient, it is advisable to mention the condition known as baby-bottle tooth decay (BBTD) for the benefit of the mother and other caregivers. Baby-bottle tooth decay is an easily preventable condition affecting primary teeth. It is caused by frequent and prolonged exposure of the primary teeth to fluids containing sugars, such as milk, formula, fruit juice, and other sweetened liquids provided in baby bottles.

TABLE 9–2. Guidelines for Daily Food Choices for Pregnant Women

Breads, cereals, and other whole-grain and enriched products
- 1 slice bread
- ¹/₂ hamburger bun or English muffin
- 3–4 small or 2 large crackers
- ¹/₂ cup cooked cereal, pasta, or rice
- 1 oz ready-to-eat cereal

Fruits
2–4 servings (include at least one citrus fruit or juice)
- ³/₄ cup juice
- 1 medium apple, banana, or other fruit
- ¹/₂ cup fresh, cooked, or canned fruit

Vegetables
3–5 servings (include at least two servings of dark green leafy, yellow, or orange vegetables)
- ¹/₂ cup cooked or chopped raw vegetables
- 1 cup leafy raw vegetables

Meat, poultry, fish, and alternates
2–3 servings
- Total of 6–7 oz cooked lean meat, poultry, fish, or other protein sources daily
- 1 oz = 1 egg
- ¹/₂ cup cooked beans
- 2 tablespoons peanut butter

Milk, cheese, and yogurt
4 servings
- 1 cup milk
- 1 cup buttermilk
- 8 oz yogurt
- ¹/₂ oz Natural cheese
- 2 oz processed cheese

Fats, sweets, and alcohol
- Limited fats/sweets
- Avoid alcoholic beverages

Adapted from United States Department of Agriculture Home & Garden Bulletin No.232-8

Treatment

Elective Dental Treatment

It is prudent to avoid elective dental care other than good plaque control during the first trimester and the last half of the third trimester if possible. The first trimester is the period of organogenesis, when the fetus is highly susceptible to environmental influences. In the last half of the third trimester, there is a hazard of premature delivery because the uterus is very sensitive to external stimuli. Prolonged chair time may need to be avoided because the woman is most uncomfortable at this time. Further, there is a possibility that supine hypotensive syndrome may occur. In a semi-reclining or supine position, the great vessels, particularly the inferior vena cava, are compressed by the gravid uterus. By interfering with venous return, this compression will cause maternal hypotension, decreased cardiac output, and eventual loss of consciousness. Supine hypotensive syndrome can usually be reversed by turning the patient on her left side, thereby removing pressure on the vena cava and allowing blood to return from the lower extremities and pelvic area.

The second trimester is the safest period for providing routine dental care. The emphasis at this time is on controlling active disease and eliminating potential problems that could arise in late pregnancy. Extensive reconstruction procedures and major oral or periodontal surgery should be postponed until after delivery. Pregnancy tumors that are painful, interfere with mastication, or continue to bleed or suppurate after mechanical débridement may require excision and biopsy prior to delivery.

Emergency Dental Treatment

Dental emergencies should be dealt with as they arise throughout the entire pregnancy to manage pain and treat infection that otherwise could result in increased stress for the mother and endangerment of the fetus. Emergency treatment calling for general anesthesia necessitates consultation with the patient's obstetrician, as does any uncertainty about prescribing medication or pursuing a particular course of treatment.

Dental Radiographs

Dental radiography is one of the more controversial areas in the management of a pregnant patient. It is most desirable not to have any irradiation during pregnancy, especially during the first trimester, because the developing fetus is particularly susceptible to radiation damage.[52] However, the safety of dental radiography has been well established, provided features such as high-speed film, filtration, collimation, and lead aprons are used. Of all aids, the most important for the patient is the protective lead apron. Studies have shown that when an apron is used during contemporary dental radiography, gonadal and fetal radiation is virtually unmeasurable.[53]

Even in light of the obvious safety of dental radiography, radiographs should be used selectively during pregnancy and only when necessary and appropriate to aid in diagnosis and treatment. In most instances, only bite-wing, panoramic, or selected periapical films are indicated.

Medications

Another area of controversy involves drug therapy because drugs given to a pregnant woman can affect the fetus by diffusion across the placenta. A conservative approach is prudent, the dentist prescribing only the minimum effective dose and duration absolutely essential for the pregnant patient's well-being and only after careful consideration of potential side effects. The dentist may need to be familiar with the classification system established by the Food and Drug Administration (FDA) in 1979 to rate fetal risk levels associated with many prescription drugs (Table 9–3). The prudent practitioner should consult references such as Briggs and colleagues' *Drugs in Pregnancy and Lactation*[54] or *Drug Facts and Comparisons*[55] for information on the FDA pregnancy risk factor associated with prescription drugs. Ideally, no drug should be administered during pregnancy, especially the first trimester.[52] However, it is sometimes impossible to adhere to this rule. It is, therefore, fortunate that most of the commonly used drugs in dental practice can be given during pregnancy with relative safety although there are a few important exceptions (Tables 9–4a, 9–4b, 9–4c). The tables

of drugs presented here are considered to be general guidelines.[56] Obviously, drugs in categories A or B are preferable for prescribing. However, many drugs that fall into category C are sometimes administered during pregnancy. These drugs present the greatest challenge to the dentist and physician in terms of therapeutics and medicolegal decisions. It should be recognized that physicians may advise against the use of some of the approved drugs or conversely may suggest the use of questionable drugs. An example of the occasional use of a questionable drug would be a narcotic for a patient in severe pain. Consulting the patient's physician may be advisable prior to prescribing any medications during pregnancy.

TABLE 9–3. Food and Drug Administration Classification System*

A Controlled studies in women fail to demonstrate a risk to the fetus in the first trimester (and there is no evidence of a risk in later trimesters), and the possibility of fetal harm appears remote.

B Either animal reproduction studies have not demonstrated a fetal risk and there are no controlled studies in pregnant women, or animal reproduction studies have shown an adverse effect (other than a decrease in fertility) that was not confirmed in controlled studies in women in the first trimester (and there is no evidence of a risk in later trimesters).

C Either studies in animals have revealed adverse effects on the fetus (teratogenic or embryocidal, or other) and there are not controlled studies in women, or studies in women and animals are not available. Drugs should be given only if the potential benefit justifies the potential risk to the fetus.

D There is positive evidence of human fetal risk, but the benefits from use in pregnant women may be acceptable despite the risk (eg, if the drug is needed in a life-threatening situation or for a serious disease for which safer drugs cannot be used or are ineffective).

X Studies in animals or human beings have demonstrated fetal abnormalities or there is evidence of fetal risk based on human experience, or both, and the risk of the use of the drug in pregnant women clearly outweighs any possible benefit. The drug is contra-indicated in women who are or may become pregnant.

*The five-category system used to classify drugs based on their potential for causing birth defects.

In periodontal therapy, the use of antimicrobial agents is common. During pregnancy, the clinician must weigh the benefits and the risks to both mother and fetus. Antibiotics with systemic effects cross the placenta and reach the fetus. The effect of a particular medication on the fetus

TABLE 9–4a. Local Anesthetic/Analgesic Administration during Pregnancy

Drug	FDA Category (Prescription Drug)	During Pregnancy
Local Anesthetics *		
Lidocaine	B	Yes
Mepivacaine	C	Use with caution; consult physician
Prilocaine	B	Yes
Bupivacaine	C	Use with caution; consult physician
Etidocaine	B	Yes
Procaine	C	Use with caution; consult physician
Analgesics		
Aspirin	C/D 3rd trimester	Caution; avoid in 3rd trimester
Acetaminophen	B	Yes
Ibuprofen	B/D 3rd trimester	Caution; avoid in 3rd trimester
Codeine	C	Use with caution; consult physician
Hydrocodone	B	Use with caution; consult physician
Oxycodone	B	Use with caution; consult physician
Propoxyphene	C	Use with caution; consult physician

*Can use vasoconstrictors if necessary.
 Avoid prolonged use.

TABLE 9–4b. Antibiotic Administration during Pregnancy

Drug	FDA Category (Prescription Drug)	During Pregnancy	Risks
Penicillins	B	Yes	Diarrhea
Erythromycin	B	Yes; avoid estolate form	Intrahepatic jaundice in mother
Clindamycin	B	Yes (with caution)	Drug concentrated in fetal bone, spleen, lung, and liver
Cephalosporins	B	Yes	Limited information
Tetracycline	D	Avoid	Depression of bone growth, enamel hypoplasia, grey-brown tooth discoloration
Ciprofloxacin	C	Avoid	Possible developing cartilage erosion
Metronidazole	B	Avoid (controversial)	Theoretical carcinogenic data in animals
Gentamicin	C	Caution; consult physician	Limited information; ototoxicity
Vanocomycin	C	Caution; consult physician	Limited information
Clarithromycin	D	Avoid; use only if the potential benefit justifies the risk to the fetus	Limited information; adverse effects on pregnancy, outcome, and embryofetal development in animals

TABLE 9–4c. Sedative-Hypnotic Drug Administration during Pregnancy

Drug	FDA Category	During Pregnancy
Benzodiazepines	D	Avoid
Barbiturates	D	Avoid
Nitrous oxide	Not assigned	Avoid in 1st trimester; otherwise use with caution; consult physician

depends on the type of antimicrobial, the dosage, the trimester, and the duration of the course of therapy.[57] At this date, there is inadequate research in relation to subgingival irrigation and local site delivery in relation to the developing fetus.

Dental Drugs During Breast-Feeding

Another perplexing problem for the dentist arises when a nursing mother requires a drug during dental treatment. There is a risk that the drug can enter the breast milk and be transferred to the nursing infant, in whom exposure could have adverse effects. Unfortunately, there is little conclusive information about drug dosage and effects via breast milk. However, retrospective clinical studies and empirical observations coupled with known pharmacologic pathways allow recommendations to be made.[52] The amount of drug excreted in breast milk is usually not more than 1 to 2 percent of the maternal dose; therefore, it is highly unlikely that most drugs have any pharmacologic significance for the infant.[58,59] Tables 9–5a and 9–5b compile recommendations regarding administration of commonly used dental drugs during breast-feeding. These recommendations are general guidelines only. As with drug use in pregnancy, individual physicians may wish to modify these suggestions.

In addition to choosing drugs carefully, it is desirable for the mother to take the drug just after breast-feeding and then to avoid nursing for 4 hours or more if possible.[52,58] This markedly decreases the drug concentration in breast milk.

ORAL CONTRACEPTIVES

Periodontal Manifestations

Because oral contraceptive (OC) use mimics hormonal levels of pregnancy, clinical manifestations are similar. Gingival tissues may have an exaggerated response to local irritants. Inflammation ranges from mild edema and erythema to severe inflammation with hemorrhagic or hyperplastic gingival tissues. It has been reported that there is more exudate in inflamed gingival tissues of OC users than in those of pregnant women.[60,61]

Investigators have reported several mechanisms for the heightened response in gingival tissues. Kalkwarf reported that the response may be due to alteration of the microvasculature, increased gingival permeability, and increasing synthesis of prostaglandin.[62] Prostaglandin E2 appears to rise significantly with increasing sex hormone.

Prostaglandin E is a potent mediator of inflammation.[63] Jensen and colleagues found dramatic microbial changes in pregnant and OC user groups as compared with a nonpregnant group.[64] A 16-fold increase in *Bacteroides* species was noted in the OC user group versus the nonpregnant group despite the lack of statistically significant clinical differences in gingival index or crevicular fluid flow. The researchers state that the increased female sex hormones substituting for the napthaquinone requirement of certain *Bacteroides* species were most likely responsible for this increase in *Bacteroides*.

There have been reports that the oral contraceptive-associated gingival inflammation may become chronic (as opposed to the acute inflammation of pregnancy) due to the extended periods of time women are exposed to elevated levels of estrogen and progesterone.[65,66] Some have reported that the inflammation increases with prolonged use of OCs. Kalkwarf did not find that duration of use made a significant difference, however, the "brand" of OC caused different responses. Further studies need to be performed in relation to dosage, duration, and type of OC used in association with the periodontium. One should note that the concentration of female sex hormones in OCs of the 2000s will be significantly less than in those of the 1970s, yet the OCs of the 2000s will have the same level of contraceptive efficacy.

Other intraoral effects of oral contraceptives are changes in salivary composition. A decreased concentration of protein, sialic acid, hexosamine fucose, hydrogen ions, and total electrolytes has been reported. Salivary flow rates have been reported to be increased in one study[67] and decreased in 30 percent of subjects in another study.[68] (Note that these studies were conducted in the 1970s.)

The dental literature reports that women taking oral contraceptives experience a twofold to threefold increase in the incidence of localized osteitis following extraction of mandibular third molars.[69] The higher incidence of osteitis in these patients may be attributed to the effects of OCs (estrogens) on clotting factors. There are, however, a number of studies that refute these findings.[70] Evidence at this date is inconclusive with regard to osteitis following third molar extractions and the use of OCs.

Also, it has been reported in the medical literature that there may be a spotty melanotic pigmentation of the skin with the use of OCs. This suggests a relationship between the use of OCs and the occurrence of gingival melanosis, especially in fair-skinned individuals.[71]

Management

A comprehensive medical history and an assessment of vital signs (particularly blood pressure) are extremely important in this group of patients. Treatment of gingival inflammation exaggerated by oral contraceptives should include establishing an oral hygiene program and eliminating local predisposing factors. It is also imperative that the patient be informed of their heightened risks and the need for meticulous home care and compliance with supportive periodontal therapy visits. Periodontal surgery may be indicated if there is inadequate resolution after initial therapy (scaling and root planing). Antimicrobial mouthwashes may be indicated as part of the home care regimen. It may be advisable to perform extraction of teeth (especially of third molars) on non-estrogenic days (days 23 to 28) of the pill cycle, to reduce the risk of a postoperative localized osteitis.[72] However, evidence of this association is inconclusive and warrants further investigation.

Although the results from animal studies have demonstrated antibiotic interference adversely affecting contraceptive sex hormone levels, several studies involving human subjects have failed to support such an interaction.[73–76] This issue is controversial, and there may be a possibility that antibiotics could render oral contraceptives inefficacious in preventing pregnancies. In 1991, an ADA Health Foundation report stated that all women of childbearing age should be informed of possible reduced efficacy of oral steroid contraceptives during antibiotic therapy and advised to use additional forms of contraception during short-term antibiotic therapy. During long-term antibiotic therapy, they should consult with their physician about using high-dose oral contraceptive preparations.[77] Although research regarding oral manifestations attributed to oral contraceptives has been reported in the literature, presumably the same effects could occur with the use of contraceptive implants (eg, Norplant®). Along the same lines, the remote possibility exists of reduced efficacy of the contraceptive implant with concurrent antibiotic administration, and the same precautions can be adhered to as with oral contraceptives.

CONCLUSION

There is increasing evidence that the female patient frequently presents with unique periodontal and systemic manifestations that alter the course of conventional periodontal therapy. The cyclic nature of the female sex hormones is often reflected in gingival tissue changes. It is the responsibility of those who treat the oral cavity to realize that they are treating the total health of the patient (and possibly the unborn fetus), not just a localized site infection.

Thorough medical histories in the female patient should include questions regarding menstrual regularity, oral contraceptive use, hormone replacement therapy, fertility medications, preg-

TABLE 9–5a. Dental Drug Administration during Breast-Feeding

Drug	During Breast-Feeding
Local anesthetics	
Lidocaine	Yes
Mepivacaine	Yes
Priolocaine	Yes
Bupivacaine	Yes
Etidocaine	Yes
Procaine	Yes
Analgesics	
Aspirin	Avoid
Acetaminophen	Yes
Ibuprofen	Yes
Codeine	Yes
Hydrocodone	No data
Oxycodone	Yes
Propoxyphene	Yes

TABLE 9–5b. Dental Drug Administration during Breast-Feeding

Drug	During Breast-Feeding
Antibiotics*	
Penicillins	Yes
Erythromycin	Yes
Clindamycin	Yes (with caution)
Cephalosporins	Yes
Tetracycline	Avoid
Ciprofloxacin	Avoid
Metronidazole	Avoid
Gentamicin	Avoid
Vancomycin	Avoid
Sedative-hypnotics	
Benzodiazepines	Avoid
Barbiturates	Avoid
Nitrous oxide	Yes

*Antibiotics have the risk of diarrhea and sensitization in the mother and infant.

nancy, breast-feeding, cyclic problems that may be associated with manifestations of the sex hormones, as well as any question that may enhance the quality of care for the individual patient and determine her particular needs. It is possible to control the periodontal health of the patient by educating her about the profound effects of the sex hormones, especially progesterone, and the importance of consistent removal of local irritants.

In the late 1990s, there has been a resurgence of curiosity relating to female issues and medical/periodontal therapy. There should be light shed on the specific management and etiology of sex hormone-mediated infections in the near future. It is also imperative that we disseminate this knowledge to other health care providers and to the community.

REFERENCES

1. Kornman K, Loesche WJ. Direct interaction of estradiol and progesterone with *Bacteroides melaninogenicus*. J Dent Res 1979;58A:10.
2. Gusberti FA, Mombelli A, Lang NP, Minder CE. Changes in subgingival microbiota during puberty. J Clin Periodontal 1990;17:685–92.
3. Mombelli A, Rutar A, Lan NP. Correlation of the periodontal status 6 years after puberty with clinical and microbiological conditions during puberty. J Clin Periodontol 1995;22(4):300–5.
4. Nakagawa S, Fujii H., Machida Y, Okuda K. A longitudinal study from prepuberty to puberty of gingivitis. Correlation between the occurrence of *Prevotella intermedia* and sex hormones. J Clin Periodontal 1994;21(10):658–6.
5. American Dental Association. Women's Oral Health Issues 1995; Dec.
6. Brown S, Bonifaz DZ. An overview of anorexia and bulimia nervosa and the impact of eating disorders on the oral cavity. Compend Contin Educ Dent 1993;14(12):1594–1608.
7. Mandel L, Kaynar A. Bulimia and parotid swelling: a review and case report. J Oral Maxillofac Surg 1992;50:1122–5.
8. Lundgren D, Magnssen B, Lindhe J. Connective tissue alterations in gingiva of rats treated with estrogens and progesterone. Odontol 1973;24: 49–58.
9. Thomson ME, Pack ARC. Effects of extended systemic and topical folate supplementation on gingivitis in pregnancy. J Clin Periodontol 1982;9:275–80.
10. Pack ARC, Thomson ME. Effects of topical and systemic folic acid supplementation on gingivitis in pregnancy. J Clin Periodontol 1980;7: 402–14.
11. Miyagi M, Aoyama H, Morishita M, Iwamoto Y. Effects of sex hormones on chemotaxis of polymorphonuclear leukoctyes and monocytes. J Periodontol 1992;63:28–32.
12. Grant D, Stern J, Listgarten M. The epidemiology, etiology and public health aspects of periodontal disease. In: Grant D, Stern J, Listegarten M. editors. Periodontics. St. Louis (MO): Mosby 1988. p. 229,332–5.
13. Ferguson MM, Carter J, Boyle P. An epidemiological study of factors associated with recurrent apthae in women. J Oral Med 1984:39(4):212.
14. Robb-Nicholson C. PMS: it's real. Harvard Women's Health Watch 1994; July 1(11):2–3.
15. Robb-Nicholson C. Gastroesophageal reflux disease. Harvard Women's Health Watch;4(6):4–5.
16. Pinard A. Gingivitis in pregnancy. Dent Register 1877;31:258–9.
17. Levin RP. Pregnancy gingivitis. Maryland State Dental Association 1987;30:27.
18. Hanson L, Sobol SM, Abelson T. The otolaryngologic manifestations of pregnancy. J Fam Pract 1986;23:51–5.
19. DeLiefde B. The dental care of pregnant women. NZ Dent J 1984;80:41–3.
20. Löe H, Silness J. Periodontal disease in pregnancy. 1. Prevalence and severity. Acta Odontol Scand 1984;21:533–51.
21. Raber-Durlacher JE, van Steenbergen TJM, van der Velden U. Experimental gingivitis during pregnancy and post-partum; clinical, endocrinological and microbiological aspects. J Clin Periodontol 1994;21:549–58.
22. Bhashkar SN, Jacoway JR. Pyogenic granuloma: clinical features, incidence, histology, and results of treatment. Report of 242 cases. J Oral Surg 1966;24:391–8.
23. Kornman KS, Loesche WJ. The subgingival flora during pregnancy. J Periodontol 1980;15: 111–22.
24. Aboul-Dahab OM, el-Sherbiny MM, Abdel-Rahman R, Shoeb M. Identification of lymphocytes subsets in pregnancy. Egyptian Dental J 1994; 40(1):653–6.
25. Raber-Durlacher JE, Leene W, Palmer-Bouva CCR, et al. Experimental gingivitis during pregnancy and post partum: immunohistochemical aspects. J Periodontol 1993;64:211–18.
26. O'Neil TCA. Maternal T-lymphocyte response and gingivitis in pregnancy. J Periodontol 1979;50: 178.

27. Brabin, BJ. Epidemiology of infection in pregnancy. Rev Infect Dis 1985;7:579.

28. Lopatin DE, Kornman KS, Loesche WJ. Modulation of immunoreactivity to periodontal disease-associated microorganisms during pregnancy. Infect Immun 1980;28:713–18.

29. Sridama V, Pacini F, Yang SL, et al. Decreased levels of helper T cells. A possible cause of immunodeficiency in pregnancy. N Engl J Med 1982; 307:352.

30. Raber-Durlacher JE, Zeylemaker WP, Meinesz AAP, Abraham-Lipijn L. CD4 to CD8 ratio and in vitro lymphoproliferative responses during experimental gingivitis in pregnancy and postpartum. J Periodontol 1991;62:663–7.

31. Lapp CA, Thomas ME, Lewis JB. Modulation by progesterone of interleukin-6 production by gingival fibroblasts. J Periodontol 1995;66(4): 279–84.

32. El-Attar TMA. Prostaglandins F2 in human gingiva in health and disease and its stimulation by female sex steroids. Prostaglandins 1976;1:331–41.

33. Ojanotko-Harri AO, Harri MOP, Hurrita HP. Altered tissue metabolism of progesterone in pregnancy gingivitis and granuloma. J Clin Periodontol 1991;8:262–6.

34. Kinnby B, Matsson L, Astedt B. Aggravation of gingival inflammatory symptoms during pregnancy associated with the concentration of activator inhibitor type 2 (PAI-2) in gingival fluid. J Periodontal Res 1996;31(4):271–7.

35. Lindhe J, Branemark P. Changes in vascular permeability after local application of sex hormones. J Periodontal Res 1967b;2:259–265.

36. Lindhe J, Branemark P. Changes in microcirculation after local application of sex hormones. J Periodontal Res 1967a;2:185–93.

37. Zachariasen RD. Ovarian hormones and oral health: pregnancy gingivitis. Compend Contin Educ Dent 1989;10(9):508–12.

38. Vittek J, Gordon G, Rappaport C, Munangi P, Southern A. Specific progesterone receptors in rabbit gingiva. J Periodontal Res 1982;17:657.

39. Muramatsu Y, Takaesu Y. Oral health status related to subgingival bacterial flora and sex hormones in saliva during pregnancy. Bull Tokyo Dent College 1994;35(3):139–51.

40. Offenbacher S, Katz V, Fertik G, et al. Periodontal infection as a possible risk factor for preterm low birthweight. J Periodontol 1996;67(10 Suppl): 1103–13.

41. Gibbs RS, Romero R, Hillier SL, et al. A review of premature birth and subclinical infections. Am J Obstet 1992;166:1515–28.

42. American Academy of Periodontology Position Paper. Periodontal disease as a potential risk factor for systemic disease. J Periodontol 1998; 69(7):841–50.

43. Damare SM, Wells S, Offenbacher S. Eicosanoids in periodontal diseases: potential for systemic involvement. Adv Exp Med Bio 1997;433:23–5.

44. Davenport ES, Williams CE, Sterne JA, et al. The East London study of maternal chronic periodontal disease and preterm low birth weight infants: study design and prevalence. Ann Periodontol 1998;3(1):213–21.

45. Dasanayake AP. Poor periodontal health of the pregnant woman as a risk. Ann Periodontol 1998;3(1):206–12.

46. Offenbacher S, Jared HL, O'Reilly PG, et al. Potential pathogenic mechanisms of periodontitis associated pregnancy complications. Ann Periodontol 1998;3(1):233–50.

47. El-Ashiry G. Comparative study of the influence of pregnancy and oral contraceptives on the gingivae. Oral Surg 1970;30:472–5.

48. Cruikshank O, Hayes PM. Maternal physiology. In: Gabbe S, Niebyl JR, Simpson JL, editors. Pregnancy in obstetrics: normal and problem pregnancies. Livingstone (NY): Churchill Livingstone; 1986.

49. Glenn FB. Immunity conveyed by a fluoride supplement during pregnancy. J Dent Child 1977; 44:391–5.

50. Glenn FB, Glenn WD III, Duncan RC. Fluoride tablet supplementation during pregnancy for caries immunity: a study of the offspring produced. Am J Obstet Gynecol 1982;143:560–4.

51. Reference manual. Pediatr Dent 1994–95:16(7).

52. Little JW, Falace DA. Dental management of the medically compromised patient. 4th edition. St. Louis (MO): Mosby;1993:383–9.

53. Bean LR Jr, Devore WD. The effects of protective aprons in dental roentgenography. 1969;28: 505–8.

54. Briggs GG, Freeman RK, Yaffe SJ. Drugs in pregnancy and lactation. 4th ed. Baltimore (MD): Williams and Wilkins;1994.

55. Olin BR, editor. Drug facts and comparisons. St. Louis (MO): Walters Kluwer; 1994.

56. Reese RE, Betts RF. Handbook of antibiotics. 2nd ed. Boston (MA): Little, Brown, and Co.:1993.

57. Otomo-Corgel J. Systemic considerations for female patients. In: Antibiotics/antimicrobial use in dental practice. Tokyo: Quintessence Publishing Co.; 1990. p. 217–21.

58. Steinberg, BJ. Sex hormonal alterations. In: Rose LD, Kay D, editors. Internal medicine for dentistry. 2nd ed. St. Louis (MO): Mosby;1990. p. 1073–7.

59. Wilson JT, Brown RD, Cherek DR, et al. Drug excretion in human breast milk: principles, pharmacokinetics and projects consequences. Clin Pharmacokinet 1980;5:1–66.

60. Zachariasen, RD. The effects of elevated ovarian hormones on periodontal health: oral contraceptives and pregnancy. Women Health 1993; 20(2):21–30.

61. Sooriyamoorthy M, Gower DB. Hormonal influences on gingival tissues: relationship to periodontal disease. J Clin Periodontol 1989;16: 201–8.

62. Kalkwarf KL. Effect of oral contraceptive therapy on gingival inflammation in humans. J Periodontol 1978;49:560–3.

63. El-Attar TMA, Roth GD, Hugoson A. Comparative metabolism of 4-C progesterone in normal and chronically inflamed human gingival tissue. J Periodontol Res 1973;8:79.

64. Jensen J, Lilijmack W, Blookquist C. The effect of female sex hormones on subgingival plaque. J Periodontol 1981;52(10):599–602.

65. Knight GM, Wade AB. The effects of oral contraceptives on the human periodontium. J Periodontal Res 1974;9:18–22.

66. Pankhurst CL. The influence of oral contraceptive therapy on the periodontium—duration of drug therapy. J Periodontol 1981;52:617–620.

67. Magnusson T, Ericson T, Hugoson A. The effect of oral contraceptives on some salivary substance in women. Arch Oral Biol 1975;20:119.

68. El-Ashiry G, El-Kafrawy AH, Nasr MF, Younis N. Effects of oral contraceptives on the gingiva. J Periodontol 1971; 42:273–5.

69. Sweet JB, Butler DP. Increased incidence of postoperative localized osteitis in mandibular 3rd molar surgery associated with patients using oral contraceptives. Am J Obstet Gynecol 1977;127:518.

70. Cohen ME, Simecek JW. Effects of gender-related factors on the incidence of localized alveolar osteitis. Oral Surg Oral Med Oral Path Oral Radiol Endod 1995;79(4):416–22.

71. Hertz RS, Beckstead PC, Brown WJ. Epithelial melanosis of the gingiva possibly resulting from the use of oral contraceptives. J Am Dent Assoc 1980;100:(5):173.

72. Fleisher AB Jr, Resnick SD. The effect of antibiotics in the efficacy of oral contraceptives. Arch Dermatol 1980;125:1582–4.

73. Back DJ, Orme MLíE. Pharmacokinetic drug interactions with oral contraceptives. Clin Pharmacokinet 1990;18(6):472–84.

74. Fraser IS, Jansen RPS. Why do inadvertent pregnancies occur in oral contraceptive users? Effectiveness of oral contraceptive regimens and interfering factors. Contraception 1983;27:531–51.

75. Murphy AA, Zacur HA, Charache P, et al. The effect of tetracycline on levels of oral contraceptives. Am J Obstet Gynecol 1991;164:28–33.

76. Neely JL, Abate M, Swinker M, et al. The effect of doxycycline on serum levels on ethinyl estradiol, norethindrone, and endogenous progesterone. Obstet Gynecol 1991;77:410–16.

77. Antibiotic interference with oral contraceptives. J Am Dent Assoc 1991;122:79.

CHAPTER 10

OSTEOPENIA, OSTEOPOROSIS AND ORAL DISEASE

Sara G. Grossi, DDS, MS
Marjorie K. Jeffcoat, DMD
Robert J. Genco, DDS, PhD

Normal bone is among the most metabolically active of human tissues. Once formed, bone is continuously changing throughout life, constantly responding to various metabolic demands. In a process known as remodeling, bone shapes itself, creating an organ with maximal compressive strength, able to fulfill its role as the load-bearing structure of the body. The human skeleton consists of two different tissues: *trabecular bone*, concentrated mostly in vertebrae, the pelvis and other flat bones, and *cortical bone,* which overlays trabecular bone and occupies mostly the shafts of long bones.[1] Cortical bone is a more dense tissue than trabecular bone, as the cells are in closer proximity with less intercellular space and matrix. Trabecular bone is metabolically more active than cortical bone, likely because of its greater surface-to-volume ratio.

To maintain this phenomenally strong load-bearing structure, young bone is constantly renewing itself. That is, "old" bone is constantly removed and replaced with "new bone," a process known as bone remodeling. In this process, bone is constantly resorbed on a particular bony surface, followed by a phase of bone formation. It is etimated that the entire skeleton is completely turned over every 7 to 10 years. Remodeling occurs at both trabecular and cortical sites. In the normal adult skeleton, bone resorption is coupled with bone formation, so that bone balance is maintained.[2] In this manner, the skeleton is maintained throughout the life of the individual.

BONE REMODELING

Bone remodeling is a complex and dynamic process aimed at the maintenance of a mineralized bone matrix. It involves a number of cellular func-tions, including replication of undifferentiated cells and recruitment and cell differentiation in both cortical and trabecular bone.[3] This concert of bone cells is referred to as the basic multicellular unit (BMU) or bone remodeling unit and constitutes the smallest functional unit of bone cells capable of undergoing the remodelling process.[4] Four distinct phases are recognizable in the bone remodeling cycle: activation, resorption, reversal, and formation. A cycle is completed in approximately 8 months. The process is under tight control by both systemic and local factors.

Systemic factors regulating bone remodeling include: (1) the calcium-regulating hormones: parathyroid hormone (PTH), 1,25-dihydroxyvitamin D $(1,25(OH)_2D_3)$, and calcitonin (CT); and (2) the systemic growth-regulating hormones: growth hormone, glucocorticoids, thyroid hormone, and sex hormones.[5] Parathyroid hormone is a polypeptide with complex effects on bone metabolism. The most important function of PTH is to maintain serum ionized calcium concentration, accomplished by stimulation of bone resorption, renal resorption of calcium, and increased synthesis of $1,25(OH)_2D_3$, which, in turn, results in increased intestinal calcium absorption.[6] Parathyroid hormone has a dual effect on bone metabolism, stimulating both resorption and formation.[5,6] The bone resorbing effect is dependent on the presence of osteoblasts or osteoblast-derived factors. Vitamin D $(1,25(OH)_2D_3)$, a hormone synthesized primarily by the kidney, has similar functions as PTH. It stimulates bone resorption and has effects on bone formation.[7] The major function of vitamin D, however, is to maintain the supply of calcium and phosphate by stimulating intestinal absorption.[8] Vitamin D is important in cell differentiation, formation of osteoclasts, and the differentiated function of osteoblasts. Calcitonin is a potent inhibitor of bone resorption. Unlike PTH, the effect of calcitonin on bone metabolism is independent from osteoblasts. Accordingly, osteoclasts express receptors for calcitonin on their membrane and not for PTH.[6]

Insulin and growth hormone (GH) are polypeptide hormones with counter-regulation. While GH is the major regulator of somatic growth, it acts indirectly by stimulating the production of circulating and local insulin-like growth factor (IGF-I) by skeletal cells,[9] which, in turn, mediates some of the effects of insulin on bone metabolism and skeletal growth.[10] Insulin stimulates bone matrix formation and mineralization. This stimulatory effect on matrix synthesis is due to an effect on osteoblast differentiation rather than an increase in collagen-producing cells.[11]

Glucocorticoids are steroid hormones with direct and indirect effects on bone metabolism. The indirect effects include inhibition of intestinal absorption of calcium and GH secretion. The direct effects include inhibition of bone collagen synthesis, probably due to a decrease in osteoblast replication,[5] and increased response to other systemic hormones such as PTH and IGF,[6] possibly by increasing receptor binding. This could be one of the mechanisms involved in steroid-induced osteoporosis.[12]

Sex hormones, both estrogen and androgens, play a central role in skeletal development and bone loss. The increase in sex hormones at puberty is partly responsible for the events leading to acceleration of cartilage growth, increased bone turnover, and increased bone mass. Both estrogen and androgen receptors are present in bone cells, pointing to the direct effects of these hormones on bone metabolism as well. Estrogen regulates bone remodeling by modulating the production of cytokines and growth factors, which, in turn, act as local regulators of the remodeling process. Cytokines under estrogen regulation with direct effects on bone cells include interleukin-1 (IL-1), tumor necrosis factor-α (TNF-α), granulocyte-macrophage colony–stimulating factor (GM-CSF) secreted by monocytes, and IL-6 and colony-stimulating factor (CSF) secreted by osteoblasts.[13] Interleukin-1 induces the synthesis of IL-6, which increases bone resorption through osteoclast recruitment. Colony-stimulating factor plays a role in the maturation of osteoclasts. Interleukin-1β and TNF-α stimulate mature osteoclasts, modulate bone cell proliferation, and induce bone resorption in vivo.[14,15] In addition, IL-1, TNF-α, and GM-CSF contribute to bone resorption by promoting osteoclast recruitment and differentiation from bone marrow precursors. Moreover, 17-B estradiol appears to stimulate the production of alkaline phosphatase and collagen IGF-1 by bone cells.[16] In addition, estrogen may affect bone turnover indirectly by acting as an antagonist to PTH. The bone-sparing effect of estrogen may be explained by its fundamental ability to interact with bone cells and modulate the cytokine circuitry that controls bone remodeling.[17]

Other local factors regulating bone remodeling are synthesized by skeletal cells and include growth factors and prostaglandins. Polypeptide growth factors include IGF-1 and -2,[18] TGF-β,[19] fibroblast growth factor (FGF),[20] platelet-derived growth factor (PDGF),[21] and bone morphogenic proteins (BMPs).[22] These factors have effects on cells of the same class (autocrine effect) or other cells within the tissue (paracrine effect). Prostaglandins are currently the only known regulators of bone remodeling that do not have a polypeptide structure.

Growth factors are also present in circulation and may act as systemic regulators of skeletal and nonskeletal metabolism but the locally produced factor has a more direct and possibly important function in cell growth. Circulating hormones may act on skeletal cells either directly or indirectly, modulating the synthesis, activation, and receptor binding of local growth factor. This, in turn, stimulates or inhibits bone formation or bone resorption. It is likely that hormones are important in the targeting of growth factors to tissues expressing specific hormonal receptors. Growth factors may play a critical role in the coupling of bone formation with bone resorption and possibly in pathophysiologic processes.[23]

Peak Bone Mass

Bone mass increases during early childhood and adolescence by linear growth of the endochondrial growth plates and by radial growth due to periosteal apposition. After closure of the growth plate around age 20 years, radial growth continues for about 10 to 15 years. Peak bone mass is therefore reached sometime between the third and early part of the fourth decade of life, declining progressively thereafter (Figure 10–1).[1,2] Peak bone mass constitutes the summation of growth and turnover during what is known as the "calcium building years." Sometime after age 40 years, a slow age-dependent phase of bone loss ensues. This calcium depletion phase results in similar losses of cortical and trabecular bone, with roughly similar rates in men and women.

In addition, postmenopausal women experience yet another phase of bone loss, that is, an accelerated loss as a consequence of the estrogen deficiency associated with menopause. Trabecular bone, being more metabolically active than cortical bone, is lost at a disproportionately faster rate during this postmenopausal phase of bone loss.

Peak bone mass has strong genetic determinants. Morrison and colleagues[24] have shown that bone mass, one of the main determinants of osteoporotic fractures, has a genetic component linked to an allelic change in the receptor for vitamin D, one of the hormones controlling calcium metabolism. However, nutritional factors, such as level of dietary calcium during skeletal growth, and environmental factors, such as physical activity, modulate the genetic disposition and contribute to the achievement of peak bone mass.[25] Failure to achieve peak bone mass predisposes to fractures later in life as age-related bone loss ensues. Genetically determined differences in peak bone mass may explain, in part, the racial and gender differences in the incidence of osteoporosis. Caucasian women have the least bone mass and African American men have the most, while Caucasian men and African American women have intermediate bone mass. Thus, assuming a constant rate of bone loss with age, Caucasian women with the lowest peak bone mass are at greatest risk for osteoporosis and fractures later in life.[1,2]

OSTEOPOROSIS

Osteoporosis means literally "porous bone," a condition where there is "too little bone" to provide mechanical support. Osteopenia, on the other hand, is a reduction in bone mineral density (BMD) below a predefined level. Osteoporosis is characterized by a reduction in BMD to a level below what is required for mechanical support.[26,27]

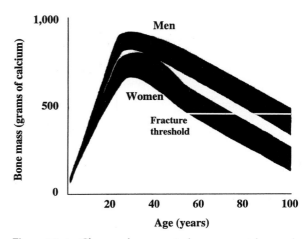

Figure 10–1. Changes that occur in bone mass with growth and aging in men and women. Factors involved in determining peak bone mass are genetic and nongenetic (nutrition, smoking, exercise). Factors increasing rate of bone loss later in life include aging, estrogen deficiency, and lifestyle factors (smoking, alcohol). Results of Morrison and colleagues (1994) suggest that bone mass is under genetic control, linked to polymorphism in the gene for vitamin D receptor.

A Consensus Development Conference defined osteoporosis as "a systemic skeletal disease characterized by low bone mass and microarchitectural deterioration with a consequent increase in bone fragility and susceptibility to fracture."[28] This definition, though descriptive, provides little usefulness for diagnosis and clinical management. Microarchitectural deterioration is not amenable to clinical measurement, whereas bone mass can be measured with accuracy and precision with dual x-ray absorptiometry (DXA). Thus, a World Health Organization panel has operationally defined osteoporosis as a BMD (T score) that is 2.5 SD below the mean peak value in young adults (Table 10–1).[29] This definition too, has limitations since BMD values are applicable to Caucasian women

---

TABLE 10–1. World Health Organization (WHO) Diagnostic Guidelines for Interpretation of Bone Mass Measurements in Caucasian Women

Severe osteoporosis
  Bone mineral density (BMD) more than 2.5 standard deviations (SD) below the mean value of peak bone mass in young normal women and the presence of fractures.
Osteoporosis
  BMD more than 2.5 SD below the mean value of peak bone mass in young normal women.
Low bone mass (osteopenia)
  BMD within –1 SD and –2.5 SD of the mean value of peak bone mass in normal young women.
Normal
  BMD not more than 1SD below mean value of peak bone mass in young normal women.

TABLE 10–2. Classification of Osteoporosis

Primary	
Idiopathic	Juvenile
	Adult
Involutional	Type I (postmenopausal)
	Type II (age-related)
Secondary	
Endocrine disorders	
Diabetes mellitus	
Gastrointestinal and malabsorption syndromes	
Myeloproliferative disorders	
Multiple myeloma	
Connective tissue diseases	
Marfan syndrome	
Ehlers-Danlos syndrome	
Chronic obstructive pulmonary disease	

only. Their relevance to other ethnic groups and to men is currently unknown.

Osteoporosis affects more than 25 million people in the United States (about 10% of the total population), including 1 in 3 postmenopausal women, and a substantial number of men. It is responsible for more than 2 million fractures annually, resulting in health-care costs in excess of 20 billion U.S. dollars. The major portion of the social and economic burden caused by fractures is due to hip fracture. The intangible costs to society due to pain and suffering associated with morbidity, need for long-term care, and mortality as a result of osteoporotic fractures add to the financial burden. Osteoporosis is clearly a major public health problem.

Classification

Osteoporosis occurs either as a primary disorder, or it may be secondary to other diseases or conditions (Table 10–2).[1] Primary osteoporosis includes idiopathic (juvenile or adult) and involutional forms. Idiopathic forms of osteoporosis are rare and affect men and women equally. Involutional osteoporosis, by far the most common form, includes two patterns: type I (postmenopausal) and type II (age-related) osteoporosis.

Type I (postmenopausal) osteoporosis occurs in peri- and postmenopausal women. Bone loss in premenopausal women is slow and approximately equal to that of men (0.3 to 0.5% per year). With the onset of menopause in females, an accelerated rate of cortical bone loss of 2 to 3% per year ensues for about 8 to 10 years. Trabecular bone is lost at a rate of about 5% per year during the first 5 to 8 years

after menopause (see Figure 10–1). Thus, type 1 osteoporosis is characterized by a disproportionate loss of trabecular bone resulting in fractures at those skeletal sites with a high volume of trabecular bone, including the vertebrae, distal forearm (Colles' fractures), and distal ankle. Clinical symptoms of the disease include bone pain (mostly from vertebral compression), loss of height and consequent deformation of the skeleton leading to dorsal kyphosis ("dowager's hump").

Type I osteoporosis is related to the estrogen deficiency associated with menopause, leading to a cascade of accelerated bone loss, decreased secretion of parathyroid hormone, increased secretion of calcitonin, and decreased calcium absorption, which further aggravates bone loss. In addition, patients with type I osteoporosis and high bone turnover have increased production of IL-1 by stimulated monocytes, as compared with age-matched controls, which also contributes to increased bone resorption.

Type II (age-related) osteoporosis appears to affect virtually the entire population of aging men and women, although it is twice as common in women. Bone loss starts around the third decade and continues through life and is characeized by slow bone loss due to decreased calcium absorption and secondary hyperparathyroidism. Bone loss affects cortical and trabecular bone equally with a rate of about 0.3 to 0.5% per year (see Figure 10–1). These two types of bone loss result in distinct fracture patterns. While postmenopausal osteoporosis manifests mostly in Colles' and vertebral fractures, age-related osteoporosis results in hip fractures in both men and women of older age. However, fractures of the humerus, proximal fibula, and pelvis are also common.

Secondary Osteoporosis

Osteoporosis may be associated with a number of endocrine diseases. Hypogonadism in either sex increases the incidence of osteoporosis. Hyperthyroidism consistently increases bone turnover but in most patients, formation and resorption remain coupled. Osteoporosis may also be associated with gastrointestinal diseases, and malabsorption syndromes that impair absorption of calcium and vitamin D. Multiple myeloma and other myeloproliferative disorders produce diffuse osteoporosis in about 10% of patients. Diffuse osteoporosis may also occur when disseminated carcinoma invades the bone marrow. An unusually severe form of osteoporosis may occur in connective tissue diseases such as osteogenesis imperfecta. Marfan and Ehlers-Danlos syndromes may also be associated with vertebral osteopenia, but less frequently include vertebral fractures.

Other causes of osteoporosis include total immobilization, such as in traumatic quadriplegia. Significant bone loss also occurs during total bed rest among nonparalyzed individuals and in astronauts during gravitational weightlessness. Osteoporosis is also associated with chronic obstructive pulmonary disease. Whether this is related to the underlying consumption of tobacco or to the pulmonary disease itself is unknown.

Pathophysiology

The pathophysiology of osteoporosis is poorly understood. Bone mass at any given time is related to peak bone mass and bone loss that has occurred since peak mass was attained. Bone is continuously remodeled throughout the life of an individual, and the rate of remodeling is increased in older adults. With the increased rate of remodeling in older age, there is uncoupling of the remodeling cycle, that is, the rate of resorption exceeds the rate of formation.[30,31] This results in a remodeling imbalance with net bone loss, lower bone mass, and ultimately increased risk for fractures. Such an imbalance would be even greater if the rate of initiation of new bone remodeling cycles were to increase. Therefore, genetically determined bone mass and age constitute the major determinants of risk of osteoporosis and osteoporotic fractures.

ORAL BONE AND OSTEOPENIA/OSTEOPOROSIS

After having reviewed the biology of bone remodeling and the basis of imbalance in coupling responsible for the onset of skeletal osteopenia and ultimately osteoporosis, the implicit question is, to what extent is oral bone affected by remodeling imbalance, and does it contribute to oral bone loss? In addition to the academic relevance of this question, it is fundamental to proper clinical management of dentate and edentulous patients suffering from both osteopenia and osteoporosis. A rational dental treatment plan in such patients is not complete if proper management of systemic bone loss is not included.

Relationship of Skeletal Osteopenia to Mandibular Bone Density

It has long been postulated that mandibular bone density may be indicative of systemic bone mineral density. In a classic series of studies, Kribbs and colleagues (Table 10–3) addressed this relationship in both normal and osteoporotic women. In an early study,[32] total body calcium as assessed by neutron activation analysis, was found to be associated with mandibular density as measured by quantitative analysis of intraoral radiographs. A later study[33] in normal, nonosteoporotic women, revealed that bone mass was not affected by age but was significantly associated with skeletal bone mass

TABLE 10–3. Relationship between Systemic and Mandibular Bone Mineral Density

Authors	Population	Major Result	Type of Study
Jeffcoat et al, [In press]	200 subjects from Women's Health Initiative Postmenopausal women	Correlation between basal bone mineral density and hip bone mineral density	Baseline data from longitudinal study
Von Wowern et al, 1994	12 women with osteoporotic fracture 14 normal women	Osteoporotic subjects had less bone mineral content and more loss of attachment compared with normals	Cross-sectional study
Kribbs et al, 1990	50 normal women, aged 20 to 90 years	Mandibular bone mass correlated with bone mass as spine and wrist	Cross-sectional study
Kribbs et al, 1990	85 osteoporotic and 27 normal women, aged 50 to 85 years	Osteoporotic group had less mandibular bone mass and density	Cross-sectional study
Kribbs et al, 1989	85 osteoporotic women	Total body calcium, bone mass at radius, and bone density at spine correlated with mandibular mass	Cross-sectional study
Kribbs et al, 1983	30 postmenopausal women	Total body calcium associated with mandibular bone density	Cross-sectional study

at the spine and wrist. A comparison of 85 osteo-porotic women with 27 normal women showed less mandibular bone mass and density and a thinner cortex at the gonion in osteoporotic compared with nonosteoporotic women.[34,35] Similarly, von Wowern and colleagues[36] reported that 12 osteoporotic subjects with a history of fractures had less mandibular bone mineral content as measured by dual photon absorptiometry than 14 normal women. It is noteworthy that all reports Kribbs and colleagues[32–35] and von Wowern and colleagues[36] described are cross-sectional studies.

The Women's Health Initiative (WHI), in the United States, is an unprecedented study of women's health after menopause. Specific risk factors for diseases including heart disease and osteoporosis are being addressed nationwide. The University of Alabama at Birmingham and the State University of New York at Buffalo are conducting oral studies ancillary to the WHI to determine whether image analysis of intraoral radiographs could be used to determine if basal mandibular BMD is correlated with hip BMD determined by DXA. Comprehensive medical histories and examinations performed as part of the parent study were linked with results of oral examinations and quantitative digital intraoral radiography.[37,38] A region of interest in the area of the basal bone of the first mandibular molar was selected for measurements of mandibular BMD. General linear models of mandibular basal BMD, hip BMD, midroot density, age, race, hormone replacement therapy, and calcium supplements were created. Preliminary analyses from the University of Alabama cohort used data from the first 200 subjects in the study.[39] Significant correlations were found between mandibular basal BMD and hip BMD (r = 0.74, $p < .001$). These findings are consistent with evidence that supports the concept that BMD of the mandible is indeed correlated with skeletal BMD.

Tooth Loss and Osteoporosis

Several studies have demonstrated a relationship between tooth loss and systemic osteoporosis in both dentate and edentulous individuals. Daniell and colleagues[40] suggested that systemic bone loss was a risk factor for edentulism. Women with severe osteoporosis, defined as extreme thinning of the metacarpal cortical area, were three times more likely (44% versus 15%) to have no teeth compared with healthy, age-matched controls. Taguchi and colleagues[41] showed that a decrease in mandibular bone density, estimated as mandibular cortical width, cor-related with tooth loss for women in their sixties. In a study of 329 healthy postmenopausal women, for each additional tooth present, spinal BMD increased 0.003 g per cm^2.[42] In a 7-year longitudinal study, rate of systemic bone loss was a predictor of tooth loss in postmenopausal women.[43] For each 1% per year decrease in whole body BMD, the risk for tooth loss more than quadrupled. Decreases in BMD at the femoral neck and spine resulted in a 50% and 45% increased risk of tooth loss respectively. Collectively, this evidence indicates that osteoporotic women have lost significantly more teeth, and more are edentulous compared with nonosteoporotic women.[40–44] Thus, women that are at risk for or suffer from osteoporosis are also at risk for tooth loss.

Periodontal Disease and Osteopenia/Osteoporosis

Unlike the clear relationship between osteoporosis and tooth loss, controversy still exists concerning the association between osteopenia/osteoporosis and periodontal disease. Conflicting results among different studies account for much of the controversy. Small sample size and fundamental differences in study design, population examined (ie, women only versus men and women), age of population studied, and methodology to assess periodontal disease and skeletal osteopenia and osteoporosis prevent interpretation and comparability of results.

Wactawski-Wende and colleagues,[45] in a study of 70 postmenopausal women, found a significant relationship between alveolar crestal bone height as a measure of periodontitis and skeletal osteopenia (femur and lumbar spine) measured by DXA. This relationship was seen after controlling for possible confounders such as dental plaque, years of menopause, and smoking. In addition, there was a relationship between osteopenia at the hip and probing attachment loss in this same group. Similarly, von Wowern and colleagues,[36] in a case-control study comparing 12 female patients with osteoporotic fractures and 14 normal women, reported significantly greater periodontal attachment loss in the osteoporotic women compared with the normal women. They found that the osteoporotic women had less mandibular bone mineral content, as measured by dual photon absorptiometry, than the 14 normal women. The mandibular bone mineral content values were 2 SD below the mandibular bone content for young reference (normal) women in 92% of the osteoporotic group and in 64% of the control group, suggesting that a high proportion of the control group also suffered from mandibular osteopenia. The relationship between osteopenia and severity of periodontal disease was also examined in a sample from the Third National Health and Nutrition Examination Survey (NHANES III) of 11,247 individuals 20 to 90 years of age.[46] Osteopenia of the hip was significantly associated with severity of periodontal disease (mean attachment loss ≥ 1.5 mm) in females and males alike (Figure 10–2), independently of the confounding effects of age, gender, smoking, or intake of dietary calcium. This association was increased even further in postmenopausal females. Hence, though limited, the evidence suggests an association between osteopenia, osteoporosis, and periodontal disease. Estrogen deficiency may explain, in part, the nature of this association.

CO–RISK FACTORS FOR OSTEOPOROSIS AND PERIODONTAL DISEASE

Osteoporosis and periodontal disease are chronic, multifactorial diseases. It is not surprising, therefore, that both diseases share common risk factors. Risk factors common to both osteoporosis and periodontal disease are listed under the categories of genetic, dietary, environmental, and systemic factors (Table 10–4). Strong evidence indicates that genetic and lifestyle factors are important risk factors for osteoporosis.[47–49] Family history of osteoporosis or fractures, thin body build, genetics, race, and advancing age constitute nonmodifiable risk factors for osteoporosis.

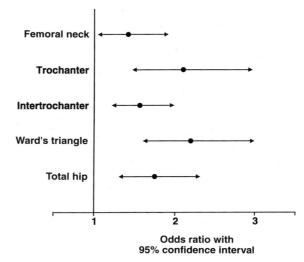

Figure 10–2. Results from the NHANES III including 11,247 individuals 20 to 90 years old indicate that BMD of the femoral neck, trochanter, intertrochanter, Ward's triangle, and total hip is a significant predictor for severe periodontal disease in men and woman alike, independently of the confounding effect of age, smoking, or intake of dietary calcium.

Skeletal bone loss can be slowed or even reversed if modifiable environmental and dietary risk factors, such as physical inactivity, cigarette smoking, low dietary calcium intake, and excessive use of caffeine and alcohol, are identified and reversed. A report from the National Osteoporosis Foundation concluded that the following factors were useful in identifying women at risk for fracture: low body weight (< 58 kg), current smoking, first-degree relative with low-trauma fracture, and per-

TABLE 10–4. Risk Factors for Osteoporosis and Periodontal Disease

	Osteoporosis	*Periodontal Disease*
Hereditary/genetics	Female gender	Age
	Caucasian or Asian race	Race
	Family history	Familial aggregation
	Menopause	IL-1 polymorphism
	Petite body build	
	Suboptimal peak bone	
Dietary factors	Low intake calcium	Low intake calcium
	Low intake vitamin D	Low intake vitamins C, E, A, selenium
	High intake caffeine, protein, salt, phosphate	
Environment	Smoking	Smoking
	Alcohol	Alcohol
	Physical inactivity	Stress
Systemic factors	Diabetes mellitus	Diabetes mellitus
	Multiple myeloma	Osteoporosis
	Connective tissue diseases	Hormone changes

TABLE 10–5. Risk Factors to Identify Women at Risk for Fracture (Recommended by the National Osteoporosis Foundation)

Low body weight (< 58 kg)
Current smoking
First-degree relative with low-trauma fracture
Personal history of low-trauma fracture

sonal history of low-trauma fracture (Table 10–5). These risk factors are simple and easy to ascertain and effective in identifying women at increased risk.

Recent evidence indicates that genetics may play an important role in the severity of periodontal disease as well.[50] Environmental factors such as smoking and excessive alcohol consumption are important modifiable risk factors for periodontal disease.[51,52] Stress and inadequate coping are also equally predictive for both periodontal disease and osteoporosis.[53] Largescale population-based studies indicate that inadequate intake of specific nutrients is also associated with severe periodontal disease.[54,55]

Estrogen Deficiency

Estrogen deficiency is the factor most closely associated with postmenopausal osteoporosis.[48,49] Deficiency of estradiol in postmenopausal and oophorectomized women is associated with decreased lumbar spine bone mineral density and increased incidence of fractures of the vertebrae and hip.[56–58] Estrogen regulates bone remodeling by modulating the production of cytokines and growth factors, especially IL-1β, TNF-α, GM-CSF, and M-CSF from bone cells.[13] Interleukin-1β and TNF-α stimulate mature osteoclasts, modulate bone cell proliferation, and induce bone resorption in vivo.[14,15] In addition, IL-1, TNF-α, and GM-CSF contribute to bone resorption by promoting osteoclast recruitment and differentiation from bone marrow precursors. Osteoblast precursors respond to the loss of estrogen by secreting IL-6, which then induces osteoclastogenesis.[16] The loss of estrogen accompanying menopause results in an increase of cytokines in the bone remodeling circuitry. Subjects with "high turnover" osteoporosis secrete increased amounts of IL-1 that is blocked by estrogen/progesterone therapy.[59] This association, apparently, is not restricted to IL-1 but also affects other major mononuclear cell secretory products, such as TNF-α and GM-CSF. Cytokine production by peripheral blood monocytes (PBM) from ovariectomized women that receive no estrogen therapy steadily increases. Moreover, in vitro treatment of human monocytes with estrogen has been shown to regulate both IL-1 and TNF.[60] Accordingly, Horowitz[61] proposed that the antiosteoporotic effect of estrogen is exerted through downregulation of cytokine synthesis and secretion by osteoblasts and other cells.

TABLE 10–6. Relationship between Estrogen Status and Periodontal Disease

Authors	Study Design/Population	Results	Conclusion
Norderyd et al, 1993	Cross-sectional 234 postmenopausal women (57 ERT; 177 non-ERT)	Gingival bleeding significantly lower in ERT vs. non-ERT. Lower levels of plaque and *Capnocytophaga* sp. Less attachment loss in ERT group vs. non-ERT	ERT associated with less gingivitis in postmenopausal women
Payne et al, 1997	Longitudinal 1 year 24 postmenopausal women (10 estrogen sufficient; 14 estrogen deficient)	Estrogen-sufficient group showed mean net gain in alveolar bone density. Estrogen-deficient group showed mean net loss in alveolar bone density	Estrogen status may influence alveolar bone density status
Jacobs et al, 1996	Longitudinal 5 years 69 women, 36 to 64 years old Natural and surgical menopause Receive estrogen therapy	Moderate relationship between BMC of mandible and lumbar spine. Positive effect of estrogen therapy on mandibular bone mass	Estrogen status directly related to mandibular bone mass

ERT = estrogen replacement therapy; BMC = bone mineral content.

Three studies have directly examined the relationship of estrogen status/deficiency and periodontal disease (Table 10–6). Norderyd and colleagues[62] reported lower, although not statistically significant, levels of clinical attachment loss in postmenopausal women receiving estrogen supplementation compared with estrogen-deficient postmenopausal women. In addition, gingival bleeding was statistically significantly reduced in the estrogen-treated postmenopausal women compared with the estrogen-deficient group, after controlling for levels of supragingival plaque and frequency of dental treatment. A 5-year longitudinal study of 69 women with surgical or natural menopause receiving hormone replacement therapy compared lumbar spine BMD, measured by dual photon absorptiometry, with mandibular bone mass assessed by quantitative measures of standardized intraoral radiographs.[63] A statistically significant but moderate correlation was observed between mandibular and lumbar spine bone mass and that estrogen replacement therapy after surgical or natural menopause had a positive effect on bone mass not only of the lumbar spine but the mandible as well.[63] Payne and colleagues[64] showed, in a 1-year longitudinal study of 24 postmenopausal women, that estrogen-deficient women displayed a mean net loss in alveolar bone density compared with estrogen-sufficient women, who displayed a mean net gain in alveolar bone density. The authors proposed estrogen defieciency as a risk factor for alveolar bone density loss. Thus, in the estrogen deficient state, the governor controlling cytokines and bone remodelling is lost, resulting in increased bone resorption and net skeletal and alveolar bone loss.

Hence, consistent evidence supports the relationship between estrogen status, periodontal disease, and mandibular bone density. Results from three independent studies clearly suggest that estrogen deficiency plays an important role in mandibular bone loss and is likely an important factor modifying the severity of periodontal disease in postmenopausal women.

Smoking

A meta-analysis of 29 studies including 2,156 smokers and 9,750 nonsmokers examined the effect of cigarette smoking on skeletal bone mineral density.[65] While bone density in premenopausal women was comparable in smokers and nonsmokers, in postmenopausal women bone loss was greater in current smokers compared with nonsmokers. The cumulative risk for hip fractures in women was 19% in smokers and 12% in nonsmokers. Among all women, one in eight hip fractures was attributable to smoking. Limited data was available for men; however, a similar proportionate effect of smoking was observed. The meta-analysis concluded that smoking may have a direct effect on bone metabo-

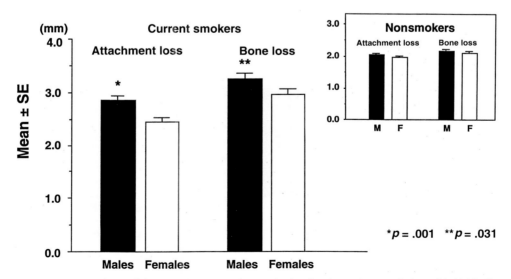

Figure 10–3. Analysis of the Erie County Study reveals that for the entire population of 1,426 individuals 25 to 74 years old, men show more severe periodontal disease than women. However, male and female nonsmokers have the same levels of alveolar bone loss. Among current smokers, on the other hand, males have significantly ($p = .03$) more alveolar bone loss compared with females, suggesting that the difference in disease severity is explained, in part, by a reduced response to smoking in females, mediated possibly by estrogen status.

lism, since the association between smoking and BMD was not explained by smokers being thinner, younger at menopause, exercising less, or tobacco smoke having a direct effect on estrogen.

The direct effect of smoking on skeletal bone is modulated by gender and estrogen. Analysis of BMD at the hip, spine, and radius of the Framingham cohort showed that men smokers had 4 to 15% lower BMD compared with nonsmokers, independent of weight, alcohol, or caffeine use,[66] implying other mechanisms for the effect of smoking on bone. Smoking did not affect skeletal BMD in women that had not taken estrogen. However, lower BMD was seen among women that had taken estrogen supplementation and were smokers compared with nonsmokers, suggesting that smoking negates the bone-sparing effect of estrogen. Smoking also accelerated the rate of bone loss at the femoral neck and total body in some elderly men and women, who participated in a 3-year placebo-controlled study of calcium and vitamin D supplementation.[67] Less efficient absorption of calcium was proposed as a possible mechanism for the smoking-related accelerated bone loss.

Smoking is the single most important modifiable risk factor for periodontal disease and osteoporosis. A meta-analysis of available literature indicates that smokers have 2.5 times the risk for severe periodontal disease compared with nonsmokers, independent of the effects of age, socioeconomic factors, diabetes mellitus, or dental plaque.[68] Furthermore, the risk is cumulative and dose dependent in that the severity of periodontal disease is related to the duration and amount of smoking.[51] When alveolar bone loss is used as the outcome measure, the risk is even greater.[69] This increased negative effect on alveolar bone may be explained by the direct effect of smoking on bone metabolism and bone resorption. In a manner similar to skeletal BMD, the effect of smoking on alveolar bone is modulated by gender and estrogen.

Analysis of the Erie County Study cohort reveals that the greater severity in periodontal disease seen in males is explained in part by smoking. That is, if only nonsmokers are examined, disease levels measured as alveolar bone loss are comparable between both genders. However, when only smokers are examined, males exhibit greater alveolar bone loss compared with females (Figure 10–3). Therefore, the greater severity of periodontal disease seen in males appears to be related to a gender response to smoking. The lesser severity of periodontal disease in premenopausal women that smoke could be explained by the bone protective effects of estrogen. When the levels of periodontal disease in postmenopausal women are examined, nonsmoking women that receive estrogen supplementation through hormone replacement therapy (HRT) exhibit less alveolar

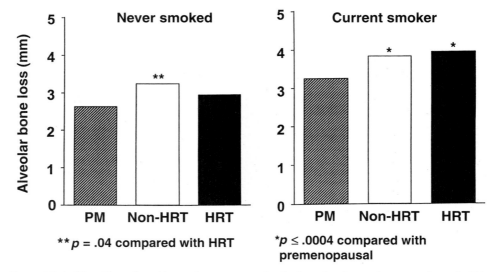

Figure 10–4. The effect of smoking and estrogen on alveolar bone loss is seen in women from the Erie County Study. Among nonsmokers, postmenopausal HRT women have levels of alveolar bone loss no different compared with premenopausal (PM) women. Non-HRT women, on the other hand, have bone loss levels significantly greater (p = .04) than PM and HRT counterparts, suggesting a protective effect of estrogen on alveolar bone loss. Among women who smoke, however, both HRT and non-HRT groups have levels of bone loss significantly greater than premenopausal women, suggesting that smoking reduces the protective effect of estrogen. HRT = hormone replacement therapy; PM = premenopausal.

bone loss compared with women that do not take estrogen (non-HRT) (Figure 10–4).[70] In fact, alveolar bone loss levels in postmenopausal women taking HRT are no different from the levels in premenopausal women. Postmenopausal women that smoke and take HRT have levels of alveolar bone loss comparable with those women that do not take HRT. Thus, in a manner analogous to skeletal bone density, estrogen has a bone-sparing effect on alveolar bone, which is negated by current smoking (see Figure 10–4). Similar findings are evident when tooth loss is examined in this population of women, that is, estrogen supplementation is protective in postmenopausal tooth loss, and current smoking negates this protective effect as well.[71]

Dietary Factors

Peak bone mass is attained at around 30 to 35 years of age as the summation of genetically determined factors modulated by dietary and environmental factors.[72] Adequate dietary calcium is essential for the growth and development of a normal skeleton.[73] Insufficient calcium intake during childhood and adolescence can reduce peak bone mass and enhance postmenopausal and age-related osteoporosis.[74] Dietary calcium supplementation has been shown to increase bone mass in children and adolescents and to reduce age-associated bone loss.

Not surprisingly, osteoporosis has been defined as a "pediatric disease." Radial BMD was correlated with current calcium intake in young women (20 to 23 years old).[75] A study of young women failed to find an association between BMD and calcium intake.[76] However, the mean calcium intake for the study group was 909 mg, high enough to obscure any possible difference. A study of about 18,000 Japanese men and women, 30 to 69 years old, found that even one glass of milk per day was protective against osteoporosis in calcium-deficient individuals.[77] The National Institutes of Health (NIH), 1994 Conference on Optimal Calcium recommends a dose of 1,000 mg per day for premenopausal women, and 1,500 mg per day for estrogen-deficient women (Table 10–7). These recommendations are for Caucasians. Requirements for other ethnic groups, as well as for persons with lower protein intakes and small skeletal size may differ.

The role of phosphorous, vitamin D, protein, fluoride, and caffeine on bone mass have been studied as well.[78] Vitamin D or its metabolites increase intestinal calcium absorption, suppress PTH levels, and increase bone density; their amount and action decrease with age. Osteoblasts have receptors for $1,25(OH)_2D_3$, which is the final product of vitamin D metabolism. Excess protein intake is related to increased calcium excretion. Fluoride is a powerful stimulator of bone formation, resulting in a major increase in trabecular bone mass. However, cortical fractures have been associated with high fluoride levels, which may be related to the fact that fluoride decreases the elasticity of bone. Caffeine is correlated with decreased bone density. In addition, studies in ovariectomized Sprague-Dawley rats fed a soy-protein diet showed a bone-sparing effect mediated by isoflavones in soy-protein.[79]

A series of recent studies examining the data from NHANES III demonstrate the significant effect of nutrition as a risk factor for periodontal disease. Trained nutritionists conducted interviews on a 24-hour diet recall on a nationwide probability sample of approximately 40,000 individuals 1 to 90+ years old. Individuals with diets deficient in calcium had statistically higher levels of periodontal disease compared with those with calcium sufficient diets.[54] This association was especially strong in younger and premenopausal women. Individuals with diets deficient in vitamins C, A, alpha-carotenoids, selenium, and lutein also showed increased risk for periodontal disease, independently of the confounding effects of age, dental plaque, and smoking.[55] Therefore, a diet complete in vitamins and minerals plays an important role, not only in ensuring achievement of peak bone mass and protection from age-related bone loss, but it also likely protects against the destruction of connective tissue and alveolar bone resulting from periodontal infection.

Genetic Factors

Osteoporosis is likely a multifactorial, polygenic condition involving mutiple genes regulating the attainment of peak bone mass and possibly the control of

TABLE 10–7. National Institutes of Health (NIH) Consensus Conference Recommendation for Optimum Calcium Intake

Premenopausal women (25 to 50 years old)	1,000 mg/d
Postmenopausal women (estrogen therapy)	1,000 mg/d
Postmenopausal women (no estrogen therapy)	1,500 mg/d
Men (25 to 65 years old)	1,000 mg/d
Women and men > 65 years old	1,500 mg/d

turnover. Early studies showed that monozygotic twins exhibited less variation in bone mass than dizygotic twins.[80] A landmark study by Morrison and colleagues[24] reported that bone mass had a genetic component that could be ascribed to an allelic change in the receptor for 1,25 dihydroxy vitamin D. The vitamin D receptor (VDR) is required for normal calcium absorption from the gut. It is estimated that common allelic variants in the gene encoding the VDR account for up to 75% of the total genetic effect on bone density in healthy Caucasian adults[24] and predicts the density of femoral and vertebral bone in prepubertal American girls of Mexican descent.[81] Other polymorphisms imparting susceptibility to osteoporosis include the binding site in collagen type I alpha 1 (COLIA 1) gene,[82,83] transforming growth factor-beta (TGF-β) gene,[84] the estrogen receptor,[85] the vitamin D promoter region of the osteocalcin gene,[86] as well as genes regulating cytokines involved in bone turnover.

Susceptibility to periodontal infection and the inflammatory responses to the infecting organism appear to be under genetic regulation as well.[87] It is possible that periodontal disease is also a polygenic condition. Candidate genes for susceptibility to periodontal disease include genes defining the FcγRII receptor, genes regulating immunoglobulin synthesis, especially IgG$_2$, and genes regulating cytokine synthesis. Specific genotypes of polymorphic IL-1β genes are associated with increased IL-1 production and associated with severity of periodontal disease in nonsmokers.[50] This IL-1 genotype was found to accurately predict prognosis and tooth survival in individuals affected by periodontal disease.[88] Current predictive models for both periodontal disease and osteoporosis do not account for all the observed variability in disease expresssion. Genetically determined individual susceptibility to both conditions may in part explain some of the unaccounted variability.

COMMON TREATMENT STRATEGIES FOR OSTEOPOROSIS AND PERIODONTAL DISEASE

Avoidance of the morbidity of osteoporosis begins with prevention. Adequate calcium intake during adolescence and early adulthood is critical to forming peak bone mass. The 1994 NIH Conference on Optimal Calcium Intake recommended that daily calcium intake of 1,000 mg of calcium per day for premenopausal, and 1,500 mg per day for postmenopausal women (see Table 10–7) should be maintained until additional research warrants revisions to such recommendations. To maximize the likelihood that bone mass is maintained over a lifetime, load-bearing exercise is also necessary. Like periodontal disease, smoking is a major risk factor for osteoporosis and avoidance of smoking or smoking cessation contributes to osseous health.

There is a limited amount of evidence that calcium supplementation may be beneficial in reducing tooth loss. In a 7-year study of 189 postmenopausal women not taking HRT, subjects were assigned to receive either placebo, calcium supplementation, or vitamin D plus calcium supplementation.[89] Four times as many (12%) placebo-treated women lost teeth during the study period compared with 3% in the calcium-supplemented group. No effect was observed with vitamin D.

Bone loss in women occurs most rapidly in the years immediately following menopause when natural levels of estrogen are greatly reduced. Hormone replacement therapy is designed to replace estrogen after menopause since this immediate postmenopausal period is a time of rapid loss of bone mineral density.[90–94] For women with a uterus, a combination of estrogen and progesterone is used; while in women without a uterus, estrogen replacement therapy (ERT) alone is employed. Many studies have reported that HRT and ERT are efficacious in sparing bone mineral and reducing fractures.[90–94]

Few studies have directly assessed the relationship between periodontal disease and its sequelae in women receiving HRT. Most of these studies have involved HRT with either estrogen or estrogen plus progesterone, and assessed tooth loss, alveolar bone loss, or other measures of periodontal health. In a longitudinal, unblinded study of 69 women receiving HRT, Jacobs and colleagues[63] compared lumbar spine bone mineral density, measured by dual photon absorptiometry, with mandibular bone mass assessed by quantitative measures of standardized intraoral radiographs. The average length of study was 5.1 years. A significant but moderate correlation was observed at the second examination. Estrogen replacement therapy was associated with less gingival bleeding after correcting for age,[62] less alveolar bone loss,[70] and less tooth loss[71] than in women without estrogen supplementation.

Major cohorts of women have been examined in two longitudinal studies in an attempt to determine if HRT has reduced the number of lost teeth in postmenopausal women. These include the 3-year study of 42,171 postmenopausal women in the Nurses Health Cohort[95] and the 10-year study of 3,921 women living in a retirement community in the Leisure World Cohort.[96] The Leisure World Cohort taking estrogen experienced a 36% reduction in tooth loss and the Nurses Health Cohort showed an inverse relationship between HRT and loss of teeth, after correcting for smoking and age. One potential source of bias in these studies (and, in fact, addressed in the reports) is the fact that the same patients that seek to prevent osteoporosis may seek preventive dental care as well. Both these populations are large but composed of relatively well-educated, higher socioeconomic groups. In a third study, 488 women aged 72 to 95 years participating in the Framingham Heart Study were examined.[97] Estrogen users had more teeth remining than had nonusers, after controlling for age, smoking status, and education.

Therapy for osteoporosis is a rapidly changing field. The latest generation of bisphosphonate drugs, such as alendronate, deposit onto bone decreasing osteoclast numbers and activity, thereby decreasing bone resorption. Alendronate has been shown to inhibit loss of bone density and decrease the risk of fracture, without disturbance of bone healing observed with earlier drugs.[98] In a pilot clinical trial, the efficacy of alendronate in slowing alveolar bone loss due to periodontitis was investigated.[38] This 9-month, double-blind, placebo-controlled, randomized clinical trial (RCT) measured loss of bone height and density using digital subtraction radiography. Alendronate reduced the risk of progressive loss of alveolar bone. The relative risk of progressive loss of bone height and density was 0.45 for the alendronate-treated patients compared with placebo-treated patients.

FUTURE RESEARCH

Although considerable research has been done in the last 10 years in understanding the functions and control mechanisms of bone cells, much work still remains to be done in the field of bone cell biology. New treatments addressing the multifactorial nature of osteoporosis will require fundamental advances in knowledge in the field of bone cell and molecular biology.

Further research is needed on the therapeutic control of bone resorption, including the nature of the cellular and molecular mechanisms by which osteoblast/ stromal cells influence progression from hematopoietic precursors to differentiated osteoclasts. Either the factor(s) responsible or the cascade of events leading to this differentiation will provide important therapeutic alternatives. Substantial evidence supports the antiosteoporotic effect of estrogen. However, significant research interest exists in

partial agonist/antagonists of estrogen, which could uniquely influence receptor conformation. Thus, research to elucidate the tertiary structure of estrogen receptors will aid in developing "designer estrogens." Clearly, much more research into the bone formation process is needed as well, with the ultimate goal of identifying agents capable of promoting bone formation. Suitable agents at present are fluoride and PTH, each of which is a substantial promoter of bone formation.

Longitudinal studies are needed to definitively elucidate the contribution of systemic osteopenia to periodontal disease, alveolar bone loss, alveolar ridge resorption, and tooth loss. Additional research is needed to identify and test, in clinical trials, agents with effects on reducing skeletal and oral bone resorption. Evidence-based treatment approaches to manage individuals suffering from both periodontal disease and systemic osteopenia are urgently needed. Preservation of alveolar bone and alveolar ridge in combination with the prevention of fracture is essential to provide the quality of life in our older population. Biomedical research needs to ensure that the quality of life and well being of this rapidly growing segment of our population will continue well into older age.

Finally, the first genetic clue to susceptibility to osteoporosis came from work with the vitamin D receptor gene. Since then, other candidate genes and genetic polymorphisms conferring susceptibility to osteoporosis have been identified, establishing osteoporosis as a polygenic disease. Additional research is needed to fully unravel the genetic make-up of osteopenia/osteoporosis. Additionally, interactions between genetic, nutritional, and lifestyle factors, such as smoking and alcohol intake, are important targets for future research. Genetic studies in osteoporosis and periodontal disease will lead to ways of not only identifying individuals susceptible to these two crippling diseases but also to understanding how the environment may contribute to modulating the susceptibility to both diseases. Future research will provide ways of identifying susceptible individuals likely to benefit from prevention of both osteopenia/osteoposis and periodontal disease.

REFERENCES

1. Riggs BL. Overview of osteoporosis. West J Med 1991;154:63–77.
2. Parfitt AM. Bone remodeling: relationship to the amount and structure for bone, and the patho-

genesis and prevention of fractures. In: Riggs BL, Melton LJ III, editors. Osteoporosis: etiology, diagnosis and management. New York: Raven Press; 1988. p. 45–93.

3. Vaananen HK. Mechanisms of bone turnover. Ann Med 1995;25:353–9.

4. Parfitt AM. The physiological and clinical significance of bone histomorphometric data. Bone histomorphometry: techniques and interpretation. Boca Raton, FL; 1983. p. 143–223.

5. Canalis E. The hormonal and local regulation of bone formation. Endocr Rev 1983;4:62–77.

6. Raisz LG. Local and systemic factors in the pathogenesis of osteoporosis. N Engl J Med 1988;318: 818–27.

7. DeLuca H. Vitamin D visited. Clin Endocrinol Metab 1980;9:1–26.

8. Raisz LG, Kream BE. Regulation of bone formation. N Engl J Med 1983:309:29–35.

9. Raisz LG. Recent advances in bone cell biology: interactions of vitamin D with other local and systemic factors. Bone Mineral 1990;9:191–7.

10. Canalis E, Centrella M, Burch W, McCarthy T. Insulin-like growth factor I mediates selective anabolic effects of parathyroid hormone in bone cultures. J Clin Invest 1989;83:60–5.

11. McCarthy T, Centrella M, Canalis E. Regulatory effects of insulin-like growth factor I and II on bone collagen synthesis in rat calvarial cultures. Endocrinology 1989;124:301–9.

12. Lukert BP, Raisz LG. Glucocorticoid-induced osteoporosis: pathogenesis and management. Ann Intern Med 1990;112:352–64.

13. Pacifici R. Estrogen, cytokines and pathogenesis of postmenopausal osteoporosis. J Bone Miner Res 1996;11:1043–51.

14. Pacifici R. Is there a causal role for IL-1 in postmenopausal bone loss? Calcif Tissue Int 1992; 50:295–9.

15. Tatakis DN. Interleukin-1 and bone metabolism. A review. J Periodontol 1993;64:416–31.

16. Girasole G, Jilka RL, Passeri G, et al. 17b-Estradiol inhibits interleukin-6 production by bone marrow-derived stromal cells and osteoblasts in vitro: a potential mechanism for the antiosteoporotic effect of estrogens. J Clin Invest 1992; 89:883–91.

17. Horowitz MC. Cytokines and estrogen in bone: anti-osteoporotic effects. Science 1993;260: 626–7.

18. McCarthy T, Centrella M, Canalis E. Cortisol inhibits the synthesis of insulin-like growth factor I in skeletal cells. Endocrinology 1990;126: 1569–75.

19. Centrella M, McCarthy T, Canalis E. Transforming growth factor beta is a bifunctional regulator of replication and collagen synthesis in osteoblast-enriched cell cultures from fetal rat bone. J Biol Chem 1987;262:2869–74.

20. Canalis E, Centrella M, McCarthy T. Effects of basic fibroblast growth factor on bone formation in vitro. J Clin Inv 1988;81:1572–7.

21. Canalis E, Centrella M, McCarthy T. Effects of platelet-derived growth factor on bone formation in vitro. J Cell Physiol 1989;140:530–7.

22. Wozney M, Rosen V, Celeste A, et al. Novel regulators of bone formation; molecular clones and activities. Science 1988;242:1528–34.

23. Canalis E, McCarthy T, Centrella M. Growth factors and cytokines in bone cell metabolism. Ann Rev Med 1991;42:17–24.

24. Morrison NA, Qi JC, Tokita A, et al. Prediction of bone density from vitamin D receptor alleles. Nature 1994;367:284–7.

25. Nordin BEC, Morris HA. The calcium deficiency model for osteoporosis. Nutr Rev 1989;47: 65–72.

26. Marcus R. The nature of osteoporosis. J Clin Endocrinol Metab 1995;81(1):1–5.

27. Kanis JA, et al. The diagnosis of osteoporosis. J Bone Miner Res 1994;9(8):1137–41.

28. Conference Report. Consensus Development Conference: diagnosis, prophylaxsis, and treatment of osteoporosis. Am J Med 1993;94:646–50.

29. World Health Organization. Assessment of fracture risk and its application to screening for postmenopusal osteoporosis. Technical Report Series. Geneva: WHO; 1994.

30. Parfitt AM. Trabecular bone architecture in the pathogenesis and prevention of fracture. Am J Med 1987;82:68–72.

31. Eriksen EF. Normal and pathological remodeling of human trabecular bone: threee dimensional reconstruction of the remodeling sequence in normal and in metabolic disease. Endocr Rev 1986;7:379–408.

32. Kribbs PJ, Smith DE, Chesnut CH. Oral findings in osteoporosis. Part II. Relationship between residual ridge and alveolar bone resorption and generalized skeletal osteopenia. J Prosthet Dent 1983;50:719–24.

33. Kribbs PJ, Chesnut CH, Ott SM, Kilcyne RF. Relationships between mandibular and skeletal bone in a population of normal women. J Prosthet Dent 1990;63:86–9.

34. Kribbs PJ, Chesnut CH. Relationships between mandibular and skeletal bone in an osteoporotic population. J Prosthet Dent 1989;62:703–7.

35. Kribbs PJ. Comparison of mandibular bone in normal and osteoporotic women. J Prosthet Dent 1990;63:218–22.

36. von Wowern N, Klausen B, Kollerup G. Osteo-

porosis: a risk factor in periodontal disease. J Periodontol 1994;65:1134–8.

37. Jeffcoat MK, Reddy MS, Magnusson I, et al. Efficacy of quantitative digital subtraction radiography using radiographs exposed in a multicenter trial. J Periodontal Res 1996;31:157–60.

38. Jeffcoat MK, Reddy MS. Alveolar bone loss and osteoporosis: evidence for a common mode of therapy using the bisphonate alendronate. In: Davidovitch Z, editor. The biologic mechanism of tooth resorption and replacement by implants. Boston: Harvard Society for the Advancement of Orthodontics; 1996.

39. Jeffcoat MK, Lewis CE, Reddy MS, et al. Postmenopausal bone loss and its relationship to oral bone loss. Periodontol 2000. [In press]

40. Daniell HW. Postmenopausal tooth loss. Contributions to edentulism by osteoporosis and cigarette smoking. Arch Intern Med 1983;143:1678–82.

41. Taguchi A, Tanimoto K, Suei Y et al. Tooth loss and mandibular osteopenia. Oral Surg Oral Med Oral Pathol Oral Radiol Endod 1995;79: 127–32.

42. Krall EA, Dawson-Hughes B, Papas A, et al. Tooth loss and skeletal bone density in healthy postmenopausal women. Osteoporosis Int 1994;4: 104–9.

43. Krall EA, Garcia RI, Dawson-Hughes B. Increased risk of tooth loss is related to bone loss at the whole body, hip, and spine. Calcif Tissue Int 1996;59:433–7.

44. Hirai T, Ishijima T, Hashikawa Y, et al. Osteoporosis and reduction of residual ridge in edentolous patients. J Prosthet Dent 1993;69:49–56.

45. Wactawski-Wende J, Grossi SG, Trevisan M, et al. The role of osteopenia in periodontal disease. J Periodontol 1996;67:1076–84.

46. Grossi SG, Nishida M, Wactawski-Wende J, et al. Skeletal osteopenia increases the risk for periodontal disease. J Dent Res 1998;77:Abstract #2140.

47. Kanis JA, McCloskey. Risk factors in osteoporosis. Maturitas 1998;30(3):229–33.

48. Ross PD. Risk factors for osteoporotic fracture. Endocrinol Metab Clin North Am 1998;27(2): 289–301.

49. Cumming SR. Treatable and untreatable risk factors for hip fracture. Bone 1996;18(3 Suppl): 165S–167S.

50. Kornman KS, Crane A, Wang H-Y, et al. The interleukin-1 genotype as a severity factor in adult periodontal disease. J Clin Periodontol 1997; 24:72–7.

51. Grossi SG, Zambon JJ, Ho AW, et al. Assessment of risk for periodontal disease. I. Risk indicators for attachment loss. J Periodontol 1994;65:260–7.

52. Tezal M, Grossi SG, Ho AW, Genco RJ. The effcet

53. Genco RJ, Ho AW, Kopman J, et al. Models to evaluate the role of stress in periodontal disease. Ann Periodontol 1998;3(1):288–302.

54. Nishida M, Grossi SG, Dunford RG, et al. Nutrition and risk for periodontal disease. I. Dietary and serum calcium. J Periodontol 1999. [In Press]

55. Nishida M, Grossi SG, Dunford RG, et al. Nutrition and risk for periodontal disease. II .Dietary vitamin C. J Periodontol 1999. [In Press]

56. Utian WH. Biosynthesis and physiologic effects of estrogen and pathophysiologic effects of estrogen deficiency: a review. Am J Obstet Gynecol 1989;161:1828–31.

57. Lindsay R, Aitken J, Anderson J. Long term prevention of postmenopausal osteoporosis by estrogen. Lancet 1976;1:1038–41.

58. Horsman A, Jones M, Francis R. The effect of estrogen dose on postmenopausal bone loss. N Engl J Med 1983;309:1404–7.

59. Pacifici R, Brown C, Puscheck E, et al. Effect of surgical menopause and estrogen replacement on cytokine release from human blood mononuclear cells. Proc Natl Acad Sci U S A 1991;88: 5134–8.

60. Cohen-Solal ME, Graulet AM, Denne MA, et al. Peripheral monocyte culture supernatants of menopausal women can induce bone resorption: involvement of cytokines. J Clin Endocrinol Metab 1993;77:1648–53.

61. Horowitz MC. Cytokines and estrogen in bone: antiosteoporotic effects. Science 1993;260:626–7.

62. Norderyd OM, Grossi SG, Machtei EE, et al. Periodontal status of women taking postmenopausal estrogen supplementation. J Periodontol 1993;64:957–62.

63. Jacobs R, Ghyselen J, Koninckx P, van Steenberghe D. Long term bone mass evaluation of mandible and lumbar spine in a group of women receiving hormone replacement therapy. Eur J Oral Sci 1996;104:10–6.

64. Payne JB, Zachs NR, Reinhardt RA, et al. The association between estrogen status and alveolar bone density changes in postmenopausal women with a history of periodontitis. J Periodontol 1997;68:24–31.

65. Law MR, Hackshaw AK. A meta-analysis of cigarette smoking, bone mineral density and risk of hip fracture: recognition of a major effect. BMJ 1997;315:841–6.

66. Kiel DP, Zhang Y, Hannan MT, et al. The effect of smoking at different life stages on bone mineral density in elderly men and women. Osteoporosis Int 1996;6:240–8.

67. Krall EA, Dawson-Hughes B. Smoking increases

bone loss and decreases intestinal calcium absorption. J Bone Miner Res 1999;14(2):215–20.

68. Papapanou PN. Periodontal diseases; epidemiology. Ann Periodontol 1996;1:1–36.

69. Grossi, SG, Genco RJ, Machtei EE, et al. Assessment of risk for periodontal disease. II. Risk indicators for alveolar bone loss. J Periodontol 1995;66:23–9.

70. El-Ghorab N, Grossi SG, Dunford R, et al. Effect of smoking and estrogen supplementation on interproximal alveolar bone loss in women. J Dent Res 1996;75:Abstract 244.

71. Ferreira C, Grossi SG, Ho AW, et al. Tooth loss in women: relationship to estrogen supplementation and smoking. J Dent Res 1996:75:Abstract 245.

72. Eisman JA. Genetics, calcium intake and osteoporosis. Proc Nutr Soc 1998;57(2):187–93.

73. Faine MP. Dietary factors related to preservation of oral and skeletal bone mass in women. J Prosthet Dent 1995;73(1):65–72.

74. National Institutes of Health. Consensus Development Conference. JAMA 1984;252:799–802.

75. Fehily AM, Coles RJ, William DE, Elwood PC. Factors affecting bone density in young adults. Am J Clin Nutr 1992;56:579–86.

76. Mazess RB, Barden HS. Bone density in premenopausal women: effect of age, dietary intake, physical activity, smoking and birth control pills. Am J Clin Nutr 1991;53:132–42.

77. Yoshida H, Nagaya T, Hayashi T, et al. Milk consumption decreases activity of human serum alkaline phosphatase: a cross-sectional study. Metab Clin Exp 1995;44(9):1190–3.

78. Heaney RP, Recker RR. Effects of nitrogen, phosphorus and caffeine on calcium balance in women. J Lab Clin Med 1982;99:46–55.

79. Arjmandi BH, Birnbaum R, Goyal NV, et al. Bone sparing effect of soy protein in ovarian hormone-deficient rats is related to its isoflavone content. Am J Clin Nutr 1998;68(6 Suppl):1364S–8S.

80. Pocock N, Eisman J, Mazess R. Genetic determinants of bone mass in adults: a twin study. J Clin Invest 1987;80:706–10.

81. Sainz J, Van Tornout JM, Loro ML, et al. Vitamin-D receptor gene polymorphisms and bone density in prepubertal American girls of Mexican descent. N Engl J Med 1997;337:77–82.

82. Langdahl BL, Ralston SH, Grant SF, Erikson EF. An Sp1 binding site polymorphism in the COLIA1 gene predicts osteoporotic fractures in both men and women. J Bone Miner Res 1998;13(9):1384–9.

83. Hampson G, et al. Bone mineral density, collagen type 1 alpha 1 genotypes and bone turnover in premenopausal women with diabetes mellitus. Diabetologia 1998;41(11):1314–20.

84. Yamada Y, Miyauchi A, Goto J, et al. Association of polymorphism of the transforming growth factor beta 1 gene with genetic susceptibility to osteoporosis in postmenopausal Japanese women. J Bone Miner Res 1998;13(10);1569–76.

85. Grant SFA, Ralston SH. Genes and osteoporosis. Trends Endocrinol Metab 1997;8:232–6.

86. Wood RJ, Fleet JC. The genetics of osteoporosis: vitamin D receptor. Ann Rev Nutr 1998;18:223–58.

87. Michalowicz BS. Genetic and heritable risk factors in periodontal disease. J Periodontol 1994;65:479–88.

88. McGuire MK, Nunn ME. Prognosis vs. actual outcome. IV. The effectiveness of clinical parameters and IL-1 genotype in accurately predicting prognoses and tooth survival. J Periodontol 1999;70:49–56.

89. Krall EA, Garcia RI, Dawson-Hughes B. Increased risk of tooth loss is related to bone loss at the whole body, hip and spine. Calcif Tissue Int 1996;59:433–7.

90. Christiansen C, Christensen MS, Transbol I. Bone mass in postmenopausal women after withdrawal of oestrogen/gestagen replacement therapy. Lancet 1981;i:459–61.

91. Ettinger B, Genant HK, Cann C. Long-term estrogen replacement therapy prevents bone loss and fractures. Ann Intern Med 1985;102:319–24.

92. Felson DT, Zhang Y, Hannan MT, et al. The effect of postmenopausal estrogen therapy on bone density in elderly women. N Engl J Med 1993;329:1141–46.

93. Lindsay R. Estrogens, bone mass and osteoporotic fracture. Am J Med 1991;91:10S–13S.

94. Naessen T, Persson I, Adami HO, et al. Hormone replacement therapy and the risk for first hip fracture. A prospective, population-based cohort study. Ann Intern Med 1990;113:95–103.

95. Grodstein F, Colditz G, Stampfer G. Postmenopausal homone use and tooth loss: a prospective study. J Am Dent Assoc 1996;127:370–7.

96. Paganini-Hill A. Benefits of estrogen replacement therapy on oral health: the leisure world cohort. Arch Intern Med 1995;155:2325–9.

97. Krall E, Dawson-Hughes B, Hannan M, et al. Postmenopausal estrogen replacement and tooth retention. Am J Med 1997;102:536–42.

98. Papapoulos SE. Bisphosphonates. Pharmacology and use in the treatment of osteoporosis. In Marcus RE, Feldman D, Kelsey J, editors. Osteoporosis. San Diego: Academic Press; 1996.

CHAPTER 11

HIV INFECTION AND PERIODONTAL DISEASES

Michael Glick, DMD

Palle Holmstrup, PhD, Dr. Odont

The human immunodeficiency virus (HIV) epidemic is not abating. By the end of 1998, an estimated 34 million individuals worldwide were infected. Eleven men, women, and children, half of these aged 15 to 24 years, acquire a new infection every minute. Approximately four people succumb to this disease every minute. Although the death rate from HIV infection has slowed down in the United States and Western Europe due to new and improved therapies, 75,000 new infections are still recorded annually.[1] This changing face of the epidemic suggests an increasing number of people living with HIV disease requiring health services. As with all chronic diseases, a multidisciplinary approach to care results in improved quality of life and decreased morbidity and mortality. This chapter focuses on oral lesions and conditions affecting the periodontium that are found in individuals with HIV infection and also explores the possible connection between the propagation of periodontal infection and the propagation of HIV infection.

As periodontal manifestations have shown to be markers for immune deterioration and HIV disease progression, early recognition of these lesions and an understanding of their significance in the course of HIV disease will impact on the overall systemic care for infected individuals. New insights into the pathogenesis of HIV infection have revealed much about the fate of, as well as the immune response to, the virus. Until recently, it was generally believed that HIV was constantly replicating, notwithstanding clinical asymptomatic periods. Therapeutic interventions focused on slowing down the replication rate as well as the transcription of viral proteins. However, new research has discovered the existence of latently infected CD4+ T cells.[2,3] This phenomenon poses a significant problem both for an effective immune response and for drug therapy.

The body's natural immune system cannot detect and eliminate cells latently infected with HIV, as these cells lack the expression of viral antigens on the cell surface. Furthermore, as the proviral DNA is already integrated into the cellular genome, it cannot be targeted by existing antiretroviral medications which inhibit the RNA reverse transcriptase of HIV. Therefore, elimination of HIV can only be accomplished by activating latently infected cells in combination with potent antiretroviral therapy. This will create a situation where latently infected cells are induced into a state of productive infection and die, while the antiretroviral therapy prevents infectious viruses released from these cells from infecting new cells.

Another concern for infected individuals is the state of their debilitated immune system. Thus, in concert with targeting infected cells, immune reconstitution also needs to be addressed. The hallmark of HIV disease is the infection and subsequent depletion of CD4+ T cells. After successful institution of antiretroviral therapy, a sharp rise of CD4+ T cells can be noticed.[4] However, this increase apparently occurs as a result of the redistribution of memory cells. These T cells are severely limited in their ability to recognize different antigens. The appearance of naïve CD4+ T cells, with specificities that had previously been lost, may occur only after several months. Thus, the immunologic repertoire during the course of HIV disease predisposes to increased susceptibility to opportunistic infections. The level of immune deterioration or reconstitution determines the individual's susceptibility to specific infections. The influence of periodontal infection on the pathogenesis of HIV disease has not been elucidated. However, the immune system weakened by HIV may have a direct influence on the pathogenesis of periodontal disease.

Individuals infected with HIV exhibit oral conditions and lesions often associated with immune suppression.[5] These oral manifestations may reflect systemic conditions or could complicate systemic disease. Among HIV-infected individuals, no oral lesions are found that are directly caused by HIV. Instead, lesions are mostly associated with immune suppression and opportunistic pathogens and can therefore be found among other immunosuppressed individuals as well. For a lesion to be classified as "HIV-associated," the lesion needs to be more common or exhibit a different clinical course and appearance than those in individuals not infected with HIV.

A multitude of lesions that affect the periodontium have been described. Moreover, aggressive periodontal lesions may be the first clinical expression of the HIV infection.[5–11] Bacterial, viral, fungal, or parasitic infections can all affect the course of HIV disease as well as take on different clinical manifestations and severity or require different treatment modalities than in non-HIV-infected individuals. Due to the impaired immune system characteristic of HIV disease, infections often present a more serious course compared with immunocompetent individuals. This is also found with infections of the periodontal tissues. Comparative studies attempting to assess the association of periodontal disease entities with HIV infection are often limited by several factors. They include the lack of specific diagnostic criteria, the use of various HIV treatment regimens, and lack of information on the immune status of the HIV-infected individual. An additional problem is biased study populations, frequently selected on the basis of institutional affiliation. This means that usually the groups of HIV-infected subjects under investigation are more seriously affected by HIV disease than the entire group of HIV-infected individuals.

TERMINOLOGY

A wide spectrum of terms have been used to describe soft and hard tissue inflammatory and/or destructive conditions of the periodontium, presumably associated with HIV infection.[12–14] An internationally accepted classification of the oral manifestations of HIV infection and their diagnostic criteria has been established by the EC-Clearinghouse on Oral Problems Related to HIV Infection and the WHO Collaborating Centre on Oral Manifestations of the Immunodeficiency Virus (EC-WHO) at a meeting in 1993.[15]

The classification includes three groups of lesions (Table 11–1): (1) lesions strongly associated with HIV infection, (2) lesions less commonly associated with HIV infection, and (3) lesions seen in HIV infection.[15] Most characteristic among the lesions listed in the latter category are the types of infection which are extremely rare in noninfected individuals. These include *Histoplasma capsulatum* and fungal infections other than candidiasis. Although a number of these diseases may affect the periodontal tissues, they are outside the scope of the present chapter. However, conventional forms of periodontal diseases affect HIV-infected individuals but may differ in their clinical course. This aspect will be discussed below in the section "lesions seen in HIV infection."

LESIONS STRONGLY ASSOCIATED WITH HIV INFECTION

Three periodontal disease entities can be considered to be strongly associated with HIV infection. These are linear gingival erythema (LGE), necrotizing gingivitis (NG) or necrotizing ulcerative gingivitis (NUG), and necrotizing periodontitis (NP) or necrotizing ulcerative periodontitis (NUP).[15] It is important to note that similar lesions may occur in non-HIV-infected individuals[16–18] even with similar prevalence.[19–23] Consequently, although the initial descriptions of these lesions referred to them as HIV-associated gingivitis and HIV-associated periodontitis, the more descriptive terminology of the lesions is used today. In the list of lesions strongly associated with HIV (Table 11–1), a few supplementary disease entities that may also affect the periodontium are included. These entities are candidiasis, Kaposi's sarcoma, and non-Hodgkin's lymphoma.

Linear Gingival Erythema

Diagnosis and Clinical Presentation
Linear gingival erythema presents as a fiery red band of the marginal gingiva, characterized by a disproportional inflammatory intensity in relation to the amount of plaque present. There are no ulcerations and no evidence of pocketing or attachment loss. A further characteristic of this type of lesion is its lack of response to improved oral hygiene and to scaling.[15]

The first description of LGE included a distinctive erythema of the free gingiva, attached gingiva, and alveolar mucosa in individuals with HIV

TABLE 11–1. Revised Classification of Oral Lesions Associated with HIV Infection

Group 1: Lesions strongly associated with HIV infection
    Candidiasis
        Erythematous
        Pseudomembranous
    Hairy leukoplakia
    Kaposi's sarcoma
    Non-Hodgkin's lymphoma
    Periodontal disease
        Linear gingival erythema
        Necrotizing (ulcerative) gingivitis
        Necrotizing (ulcerative) periodontitis

Group 2: Lesions less commonly associated with HIV infection
    Bacterial infections
        Mycobacterium avium-intracellulare
        Mycobacterium tuberculosis
    Melanotic hyperpigmentation
    Necrotizing (ulcerative) stomatitis
    Salivary gland disease
        Dry mouth due to decreased salivary flow rate
        Unilateral or bilateral swelling of major salivary glands
    Thrombocytopenic purpura
    Ulceration NOS (not otherwise specified)
    Viral infections
        Herpes simplex virus
        Human papillomavirus (warty-like lesions)
          Condyloma acuminatum
          Focal epithelial hyperplasia
          Verruca vulgaris
        Varicella-zoster virus
          Herpes zoster
          Varicella

Group 3: Lesions seen in HIV infection
    Bacterial infections
        Actinomyces israelii
        Escherichia coli
        Klebsiella pneumoniae
    Cat-scratch disease
    Drug reactions (ulcerative, erythema, multiforme, lichenoid, toxic epidermolysis)
    Epithelioid (bacillary) angiomatosis
    Fungal infection other than candidiasis
        Cryptococcus neoformans
        Geotrichum candidum
        Histoplasma capsulatum
        Mucoraceae (Mucormycosis/zygomycosis)
        Asperigillus flavus
    Neurologic disturbances
        Facial palsy
        Trigeminal neuralgia
    Recurrent aphthous stomatitis
    Viral infections
        Cytomegalovirus
        Molluscum contagiosum

With permission from EC-Clearinghouse on Oral Problems Related to HIV Infection and WHO Collaborating Centre on Oral Manifestations of the Immunodeficiency Virus. Classification and diagnostic criteria for oral lesions in HIV infection. J Oral Pathol Med 1993;22:289–91.

disease.[24] Free gingival erythema, appearing as an intense linear band extending 2 to 3 mm apically from the free gingival margin was seen in more than 50% of cases. Punctate or diffuse erythema of the attached gingiva was another prominent feature. The lesions were associated with pain in some instances and most frequently involved the entire mouth with an equal distribution to all quadrants. Sometimes they were limited to one or two teeth, and the changes were present even with little or no plaque accumulations. The extent of gingival banding measured by the number of affected sites was later suggested to depend on tobacco usage.[25] While 15% of affected sites were originally reported to bleed on probing and 11% exhibited spontaneous bleeding,[24] a key feature of linear gingival erythema is now considered to be lack of bleeding on probing.[14]

Prevalence

A few studies of unbiased groups of patients have indicated that gingivitis with bank-shaped or punctate marginal erythema may be relatively rare in HIV-infected patients and probably represents a clinical finding which is not more frequent than in the general population.[20,21] Other studies of various groups of HIV-infected patients have revealed the prevalence of gingivitis with band-shaped patterns in 0.5 to 49%.[25–29] These prevalence values reflect some of the problems with non-standardized diagnosis and selection of study groups as mentioned above. There is no doubt that several studies comprise cohorts of patients with poor oral hygiene,[26,27] and the degree to which the reported inflammatory processes respond to conventional therapy is currently unknown. A preponderance of HIV-associated red banding was not noted in a recent British study, while diffuse and punctate erythema was significantly more prevalent in HIV-infected than in non-HIV-infected individuals.[23] Red gingival banding as a clinical feature alone is, therefore, not strongly associated with HIV infection.

While several studies are available on HIV-infected adults, few reports describe HIV-related diseases among children. In two studies, however, as many as 30% and 37%, respectively, were diagnosed with so-called HIV-gingivitis, which is synonymous with LGE.[30,31]

Etiology and Pathogenesis

There are suggestions that candidal infection is the etiologic agent in some cases of gingival inflammation, including LGE.[23,24,32] However, some studies have revealed microflora comprising both *Candida albicans* and a number of periodontopathic bacteria consistent with those seen in conventional periodontitis, that is, *Porphyromonas gingivalis, Prevotella intermedia, Actinobacillus actinomycetemcomitans, Fusobacterium nucleatum,* and *Campylobacter rectus.*[33,34] Studies using DNA probes have suggested the percentage of *A. actinomycetemcomitans*-positive sites in HIV-associated gingivitis and matched gingivitis sites of HIV-seronegative patients to be 23% and 7%, respectively. Furthermore, positive sites were 52% and 17% for *P. gingivalis*, 63% and 29% for *P. intermedia*, and 50% and 14% for *C. rectus*, respectively.[33,34] *C. albicans* has been isolated by culture in about 50% of HIV-associated gingivitis sites, in 26% of unaffected sites of HIV-seropositive patients, and in 3% of healthy sites of HIV-seronegative patients. The frequent isolation and the pathogenic role of *C. albicans* may be related to the high levels of the yeast in the saliva and oral mucosa of HIV-infected patients.[35]

The significance of CD4+ T cell depletion in the pathogenesis of LGE is uncertain. A study of 25 patients with so-called HIV-associated gingivitis showed CD4/CD8 ratios within the low normal range.[24] In another study of the red banding of the gingiva, it was concluded that the condition was not related to immunosuppression, as equal number of cases had CD4+ T cell counts above and below 400/mm^3.[19] A similar result has been obtained by others.[25] However, a more recent study comprising 396 HIV-seropositive individuals classified according to their peripheral CD4+ lymphocyte counts revealed linear gingival erythema in 2 patients with less than 200 CD4 cells/mm^3 as opposed to none among patients with 200 CD4 cells/mm^3 or more.[6]

An interesting histopathologic finding in biopsy specimens from the banding zone has revealed no inflammatory infiltrate but an increased number of blood vessels, which explains the red color of the lesions.[36] The incomplete inflammatory reaction of the host tissue may be the cause of the lack of response to conventional treatment.

Differential Diagnosis

A number of diseases present clinical features resembling those described above and which, accordingly, do not resolve after improved oral hygiene and débridement. Oral lichen planus is frequently associated with a similar inflammatory red band of the attached gingiva,[37] and mucous membrane pemphigoid may also have this appearance.[38] *Geotrichum candidum* infection[39] and hypersensitivity reactions manifesting as plasma cell gingivitis[40] are other rare differential diagnoses. In rare instances, gingivitis-like changes may also be the result of thrombocytopenia.[41]

Treatment

Important characteristics of the originally described entity of LGE included a temporal lack of response to plaque removal and an erythematous appearance disproportional to the amount of plaque. Reports of different therapeutic results may be due to the varied definition of LGE. Conventional therapy with 0.12% chlorhexidine gluconate mouth rinses twice daily has been reported to show significant improvement after 3 months.[42] However, HIV-associated free gingival erythema did not respond to removal of plaque by intense scaling and root planing and improved plaque control measures, alone or supplemented with povidone-iodine irrigation 3 to 5 times daily. There was no significant improvement in clinical features or indices after 1 and 3 months of treatment. However, the povidone-iodine irrigation substantially reduced pain reported to be associated with the lesions examined.[11]

As mentioned above, LGE may in some cases be related to the presence of *C. albicans*. In accordance with this finding, clinical observations indicate that improvement is frequently dependent on successful eradication of intraoral *C. albicans*, which results in the disappearance of the characteristic features.[24] Consequently, attempts to identify the presence of fungal infection either by culture or smear are recommended, followed by antimycotic therapy in *C. albicans*-positive cases.

Necrotizing (Ulcerative) Gingivitis and Periodontitis

Diagnosis and Clinical Presentation

The necrotizing (ulcerative) diseases NG, NP, and necrotizing stomatis (NS) are the most severe periodontal disorders, presumably caused by bacteria. These entities may represent various stages of similar disease process.[43] The distinction between NG and periodontitis is parallel to the distinction between gingivitis and periodontitis. Thus, NG should be limited to lesions only involving gingival tissue with no loss of periodontal attachment.[29] In most patients, however, the disease process rapidly results in loss of attachment, in which case NP is the correct terminology. Previously, progression of the disease process across the

mucogingival junction would have qualified for the diagnosis of NS,[41] but the description of NP as proposed by EC-WHO incorporates tissue destruction extending across the mucogingival border. Consequently, the differential diagnosis between NP and NS is not always clear, as NS is sometimes described as extending from areas of NP.[15] Necrotizing stomatitis is mentioned below in the section on "lesions less commonly associated with HIV infection."

There is considerable variation in the clinical manifestations ranging from initial lesions with necrosis limited to the top of the interdental papillae, to moderate manifestations with involvement of the entire attached gingiva with tooth mobility and sequestration of parts of the crestal bone, to severe cases with extensive bone loss and necrosis of supporting tissues. Fetor oris evolves in most cases as a characteristic feature.

The initial lesion typically presents with changes in gingival contour, such as interproximal necrosis, ulceration, and cratering. The most distinguishing feature is soft tissue necrosis and the rapid destruction of periodontal attachment and bone. Severe cases can affect all teeth, but more frequently, several localized areas are affected independently, and all regions appear to have similar chances of being affected. The lesions are not always associated with deep pocket formation, as extensive gingival necrosis often coincides with loss of crestal alveolar bone. On the other hand, the rapid progression of the soft tissue necrosis sometimes leads to the exposure of the alveolar bone, which becomes sequestrated and leaves deep interdental craters.[23] Frequently, such defects are located in the molar/premolar region.

Severe pain has been mentioned as a distinguishing feature of HIV-associated periodontitis[15,23,41,44] and the chief reason for patients seeking treatment. Bleeding on probing is a prominent feature, and about 50% of involved sites bleed spontaneously.[23] The number of sites affected by papillary destruction have been shown to be significantly determined by tobacco usage.[25] About 85% of individuals with HIV-associated periodontitis lesions have been described to be aware of their serostatus at their initial visit.[23]

Prevalence

Meaningful comparisons of prevalence data among the available studies remain unavailable because of the diversity in the study methods and diagnostic criteria and the variance in groups under investigation. One major problem is the lack of a clear distinction between NG and NP in the majority of the literature. However, even taking these limitations into account, studies show that NG is more common among HIV-seropositive individuals than in the general population. The prevalence in these studies ranges from 5 to 11%.[8,19,27,45–47] In contrast, other more recent studies have either found low prevalence (0 to 0.7%)[23,29,48] or no significant difference between cohorts of HIV-seropositive and HIV-negative patients.[22] The anterior gingiva is most commonly affected,[44] which agrees with NG in HIV-seronegative patients.[49] Gingival ulceration may affect individual teeth or extend to several areas of the jaws.[8]

Necrotizing periodontitis has been described in 88% among 136 HIV-infected patients.[28] However, most studies have shown considerably lower prevalence values of NP among HIV-infected individuals, such as 6.3% of 700 HIV-seropositive patients[50] and in 1% of 200 HIV-seropositive patients.[29] Yet, other studies have suggested that HIV-associated periodontitis with ulceration and tissue necrosis may be relatively rare and that the prevalence may, in fact, not differ significantly from that of similar lesions of the general population.[17–21]

Etiology and Pathogenesis

Established knowledge of the pathogenic background of tissue necrosis in NG and NP is limited. One of the most interesting questions is whether less pathogenic organisms can cause tissue necrosis in HIV-infected as compared with non-HIV-infected individuals. Data on the microflora associated with necrotic periodontal lesions are unfortunately compromised by frequent lack of precise description of the sites from which the microbiologic samples were obtained. There is no doubt that many samples are obtained from deep pockets, and consequently, the findings may not be directly related to tissue necrosis. No clear distinction can therefore be drawn between NP and other forms of HIV-associated periodontitis in the description of the microbiologic profile. A further complication is that the available information on the microbiology of HIV-associated NG is very limited. The isolated organisms include *Borrelia*, gram-positive cocci, β-hemolytic streptococci, and *C. albicans*.[8]

The occurrence of *P. gingivalis*, spirochetes, and motile eubacteria in periodonitis has been found to be the same in HIV-infected patients and in systemically healthy adults.[51] Also, the microflora isolated from HIV-associated periodontitis was similar to that of classic adult periodontitis, except

that *P. gingivalis* was more prevalent in conventional periodontitis.[33,34,52] Greater numbers of *P. gingivalis* have been revealed in samples from non-HIV-infected subjects with healthy periodontium than in samples from HIV-associated periodontitis.[51] Other findings have indicated that subgingival plaque in acquired immunodeficiency syndrome (AIDS) patients with periodontitis can harbor high proportions of the same periodontal pathogens as are associated with periodontitis in non-HIV-infected individuals, but additional high proportions of other opportunistic pathogens like *Clostridium*, *Enterococcus*, and *C. albicans*.[52] The suggestion that the predominant subgingival microflora in HIV-associated periodontitis is in many ways similar to that of progressing periodontitis lesions in systemically healthy adults has been supported by others.[53] On the other hand, this investigation of HIV-associated periodontitis lesions also revealed organisms rarely associated with common types of periodontitis. Higher proportions of *C. albicans* and *C. rectus* were characteristic of HIV-associated periodontitis, the qualitative profiles of HIV-associated gingivitis and HIV-associated periodontitis being similar and only *C. rectus* showing major quantitative differences. None of the available studies answer the important question whether other pathogens cause tissue breakdown in HIV-associated disease unlike in non-HIV associated disease. Necrotizing gingivitis has been associated with peripheral CD4+ lymphocyte depletion in a few studies.[6,47] However, the disease has also been found to be unrelated to immunosuppression, with equal numbers of patients having CD4+ T cell counts above and below 400/mm³.[19]

The severity of periodontal destruction has been associated with the progression of HIV disease in several studies.[20,21,24,25,28,50,54–56] The cause mentioned in these studies is that the progressive depletion of immune effector and regulatory cells in HIV-seropositive patients compromises the local host defense to such an extent that the susceptibility to periodontal disease increases. One study even suggested that NP was a stronger predicator of HIV disease progression and immune suppression than established AIDS defining illnesses.[50] A temporal relationship between NP and poor survival was also suggested, where almost 60% of patients with NP died within 18 months of the periodontal diagnosis. However, other studies have indicated that the association between HIV-related immune depletion and periodontal destruction is less strong.[57–59]

Differential Diagnosis

A number of oral mucosal diseases can be confused with NG and NP. These include bullous lesions of benign mucous membrane pemphigoid and erythema multiforme exudativum, but the progressive nature and the localized occurrence of NG and NP usually distinguish these diseases from bullous mucosal diseases. Acute forms of leukemia may be associated with necrotizing gingival ulcers of the oral mucosa, which sometimes manifest in the marginal gingiva.[17,18] The gingival lesions are often bluish red and edematous. Medical examination will reveal the cause in suspect cases. Since serologic/hematologic examination usually is necessary for patients unaware of a possible HIV infection or another cause of the necrotizing periodontal disease, a possible supplementary blood examination to look for leukemia is justifiable.

Treatment

The treatment aspects of NG and NP are similar. In HIV-infected patients, the diseases do not routinely respond to conventional treatment with scaling and improved oral hygiene.[24] However, the adjunctive use of metronidazole in these patients is reported to be extremely effective in reducing acute pain and promoting rapid healing.[50,60] Due to the susceptibility of HIV-infected patients to candidal infections,[61] simultaneous treatment with appropriate antimycotic agents may be necessary. Although it has been postulated that healing is delayed in HIV-infected patients and pain may be prolonged,[8] other studies did not reveal increased incidence of delayed healing after extraction or other complications even in severely immunocompromised individuals. Therefore, prophylactic antimicrobials were not recommended.[62,63] Frequent use of antibiotics may give rise to problems due to microbial resistance; hence a restrictive attitude is important.

Follow-up care for HIV-associated necrotizing periodontal diseases is essential to ensure success in treatment. Inadequate plaque control in sites affected by NP is often associated with delayed healing and continued rapid destruction.[11] In many cases, extensive tissue destruction results in residual defects, which may make it very difficult for the patient to maintain oral hygiene. Oral hygiene in these areas often requires the use of interproximal devices and soft, smaller brushes. Antibiotic prophylaxis may not be necessary in relation to scaling, since bacteria were recovered from venipuncture 15 minutes after scaling but

were not detectable in samples obtained at 30 minutes.[64] Removal of sequestra does not always appear to require antibiotic coverage.[65]

LESIONS LESS COMMONLY ASSOCIATED WITH HIV INFECTION

A number of lesions less commonly associated with HIV infection may affect the periodontal tissues. Necrotizing stomatitis is among the most serious, but other important diseases are lesions caused by herpes simplex virus, human papilloma virus, and varicella-zoster virus. These lesions, however, are not included in this chapter.

Necrotizing Stomatitis

Necrotizing stomatitis (NS) is defined as a localized, acutely painful ulceronecrotic lesion of the oral mucosa, exposing underlying bone or penetrating or extending into contiguous tissues. The lesions may extend from areas of NP.[15]

Diagnosis and Clinical Presentation

The clinical aspects of NS resemble those of NG and NP. Necrotizing stomatitis is the most severe and is not as common as NG and NP.[5] The extensively destructive lesions are rapidly progressive, ulcerative, and necrotizing. In most cases, the lesions extend from the gingiva into the adjacent mucosa and bone, causing destruction of both oral soft tissues and underlying bone. The disease appears to be related to the immune depletion caused by HIV infection.[66] Importantly, it may be life threatening,[67] and the clinical features of NS resemble noma as described by Tempest.[68] Progression of NP to NS may result in progressive osseous destruction,[69] with sequestration and/or the development of oroantral fistula and osteitis.[70] The differential diagnostic and treatment aspects for NS are similar to those of NG and NP.[67]

LESIONS SEEN IN HIV INFECTION

Individuals infected by HIV may suffer from common forms of periodontal diseases without tissue necrosis or other characteristic features of HIV infection as described above. These diseases with less dramatic clinical features include adult periodontitis[20,21] and rapidly progressive periodontitis.[8] The most interesting aspect of these diseases in HIV-infected populations is whether their prevalence figures and progression of attachment loss are similar to those encountered in non-HIV-infected individuals.

Conventional Adult Periodontitis/ Rapidly Progressive Periodontitis

Prevalence

A number of studies among HIV-seropositive individuals have reported high prevalence figures of severe attachment loss, but others have failed to show differences between HIV-seropositive and HIV-seronegative individuals.[32] The reported prevalence figures of periodontitis among HIV-seropositive patients show considerable variation (5 to 69%), the variation being due to differences in study groups. For instance, several studies comprise groups of patients who are selected on the basis of admission to hospitals or to the dental setting, but it is not possible to identify mechanisms of selection in all referred studies.

Severe periodontal destruction was revealed in 11% of 44 HIV-seropositive patients[45] and progressive periodontitis comparable with rapidly progressive periodontitis[71] was diagnosed with similar frequency among 110 HIV-seropositive patients.[8] Twenty-seven percent of 200 HIV-seropositive patients had moderate or advanced adult periodontitis.[29] In a study of 181 heterosexual men and women with AIDS, 92% of the patients being intravenous drug users, the prevalence was much higher than in other studies. The clinical features were not reported in detail, and figures for patients without tissue necrosis could not be identified. Early periodontitis was found in 24%, moderate in 23%, and advanced in 22%. Significantly increased severity of periodontitis was seen in women as compared with men.[26]

A number of studies have shown limited prevalence figures. Among 141 HIV-seropositive homosexual males, 5% had severe periodontitis as compared with 0.2% among 606 seronegative homosexual males. The reported prevalence was markedly lower than that reported for severe periodontitis in adult males in the United States. No radiographic examination was available.[22] Studies based on the registration of periodontal indices have shown that loss of attachment associated with HIV infection is a relatively rare condition, at least in some cohorts of patients.[20,21] One of the most recent studies revealed no significant differences in bleeding on probing, pocket formation, or attachment loss among HIV-seronegative and HIV-seropositive individuals and AIDS patients in Tan-

zania.[52] However, when using clinical attachment loss and radiographic assessment of alveolar bone loss, definite trends are evident pointing to HIV infection being a risk indicator for progression of periodontitis.[32]

Etiology and Pathogenesis

Reports of the microbiology of HIV-associated periodontitis do not always state whether microbial samples have been obtained from lesions with or without necrosis. The available microbiologic data are described above in relation to NG and NP.

The reports on the significance of HIV-related immune deterioration and loss of attachment are conflicting. However, most studies have revealed an association between progression of periodontitis and decreased number of peripheral T-helper cells. One study has shown that periodontitis in patients with more advanced stages of HIV infection was related to severity of systemic disease and to decreasing numbers of CD4+ lymphocytes but not to visible plaque index or occurrence of periodontal pathogenic microorganisms.[54] A 20-month follow-up study of 114 homosexual and bisexual men showed relative attachment loss of 3 mm or more occurring 6.16 times more frequently among subjects with CD4+ counts < 200 compared with subjects with counts of 200 or more. Among individuals aged 35 years and over, the incidence (33%) of relative attachment loss of 3 mm or more was significantly higher in more immunosuppressed individuals compared with the incidence (5%) in less immunosuppressed subjects. In 78 individuals seen at follow-up visits, mean gingival indices increased and were significantly higher in the seropositive subjects compared with the seronegative ones, but gingival indices were not related to CD4+ T cell counts within the seropositive group. The study suggested a greater sensitivity to plaque in the seropositive group. The authors concluded that immunosuppression, especially in combination with older age, may be a risk for attachment loss, and HIV seropositivity, independent of CD4+ T cell counts, may be a risk factor for gingival inflammation.[19] In a study of 29 HIV-seropositive patients and 27 control patients, the HIV-seropositive patients had a higher mean percent of sites exhibiting suppuration than the control group.[59] Among 312 men with HIV infection, decreased CD4 lymphocyte counts predicted the extent and severity of periodontal attachment loss but not pocketing, which was only related to HIV infection when compared with 260 men without HIV.[22] In contrast, a recent report from Tanzania did not reveal any significant associations between periodontal indicies with regard to lymphocyte and CD4+ T cell counts among the HIV-infected individuals including AIDS patients.[58]

Treatment

Since deterioration of the immune deficiency may be a risk factor for attachment loss, and HIV-seropositivity may be a risk factor for gingival inflammation, it is particularly important that HIV-infected individuals practice intensive oral hygiene and receive frequent professional preventive dental treatment.[19] This supports the idea of providing intensive oral care programs to be initiated as soon as the diagnosis of HIV infection is established.

REFERENCES

1. WHO End of year annual report on HIV and AIDS. Geneva: WHO; 1998.
2. Chun TW, Stuyer L, Mizell SB, et al. Presence of inducible HIV-1 latent reservoir during highly active antiretroviral therapy. Proc Natl Acad Sci 1997;94:13193–7.
3. Finzi D, Hermankova M, Peirson T, et al. Identification of a reservoir for HIV-1 in patients on highly active antiretroviral therapy. Science 1997;278:1295–300.
4. Leandersson AC, Bratt G, Fredrikson M, et al. Specific T-cell responses in HIV-infected patients after highly active antiretroviral therapy (HAART). Abstract 31142. Geneva: 12th World AIDS Conference; 1998.
5. Glick M, Muzyka BC, Lurie D, Salkin LM. Oral manifestations associated with HIV disease as markers for immune suppression and AIDS. Oral Surg Oral Med Oral Pathol 1994;77:344–9.
6. Ceballos-Salobrena A, Aguirre-Urizar JM, Bagan-Sebastian JV. Oral manifestations associated with human immunodeficiency virus infection in a Spanish population. J Oral Pathol Med 1996;25:523–6.
7. Ficarra G, Berson AM, Silverman S, et al. Kaposi's sarcoma of the oral cavity: a study of 134 patients with a review of the pathogenesis, epidemiology, clinical aspects and treatment. Oral Surg Oral Med Oral Pathol 1988;66:543–50.
8. Reichart PA, Gelderblom HR, Becker J, Kuntz A. AIDS and the oral cavity. The HIV-infection: virology, etiology, origin, immunology, precautions and clinical observations in 110 patients. Int J Oral Maxillofac Surg 1987;16:129–53.
9. Schiøt M, Pindborg JJ. AIDS and the oral cavity. Epidemiology and clinical oral manifestations of human immune deficiency virus infection: a review. Int J Oral Maxillofac Surg 1987;16:1–14.
10. Scully C, Laskaris G, Pindborg JJ, et al. Oral manifestations of HIV infection and their management. I. More common lesions. Oral Surg Oral Med Oral Pathol 1991;71:158–66.
11. Winkler JR, Robertson PB. Periodontal disease associated with HIV-infection. Oral Surg Oral Med Oral Pathol 1992;73:145–50.
12. Holmstrup P, Westergaard J. Periodontal diseases in HIV-infected patients. J Clin Periodontol 1994;21:270–80.
13. Holmstrup P, Westergaard J. HIV infection and periodontal diseases. Periodontol 2000 1998;18:37–46.
14. Robinson PG, Winkler JR, Palmer G, et al. The diagnosis of periodontal conditions associated with HIV infection. J Periodontol 1994;65:236–43.
15. EC-Clearinghouse on Oral Problems Related to HIV Infection and WHO Collaborating Centre on Oral Manifestations of the Immunodeficiency Virus. Classification and diagnostic criteria for oral lesions in HIV infection. J Oral Pathol Med 1993;22:289–91.
16. Mealey BL. Periodontal implications: medically compromised patients. Ann Periodontol 1996;1:256–321.
17. Glick M, Garfunkel AA. Common oral findings in two different diseases—leukemia and AIDS. Part I. Compend Contin Educ Dent 1992;13:432–50.
18. Garfunkel AA, Glick M. Common oral findings in two different diseases—leukemia and AIDS. Part II. Compend Contin Educ Dent 1992;13:550–62.
19. Barr C, Lopez MR, Rua-Dobles A. Periodontal changes by HIV serostatus in a cohort of homosexual and bisexual men. J Clin Periodontol 1992;19:794–801.
20. Drinkard CR, Decker L, Little JW, et al. Periodontal status of individuals in early stages of human immunodeficiency virus infection. Comm Dent Oral Epidemiol 1991;19:281–5.
21. Friedman RB, Gunsolley J, Gentry A, et al. Periodontal status of HIV-seropositive and AIDS patients. J Periodontol 1991;62:623–7.
22. Melnick SL, Engel D, Truelove E, et al. Oral mucosal lesions: association with the presence of antibodies to the human immunodeficiency virus. Oral Surg Oral Med Oral Pathol 1989;68:37–43.

23. Robinson PG, Sheiham A, Challacombe SJ, Zakrzewska JM. The periodontal health of homosexual men with HIV infection: a controlled study. Oral Dis 1996;2:45–52.

24. Winkler JR, Grassi M, Murray PA. Clinical description and etiology of HIV-associated periodontal disease. In: Robertson PB, Greenspan JS, editors. Oral manifestations of AIDS. Proceedings of First International Symposium on Oral Manifestations of AIDS. Littleton: PSG Publishing Company; 1988. p.49.

25. Swango PA, Kleinman DV, Konzelman JL. HIV and periodontal health. A study of military personnel with HIV. J Am Dent Assoc 1991;122:49–54.

26. Klein RS, Quart AM, Small CB. Periodontal disease in heterosexuals with acquired immuno-deficiency syndrome. J Periodontol 1990;62:535–40.

27. Laskaris G, Hadjivassiliou M, Stratigos J. Oral signs and symptoms in 160 Greek HIV-infected patients. J Oral Pathol Med 1992;21:120–3.

28. Masouredis CM, Katz MH, Greenspan D, et al. Prevalence of HIV-associated periodontitis and gingivitis in HIV-infected patients attending an AIDS clinic. J Acquir Immune Defic Syndr 1992;5:479–83.

29. Riley C, London JP, Burmeister JA. Periodontal health in 200 HIV-positive patients. J Oral Pathol Med 1992;21:124–7.

30. San Martin T, Jandinski JJ, Palumbo P. Periodontal diseases in children infected with HIV [abstract]. J Dent Res 1992;71:366A.

31. Schoen D, Murray P, Jandinski J. Periodontal status of HIV-positive children [abstract]. J Dent Res 1994;73:2003A.

32. Lamster IB, Grbic JT, Mitchell-Lewiss DA, et al. New concepts regarding the pathogenesis of periodontal disease in HIV infection. Ann Periodontol 1998;3:62–75.

33. Murray PA, Grassi M, Winkler JR. The microbiology of HIV-associated periodontal lesions. J Clin Periodontol 1989;16:636–42.

34. Murray PA, Winkler JR, Peros WJ, et al. DNA probe detection of periodontal pathogens in HIV-associated periodontal lesions. Oral Microbiol Immunol 1991;6:34–40.

35. Tylenda CA, Larsen J, Yeh C-K, et al. High levels of oral yeasts in early HIV-infection. J Oral Pathol Med 1989;18:520–4.

36. Glick M, Pliskin ME, Weiss RC. The clinical and histologic appearance of HIV-associated gingivitis. Oral Surg Oral Med Oral Pathol 1990;69:395–8.

37. Holmstrup P, Schiøtz AW, Westergaard J. Effect of dental plaque control on gingival lichen planus. Oral Surg Oral Med Oral Pathol 1989;69:585–90.

38. Pindborg JJ. Atlas of diseases of the oral mucosa. 5th ed. Copenhagen: Munksgaard; 1992. p.246.

39. Heinic GS, Greenspan D, MacPhail LA, Greenspan JS. Oral *Geotrichum candidum* infection associated with HIV-infection. A case report. Oral Surg Oral Med Oral Pathol 1992;73:726–8.

40. Serio FG, Siegel MA, Slade BE. Plasma cell gingivitis of unusual origin. A case report. J Periodontol 1991;62:390–3.

41. EC-Clearinghouse on Oral Problems Related to HIV Infection and WHO Collaborating Centre on Oral Manifestations of the Human Immunodeficiency Virus. An update of the classification and diagnostic criteria of oral lesions in HIV-infection. J Oral Pathol Med 1991;20:97–100.

42. Grassi M, Williams, CA, Winkler JR, Murray PA. Management of HIV-associated periodontal diseases. In: Robertson PB, Greenspan JS, editors. Perspectives on oral manifestations of AIDS. Proceedings of First International Symposium on oral manifestations of AIDS. Littleton: PSG Publishing Company; 1988. p.119.

43. Horning GM, Cohen ME. Necrotizing ulcerative gingivitis, periodontitis, and stomatitis: clinical staging and predisposing factors. J Periodontol 1995;66:990–8.

44. Greenspan D, Schiødt M, Greenspan J, Pindborg JJ. AIDS and the mouth. Copenhagen: Munksgaard; 1990.

45. Porter SA, Luker J, Scully C, et al. Orofacial manifestations of a group of British patients infected with HIV-1. J Oral Pathol Med 1989;18:47–8.

46. Schulten EJAM, ten Kate RW, van der Waal I. Oral manifestations of HIV-infection in 75 Dutch patients. J Oral Pathol Med 1989;18:42–6.

47. Thompson SH, Charles GA, Craig DB. Correlation of oral disease with the Walter Reed staging scheme for HIV-1–seropositive patients. Oral Surg Oral Med Oral Pathol 1992;73:289–92.

48. Moniaci D, Greco D, Flecchia G, et al. Epidemiology, clinical features and prognostic value of HIV-1 related oral lesions. J Oral Pathol Med 1990;19:477–81.

49. Barnes GP, Bowles WF, Carter HG. Acute necrotizing ulcerative gingivitis: a survey of 218 cases. J Periodontol 1973;44:35–42.

50. Glick M, Muzyka BC, Salkin LM, Lurie D. Necrotizing ulcerative periodontitis: a marker for immune deterioration and a predictor of the diagnosis of AIDS. J Periodontol 1994;65:393–7.

51. Gornitsky M, Clark DC, Siboo R, et al. Clinical documentation and occurrence of putative periodontopathic bacteria in human immunodeficiency virus-associated periodontol disease. J Periodontol 1991;62:576–85.

52. Zambon JJ, Reynolds HS, Genco RJ. Studies of the subgingival microflora in patients with acquired immunodeficiency syndrome. J Periodontol 1990;61:699–704.

53. Rams TE, Andriolo M, Feik D, et al. Microbiological study of HIV-related periodontitis. J Periodontol 1991;62:74–81.

54. Lucht E, Heimdahl A, Nord CE. Periodontal disease in HIV-infected patients in relation to lymphocyte subsets and specific micro-organisms. J Clin Periodontol 1991;18:252–6.

55. Steigley KE, Thompson SH, McQuade MJ, et al. A comparison of T4:T8 lymphocyte ratio in the periodontal lesion of healthy and HIV-positive patients. J Periodontol 1992;63:753–6.

56. Tomar SL, Swango PA, Kleinman DV, Burt B. Loss of periodontal attachment in HIV-seropositive military personnel. J Periodontol 1995;66:421–8.

57. Martinez-Canut P, Guarinos J, Bagán JV. Periodontal disease in HIV seropositive patients and its relation to lymphocyte subsets. J Periodontol 1996;67:33–6.

58. Scheutz F, Matee MIN, Andsager L, et al. Is there an association between periodontal condition and HIV infection? J Clin Periodontol 1997;24:580–7.

59. Smith GLF, Cross DL, Wray D. Comparison of periodontal disease in HIV seropositive subjects and controls. I. Clinical features. J Clin Periodontol 1995;22:558–68.

60. Scully C, Porter SR, Luker J. An ABC of oral health care in patients with HIV-infection. Brit Dent J 1991;171:149–50.

61. Holmstrup P, Samaranayake LP. Acute and AIDS-related oral candidoses. In: Samaranayake LP, MacFarlane TW, editors. Oral candidosis. London: Wright; 1990. p.133.

62. Robinson PG, Cooper H, Hatt J. Healing after dental extractions in men with HIV-infection. Oral Surg Oral Med Oral Pathol 1992;74:426–30.

63. Glick M, Abel SN, Muzyka BC, DeLorenzo M. Dental complications after dental treatment of patients with AIDS. J Am Dent Assoc 1994;125:296–301.

64. Lucartorto FM, Franker CK, Maza J. Postscaling bacteremia in HIV-associated gingivitis and periodontitis. Oral Surg Oral Med Oral Pathol 1992;73:550–4.

65. Robinson P. The management of HIV. Brit Dent J 1991;171:287.

66. Muzyka BC, Glick M. Necrotizing stomatitis and AIDS. Gen Dent 1994;42:66–8.

67. Williams CA, Winkler JR, Grassi M, Murray PA. HIV-associated periodontitis complicated by necrotizing stomatitis. Oral Surg Oral Med Oral Pathol 1990;69:351–5.

68. Tempest MN. Cancrum oris. Br J Surg 1966;53:949–53.

69. SanGiacomo TR, Tan PM, Loggi DG, Itkin AB. Progressive osseous destruction as a complication of HIV-periodontitis. Oral Surg Oral Med Oral Pathol 1990;70:476–9.

70. Felix DH, Wray D, Smith GLF, Jones GA. Oroantral fistula: an unusual complication of HIV-associated periodontal disease. Br Dent J 1991;171:61–2.

71. Page RC, Altman LC, Ebersole JL, et al. Rapidly progressive periodontitis. A distinct clinical condition. J Periodontol 1983;54:197–209.

CHAPTER 12

PERIODONTAL DISEASE AND PERIODONTAL MANAGEMENT IN PATIENTS WITH CANCER

Joel B. Epstein, DMD, MSD, FRCD(C)

PATIENTS WITH HEAD AND NECK CANCER

Radiation therapy that includes the oral cavity and salivary glands may have dramatic effects upon oral health. The acute effects of radiation therapy include mucositis, altered salivary gland function, and risk of mucosal infection. The long-term effects include alteration in the vascularity of soft tissue and bone, salivary gland damage, reduction in the cellularity of bone and connective tissue, and risk of increased collagen synthesis resulting in fibrosis (Figure 12–1). Cellular damage may lead to reduction in cellularity of tissue, fibrosis of connective tissue, and vascular changes with intimal thickening, endarteritis, and thrombosis. These changes result in hypovascular, hypocellular, and hypoxic tissue.[1–4] The affected bone has a reduced capacity to remodel and may be at increased risk of infection.

The periodontium is sensitive to the effects of radiation at high doses.[1–11] Blood vessels in the periodontium, periosteum, and the periodontal ligament[1,3,7,8] may be affected, leading to widening of the periodontal ligament space.[9–11] These changes may result in increased risk of periodontal disease and altered healing with impaired capacity of bone remodeling and repair.[1,12,13] Rampant periodontal destruction may occur in the absence of good oral hygiene.[12] Because of the effects of therapeutic radiation, periodontal involvement of teeth to be included in the high-dose fields must be assessed prior to radiation therapy to identify teeth that cannot be maintained for a lifetime and may require extraction prior to irradiation.[14,15] It has been shown that preradiation extraction of teeth carries a lower risk of osteonecrosis than extraction of teeth following radiation therapy.[16]

An additional consideration in preradiation treatment planning is the finding that periodontal involvement of teeth in high-dose radiation of some sites can lead to the development of osteonecrosis.[17] Periodontal attachment loss, particularly on the buccal aspect of teeth in a high-dose radiated field, has been reported to represent a risk factor for the development of osteonecrosis.[18]

It is important to realize that periodontal attachment loss is greater in teeth in irradiated sites;[18] therefore, preradiation treatment planning should include consideration of the impact of additional attachment loss over time on the ability to retain teeth and, in particular, to maintain teeth that may serve as abutment teeth for dental prostheses. Statistically significant increase in attachment loss occurs in teeth in the sites of high-dose irradiation and is reflected in increased mobility of

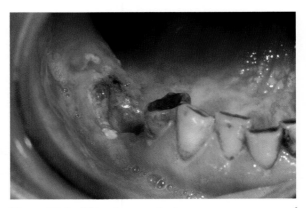

Figure 12–1. This photograph demonstrates exposure of bone in a patient following head and neck radiation therapy. Radiation changes are seen involving the gingival tissues extending into the floor of the mouth, and the necrotic, stained area of the bone is exposed in the molar region.

TABLE 12–1. Considerations for Preradiation Extraction of Teeth in the High-Dose Fraction

Caries: nonrestorable teeth
Active periapical disease: symptomatic teeth
Moderate to advanced periodontal disease
Lack of opposing teeth, compromised hygiene
Partial impaction or incomplete eruption of teeth
Extensive periapical lesions (not if chronic or well localized)

these teeth in irradiated fields.[18] Also, following radiation therapy, tooth loss is greater in fields of irradiation. The increased periodontal involvement and loss of teeth in the high-dose fraction indicates a local effect on the tissue, likely due to changes in the cellularity, vascularity, and reduced healing/remodeling potential of the periodontium.

Similarly, decreased saliva volume has been shown in patients with Sjögren's syndrome to result in increased risk of alveolar bone loss, attachment loss, and increased distance between the cemento-enamel junction and the alveolar bone crest.[19] In patients with head and neck cancer and xerostomia, the periodontal breakdown was comparable with the results reported in those with Sjögren's syndrome.[18] However, more significant periodontal destruction was noted in the teeth within the irradiated bone, supporting the potential for irradiation-induced changes in the periodontium to influence progression of periodontal involvement. Of course, the progression of the periodontal condition is also related to the patient's home care.

The patient's current periodontal status and the probability of continuing loss of periodontal attachment in general and greater attachment loss within the fields of high-dose irradiation should be considered in dental treatment planning prior to radiation therapy. A UK study found that only 11.2% of patients who reported regular dental office attendance prior to a diagnosis of oral cancer had no dental conditions that required treatment before radiation therapy.[20] The provider must be knowledgeable and understand the basis of radiation therapy, the nature of the planned radiation treatment for each patient (radiation dose, schedule, and fields) and the oral/dental/periodontal status in order to develop the best preradiation treatment plan.[21]

Teeth in the high-dose radiation field that should be extracted prior to radiation therapy are those that are nonrestorable, and those with moderate to severe periodontal disease that makes their long-term prognosis questionable or poor (Table 12–1). Periodontal considerations suggesting the possible need for extraction include probing depths or attachment loss of > 5 mm, moderate to advanced alveolar bone loss, or advanced recession with or without mucogingival involvement. In patients with limited past dental care, poor oral hygiene, and evidence of past dental/periodontal disease, more aggressive management should be considered. The recommendation for pretreatment extractions may be modified on the basis of the position of the teeth in question and should take into consideration the relative importance of individual teeth for future restoration and function, such as teeth that may serve as abutments for prostheses.

Following radiation therapy, good oral care and compliance with recommendations for oral care are improved with regular post-treatment dental visits for reinforcement of oral maintenance.[22] Periodontal treatment following radiation therapy must be provided with knowledge of fields of irradiation. Despite the potential for the development of osteonecrosis in high-dose volumes, if surgical intervention is considered, it has been shown that treatment including periodontal surgery is possible, if necessary, and may be more easily tolerated than extraction.[23]

PATIENTS RECEIVING HIGH-DOSE CHEMOTHERAPY AND/OR BONE MARROW TRANSPLANT

Periodontal manifestations of leukemia occur in some patients prior to the diagnosis of leukemia. The periodontal findings may occur as early manifestations of disease or may develop during cancer therapy (Figures 12–2, 12–3). Patients, especially those with significant platelet dysfunction, may present with gingival bleeding. In some patients, and more commonly in those with monocytic and myelomonocytic leukemia, gingival infiltration may be seen (Figure 12–4). In patients with neutrophil dysfunction or neutropenia, the inflammatory response may be blunted or not seen, leading to nonhealing gingival ulceration and poor response to tissue therapy following dental procedures. In patients with reduced red cell production, the oral tissues may appear pale (Figure 12–5). Thus, the presentation prior to diagnosis and during treatment of leukemia may be variable, ranging from significant oral changes that may lead to the diagnosis of leukemia to minimal findings that are not suggestive of an underlying disease.

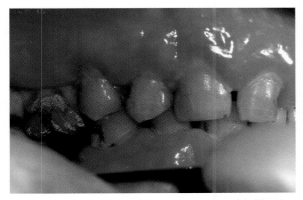

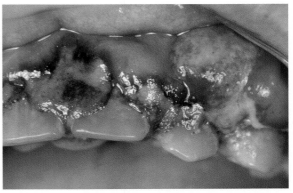

Figure 12–2. This figure demonstrates gingival infiltration with minimal inflammatory response and some tissue pallor in a patient with progressive chronic lymphocytic leukemia.

Figure 12–3. This figure represents gingival infiltration with soft tissue necrosis, minimal inflammatory response and some bleeding into tissues in a patient with progressing myelodysplastic syndrome, later diagnosed as chronic myelogenous leukemia.

Prior to medical management, oral health assessment is conducted to identify oral conditions that may become symptomatic during medical therapy, particularly those that may represent risk sites of infection. Studies have shown that oral and periodontal assessment and management reduce the risk of infection and fever associated with oral conditions.[24–28] The clinical diagnosis of oral infection depends upon an accurate history of oral symptoms and a thorough examination. Signs and symptoms may be minimized in neutropenic patients, with reduced erythema, swelling, and pain in sites of infection. Careful appraisal of the patient with cancer is needed, with understanding of pre-existing sites of periodontal involvement and careful evaluation that includes an assessment of tissue tenderness. While some have empirically raised concerns that periodontal probing and periodontal maintenance procedures may increase the risk of bacteremia in leukemic patients prior to medical management, this has not been seen in studies assessing the risk of fever or bacteremia following such procedures.[24,25,27,29] Patients may be febrile during neutropenia, and potential oral sources of infection must be carefully considered.

The patient's underlying systemic disease and its medical management are critical factors in determining the risk for infection. Oral infection is seen in approximately one-third of patients with acute leukemia or chronic leukemia in the blast phase.[30] In patients receiving chemotherapy for solid tumors, 10% may develop oral infection.[31,32] The complications common in patients on intensive chemotherapy protocols for breast cancer (methotrexate, 5-fluorouracil, vincristine, and prednisone) include neurotoxicity (65%), mucositis (21%, often associated with neutropenia), and candidiasis.[32] In immuno-compromised patients with blood dyscrasias, the frequency and severity of infection increases with the severity and duration of granulocytopenia.[33–35] Fifty-four percent of adult patients with leukemia develop oral lesions during chemotherapy.[34] The length of hospital stay is greater in patients who develop oral lesions, and in 25% of patients with positive blood cultures, an oral source is probable. Increased length of hospitalization and alpha-hemolytic streptococcal septicemia have been reported in patients with oral ulcerative mucositis consistent with an oral source of infection.[36] Thus, the oral cavity is a site of potential systemic infection in neutropenic patients.

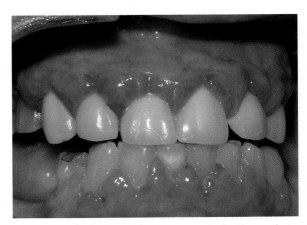

Figure 12–4. This figure demonstrates gingival hyperplasia, with bleeding into the gingival margins, particularly at interdental papillae. This was an individual with previous diagnosis of myelodysplastic syndrome and the gingival involvement was the initial finding of progression to acute myelogenous leukemia.

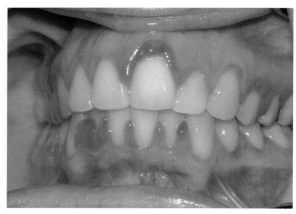

Figure 12–5. This photograph demonstrates mild gingival hyperplasia in interdental regions and isolated areas of the gingival margins. There is tissue pallor and no evidence of hemorrhage. This patient was diagnosed with acute myelogenous leukemia (AML) type 4.

Bacteremia due to oral sources has been well documented in immunosuppressed patients.[25,26,30,31,34,36] Bacterial infections may arise from oral sources in one-third of patients with acute leukemia. The bacteria implicated include periodontal flora, streptococci, and staphylococci (Figure 12–6). More recently, an increase in streptococcal bacteremia has been reported in leukemic patients.[34,36,37–41] The shift in the organisms identified in bacteremia may be due to use of systemic antibacterial prophylaxis with improved coverage of gram-negative organisms. Current antibiotic coverage may have an impact on the potential for exacerbation of pre-existing periodontal disease. Gingivitis and periodontitis due to mixed bacterial infections are also common and have been reported in up to 25% of all infections in patients with acute nonlymphocytic leukemia.[26]

Patients with chronic periodontal disease receiving high-dose chemotherapy may develop acute exacerbations at pre-existing sites of disease during periods of neutropenia.[42–45] Assessment of the periodontal flora during chemotherapy showed that a shift in the flora to increased gram-negative bacilli occurred in less than 50% of patients.[46,47] Of these, the *Pseudomonas* species predominated although *Klebsiella pneumoniae* was also present.[48] Periodontal disease and attachment loss was associated with recovery of staphylococci from supragingival sites but no correlation with yeast colonization was seen. In another study, the periodontal flora in leukemic patients were assessed in sites of exacerbation of periodontal disease.[44] In 24 patients, exacerbations developed during neutropenia in all but 2 cases. The potential pathogens identified were *Staphylococcus epidermidis, Candida albicans, Staphylococcus aureus,* and *Pseudomonas aeruginosa* in primary infection or mixed culture. The subgingival flora associated with these exacerbations were indigenous when compared with noncancer patients. In these patients, inflammatory signs were suppressed, making detection difficult.[49,50]

Thus, pre-existing periodontal disease may serve as a site for the development of infection in neutropenic patients.[25,47,51] An oral source of septicemia was suspected in 25% of patients with acute leukemia who received dental care and scaling prior to chemotherapy, compared with 77% of patients without such dental care prior to chemotherapy.[25] The primary sources were pericoronitis or pre-existing periodontal infections. In a study of fever following oral examination with and without periodontal probing and scaling in leukemic patients, no differences were seen in the incidence of fever or bacteremia between groups.[29] Oral preventive care has been shown to not result in increased risk of bacteremia or in fever and is associated with less severe oral mucositis.[24] Thus, periodontal evaluation and treatment may reduce the potential for septicemia from periodontal sources.

In patients who will become neutropenic, dental and periodontal treatment should be completed prior to chemotherapy. It is desirable to have a 2-week healing period prior to the anticipated onset of neutropenia. In patients with solid tumors treated with chemotherapy, the treatment schedules are provided in a planned series, often on a 3 to 4 week

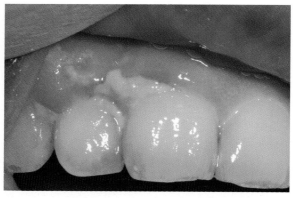

Figure 12–6. This patient was undergoing chemotherapy for acute myelogenous leukemia and developed an area of tenderness between the incisors. Clinically, ulceration of the interdental papillae with minimal erythematous reaction and possible extension of the ulceration along the attached gingival tissue is seen. A culture identified *Staphylococcus* bacteria in this region.

basis for a number of treatments. In patients with solid tumors, chemotherapy may result in a short-term depression in white cell counts. Typically, blood counts improve prior to the next course of chemotherapy. Dental and periodontal treatment should be provided when the white cell counts are not suppressed, which is typically 2 to 3 weeks following a course of chemotherapy, just prior to the next dose of chemotherapy. Antibiotic coverage may be considered when the neutrophil counts are less than 500 cells/mL, if the treatment cannot be delayed until counts are higher than 1,000 cells/mL.

Empiric antibiotic therapy for management of the febrile neutropenic patient is well established. The antibiotic must be broad spectrum, bacteriocidal, and given in appropriate dose and schedule. Metronidazole appears to be an important antimicrobial in the management of oral infection associated with fever in neutropenic patients.[52] In leukemic patients, who remain febrile despite broad-spectrum antibiotics, defervescence may occur when metronidazole is added to the antibiotic regimen.[52]

The use of topical agents has not yet been shown to be effective in the prevention of colonization of the oropharynx and in the prevention of oromucosal infections. Chlorhexidine has been shown to reduce plaque formation and disperse established plaque; the agent may assist in managing gingivitis and periodontal involvement, reduce caries risk, and may decrease oral colonization by *Candida*.[53,54]

In patients who will become neutropenic, prior to myelosuppressive chemotherapy, elimination of pre-existing foci of infection is desired. The oral cavity, dentition, and periodontium must be examined thoroughly, including radiographic evaluation, when indicated, on the basis of the findings of the examination. If necessary, delaying the myelosuppressive therapy should be considered in order to manage a symptomatic dental infection. If asymptomatic periapical pathosis is present, dental treatment may be completed after chemotherapy, and the patient should be covered by appropriate systemic antibiotic therapy during myelosuppression.[55–57] Local irritants such as calculus and rough irregular dental surfaces should be managed to reduce local tissue irritation. Dentures should be cleaned regularly, and removal of the appliance at night is recommended due to microbial colonization of the denture surface.[58] In cancer patients, pretreatment oral/dental management has been shown to decrease the length of hospital stay, and to be associated with reduced oral complications.[58,59–61] Good oral hygiene has been reported

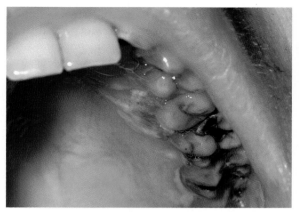

Figure 12–7. This patient felt discomfort in the palatal gingival tissues. The clinical diagnosis was herpes simplex virus, and increasing acyclovir dose led to resolution. These lesions were confirmed as HSV on viral culture, and exfoliative cytology demonstrated the presence of HSV-like inclusions.

to reduce the risk of mucositis and not increase the risk of fever or bacteremia.[24]

In leukemia/bone marrow transplant (BMT) patients, reactivation of latent herpes simplex virus (HSV) infection occurs in the majority of carriers in the "absence" of viral prophylaxis.[62–64] In the mouth, the lesions most commonly affect the keratinized mucosa of the gingiva, the palate, and the tongue, frequently beginning on the attached gingiva as 1- to 2-mm, rounded ulcerations that can extend to form large confluent lesions (Figures 12–7, 12–8). A patient seropositive for HSV has a

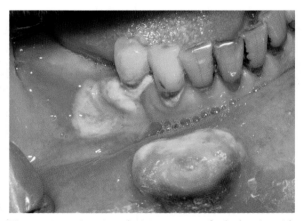

Figure 12–8. A patient during treatment for leukemia, with ulceration involving the gingival tissues, extending from the margin into the vestibular mucosa and bicuspid region, and an extensive ulceration with the development of exophytic mass on the lip. Culture and tissue sampling identified herpes simplex virus, and treatment with acyclovir was associated with improvement in the lesions.

high probability of viral reactivation during induction chemotherapy for leukemia or during BMT.[65-67] Since HSV infections in immunocompromised patients are severe and can be associated with high morbidity and mortality, chemoprophylaxis with acyclovir and its analogs has become standard for seropositive patients during BMT.[68-72] Acyclovir-resistant HSV during prolonged treatment has been reported although when this occurs, increasing the dose of acyclovir or its analogs may be effective, and foscarnet is also available.[62,65,72-77] Other antivirals are under development.[72,76]

Varicella-zoster infection is also common in immunocompromised patients, with the lesions initially confined to the dermatome distribution of the involved nerve branches. Cytomegalovirus (CMV) causes up to 20% of post-transplant deaths, and reactivation occurs in up to 70% of seropositive patients.[78] Cytomegalovirus can present as persisting oral mucosal ulcers and has been reported to cause gingival enlargement.[79-82] Diagnosis requires suspicion of the potential causes of the lesion and is based on clinical findings and positive virus identification in the involved tissue.

Periodontal disease should be assessed and managed prior to medical treatment of oropharyngeal cancer and in patients in whom neutropenia may develop during treatment. Oral and periodontal infection may exacerbate during cancer therapy and may result in oral pain and infection as well as systemic infection that results in morbidity and can lead to mortality. Pretreatment assessment and management and maintenance of oral hygiene have been shown to be effective in preventing oral and systemic complications during treatment of patients with cancer.

REFERENCES

1. Guglielmotti MB, Ubios AM, Cabrini RL. Alveolar wound healing after x-irradiation: a histologic, radiographic and histometric study. J Oral Maxillofac Surg 1986;44:972–6.

2. Wright WE. Periodontium destruction with oncology therapy. Five case reports. J Periodontol 1987; 58:559–63.

3. Marx RE. Osteoradionecrosis: a new concept of its pathophysiology. J Oral Maxillofac Surg 1983; 41:351–7.

4. Marx RE, Johnson RP. Studies on the radiobiology of osteoradionecrosis and their clinical significance. Oral Surg Oral Med Oral Pathol 1987; 64:379–90.

5. Arcuri MR, Schneider RL. The physiological effects of radiotherapy on oral tissue. J Prosthodont 1992;1:37–41.

6. Fattore D, Straus R, Bruno J. The management of periodontal disease in patients who have received radiation therapy for head and neck cancer. Spec Care Dent 1987;7:120–3.

7. Pappas GC. Bone changes in osteoradionecrosis and their clinical significance. Oral Surg Oral Med Oral Pathol 1987;64:379–90.

8. Beumer J, Curtis TZ. Radiation therapy of head and neck tumors. In: Beumer J, Curtis TA, Firtell DW, editors. Maxillofacial Rehabilitation. St Louis: CV Mosby, 1979. p. 43–89.

9. Fujita M, Tanimoto K, Wada T. Early radiographic changes in radiation bone injury. Oral Surg Oral Med Oral Pathol 1986;61:641–4.

10. Medak H, Burnett GW. The effect of x-ray irradiation on the oral tissues of the Macacus rhesus monkey. Oral Surg Oral Med Oral Pathol 1954; 7:778–86.

11. Chambers F, Ng E, Ogden H, et al. Mandibular osteomyelitis in dogs following irradiation. Oral Surg Oral Med Oral Pathol 1958;11:843–59.

12. Silverman S, Chierici G. Radiation therapy of oral carcinomas. I. Effects on oral tissues and management of the periodontium. J Periodontol 1965;36:478–84.

13. Joyston-Bechal S. Prevention of dental diseases following radiotherapy and chemotherapy. Int Dent J 1992;42:47–53.

14. Consensus Development Panel. Consensus statement: oral complications of cancer therapies. NCI Monogr 1990;9:3–8.

15. Sonis ST, Woods PD, White A. Pretreatment oral assessment. NCI Monogr 1990;9:37–42.

16. Epstein JB, Rea G, Wong FLW, et al. Osteonecrosis: study of the relationship of dental extraction in patients receiving radiotherapy. Head Neck Surg 1987;10:48–54.

17. Galler C, Epstein JB, Guze KA, et al. The development of osteoradionecrosis from sites of periodontal disease activity: report of 3 cases. J Periodontol 1992;63:310–6.

18. Epstein JB, Lunn R, Le N, Stevenson-Moore P. Periodontal attachment loss in patients following head and neck radiation therapy. Oral Surg Oral Med Oral Pathol Oral Radiol Endod 1998;86(6): 673–7.

19. Najera MP, Al-Hashimi I, Plemons JM, et al. Prevalence of periodontal disease in patients with Sjögren's syndrome. Oral Surg Oral Med Oral Pathol Oral Radiol Endod 1997;83: 453–7.

20. Lizi EC. A case for a dental surgeon at regional radiotherapy centres. Brit Dent J 1992;173:24–6.

21. Stevenson-Moore P. Essential aspects of a pretreatment oral examination. NCI Monogr 1990;9:33–6.

22. Epstein JB, van der Meij EH, Lunn R, et al. Effects of compliance with fluoride gel application on caries and caries risk in patients after radiation therapy for head and neck cancer. Oral Surg Oral Med Oral Pathol Oral Radiol Endod 1996;82:268–75.

23. Epstein JB, Corbett T, Galler C, Stevenson-Moore P. Surgical periodontal treatment in radiotherapy-treated head and neck cancer patient. Spec Care Dent 1994;14:182–7.

24. Borowski B, Benhamou E, Pico JL, et al. Prevention of oral mucositis in patients treated with high-dose chemotherapy and bone marrow transplantation: a randomised controlled trial comparing two protocols of dental care. Europ J Cancer, Oral Oncol 1994;30(B):93–7.

25. Greenberg MA, Cohen SG, McKitrick JC, Cassileth PA. The oral flora as a source of septicemia in patients with acute leukemia. Oral Surg Oral Med Oral Pathol 1982;53:32–6.

26. Overholser CD, Peterson DE, Williams LT, Schimpff SC. Periodontal infection in patients with acute nonlymphocytic leukemia: prevalence of acute exacerbations. Arch Intern Med 1982;142:551–4.

27. Peterson DE, Overholser CD, Schimpff SC, et al. Relationship of intensive oral hygiene to systemic complications in acute nonlymphocytic leukemia. Proc Am Fed Clin Res 1981;29:440A.

28. Levy-Polack MP, Sebelli P, Polack NL. Incidence of oral complications and application of a preventive protocol in children with acute leukemia. Spec Care Dent 1998;18:189–93.

29. Weikel DS, Peterson DE, Rubinstein LE, et al. Incidence of fever following invasive oral interventions in the myelosuppressed cancer patient. Cancer Nurs 1989;12:265–70.

30. Dreizen S, McCredie KB, Keating MJ, Bodey GP. Oral infections associated with chemotherapy in adults with acute leukemia. Postgrad Med 1982;71:133–46.

31. Dreizen S, Bodey GP, Valdivieso M. Chemotherapy-associated oral infections in adults with solid tumors. Oral Surg Oral Med Oral Pathol 1983;55:113–20.

32. McCarthy GM, Skillings JR. Orofacial complications of chemotherapy for breast cancer. Oral Surg Oral Med Oral Pathol 1992;74:172–8.

33. Dreizen S, McCredie KB, Bodey GP, Keating MJ. Quantitative analysis of the oral complications of antileukemia chemotherapy. Oral Surg Oral Med Oral Pathol 1986;62:650–3.

34. Epstein JB, Gangbar SJ. Oral mucosal lesions in patients undergoing treatment for leukemia. J Oral Med 1987;43:132–7.

35. Navari RM, Buckner CD, Clift RA, et al. Prophylaxis of infection in patients with aplastic anemia receiving allogeneic marrow transplants. Am J Med 1984;76:564–72.

36. Ruescher TJ, Sodeifi A, Scrivani SJ, et al. The impact of mucositis on alpha-hemolytic streptococcal infection in patients undergoing autologous bone marrow transplantation for hematologic malignancies. Cancer 1998;82:2275–81.

37. Donnelly JP. Bacterial complications of transplantation: diagnosis and treatment. J Antimicrob Chemother 1995;36(B):59–72.

38. Donnelly JP, Muus P, Horrevorts AM, et al. Failure of clindamycin to influence the course of severe oromucositis associated with streptococcal bacteraemia in allogeneic bone marrow transplant recipients. Scand J Infect Dis 1993;25:43–50.

39. Donnelly JP, Muus P, Schattenberg A, et al. A scheme for daily monitoring of oral mucositis in allogeneic BMT recipients. Bone Marrow Transplant 1992;9:409–13.

40. Mossad SB, Longworth DL, Goormastic M, et al. Early infectious complications in autologous bone marrow transplantation: a review of 219 patients. Bone Marrow Transplant 1996;18:265–71.

41. Channock SJ, Pizzo PA. Infectious complications of patients undergoing therapy for acute leukemia: current status and future prospects. Semin Oncol 1997;24:132–40.

42. Peterson DE. Pretreatment strategies for infection prevention in chemotherapy patients. NCI Monogr 1990;9:61–71.

43. Overholser CD, Peterson DE, Williams LT, Schimff SC. Periodontal infection in patients with acute nonlymphocytic leukemia: prevalence of acute exacerbations. Arch Intern Med 1982;142:551–4.

44. Peterson DE, Minah GE, Overholser CD, et al. Microbiology of acute periodontal infection in myelosuppressed cancer patients. J Clin Oncol 1987;5:1461–8.

45. Stansbury DM, Peterson DE, Suzuki JB. Rapidly progressive acute periodontal infection in a patient with acute leukemia. J Periodontol 1988;59:544–7.

46. Minah GE, Rednor JL, Peterson DE, et al. Oral succession of gram-negative bacilli in myelosup-

pressed cancer patients. J Clin Microbiol 1986; 24:210–13.

47. Moore WEC, Holdeman LV, Cato EP, et al. Bacteriology of moderate (chronic) periodontitis in mature adult humans. Infect Immun 1983;42: 510–155.

48. Reynolds MA, Minah GE, Peterson DE, et al. Periodontal disease and oral microbial successions during myelosuppressive cancer chemotherapy. J Clin Periodontol 1989;16:185–9.

49. Bodey GP, Buckley M, Sathe YS, Freireich EJ. Quantitative relationships between circulating leukocytes and infection in patients with acute leukemia. Ann Intern Med 1966;64:328–40.

50. Sickles EZ, Greene WH, Wiernik PH. Clinical presentation of infection in granulocytopenic patients. Arch Intern Med 1975;135:715–9.

51. Bergman OJ. Oral infections and septicemia in immunocompromised patients with hematologic malignancies. J Clin Microbiol 1988;26: 2105–9.

52. Barrett AP, Schifter M. Antibiotic strategy in orofacial/ head and neck infections in severe neutropenia. Oral Surg Oral Med Oral Pathol 1994;77:350–5.

53. Fardal O, Turnbull RS. A review of the literature on use of chlorhexidine in dentistry. J Am Dent Assoc 1986;112:863–9.

54. Langslet A, Olsen I, Lie SO, Lokken NP. Chlorhexidine treatment of oral candidiasis in seriously diseased children. Acta Paediatr Scand 1974;63: 809–11.

55. Overholser CD, Peterson DE, Bergman SA, Williams LT. Dental extractions in patients with acute nonlymphocytic leukemia. J Oral Surg 1982; 40:296–8.

56. Peterson DE, Overholser CD, Williams LT. Endodontic therapy in patients receiving myelosuppressive chemotherapy. Proc J Dent Res 1982; 61:276.

57. Peters E, Monopoli M, Woo SB, Sonis S. Assessment of the need for treatment of postendodontic asymptomatic periapical radiolucencies in bone marrow transplant recipients. Oral Surg Oral Med Oral Pathol 1993;76:45–8.

58. De Paola LG, Minah GE. Isolation of pathogenic microorganisms from dentures and denture soaking containers of myelosuppresed cancer patients. J Prosthet Dent 1983;49:20–4.

59. Epstein JB, Chin EA, Jacobson JJ, et al. The relationship among fluoride, cariogenic oral flora, and salivary flow rate during radiation therapy. Oral Surg Oral Med Oral Pathol Oral Radiol Endod 1998;86:286–92.

60. Sonis S. Mucositis as a biological process: a new hypothesis for the development of chemotherapy-induced stomatotoxicity. Oral Oncol 1998;34: 39–34.

61. Sonis S, Kunz A. Impact of improved dental services on the frequency of oral complications of cancer therapy for patients with non-head-and-neck malignancies. Oral Surg Oral Med Oral Pathol 1988;65:19–22.

62. Epstein JB, Sherlock C, Page JL, et al. Clinical study of herpes virus infection in leukemia. Oral Surg Oral Med Oral Pathol 1990;70:38–43.

63. Epstein JB, Scully C. Herpes simplex virus in immunocompromised patients: growing evidence of drug resistance. Oral Surg Oral Med Oral Pathol 1991;72:47–50.

64. Epstein JB, Ransier A, Sherlock CH, et al. Acyclovir prophylaxis of oral herpes virus during bone marrow transplantation. Oral Oncol, Eur J Cancer 1996;32(b):158–62.

65. Barrett AP. A long-term prospective clinical study of oral complications during conventional chemotherapy for acute leukemia. Oral Surg Oral Med Oral Pathol 1987;63:313–6.

66. Meyers JD, Flournoy N, Thomas ED. Infection with herpes simplex virus and cell-mediated immunity after marrow transplant. J Infect Dis 1980; 142:338.

67. Saral R, Ambinder RF, Burns WH, et al. Acyclovir prophylaxis against recrudescent herpes simplex virus infections in leukemia patients: a randomized double-blind placebo controlled study. Ann Intern Med 1983;99:773–7.

69. Lam MT, Pazin GJ, Armstrong JA, Ho M. Herpes simplex infection in acute myelogenous leukemia and other hematologic malignancies: a prospective study. Cancer 1981;48:2168–71.

70. Rand KH, Kramer B, Johnson AC. Cancer chemotherapy-associated symptomatic stomatitis: role of herpes simplex virus (HSV). Cancer 1982; 50:1262–5.

71. Wade JC, Newton B, Flournoy N, Meyers JD. Oral acyclovir prophylaxis of herpes simplex virus infection after marrow transplant. Ann Intern Med 1984;100:823–7.

72. Cassady KA, Whitley RJ. New therapeutic approaches to alpha-herpesvirus infections. J Antimicrob 1997;39:119–28.

73. Oakley C, Epstein JB, Sherlock CH. Reactivation of oral herpes simplex virus. Implications for clinical management of herpes simplex virus recurrence during radiotherapy. Oral Surg Oral Med Oral Pathol 1997;84:272–8.

74. Burns WH, Santos GW, Saral R, et al. Isolation and characterization of resistant herpes simplex virus after acyclovir therapy. Lancet 1982;1:421–3.

75. Crumpacker CS, Schnipper LE, Marlowe SI, et al. Resistance to anti-viral drugs of herpes simplex virus isolated from a patient treated with acyclovir. N Engl J Med 1982;306:343–6.

76. de Clerq E. In search of a selective antiviral chemotherapy. Clin Microbial Rev 1997;10:674–93.

77. Wagstaff AJ, Bryson HM. Foscarnet. A reappraisal of its antiviral activity, pharmacokinetic properties and therapeutic use in immunocompromised patients with viral infections. Drugs 1994;48:199–226.

79. Zaia JA, Forman SJ. Cytomegalovirus infection in the bone marrow transplant recipient. Infect Dis Clinics N Am 1995;9:879–900.

80. Scully C, Epstein J, Porter S, Cox M. Viruses and chronic disorders involving the human oral mucosa. Oral Surg Oral Med Oral Pathol 1991; 72:537–44.

81. Schubert MM, Epstein JB, Lloid ME, Cooney E. Oral infection due to cytomegalovirus in immunocompromised patients. J Oral Pathol Med 1993; 22:268–73.

82. Epstein JB, Sherlock CH, Wolber RA. Oral manifestations of cytomegalovirus infection. Oral Surg Oral Med Oral Pathol 1993;75:443–51.

CHAPTER 13

PERIODONTAL CONSIDERATIONS IN PATIENTS WITH BONE MARROW OR SOLID ORGAN TRANSPLANTS

Terry D. Rees, DDS, MSD

The science of organ and bone marrow transplantation has evolved over the past 30 to 40 years from last-ditch desperate efforts to briefly prolong life, or improve the quality of life, to a sophisticated treatment modality that is preferred in the management of a variety of diseases.[1] In most instances, the various diseases and disorders which lead to a need for transplantation have oral manifestations, which may cause the alert dental practitioner to refer the affected patient for medical evaluation and appropriate treatment, including transplantation. Improved prognosis following organ transplantation is the direct result of the development of superior methods for obtaining donor-patient tissue matches, transportation solutions, and the effective use of immunosuppressant drugs.[2] Although transplantation procedures are often beneficial, they are not without complications, which range from life-threatening infections to rejection of the grafted organ. Safe and effective dental therapy in these patients requires an understanding of the diseases that are best treated by transplantation, their complications, and the after effects of the transplantation procedure. In each circumstance, careful dental protocols must be followed in order to provide this safe and effective care for patients.[3] Dental infections and manipulation of oral tissues may subject immunosuppressed patients to infections, which can lead to organ rejection, compromise of other body systems, or even death. This paper will review the systemic conditions that may result in a need for organ or bone marrow transplantation, discuss systemic and oral complications associated with the diseases and their treatment, and provide a protocol for the management of patients who are transplant recipients.

KIDNEY TRANSPLANTATION

Acute and Chronic Renal Failure

Renal failure is a major complication of kidney disease and transplantations, and failure in both native and transplanted kidneys most commonly occurs as a result of chronic renal disease. Progressive end-stage renal disease may develop rapidly or may occur many years after the onset of the initiating condition. Essentially, renal failure occurs as a result of the accumulation of circulating serum proteins, which, in turn, induce endocytosis of renal vascular epithelial cells and a nephrotoxic effect due to the release of vasoactive and inflammatory substances into the renal interstitium. Classic phases of failure include inflammation, fibrosis, atrophy, and end-organ damage.[4,5]

Glomerulonephritis in its various forms was once the most common condition leading to chronic renal failure (CRF). However, due to more success in noninvasive management of glomerulonephritis, diabetes mellitus is now the most common cause of chronic failure, followed by prolonged or progressive hypertension.[5–8]

Glomerulonephritis usually presents with manifestations of nephrotic syndrome, which may be acute or chronic in nature. This condition is characterized by massive edema, proteinuria, hypoalbuminemia, and susceptibility to intercurrent infections. Poststreptococcal glomerulonephritis is associated with an inflammatory reaction appearing after infection with group A or B hemolytic streptococci or with staphylococci. Nephritis has been associated with skin infections, but its relationship to oral streptococcal bacteremias is unknown.

Other forms of postinfectious glomerulonephritis may occur after a variety of bacterial, viral, or parasitic infections. This type of nephritis may be induced by bacterial endocarditis or infected ventriculoatrial shunts. The severity of nephritis is related to the duration of infection before appropriate antibacterial therapy is initiated. Control of the causative infection usually leads to the rapid resolution of glomerulonephritis, but irreversible renal failure can occur, especially if initiation of antimicrobial therapy has been delayed. It should be noted, however, that antimicrobial therapy itself may induce acute interstitial nephritis.

Membranoproliferative glomerulonephritis (hypocomplementemia) may occur due to inherited complement deficiencies or in conjunction with other conditions such as systemic lupus erythematosus, mixed cryoglobulinemia, systemic sclerosis, shunt infections, or bacterial endocarditis, all of which are associated with persistent immune complex formation.[9] Rapidly progressive glomerulonephritis may induce a steady alteration of renal function over a period of weeks or months, potentially leading to renal failure. This condition may also be associated with bacterial endocarditis or shunt infection.

Goodpasture's syndrome features a specific pathologic entity associated with formation of antibodies to glomerular epithelial basement membranes (GMB). Other forms of anti-GMB may be associated with pulmonary changes resulting from influenza, abuse of tobacco or illicit drugs, or other conditions that permit circulating antibody complexes access to lung alveoli.[4,10] Anti-GMB diseases usually progress to renal failure within 1 year of onset.

Fibrillary glomerulonephritis has recently been described as an idiopathic disorder which features pathognomonic fibril deposition in the glomeruli, which may induce nephrotic effects. At present, there is no known treatment for this disorder.

Immunoglobulin A (IgA) nephropathy (Berger's disease) is usually idiopathic but may occur in association with other diseases such as hepatic cirrhosis. The condition usually leads to reversible acute renal failure, but some patients experience life-threatening renal failure, sometimes over a period of 20 or more years.[4] IgA disease often recurs in patients undergoing kidney transplantation, although resultant graft rejection is rare.[11]

Hereditary nephritis (Alport's syndrome) may be accompanied by hepatic impairment. The condition is often progressive, especially in men, leading to end-stage renal failure over a period of years.

Nephrotic syndrome may occur in association with systemic conditions such as amyloidosis, systemic lupus erythematosus, and diabetes mellitus and ranges in degree from lipoid nephrosis to renal failure requiring transplantation. Unfortunately, the condition may recur in the transplanted kidney.[4] More rapid renal deterioration may occur when related to heroin abuse or acquired immunodeficiency syndrome (AIDS).[12] Corticosteroid-resistant patients with nephrotic syndrome may require cyclosporine therapy before renal transplantation. Therefore, these individuals are prone to cyclosporine-induced gingival overgrowth, together with more serious drug side-effects.[13–16] Cyclosporine may induce toxic nephropathy both before and after kidney transplantation.[4,14]

Membranous nephropathy may occur idiopathically or in association with the presence of solid tumors, systemic lupus erythematosus, hepatitis B, and occasionally hepatitis C infection, or with certain medications such as gold salts, penicillamine, or amphotericin B.[13] Nephrotic patients may be particularly susceptible to drug-induced rhabdomyolysis.[17]

Acute renal failure may be associated with elevated blood urea nitrogen (BUN) and creatinine concentrations. Acute failure may be induced by a reduction in blood volume due to hemorrhage, severe hypotension, advanced heart failure, or liver disease. Drugs such as angiotensin-converting enzyme (ACE) inhibitors or ACE receptor inhibitors may sustain renal hypotension. Ingestion of nonsteroidal anti-inflammatory drugs (NSAIDs) may produce similar effects.[18] Renal failure can occur as a complication of severe ischemia or hypovolemia or that of a major surgical procedure such as cardiac surgery and may also be induced by sepsis or by obstructive biliary cirrhosis. Acute renal tubular necrosis is generally reversible, but hemodialysis may be required.[19,20]

Chronic renal failure is a bilateral, progressive deterioration of functioning nephrons and is often insidious in progression. Acute and chronic renal failure can alter the function of virtually every organ system of the body.[8] The uremic syndrome occurs in part due to the accumulation of BUN and other metabolic waste products normally excreted by the kidneys. The condition features azotemia, impaired ability to concentrate urine, polyuria, hypokalemia, hypocalcemia, hyperphosphatemia, and metabolic acidosis in its late stages. It may be accompanied by hypertension, pericarditis, congestive heart failure, coronary artery disease, multiple neuropathies, metabolic encephalopathy, osteopenia or osteoporosis, and bleeding disorders due to anemia.[18,21]

Abnormal hemostasis occurs as a result of prolonged bleeding time, decreased activity of the platelet receptor complex, abnormal platelet aggregation and adhesiveness, and impaired prothrombin consumption. Central nervous system disturbances may first manifest as inability to concentrate, drowsiness, insomnia, memory lapses, and errors in judgment. If untreated, the condition becomes associated with hiccups, cramps, muscle twitching, asterixis, stupor, seizures, and coma.[8,22–24]

Gastrointestinal abnormalities include anorexia, nausea and vomiting, as well as uremic fetor, which is the uriniferous breath odor resulting from breakdown of the urea in saliva to ammonia. This condition may also be associated with a metallic taste sensation. Mucosal ulcerations may occur at any level of the gastrointestinal tract.

Endocrine-metabolic disturbances include altered parathyroid function, glucose intolerance, and insulin metabolism disorders. Dermatologic disorders may include the pallor of anemia, ecchymoses and hematomas due to defective hemostasis, calcium deposition in soft tissues, pruritus and excoriations related to secondary hyperparathyroidism, and/or dehydration. In some circumstances, the combination of anemia and hematologic dysfunction leads to development of a sallow, yellow cast to the skin or to slate-gray-to-bronze discoloration associated with hemochromatosis. In severe uremia, the concentration of urea in sweat and saliva may be sufficient to induce a deposition of a fine white powder (uremic frost) on the skin and mucosa as the result of evaporation.[8,21,22,23,25]

Renal osteodystrophy occurs in renal failure due to disordered calcium and phosphorus metabolism and altered vitamin D absorption and metabolism. The result is a secondary hyperparathyroidism induced by renal retention of phosphorus, which causes a compensatory release of calcium from bone in an effort to maintain the calcium-phosphorus homeostasis. Skeletal changes include altered bone remodeling, osteopenia, osteomalacia and osteoporosis, osteitis fibrosa cystica, osteosclerosis, and central giant cell tumors (the brown tumor of hyperparathyroidism).[5,8,21–23,26,27]

Individuals with renal failure exhibit increased susceptibility to infection due to altered leukocyte, monocyte, and lymphocyte function. The systemic conditions associated with end-stage renal disease (hyperglycemia, protein malnutrition, serum and tissue hyperosmolarity) further impair infection susceptibility. This susceptibility may continue in patients receiving dialysis or renal transplantation, due in part to the administration of immunosuppressant drugs.[8]

Oral Features of Renal Failure

Renal failure induces many abnormalities in the oral cavity. An increase in salivary calculus formation has been described, probably due to elevated serum calcium-phosphate levels. Conversely, caries incidence may be reduced, possibly due to plaque inhibition related to increased levels of salivary urea.[28] Uremic stomatitis occurs in two forms (1) the erythemopultaceous type, which features dry, burning, erythematous, and painful oral tissues that may be covered with a thick gray exudate; and (2) the ulcerative form, which is characterized by mucosal ulcerations. Xerostomia may be the most common oral manifestation and occurs due to altered salivary production, with or without parotid enlargement or infectious parotitis. Oral dryness may be compounded by nasal congestion resulting from insidious nasal bleeding, which, in turn, initiates mouth breathing. Insidious oral bleeding may induce gingival hemorrhage and hematoma formation in the presence of slight trauma. Enamel hypoplasia and brownish discoloration of the teeth may occur in children, and pulpal narrowing has been described. Infections may be quite frequent with candidal overgrowth being common, although bacterial, viral, and other fungal infections may also occur. Increased esophageal reflux has been described among dialysis patients, with resultant dental erosion and oral discomfort.[21–23,28,29]

Secondary hyperparathyroidism may induce fine granular metastatic calcifications in the connective tissues of the oral cavity, which may initiate mucosal swelling, pain, and ulceration. Radiographic evidence of hyperparathyroidism may include loss of lamina dura around the teeth. This is not a universal finding and may occur more often in the anterior dentition.[22,23] A reduced radiodensity of the bones of the jaws may occur in association with osteopenia. This can result in a "ground glass" radiographic osseous appearance, which may be associated with an increased possibility of spontaneous fractures of the jaws in extreme cases. Extraction sockets tend to retain the lamina dura and sclerotic radiopacities have been reported. Small unilocular or multilocular cystic lesions of the jaws may denote pseudocyst cavities or giant cell tumors (brown tumor). These lesions may induce loosening of teeth, jaw enlargement, and localized oral pain. Spontaneous gingival hemorrhage, ulcerations, and petechial lesions are common.[21–23,27,28]

Increased mobility of teeth is a common finding in osteopenic patients, even in the absence of periodontal pockets. Individuals with osteopenia experience increased tooth loss and more advanced periodontal disease. This may be reversed in women by estrogen therapy or by use of bisphonates.[30–34] Periodontal inflammation is very common among patients with renal failure, and opportunistic infections with or without blood seeding is a constant hazard.[25,35,36] Extraction of loose teeth should be avoided because of delays in wound healing. In most instances, mobile teeth can be maintained with splinting.[21–23,25,27,37]

Dialysis

Hemodialysis may be employed in the management of reversible or irreversible renal failure. Unfortunately, dialysis may also adversely affect renal function due to decreased urine output, induction of hypotension, or complement activation.[38,39]

A variety of drugs commonly used in dentistry may induce acute renal failure through tubular necrosis. These drugs include aminoglycoside antibiotics, acyclovir, sulfonamides, and acetaminophen.[17] The severity of the nephrotoxic effect may relate to dosing frequency and plasma levels achieved, especially in patients with concurrent renal ischemia.[40] The presence of sepsis or liver disease, particularly severe obstructive jaundice, may enhance drug-induced nephrotoxicity.

Accumulation of uric acid from gout or other diseases may also induce acute or chronic renal disease and failure. Chronic urate nephrotoxicity is rare today but occasionally results from deposition of sodium urate crystals in the kidney medullary interstitium.[41] Fanconi-like syndromes are possible when tetracyclines or other specific drugs are used in patients with pre-existing nephrosis.

Hemodialysis is initiated when a failing kidney cannot successfully excrete waste products, regulate acid-base balance, or maintain sodium homeostasis. In this procedure, solutes such as excessive urea or potassium are filtered out of the blood, and excessive extracellular fluid is removed. The procedure is usually performed every 2 to 3 days and requires 3 to 5 hours per session.[21] Side effects include severe hypotension, cramping, nausea, and vomiting.[42]

Vascular access is necessary to perform blood purification by dialysis. Today, this is most frequently accomplished by the creation of an arteriovenous fistula, often by anastomosis of the radial artery and cephalic vein of the arm.[39,43] To make this technique efficient, the anastomosis should be in place for 6 to 8 weeks before use to enable vessels to mature and enlarge. Consequently, this site is rarely used in the event immediate dialysis should be necessary to treat acute renal failure. In such circumstances, a double lumen catheter is inserted in the femoral, internal jugular, or subclavian vein. The dialysis equipment enables blood flow through a filtering membrane, resulting in the cleansing of the dialysate solutions. In some circumstances, the membrane may activate complement via the alternate pathway or generate interleukin-1 (IL-1), which can induce hypotension and β_2-microglobulin accumulation. These effects may be minimized by use of biocompatible membrane materials. Despite this, dialysis membranes may activate the clotting mechanism within the dialysis system itself. Intersystem clotting is controlled by administration of heparin.[39]

Indications for hemodialysis include uremia, hyperkalemia, volume overload, acidosis, uremic pericarditis, and other features of uremic syndrome. Hypotension is the major complication of hemodialysis, usually occurring as the result of excessive filtration and volume depletion. The condition is far more likely when vasoconstrictive mechanisms are impaired as a result of medications or of autonomic neuropathy such as that found in diabetics. Chronic anemia may also result due to factors such as decreased erythropoietin production, iron deficiency, folate deficiency, or hemolysis related to the dialysis process.[39]

Long-term hemodialysis patients may manifest musculoskeletal changes such as carpal tunnel syndrome, arthropathies, or amyloidosis, with or without increased tissue levels of β_2-microglobulin.[7] Encephalopathy may occur toward the end of dialysis and may persist even after completion of the therapeutic regime. Symptoms include subtle changes in personality, reduced short-term memory, slurred speech, and myoclonic spasms of the face, arms, legs, and trunk.[39]

Therapeutic outcomes of hemodialysis have remained constant over the past few years, with a mortality rate of approximately 20 to 25%. Complications include cardiovascular disease (stroke, myocardial infarction) and infections. A variety of infections occur due to protein malnutrition and inability to produce antibodies. As a consequence, hemodialysis patients are at increased risk for infectious endocarditis and endoarteritis at the shunt site. The patient's quality of life is impaired by frequent dialysis that must be performed and the amount of time required to complete the therapy although hemodialysis can be performed at home, after a reliable family member has been trained to conduct the procedure.

Peritoneal dialysis is performed by introducing dialysate solution into the peritoneal cavity. The procedure may be continuous (continuous ambulatory peritoneal dialysis) or periodic (cyclic ambulatory peritoneal dialysis). It is often the treatment of choice in acute renal failure, obviates the need for heparin, and minimizes marked changes in blood pressure, especially the hypotension associated with conventional dialysis. In this technique, the dialysis solution is infused into the abdominal cavity and drained after sufficient time for collection of toxic waste products and excess fluids. Often three to five exchanges are performed daily but the procedure can be performed at home. The primary complications are infection of the exit port within the catheter or infection in the peritoneal cavity. Other disadvantages include protein loss and glucose absorption into the bloodstream and this procedure also interferes with patient quality of life.[44]

Most peritoneal infusion infections are caused by gram-positive microorganisms such as *Staphylococcus epidermitis* and *Staphylococcus aureus*. However, peritonitis may also be induced by gram-negative anaerobic organisms including putative periodontal pathogens and by fungi.[27,28,44]

Renal Transplantation

Renal transplantation offers the best opportunity for resumption of normal daily activities and full rehabilitation in end-stage renal disease (ESRD) although graft rejection and infection remain serious problems. Both living and cadaver organs can be used; however, the best results occur when donors and recipients share compatible ABO blood groups and HLA antigens. No matching of Rh factor is required. Transplantation from identical twins offers the greatest opportunity for success, and immunosuppressant drugs are usually not required with fully compatible donor-receptors.

Improvements in immunosuppressant protocols have resulted in reduced graft rejection even in poorly matched donor-receptors. Unfortunately, immunosuppressant drugs also suppress host defenses against bacterial, viral, and fungal infections.[45] When possible, pregraft antibody titers against varicella zoster virus (VZV), cytomegalovirus (CMV), hepatitis B (HBV), and the human immunodeficiency virus (HIV) should be obtained prior to transplantation.[46] Receptor patients who are seronegative for VZV or HBV should receive vaccination prior to transplantation, although anti-CMV antibodies do not always confer protection.[44,47]

Graft rejection is mediated by both humoral and cellular mechanisms. Acute rejection may occur if the recipient patient has cytotoxic antibodies to donor blood group or HLA antigens. Chronic humoral rejection progresses more slowly but inexorably leads to graft loss.

Cardiovascular disease is one of the leading causes of morbidity and mortality in organ recipients and may include congestive heart failure, severe hypertension, or cardiac arrythmias. An increased incidence of infective endocarditis may occur even in patients without known cardiac valvar lesions.[21,48] Risk factors include pretransplant cardiovascular disease, diabetes mellitus, elevated serum lipids, hypertension, tobacco or drug abuse, and allograft dysfunction. Patients who have undergone coronary artery angioplasty or bypass surgery are at increased risk of re-stenosis.[48] Hypertension is very common after renal transplantation, most often due to the direct nephrotoxic effect of cyclosporine or possibly tacrolimus. Hypertension may lead to chronic graft rejection due to reduced renal function or renal artery stenosis.[48]

Infection is a constant hazard and most often occurs immediately following transplantation. Surgical wound infection, blood transfusions before or during organ transplantation (especially hepatitis C transmission), dialysis-related sepsis, urinary tract infection, and aspiration pneumonia infections are most common. The greatest risk of post-transplant infection occurs within the first 6 months, when immunosuppressive therapy is at its peak.[37] Delayed infections most often occur due to viral (HSV, CMV, EBV), fungal (*Candida albicans*) or other opportunistic organisms.[49–51]

Other common post-transplant complications include hyperlipidemia, which may be influenced by hyperinsulinemia or by the use of drugs such as cyclosporine or diuretics. Hyperparathyroidism may persist after renal transplantation and may require initiation of dialysis. Metabolic derangement, hyperkalemia, hypomagnesemia, hyperuricemia, and post-transfusion diabetes mellitus (PTDM) are additional risks. The last may be associated with administration of corticosteroids, but cyclosporine and tacrolimus can also be diabetogenic due to increased insulin resistance, decreased insulin secretion, or other mechanisms. Anemia and leukopenia are associated with poor renal function and deficiency in the renal production of erythropoeitin, which is essential to red blood cell development.

Liver disease is a common complication following renal transplantation. This may be drug-induced (cyclosporine, azathioprine) or due to viral hepatitis.

Immunosuppression therapy is usually provided by various combinations of glucocorticoids, azathioprine, cyclosporine, tacrolimus, monoclonal antibody OKT 3, or antilymphocyte globulin. Appropriate cyclosporine or tacrolimus serum levels are essential to prevent graft rejection although higher serum levels are associated with more severe adverse side effects. Serum levels can be unintentionally increased by simultaneous intake of drugs such as erythromycin, oral contraceptives, and some calcium channel blockers.

Rifampin, phenobarbital, phenytoin, and other anticonvulsant drugs may decrease cyclosporine levels, and aminoglycoside antibodies may promote cyclosporine nephrotoxicity. Thus, the prescription of any drug for patients receiving cyclosporine should be preceded by medical consultation.[18,48]

Cyclosporine is an excellent immunosuppressant drug, which is often prescribed following organ transplantation because it selectively suppresses cell-mediated immunity. Complications of the drug include nephrotoxicity, renal vasculopathy, hypertension, chronic renal interstitial fibrosis (which is also common in heart transplantation), neurotoxicity, gingival overgrowth, and increased susceptibility to malignancies, including B cell lymphoma, squamous cell carcinoma of the skin, lip or oral mucosa, or Kaposi's sarcoma.[23,35,52–86] Malignancy may be transmitted from the donor or it may develop de novo post-transplantation,[65,87–89] and oral malignancies have been reported within sites of cyclosporine-induced gingival overgrowth.[82,90] Cyclosporine-induced perioral dermatitis has been described and features red papules, pustules, and scaling of the chin, upper lip, and nasolabial fold.[23]

Oral hairy leukoplakia may occur in HIV-negative individuals taking cyclosporine, and gingival overgrowth is a common occurrence. This may be especially prevalent in patients with pregraft periodontitis.[91,92] Nephrotoxicity and neurotoxicity may be more severe in patients immunosuppressed with tacrolimus although gingival enlargement has not been identified in association with this drug.[93]

Recent evidence indicates that the presence or absence of pretransplant gingival hyperplasia may influence the incidence and severity of drug-induced gingival overgrowth.[92] The true incidence of cyclosporine-induced gingival enlargement is difficult to determine since the drug is often used

for organ transplant patients in combination with antihypertensive drugs such as the calcium channel blocking agent, nifedipine, also associated with gingival overgrowth.[57,94–97] Recent reports indicate that nifedipine-induced gingival overgrowth can be reversed by using alternative calcium channel blocking drugs such as amlodipine or isradipine.[98,99] Other calcium channel blockers, however, may induce increased plasma levels of cyclosporine while nifedipine does not. This may explain the frequent use of nifedipine in postrenal transplant patients.[3] Treatment for drug-induced gingival overgrowth includes establishment of effective oral hygiene and discontinuance or reduction in dosage of the causative drug, when possible. Unfortunately, surgical removal of enlarged gingivae is often necessary to facilitate patient oral hygiene measures.

New immunosuppressant drugs (sirolimus and mycophenolate mofetil) are now available as cyclosporine substitutes, when appropriate. These agents appear to induce fewer side effects, and no gingival overgrowth has been reported to date.

Dental Management

No firm protocols have been established for dental management of recipients of solid organ transplants. Periodontal disease was recently reported in 100% of 45 renal dialysis patients studied, suggesting that most patients scheduled for renal dialysis or transplantation may have oral infections which could prove life-threatening.[100] However, application of common treatment principles should facilitate safe and effective periodontal therapy. Dental and periodontal management of patients with ESRD must be carefully coordinated with the patient's physician. The dentist should participate in treatment planning and provide necessary pretreatment for patients scheduled for elective dialysis or organ transplantation. Under ideal circumstances, all potential oral foci of infection should be eliminated prior to transplant placement.[37,50,101,102] Teeth that are beyond repair and those that are suspect should be extracted although endodontic therapy may be appropriate in selected circumstances. Patients should be instructed in effective oral physiotherapy, and the use of antiseptic mouthrinses such as chlorhexidine may be appropriate.[18,28,37,103,104] Individuals who receive organ transplantation on an emergency basis and who have existing dental infection should be given antibiotics before and after the transplantation until dental treatment can be accomplished.

The potential for oral and systemic infections is quite high after transplantation because of the use of immunosuppressive drug regimens. These drugs may include cyclosporine, tacrolimus, corticosteroids, azathioprine, antilymphocyte globulin, or combinations of these. Most organ transplant recipients are maintained on immunosuppressant drugs for life to attenuate graft rejection.[3,50] Immunosuppressant drugs may mask early manifestations of oral infection, including periodontal disease.[18,23] Patients are especially susceptible to urinary tract infections with *Escherichia coli*. Most vascular access site infections occur from *S. aureus*. Occasionally, however, the oral cavity is the source of gram-negative enterococcal infections (*Pseudomonas, Proteus, Klebsiella*), fungal infections (*Candida, Aspergillus, Mucor*), or viral infections (herpes simplex, Epstein-Barr, cytomegalovirus, and others), all of which can result in life-threatening systemic sepsis.[37] Oral lesions suggestive of infection should be evaluated by cytologic examination, culture, and/or biopsy, when indicated.[105–107]

Medical complications associated with renal dialysis or transplantation must be clearly identified by obtaining a thorough medical and dental history, by evaluation of vital signs, by use of appropriate laboratory screening tests, and by medical consultation.

Drugs often used in dental practice may be retained in blood plasma for prolonged periods of time due to diminished renal function in ESRD patients. Therapeutic administration of these drugs may require adjustment of dosage or lengthening of intervals between administration. The prudent practitioner should consult the patient's physician prior to the use of any drugs.[18,28] Local anesthetics are metabolized in the liver and therefore usually safe for ESRD patients. Acetaminophen and codeine may be appropriate for postoperative analgesia, but aspirin and other NSAIDs should be avoided. Antibiotics such as aminoglycosides, tetracyclines, and polypeptides (bacitracin and polymyxin) are nephrotoxic. Potassium penicillins should not be prescribed because of their high levels of potassium salts.[27]

Patients with ESRD should be observed for signs and symptoms associated with long-term glucocorticosteroid therapy. These include excessive weight gain, moon facies, buffalo hump, abdominal striae, acne, and mental depression, or psychosis.[18] Stressful dental procedures may require corticosteroid supplementation. Recent evidence, however, suggests that the administration of low-dose corticosteroids (prednisone, 5 to 10 mg administered every other day) is not likely to induce an adrenal crisis, especially if dental procedures are performed on the alternate day. Higher levels of corticosteroids will protect the patient from adrenal deficiency and shock. Further protection against adrenal crisis may be attained by following a stress reduction protocol consisting of morning appointments, maintenance of a nonthreatening treatment environment, use of conscious sedation, attainment of profound local anesthesia, and prescription of safe and effective postoperative analgesics. Some authorities recommend doubling the usual steroid dose the day before, on the day of, and for 2 days following a stressful dental procedure. As an alternative, the dentist must be prepared to administer intravenous corticosteroid supplementation in the event of an adrenal crisis.[23,25,37]

Dental treatment should be conservative and noninvasive when possible, especially during the first 3 months after transplantation.[23] When an invasive periodontal or surgical procedure is planned, prophylactic antibiotic coverage should be considered, especially if a dialysis shunt or fistula is present.[18,23,27,28,37] Generally, the recommendations of the American Heart Association for the prevention of bacterial endocarditis are considered sufficient.[108,109] Infective endocarditis (IE) may occur in dialysis patients with no evidence of previous cardiac valvar damage.[28] Therefore, the dental practitioner should remain alert for signs and symptoms of IE, which include fever of unknown origin, malaise, unexplained elevation of white blood cells, and others.[101]

Chlorhexidine rinses prior to soft tissue manipulation may reduce the occurrence of orally induced bacteremias.[103,108,110] Several authorities have noted, however, that there are no controlled studies that establish the beneficial effect of topical or systemic prophylactic antibiotic therapy in organ transplant patients.[2,111,112] They note that antibiotic suppression of normal bacterial flora may render the patient more susceptible to enterococcal, fungal, or other opportunistic systemic infections.

Care must be taken to avoid trauma to the arteriovenous site in patients who are receiving hemodialysis either before or after renal transplantation. The arm with an anastomosis site should not be used for injection of intramuscular or intravenous medications, and the access site should not be used as a portal for injections.[23,28] Blood pressure recordings should not be obtained from the involved arm, and the arm should not be placed in a cramped position.[23,25]

The presence of a hemodialysis access site places the patient at increased risk for endarteritis induced by manipulation of periodontal tissues.

Peritoneal dialysis patients are subject to retrograde staphylococcal or streptococcal infection, but there is only a low risk of orally-induced bacteremia initiating this infection.[28,37]

Excessive and prolonged bleeding may occur in ESRD in conjunction with dialysis or following transplantation. This may be compounded in patients receiving hemodialysis because heparin is usually administered during the dialysis process to prevent clotting, and warfarin compounds (Coumadin) may be used for management of related medical complications. Patients with ESRD may have reduced platelet counts and function due to uremia, further increasing bleeding potential.[28] For these reasons, any necessary dental procedure likely to induce bleeding should be performed following medical consultation, usually on the day after dialysis to allow normal clotting, and to permit partial healing prior to the next dialysis session.[27,28] Surgical flaps should be avoided when possible, and appropriate surgical techniques should be performed (atraumatic surgery, adequate wound closure with sutures, application of postsurgical pressure with or without topical clotting agents such as gelfoam, topical thrombin, oxidized regenerated cellulose or synthetic collagen.)[18,21,25,27,28,113–115] Screening laboratory tests should be obtained prior to invasive procedures, including a complete blood count with platelets, a partial thromboplastin time, and a prothrombin time. Drugs such as 1-deamino-8-D-arginine vasopressin (DDAVP) or conjugated estrogen may be prescribed by the patient's physician to further control hemorrhage during necessary oral surgical procedures.[27,28]

Liver Diseases

Acute hepatitis may be caused by a variety of viruses, drugs, or toxins. In most circumstances, recovery occurs over time, but hepatitis B virus (HBV) infections may lead to chronic liver disease in 5 to 10% of adults and 80 to 90% of children. Chronic liver disease also develops in 70 to 90% of individuals infected with hepatitis C virus (HCV). Infection with HBV has been markedly reduced in the developed countries due to immunization against the virus, appropriate health care for infected individuals, and establishment of universal precautions against disease transmission among health care workers. Hepatitis C virus is primarily transmitted by parenteral means (blood transfusion, intravenous drug abuse, or occupational exposure to blood or blood products). In some circumstances, HCV may be community acquired in

association with risk factors such as household exposure, sexual contact, or multiple sex partners. Transmission of HCV has declined as a result of screening tests, which identify the virus in blood and blood products prior to transfusion.[116–118]

In most cases, acute viral liver infections are transient although a small percentage of infected individuals will follow a fulminant course leading to hepatic coma or death. The most significant aftermath of acute hepatic viral infection is chronic hepatic deficiency, which may lead to end-stage hepatic disease (ESHD) or development of hepatic malignancy.

Chronic hepatitis is generally described as hepatic inflammation that lasts longer than 6 months. It is most commonly caused by autoimmune hepatitis and chronic viral hepatitis.[119,120] Alternatively, the condition may be drug induced or initiated by genetic susceptibility (Wilson's disease), primary biliary cirrhosis, or primary sclerosing cholangitis. On occasion, clinical features are absent, but elevated serum aminotransferase levels may be noted. Common clinical features include fatigue, malaise, abdominal pain, and possibly jaundice. The condition may lead to liver failure, and the patient may eventually require organ transplantation. Other causes of ESHD include primary hepatocellular carcinoma without metastasis, alcoholic liver disease, acetaminophen overdose, overdose of other drugs, or toxin-induced hepatitis.[117,121]

Severe recurrent HBV infection can develop in patients suffering from chronic hepatitis B, and recurrent viremia invariably occurs in individuals who undergo transplantation due to chronic hepatitis C.[122,123] In addition to recurrent hepatitis, this often leads to liver fibrosis or cirrhosis. Recent evidence suggests that HBV is sequestered in extrahepatic tissues, especially bone marrow. This may explain why recurrent HBV occurs.[124]

Liver cirrhosis is the sequela of a wide variety of chronic progressive hepatic diseases that lead to scarring and fatty infiltration of liver tissues and disruption of normal liver architecture and function. To date, no clinical features have been recognized that invariably signify liver cirrhosis. Clinical indicators, however, include palmar erythema, spider nevi, gynecomastia, testicular atrophy, splenomegaly, ascites, esophageal varices, and xanthelasma, and the condition may ultimately lead to hepatic encephalopathy or the hepatorenal syndrome.[12,121,123] Skin bronzing is common in various types of hepatic diseases but most frequently occurs in specific forms of cirrhosis (alcoholic, primary biliary, or hemochromatosis).[123]

Liver Transplantation

Liver transplantation has become the standard of care for virtually all forms of ESHD. Absolute contraindications for transplantation include seropositivity for HIV, extrahepatic malignancy, metastatic hepatic malignancy, active sepsis, advanced cardiopulmonary disease, and active alcoholism or substance abuse.[116,117,121,123,125,126]

To avoid the need for long-term hemodialysis, patients who suffer from severe renal disease may require a combined liver-kidney transplant although individuals with severe neurologic or cardiopulmonary disease cannot withstand the stress of transplantation surgery. Increased vascular peripheral resistance may induce transient myocardial dysfunction even in individuals free of pre-existing cardiovascular disease.

Postoperative management after liver transplantation includes the use of immunosuppressant drugs (corticosteroids, azathioprine, cyclosporine, tacrolimus, or others) to help prevent organ rejection. Both cyclosporine and tacrolimus can induce nephrotoxicity, hepatotoxicity, neurotoxicity, and diabetes mellitus. Hirsutism and gingival overgrowth are not associated with tacrolimus. Patients may continue to suffer from pregraft systemic disorders such as severe cardiopulmonary disease or renal dysfunction.[127]

Complications of hepatic transplantation include nonfunction or compromised function of the implanted liver (5 to 10%), and graft rejection or infection. Candidiasis and aspergillosis infections have a high morbidity rate because they often occur in critically ill patients or those who require extremely high dosages of immunosuppressant drugs. Viral, mycobacterial, parasitic, and bacterial (*Nocardia, Legionella, Listeria*) infections become more evident a few months following transplantation, and infection with CMV is almost universal in this patient group. Immunosuppressive therapy has resulted in a marked decrease in the prevalence of irreversible graft rejection, especially if high trough levels of cyclosporine or azathioprine are sustained. Recurrent autoimmune hepatitis has been reported when immunosuppressant therapy is reduced.

Osteoporosis is common in individuals with chronic cholestatic liver disease, even following liver transplantation. Recent evidence suggests that increased bone density and elimination of vertebral fractures occurs when administration of intravenous bisphonates is initiated 3 months before transplantation and maintained for 9 months thereafter.[128]

Cyclosporine and tacrolimus are both metabolized in the liver and therefore drug interactions may occur. Ketoconazole may increase circulating levels of these immunosuppressant drugs while phenytoin reduces serum levels due to enzyme-induced enhanced metabolism. Hyperuricemia often occurs after liver transplantation, and treatment may be difficult because allopurinol alters azathioprine metabolism, and NSAIDs may adversely influence renal function.

Despite these potential complications, the 5-year survival rate for liver transplantation continues to improve. That average is currently above 80%.[125]

Dental Management

Prior to liver transplantation, the primary goal of dental intervention is to eliminate oral sepsis which could potentially lead to systemic infection and possible transplant rejection or compromise. There are many consequences of ESHD, however, which must be considered when developing a dental treatment plan for such patients. For example, the ability of the liver to metabolize drugs may be impaired. Drugs commonly used in dentistry, such as acetaminophen, narcotics, local anesthetics, benzodiazepam, barbiturates, and antibiotics (erythromycin, ampicillin), are metabolized in the liver, and these agents should be used with caution. Alternative drugs should be considered, and minimal required dosages should be administered following consultation with a physician.

Bleeding disorders are very common in patients with ESHD. This may result from a decrease in coagulation factors produced by the liver or from thrombocytopenia due to bone marrow suppression or hypersplenism. Increased clot fibrolysis may also occur. Patients with ESHD should be screened prior to invasive dental procedures by obtaining appropriate blood tests, including a complete blood count, bleeding time, prothrombin time, and partial thromboplastin time. Prothrombin times are important in evaluating the function of the clotting factors manufactured in the liver.[129] In recent years, an international reference thromboplastin (IRT) has been developed to facilitate standardized prothrombin results in all medical laboratories.[91,101,130–137] Corrected normal prothrombin time has been established with an international normalized ratio (INR) of approximately 1.0, although patients receiving anticoagulant medications may be maintained at INR levels ranging from 1.2 to 4.0.[131,132] Patients with an

INR value of 3.5 or lower can usually be managed successfully for invasive dental procedures without lowering the INR level, provided appropriate local hemostatic measures are taken.[91,130,131,134,135,137] The use of oral rinses containing tranexamic acid may be sufficient to control hemorrhage in minor surgical procedures in patients with an INR of 4.0 or less. However, extensive surgical procedures in the same patients may require additional hemostatic measures.[136,138] In ESHD patients, however, all hemorrhagic factors should be taken into consideration and those individuals with altered platelet levels (below 50,000) or INR values higher than 3.5 may need vitamin K supplementation, blood transfusion, or infusion of fresh frozen plasma or packed platelets. In all cases, selection and application of proper surgical techniques should be used as described previously.

Abnormal protein metabolism associated with hepatic failure may result in toxic levels of serum ammonia. This substance may induce asterixis, hepatic encephalopathy, coma, or death. The dental clinician must remain alert for signs or symptoms of these conditions. These may include personality changes, mood alterations, confusion and/or eventual tonic or clonic muscle activity. Altered protein metabolism may also interfere with normal wound healing. Excessive postoperative bleeding following oral procedures may induce swallowing of blood and thus a possible increase in serum ammonia levels. The patient who has undergone nonsurgical or surgical therapy should not be dismissed until clot stabilization has been achieved.[115,138]

Ascites is the accumulation of fluid in the peritoneal cavity, secondary to liver failure or portal hypertension. Bacterial peritonitis is potentially life threatening in patients with ascites and may be initiated by transient bacteremia induced by manipulation of oral soft tissues. Consequently, prophylactic antibiotic coverage is indicated for dental procedures likely to induce significant bleeding.[112,138] The antibiotic regimen recommended by the American Heart Association for prophylaxis against bacterial endocarditis is probably sufficient although some authorities recommend broad-spectrum antibiotics or metronidazole in conjunction with amoxicillin to provide protection against a broader range of bacteria.

With the exception of patients with ascites, the issue of whether or not to administer prophylactic antibiotics to patients with liver disease continues to be controversial.[2,111,112,139] No controlled studies are available to suggest that bacteremias induced by dental procedures affect the prognosis for patients with ESHD or those with liver transplants. Suppression of oral bacteria may promote sepsis from opportunistic organisms such as *Candida albicans*.[111] In any case, any oral sepsis has the potential to induce life-threatening systemic septicemia. Consequently, afflicted patients must be informed of the significance of good oral health to their survival. They must be instructed in effective oral hygiene procedures, and frequent recall intervals of 2 to 3 months should be established. These principles apply both before and after liver transplantation.

In most instances, successful organ transplantation reduces the dental treatment risks to those risks described previously in patients taking immunosuppressive drugs. It should be anticipated that solid-organ transplant patients will require these drugs indefinitely.

Pancreatic Transplantation

Pancreas transplantation is occasionally used in the treatment of type 1 diabetes mellitus. The organ is often obtained in conjunction with kidney transplantation from the same donor. Postoperative complications often occur, and the need for long-term immunosuppression adversely affects treatment outcomes.

Pancreatic transplantation may not reverse pre-existent diabetic microangiopathies, nephropathy, or retinopathy but may halt or reverse diabetic neuropathy. Under selected circumstances, the procedure may be beneficial, especially in diabetic patients who require renal hemodialysis or kidney transplantation.[140]

Lung Transplantation

Lung transplantation may be performed unilaterally, bilaterally, or as a joint heart-lung transplantation. Treatment outcomes are not yet as successful as those reported for renal and hepatic transplants although they range between 50 and 70%. Indications include emphysema, idiopathic pulmonary fibrosis, primary pulmonary hypertension, cystic fibrosis, and other rare disorders.

Availability of donor lungs is scarce, and therefore the selection of recipient candidates is restricted. Active tobacco smokers or those who inhale or smoke illicit drugs are not accepted, and no other systemic diseases should be present which may result in end-organ damage.[10,141] Potential recipients who have significant coronary artery disease, renal insufficiency, hepatic diseases, osteoporosis, or significant neurologic impairment are also excluded. Patients with a history of previous malignancy, chronic systemic illnesses (diabetes mellitus and others), or chronic unresolved infections may also be precluded from receiving lung transplantation.[142]

Heart-lung transplants may be indicated for irreparable congenital cardiac defects or simultaneous advanced heart and lung disease. Cystic fibrosis usually requires bilateral lung transplantation while unilateral organ transplants are performed when indicated for more localized pulmonary diseases.

Post-transplant complications include acute graft rejection, usually occurring within the first 3 months after placement. Bronchiolitis obliterans occurs in at least half of all patients receiving lung transplants and is the primary cause of chronic transplant rejection.[143,144] Airway stenosis may also adversely affect treatment outcomes. As in all other solid-organ transplants, infection is a major cause of mortality. This is especially true for recipients of lung transplants because the lungs are highly vulnerable to direct contact with infectious microorganisms as well as to hematologic infection. Most infections are bacterial (*Staphylococcus*), viral (CMV), or fungal (*Aspergillus*). The immunosuppressive complications previously described for other solid-organ transplants are common. These include nephrotoxicity, hypertension, hyperlipidemia, neurotoxicity, osteoporosis, and lymphoproliferative disorders. Recurrence of underlying diseases such as sarcoidosis, lymphangioleiomyomatosis, and interstitial pneumonitis have been reported.[142,145]

Dental protocols have not been established for management of post–lung transplant patients, but putative periodontal pathogenic microorganisms have been implicated in lower respiratory infections.[146] Therefore, establishment of periodontal health and elimination of any oral sepsis are imperative.[146–148] General protocols for patients using immunosuppressive drugs are also applicable.

Heart Transplantation

Cardiac transplantation is limited to patients most likely to survive the procedure and resume normal life functions. As a result, transplants are limited to individuals who have not suffered from other end-stage organ damage, those who do not have significant systemic infections (HIV seropositivity), and those without advanced systemic diseases such as diabetes mellitus or collagen vascular disease.

Tissue cross-matching between the donor and recipient is difficult due to a shortage of sufficient donors. Consequently, organ selection is based on heart size, ABO blood type matching, negative lymphocyte cross-match, and avoidance of transplantation from a CMV-positive donor to a CMV-negative recipient. As a result, prevention of organ rejection while avoiding the adverse effects of immunosuppressive drugs is essential for successful transplantation.

Transplantation may be indicated for any patient with end-stage heart disease and a prognosis for survival of 2 years or less. It is also indicated for patients with severely limited quality of life following other appropriate medical or surgical therapy. Candidates may include those with congestive heart failure, coronary artery disease (including angina pectoris and myocardial infarction), patients with hypertrophic cardiomyopathy, severe valvar defects, or intractable ventricular tachyarrhythmias.[149,150]

Exclusion criteria include individuals with active virulent infections, those with recent pulmonary infarction, severe diabetes mellitus with end-organ damage, irreversible pulmonary hypertension, active peptic ulcerations, recent or current malignancy, or cerebrovascular disease, those with active alcohol or substance abuse, or severe chronic obstructive pulmonary disease.[150]

Complications are common among post–cardiac transplant recipients. Early complications may include acute graft rejection, right side heart failure and bacterial, viral, or protozial infection. Late complications occur relative to chronic transplant rejection and lifelong administration of immunosuppressive drugs.

Chronic rejection elicits fibrointimal hyperplasia which may be aggravated by CMV infection. Successful therapeutic outcomes may allow approximately 70% restoration of maximal cardiac output during resting and exercise stages. The transplanted heart commonly remains denervated resulting in some alterations in cardiac function.[101] Angina rarely occurs during subsequent post-transplant coronary artery disease, resulting in "silent" myocardial infarction or sudden death. Less serious symptoms of immunosuppression include hypertrichosis, impotence in men, and painful menstruation in women. In general, women experience a significantly higher degree of symptomatic side effects although cyclosporine-related gingival enlargement is frequent in both sexes.[151]

Dental Management

Dental management of heart transplant patients is consistent with that previously described. However, strong evidence suggests a positive correlation between the presence of severe periodontitis and risk of myocardial infarction.[152–159] Therefore, achievement of periodontal health may be essential for successful management of recipient patients.

As discussed above, the use of immunosuppressant agents alters host response while simultaneously suppressing the inflammatory response.[11,54,160–163] Although prolonged corticosteroid therapy may lead to osteoporosis and other abnormalities in bone and periodontal fibrous tissue, available evidence suggests that destructive periodontitis is no more common among patients treated with corticosteroids than the general population. Such patients may, however, be more susceptible to primary herpetic or other viral or fungal infections.

Immunosuppression may affect bone marrow function. The resulting thrombocytopenia, anemia, and neutropenia may lead to oral hemorrhage and severe bacterial, viral, fungal, or mixed infections. The risk of infection is directly proportional to the degree and duration of the drug-induced leukopenia and anemia.[54,164–167]

Cyclosporine-induced gingival enlargement resembles other drug-induced gingival overgrowth, both clinically and histologically. The labial surfaces of anterior teeth are most frequently affected and the overgrowth usually begins within 3 months of start of treatment. The reaction may be preceded by plaque-related inflammation.[35,168] Effective plaque control and removal of local irritants, with or without the use of antimicrobial mouthrinses, may diminish the severity of cyclosporine-induced gingival enlargement,[103,104,169–172] but oral hygiene measures alone do not totally suppress gingival overgrowth.[35,61,66,82]

Prophylactic antibiotic therapy should be considered for periodontal or oral surgical procedures required during the first 6 months of recuperation following heart transplantation. If the recipient patient achieves maximal restoration of cardiac function, preventive antibiotics for dental therapy may not be required unless a requirement for a high maintenance level of immunosuppression is present.[28,112] The medical complications of organ transplantation, however, may put recipient patients at risk of orally acquired systemic sepsis. Close coordination between the patient's physician and dentist is essential; and, continuance of excellent oral health is required.[173,174]

Bone Marrow Transplantation

Bone marrow transplantation (BMT) is currently used in the treatment of leukemia, lymphoma, multiple myeloma, neuroblastoma, some solid tumors, and various forms of anemia.[76,175–181] In this procedure, autologous stem cells or bone marrow from a donor is infused into a recipient who may or may not have received chemoradiation therapy designed to eliminate the host marrow cells.

Usually, BMT grafts are obtained from a histocompatible donor, and syngeneic graft material may be taken from an identical twin. On some occasions, the patient's own marrow cells may be harvested and reimplanted following chemotherapy. It is difficult to obtain true histocompatibility in allogeneic graft procedures. Therefore, allogeneic engraftment usually initiates graft-versus-host disease (GVHD), in which the transplanted marrow cells recognize the new host as foreign and attempt rejection.[182–184]

Chemotherapy and total body irradiation may be used to destroy malignant marrow cells prior to engraftment although chemotherapy alone is currently preferred in many oncology centers. Chemoradiation therapy is usually conducted 1 to 2 weeks prior to BMT.[183,184] After infusion of donor cells, stem cells, or bone marrow, the patient is isolated for 4 to 6 weeks to minimize the risk of infection while marrow cells are revitalized and host defenses re-established.[76,179,182,185–187] Immunosuppressant drugs and granulocyte colony growth factors (GCGF) are started at the time of engraftment, and pancytopenia exists until the absolute neutrophil count exceeds 500 cells/mm^3.[188–190]

Patients who undergo BMT are at high risk for development of opportunistic viral, fungal, and bacterial infections, including putative periodontal pathogens.[191–204] Children may suffer from developmental abnormalities.[205–209] Epstein-Barr virus has been reported to induce hairy leukoplakia in HIV-negative BMT patients.[210] Recipients of BMT may also be susceptible to necrotizing ulcerative gingivitis, necrotizing stomatitis, and possibly necrotizing ulcerative periodontitis.[106] Lesions of this type during marrow suppression are best treated with gentle débridement, chlorhexidine, or povidine-iodine mouthrinses, removal of necrotic osseous and soft tissue, and antibiotic therapy administered after consultation with the oncologist.[49,169–172,195,211–213]

Graft-versus-host disease is a multisystem, potentially life-threatening phenomenon, in which the engrafted marrow reacts against the tissues of the host.[185,214] A similar condition may occasionally be induced by blood transfusion.[215–217] Up to 70% of BMT patients may be affected with acute GVHD within the first 30 days after engraftment.[218–220] Affected tissues include the liver, lungs, gastrointestinal tract, exocrine glands, skin, and mucosa.[218] Acute GVHD may induce painful, erythematous or ulcerative oral mucosal lesions. Lesions which persist for more than 1 month are considered chronic although GVHD may appear de novo months or years after engraftment.[219,221] Chronic GVHD may present with oral features suggestive of lichen planus, systemic lupus erythematosus, scleroderma, or Sjögren's syndrome.[222–224] Diagnosis is based on clinical features and biopsy findings suggestive of the mucocutaneous conditions described above.[225] Oral signs may range from mild mucosal erythema to severe mucositis, desquamative gingivitis, xerostomia, and infections.[226–229] Chemoradiation therapy–induced xerostomia may subside over time after cessation of treatment. While present, however, it may promote dental caries and mucositis.[218] On occasion, unusual oral side effects may occur, including minor salivary gland retention phenomena, verrucous xanthomas, and atypical pyogenic granulomas.[184,226,227,229,230]

Cyclosporine or tacrolimus are usually prescribed for the prevention and treatment of GVHD although successful treatment of chronic oral lesions with psoralen plus ultraviolet A (PUVA) has recently been reported.[231] It is desirable to maintain immunosuppression with the minimal quantity of drug necessary, but in the event of persistent GVHD, the dosage may be increased.

Periodontal management prior to BMT is consistent with the protocols described above. When possible, maximal oral health should be achieved prior to engraftment. However, brushing and flossing are usually discontinued immediately following chemoradiation and re-initiated only after white blood cell counts exceed 2000/mm³.[188] In the interim, oral cleansing is performed using cotton swabs, gauze sponges, soft sponge sticks, and chlorhexidine rinses.[103,232] After partial recovery, patients are managed as described for other recipients of organ transplants. Oral GVHD is usually controlled by meticulous oral hygiene, frequent dental recall visits, and use of topical or systemic corticosteroids, antifungals, and antivirals.[184,233] Mucositis may be soothed by rinsing with lukewarm saline or 5% sodium bicarbonate solution to elevate salivary pH. Other soothing mouthrinses containing kaolin, diphenhydramine, and topical anesthetics have been recommended for comfort.[234–237]

Treatment of oral infections with antibiotic combinations are often indicated to prevent gram-negative bacillary septicemia when oral or periodontal tissues must be manipulated during marrow suppression therapy. Agents such as trimethoprim and sulfamethoxazole may be recommended by the patient's oncologist.[119,237–240]

REFERENCES

1. Perlroth MG. The role of organ transplantation in medical therapy. In: Rubenstein E, Federman DD, editors. Scientific American medicine. New York: Scientific American Medicine, Inc.; 1986.
2. Glassman P, Wong C, Gish R. A review of liver transplantation for the dentist and guidelines for dental management. Spec Care Dent 1993; 13:74–80.
3. Sakurai K, Drinkwater D, Sutherland DE, et al. Dental treatment considerations for the pre- and post-organ transplant patient. J Calif Dent Assoc 1995;23:61–6.
4. Coggins CH, Rennke HG, Rose BD. Glomerulonephritis and the nephrotic syndrome. In: Dale DC, Federman DD, editors. Scientific American medicine. New York: Scientific American Medicine, Inc.; 1995.
5. Remuzzi G, Bertani T. Pathophysiology of progressive nephropathies. New Engl J Med 1998;339:1448–56.
6. Appel GB. Preventing or slowing the progression of diabetic nephropathy. BUMC Proc 1999;12:3–6.
7. Fenves AZ, Stone MJ, Johnson KB. Systemic primary amyloidosis in chronic hemodialysis. BUMC Proc 1999;12:61–4.
8. Lazarus JM, Brenner BM. Chronic renal failure. In: Harrison's Principles of internal medicine, 14th ed. New York: McGraw-Hill Co.; 1998. p. 1513–20.
9. Donohoe JF. Scleroderma and the kidney. Kidney Int 1992;41:462–77.
10. Cruz R, Davis M, O'Neil H, et al. Pulmonary manifestations of inhaled street drugs. Heart Lung 1998;27:297–305.
11. Bachman U, Biava C, Amend W, et al. The clinical course of IgA nephropathy and Henoch-Schönlein purpura following renal transplantation. Transplantation 1986;42:511–5.
12. Rees TD. Oral effects of drug abuse. Curr Rev Oral Biol Med 1992;3:163–84.
13. Butler WT, Bennett JE, Alling DW, et al. Nephrotoxicity of amphotericin B: early and late effects in 81 patients. Ann Intern Med 1964;61:175–87.
14. Lee MR. Dopamine and the kidney: ten years on. Clin Sci 1993;83:357–75.
15. Olsen NV, Hansen JM, Ladefoged SD, et al. Renal tubular resorption of sodium and water during

infusion of low-dose dopamine in normal men. Clin Sci 1990;78:503–7.

16. Zager RA. Gentamicin effects on renal ischemia/reperfusion injury. Circ Res 1992;70:20–8.

17. Black RM. Acute renal failure. In: Dale DC, Federman DD, editors. Scientific American medicine. New York: Scientific American Medicine, Inc.; 1995.

18. Naylor GD, Fredericks MR. Pharmacologic considerations in the dental management of the patient with disorders of the renal system. Dent Clin N Am 1996;40:665–83.

19. Better OS, Stein JH. Early management of shock and prophylaxis of acute renal failure in traumatic rhabdomyolysis. N Engl J Med 1990;322:825–9.

20. Zager RA, Gamelin LM. Pathogenetic mechanisms in experimental hemoglobinuric acute renal injury. Am J Physiol 1989;256:F455–66.

21. Ferguson GA, Whyman RA. Dental management of people with renal disease and renal transplants. N Z Dent J 1998;94:125–30.

22. Bookatz BN. Management of oral problems related to kidney disease and dialysis. In: McDonald RD, Hurt WC, Gilmore HW, Middleton RA, editors. Current therapy in dentistry. Vol. 7. St. Louis: C.V. Mosby Co.; 1980. p. 31–6.

23. Cohen SG. Renal disease. In: Lynch MA, Brightman VJ, Greenberg MS, editors. Burket's oral medicine, 9th ed. Philadelphia: J.B. Lippincott Co.; 1994. p. 487–509.

24. Pierce TB, Razzuk MA, Razzuk LM, Hoover SJ. A comprehensive review of the physiology of hemostasis and antithrombotic agents. BUMC Proc 1999;12:39–50.

25. Eigner TL, Jastak JT, Bennett WM. Achieving oral health in patients with renal failure and renal transplants. J Am Dent Assoc 1986;113:612–6.

26. Wactawski-Wende J, Grossi SG, Trevisan M, et al. The role of osteopenia in oral bone loss and periodontal disease. J Periodontol 1996;67:1076–84.

27. Ziccardi VB, Saini J, Demas PN, Braun TW. Management of the oral and maxillofacial surgery patient with end-stage renal disease. J Oral Maxillofac Surg 1992;50:1207–12.

28. DeRossi SS, Glick M. Dental considerations for the patient with renal disease receiving hemodialysis. J Am Dent Assoc 1996;127:211–9.

29. Glick M. Dental considerations for the patient with renal disease receiving hemodialysis. J Am Dent Assoc 1996;127:211–9.

30. Bando K, Nitta H, Matsubara M, Ishikawa I. Bone mineral density in periodontally healthy and edentulous postmenopausal women. Ann Periodontol 1998;3:322–7.

31. Grossi SG. Effect of estrogen supplementation on periodontal disease. Comp Cont Ed Dent 1998;(Suppl)22:S30–6.

32. Jeffcoat MK. Osteoporosis: a possible modifying factor in oral bone loss. Ann Periodontol 1998;3:312–21.

33. Reddy MS, Weatherford TW III, Smith CA, et al. Alendronate treatment of naturally-occurring periodontitis in beagle dogs. J Periodontol 1995;66:211–7.

34. Reeves HL, Francis RM, Manas DM, et al. Intravenous bisphosphonate prevents symptomatic osteoporotic vertebral collapse in patients after liver transplantation. Liver Transplant Surg 1998;4:404–9.

35. Seymour RA, Thomason JM, Nolan A. Oral lesions in organ transplant patients. J Oral Pathol Med 1997;26:297–304.

36. Yamalik N, Avcikurt UF, Caglayan F, Eratalay K. The importance of oral foci of infection in renal transplantation. Aust Dent J 1993;38:108–13.

37. Naylor GD, Hall EH, Terezhalmy GT. The patient with chronic renal failure who is undergoing dialysis or renal transplantation: another consideration for antimicrobial prophylaxis. Oral Surg Oral Med Oral Pathol 1988;65:116–21.

38. Alfrey AC. Phosphate, aluminum and other elements in chronic renal disease. In: Schrier RW, Gottschalk CW, editors. Diseases of the kidney, 5th ed. Boston: Little, Brown and Co.; 1991. p. 3153.

39. Tolkoff-Rubin NE. Dialysis and transplantation. In: Dale DC, Federman DD, editors. Scientific American medicine. New York: Scientific American Medicine, Inc. 1996.

40. Gotch FA, Sargent JA. A mechanistic analysis of the National Cooperative Dialysis Study. Kidney Int 1985;28:526–34.

41. Beck LH. Requiem for gouty nephropathy. Kidney Int 1986;30:280–7.

42. Schulman G, Hakim RM. Complications of hemodialysis. In: Jacobson H, Shaker K, Klahr S, editors. Principles and practice of nephrology, 2nd ed. St. Louis: C.V. Mosby Co.; 1995. p. 673.

43. Brescia MJ, Cimino JE, Appel K, Harwich BJ. Chronic hemodialysis using venipuncture and surgically created arteriovenous fistula. N Engl J Med 1966;275:1089–92.

44. Carpenter CB, Lazarus JM. Dialysis and transplantation in the treatment of renal failure. In: Fauci AS, Braunwald E, Wilson JO, et al, editors. Harrison's Principles of internal medicine, 14th ed. New York: McGraw-Hill Co.; 1998. p. 1520–9.

45. Ruskin JD, Wood RP, Bailey MR, et al. Comparative trial of oral clotrimazole and nystatin for

oropharyngeal candidiasis prophylaxis in orthotopic liver transplant patients. Oral Surg Oral Med Oral Pathol 1992;74:567–71.

46. Schubert MM, Epstein JB, Lloyd ME, Cooney E. Oral infections due to cytomegalovirus in immunocompromised patients. J Oral Pathol Med 1993;22:268–73.

47. Whitley RJ, Blum MR, Barton N, de Miranda P. Pharmacokinetics of acyclovir in humans following intravenous administration. A model for the development of parenteral antivirals. Am J Med 1982;73(Suppl 1A):165–71.

48. McCauley J. Medical complications. In: Shapiro R, Simmons RL, Starzl TE, editors. Complications of renal transplantation. Stamford, CT: Appleton & Lange; 1997. p. 299–313.

49. Finberg R, Fingeroth J. Infections in transplant recipients. In: Fauci AS, Braunwald E, Wilson JO, et al, editors. Harrison's Principles of internal medicine, 14th ed. New York: McGraw-Hill Co.; 1998. p. 840–6.

50. Kusne S, Manez R. Infectious complications. In: Shapiro R, Simmons RL, Starzl TE, editors. Complications of renal transplantation. Stamford, CT: Appleton & Lange; 1997. p. 315–32.

51. Muzyka BC, Glick M. A review of oral fungal infections and appropriate therapy. J Am Dent Assoc 1995;126:63–72.

52. Aebischer MC, Zala LB, Braathen LR. Kaposi's sarcoma as manifestation of immunosuppression in organ transplant recipients. Dermatology 1997;195:91–2.

53. al-Sulaiman MH, Mousa DH, Dhar JM, al-Khader A. Does regressed post-transplantation Kaposi's sarcoma recur following reintroduction of immunosuppression? Am J Nephrol 1992; 12:384–6.

54. Bakr MA, Sobh M, el-Agroudy A, et al. Study of malignancy among Egyptian kidney transplant recipients. Transplant Proc 1997;29:3067–70.

55. Bencini PL, Marchesi L, Cainelli T, Crosti C. Kaposi's sarcoma in kidney transplant recipients treated with cyclosporine. Br J Dermatol 1988; 118:709–14.

56. Bencini PL, Montagnino G, Sala F, et al. Cutaneous lesions in 67 cyclosporine-treated renal transplant recipients. Dermatologica 1986;172:24–30.

57. Blohme I, Larko O. No difference in skin cancer incidence with or without cyclosporine. A 5-year perspective. Transplant Proc 1992;24:313.

58. Bocchi EA, Higuchi ML, Vieira ML, et al. Higher incidence of malignant neoplasms after heart transplantation for treatment of chronic Chagas' heart disease. J Heart Lung Transplant 1998;17: 399–405.

59. Brambilla L, Boneschi V, Fossati S, et al. Vinorelbine therapy for Kaposi's sarcoma in a kidney transplant patient. Dermatology 1997;194: 281–3.

60. Bunney MH, Benton EC, Barr BB, et al. The prevalence of skin disorders in renal allograft recipients receiving cyclosporine A compared with those receiving azathioprine. Nephrol Dialysis Transplant 1990;5:379–82.

61. Eslambolchi F, Rees TD, Iacopino AM. Cyclosporine A-induced gingival enlargement. A comprehensive review. Quintessence Int 1999 [In press].

62. Euvrard S, Kanitakis J, Pouteil-Noble C, et al. Aggressive squamous cell carcinomas in organ transplant recipients. Transplant Proc 1995;27:1767–8.

63. Glover MT, Deeks JJ, Raftery MJ, et al. Immunosuppression and risk of non-melanoma skin cancer in renal transplant recipients [letter]. Lancet 1997;349:398.

64. Green C, Hawk JL. Cutaneous malignancy related to cyclosporine A therapy. Clin Exp Dermatol 1993;18:30–1.

65. Gruber SA, Gillingham K, Sothern RB, et al. De novo cancer in cyclosporine-treated and non-cyclosporine-treated adult primary renal allograft recipients. Clin Transplant 1994;8:388–95.

66. Hallmon WW, Rossmann JA. The role of drugs in the pathogenesis of gingival overgrowth. A collective review of current concepts. Periodontol 2000 1999 [In press].

67. Halmos O, Inturri P, Galligioni A, et al. Two cases of Kaposi's sarcoma in renal and liver transplant recipients treated with interferon. Clin Transplant 1996;10:374–8.

68. Hepburn DJ, Divakar D, Bailey RR, Macdonald KJ. Cutaneous manifestations of renal transplantation in a New Zealand population. N Z Med J 1994;107:497–9.

69. Hiesse C, Kriaa F, Rieu P, et al. Incidence and type of malignancies occurring after renal transplantation in conventionally and cyclosporine-treated recipients: analysis of a 20-year period in 1600 patients. Transplant Proc 1995;27:972–4.

70. Hiesse C, Larue JR, Kriaa F, et al. Incidence and type of malignancies occurring after renal transplantation in conventionally and in cyclosporine-treated recipients: single-center analysis of a 20-year period in 1600 patients. Transplant Proc 1995;27:2450–1.

71. Jordan ML. Malignancy after renal transplantation. In: Shapiro R, Simmons RL, Starzl TE, editors. Complications of renal transplantation. Stamford, CT: Appleton & Lange; 1997. p. 353–82.

72. London NJ, Farmery SM, Will EJ, et al. Risk of

neoplasia in renal transplant patients. Lancet 1995;346:403–6.

73. Margiotta V, Florena AM, Giuliana G. Primary angiosarcoma of the alveolar mucosa in a haemodialysis patient: case report and discussion. J Oral Pathol Med 1994;23:429–31.

74. Margolius I, Stein M, Spencer D, Bezwoda WR. Kaposi's sarcoma in renal transplant recipients. Experience at Johannesburg Hospital, 1966-1989. S African Med J 1994;84:16–7.

75. Masuhara M, Ogasawara H, Katyal SL, et al. Cyclosporine stimulates hepatocyte proliferation and accelerates development of hepatocellular carcinomas in rats. Carcinogenesis 1993;14:1579–84.

76. Maxymiw WG, Wood RE. The role of dentistry in patients undergoing bone marrow transplantation. Br Dent J 1989;167:229–34.

77. Maxymiw WG, Wood RE, Lee L. Primary, multifocal, non-Hodgkin's lymphoma of the jaws presenting as periodontal disease in a renal transplant patient. Int J Oral Maxillofac Surg 1991;20:69–70.

78. Merot Y, Miescher PA, Balsiger F, et al. Cutaneous malignant melanomas occurring under cyclosporine A therapy: a report of two cases. Br J Dermatol 1990;2:237–9.

79. Montagnino G, Bencini PL, Tarantino A, et al. Clinical features and course of Kaposi's sarcoma in kidney transplant patients: report of 13 cases. Am J Nephrol 1994;14: 121–6.

80. Ozen S, Saatci U, Karaduman A, et al. Kaposi's sarcoma in a paediatric renal transplant recipient. Nephrol Dialysis Transplant 1996;11:1162–3.

81. Penn I. Cancers in cyclosporine-treated vs azathioprine-treated patients. Transplant Proc 1996;28: 876–8.

82. Rees TD. Drugs and oral disorders. Periodontol 2000 1998;18:21–36.

83. Regev E, Zeltser R, Lustmann J. Lip carcinoma in renal allograft recipient with long-term immunosuppressive therapy. Oral Surg Oral Med Oral Pathol 1992;73:412–4.

84. Sabeel A, Qunibi W. Recurrent Kaposi's sarcoma in a renal transplant recipient maintained on minimum doses of immunosuppression [letter]. Neph Dialysis Transplant 1998;13:1609–10.

85. Thomas DW, Seddon SV, Shepherd JP. Systemic immunosuppression and oral malignancy: a report of a case and review of the literature. Br J Oral Maxillofac Surg 1993;31:391–3.

86. Veness MS. Cardiac transplant-related cutaneous malignancies in an Australian recipient: immunosuppression, friend or foe? Clin Oncol 1998;10:194–7.

87. Jonas S, Rayes N, Neumann U, et al. De novo malignancies after liver transplantation using tacrolimus-based protocols or cyclosporine-based quadruple immunosuppression with an interleukin-2 receptor antibody or antihymocyte globulin. Cancer 1997;6:1141–50.

88. Lipkowitz GS, Madden RL. Transmission of Kaposi's sarcoma by solid organ donation. Transplant Sci 1994;4:9–11.

89. Sheil AG, Disney AP, Mathew TH, Amiss N. De novo malignancy emerges as a major cause of morbidity and late failure in renal transplantation. Transplant Proc 1993;25:1383–4.

90. Varga E, Tyldesley WR. Carcinoma arising in cyclosporine-induced gingival hyperplasia. Br Dent J 1991;171:26–7.

91. Patton LL, Ship JA. Treatment of patients with bleeding disorders. Dent Clin North Am 1994; 38:465–82.

92. Varga E, Lennon M, Mair L. Pre-transplant gingival hyperplasia predicts severe cyclosporine-induced gingival overgrowth in renal transplant patient. J Clin Periodontol 1998;25:225–30.

93. Adams CK, Famili P. A study of the effects of FK506 on gingival tissues. Transplant Proc 1991;23:3193–4.

94. Nery E, Edson R. Prevalence of nifedipine-induced gingival hyperplasia. J Periodontol 1995;66: 572–8.

95. Ryman K, Pharm D, Gurk-Turner C. Pharmacology notes—calcium channel blocker review. BUMC Proc 1999;12:34–6.

96. Thomason JM, Seymour RA, Ellis JS, et al. Determinants of gingival overgrowth severity in organ transplant patients. An examination of the role of HLA phenotype. J Clin Periodontol 1996; 23:628–34.

97. Wilson RF, Morel A, Smith D, et al. Contribution of individual drugs to gingival overgrowth in adult and juvenile renal transplant patients treated with multiple therapy. J Clin Periodontol 1998;25:457–64.

98. Jorgensen MG. Prevalence of amlodipine-related gingival hyperplasia. J Periodontol 1997;68:676–8.

99. Westbrook P, Bednarczyk EM, Carlson M, et al. Regression of nifedipine-induced gingival hyperplasia following switch to a same class calcium channel blocker, isradipine. J Periodontol 1997;68:645–50.

100. Naugle K, Darby ML, Bauman DB, et al. The oral heath status of individuals on renal dialysis. Ann Periodontol 1998;3:197–205.

101. Rees TD, Rose LF. Periodontal management of patients with cardiovascular diseases. J Periodontol 1996;67:627–35.

102. Slots J. Casual or causal relationship between periodontal infection and non-oral disease: [guest editorial] J Dent Res 1998;77:1764–5.

103. Ciancio SG. Expanded and future uses of mouthrinses. J Am Dent Assoc 1994;125: 29S–32S.

104. Ciancio SG, Bartz NW, Lauciello FR. Cyclosporine-induced gingival hyperplasia and chlorhexidine—a case report. Int J Periodont Restor Dent 1991;11:241–5.

105. MacPhail LA, Hilton JF, Heinic GS, Greenspan D. Direct immunofluoresence vs. culture for detecting HSV in oral ulcers: a comparison. J Am Dent Assoc 1995;126:74–8.

106. Rees TD. Periodontal considerations in the management of the cancer patient. J Periodontol 1997;68:791–801.

107. Samaranayake LP, MacFarlane TW, Lamey PJ, Ferguson MM. A comparison of oral rinse and imprint sampling techniques for the detection of yeast, coliform and *Staphylococcus aureus* carriage in the oral cavity. J Oral Pathol 1986; 15:386–8.

108. Dajani AS, Taubert KA, Wilson W, et al. Prevention of bacterial endocarditis. J Am Med Assoc 1997;277:1794–801, Circulation 1997;96: 358–66.

109. Lamas WP. A study of transient bacteremia following an intraoral soft tissue biopsy [MS Thesis]. Baylor College of Dentistry; 1998.

110. Rutkauskas JS, Davis JW. Effects of chlorhexidine during immunosuppressive chemotherapy. A preliminary report. Oral Surg Oral Med Oral Pathol 1993;76:441–8.

111. Douglas LR, Douglass JB, Sieck JO, Smith PJ. Oral management of the patient with end-stage liver disease and the liver transplant patient. Oral Surg Oral Med Oral Pathol Oral Radiol Endod 1998;86:55–64.

112. Little JW, Rhodus NL. Dental treatment of the liver transplant patient. Oral Surg Oral Med Oral Pathol 1992;73:419–26.

113. Mulligan R, Weitzel KG. Pretreatment management of the patient receiving anticoagulant drugs. J Am Dent Assoc 1988;117:479–83.

114. Okamoto GU, Duperon DF. Bleeding control after extractions in a patient with aplastic anemia during bone marrow transplantation: report of case. ASDC J Dent Child 1989;56:50–5.

115. Rossmann JA, Rees TD. The use of hemostatic agents in dentistry. Postgrad Dent 1996;3(3): 3–12.

116. Keeffe EB. Chronic hepatitis. In: Dale DC, Federman DD, editors. Scientific American medicine. New York: Scientific American Medicine, Inc.; 1998.

117. Keeffe EB. Acute hepatitis. In: Dale DC, Federman DD, editors. Scientific American medicine. New York: Scientific American Medicine, Inc.; 1998.

118. Lodi G, Porter SR, Scully C. Hepatitis C virus infection: review and implications for the dentist. Oral Surg Oral Med Oral Pathol Oral Radiol Endod 1998;86:8–22.

119. Semba SE, Mealey BL, Hallmon WW. Dentistry and the cancer patient. Part 2. Oral health management of the chemotherapy patient. Comp Cont Educ Dent 1994;15:1378–88.

120. Sempoux C, Horsmans Y, Lerut J, et al. Acute lobular hepatitis as the first manifestation of recurrent autoimmune hepatitis after orthotopic liver transplantation. Liver 1997;17:311–5.

121. Keeffe EB. Cirrhosis of the liver. In: Dale DC, Federman DD, editors. Scientific American medicine. New York: Scientific American Medicine, Inc.; 1998.

122. Belli LS, Silini E, Alberti A, et al. Hepatitis C virus genotypes, hepatitis and hepatitis C virus recurrence after liver transplantation. Liver Transplant Surg 1996;2:200–5.

123. Podolsky DK, Isselbacher KJ. Major complications of cirrhosis. In: Fauci AS, Braunwald E, Wilson JO, et al, editors. Harrison's Principles of internal medicine, 14th ed. New York: McGraw-Hill Co.; 1998. p. 1710–25.

124. Ilan Y, Galun E, Nagler A, et al. Sanctuary of hepatitis B virus in bone marrow cells of patients undergoing liver transplantation. Liver Transplant Surg 1996;2:206–10.

125. Dienstag J. Liver transplantation. In: Fauci AS, Braunwald E, Wilson JO, et al, editors. Harrison's Principles of internal medicine, 14th ed. New York: McGraw-Hill Co.; 1998. p. 1721–5.

126. Isselbacher KJ, Podolsky DK. Infiltrative and metabolic diseases affecting the liver. In: Fauci AS, Braunwald E, Wilson JO, et al, editors. Harrison's Principles of internal medicine, 14th ed. New York: McGraw-Hill Co.; 1998. p. 1717–20.

127. Sampathkumar P, Lerman A, Kim BY, et al. Post-liver transplantation myocardial dysfunction. Liver Transplant Surg 1998;4:399–403.

128. Ludwig J, Hashimoto E, Porayko MK, Therneau TM. Failed allografts and causes of death after orthotopic liver transplantation from 1985 to 1995: decreasing prevalence of irreversible hepatic allograft rejection. Liver Transplant Surg 1996;2:185–91.

129. Bussey HI, Force RW, Bianco TM, Leonard AD. Reliance of prothrombin time ratios causes significant errors in anticoagulation therapy. Arch Intern Med 1992;152:278–82.

130. Carr MM, Mason RB. Dental management of anticoagulated patients. J Can Dent Assoc 1992;58:838–44.

131. DeClerck D, Vinckier F, Vermylen J. Influence of anticoagulation on blood loss following dental extractions. J Dent Res 1992;71:387–90.

132. Hirsh J, Dalen JE, Deykin D, Poller L. Oral anticoagulants. Mechanism of action, clinical effectiveness, and optimal therapeutic range. Chest 1992;102(Suppl 4):312s–326s.

133. International Committee for Standardization in Haematology and International Committee on Thrombosis and Haemostasis. ICSH/ICTH recommendations for reporting prothrombin time in oral anticoagulant control. J Clin Pathol 1985;38:133–4.

134. Lippert S, Gutschik E. Views of cardiac-valve prosthesis patients and their dentists on anticoagulation therapy. Scand J Dent Res 1994;102:168–71.

135. Martinowitz U, Mazar AL, Taicher S, et al. Dental extraction for patients on oral anticoagulant therapy. Oral Surg Oral Med Oral Pathol 1990;70:274–7.

136. Purcell CAH. Dental management of the anticoagulated patient. N Z Dent J 1997;93:87–92.

137. Ramstrom G, Sindet-Pedersen S, Hall G, et al. Prevention of postsurgical bleeding in oral surgery using tranexamic acid without dose modification of oral anticoagulants. J Oral Maxillofac Surg 1993;51:1211–6.

138. Rakocz M, Mazar A, Varon D, et al. Dental extractions in patients with bleeding disorders. Oral Surg Oral Med Oral Pathol 1993;75:280–2.

139. Cutler LS. Evaluation and management of the dental patient with a history of hepatitis, jaundice, or liver disease. J Conn State Dent Assoc 1985; 59:115–7.

140. Carithers RL, Perkins JD. Liver and pancreas transplantation. In: Dale DC, Federman DD, editors. Scientific American medicine. New York: Scientific American Medicine, Inc.; 1998.

141. Caiffa WT, Vlahov D, Graham NMH. Drug smoking, *Pneumocystis carinii* pneumonia, and immunosuppression increase risk of bacterial pneumonia in HIV-seropositive injection drug users. Am J Respir Crit Care Med 1994;150:1493–8.

142. Maurer JR. Lung transplantation. In: Fauci AS, Braunwald E, Wilson JO, et al, editors. Harrison's Principles of internal medicine, 14th ed. New York: McGraw-Hill Co.; 1998. p. 1491–3.

143. Hohlfeld J, Niedermeyer J, Hamm H, et al. Seasonal onset of bronchiolitis obliterans syndrome in lung transplant recipients. J Heart Lung Transplant 1996;15:888–94.

144. Sundaresan S, Trulock EP, Mohanakumar T, et al. Prevalence and outcome of bronchiolitis obliterans syndrome after lung transplantation. Washington University Lung Transplant Group. Ann Thorac Surg 1995;60:1341–6.

145. Maurer JR, Tewari S. Nonpulmonary medical complications in the intermediate and long-term survivor [review]. Clin Chest Med 1997; 18:367–82.

146. Scannapieco FA, Mylotte JM. Relationships between periodontal disease and bacterial pneumonia. J Periodontol 1996;67:1114–22.

147. Hayes C, Sparrow D, Cohen M, et al. The association between alveolar bone loss and pulmonary function: the VA dental longitudinal study. Ann Periodontol 1998;3:257–61.

148. Limeback H. Implications of oral infections on systemic diseases in the institutionalized elderly with a special focus on pneumonia. Ann Periodontol 1998;3:262–75.

149. Bourke JP, Loaiza A, Parry G, et al. Role of orthotopic heart transplantation in the management of patients with recurrent ventricular tachyarrhythmias following myocardial infarction. Heart 1998;80:473–8.

150. Schroeder JS. Cardiac transplantation. In: Fauci AS, Braunwald E, Wilson JO, et al, editors. Harrison's Principles of internal medicine, 14th ed. New York: McGraw-Hill Co.; 1998. p. 1298–300.

151. Moons P, De Geest S, Abraham I, et al. Symptom experience associated with maintenance immunosuppression after heart transplantation: patients' appraisal of side effects. Heart Lung 1998;27:315–25.

152. Beck JD, Offenbacher S, Williams R, et al. Periodontitis: a risk factor for coronary heart disease? Ann Periodontol 1998;3:127–41.

153. Herzberg MC, Meyer MW. Dental plaque, platelets, and cardiovascular diseases. Ann Periodontol 1998;3:151–60.

154. Herzberg MC, Meyer MW. Effects of oral flora on platelets: possible consequences in cardiovascular disease. J Periodontol 1996;67:1138–42.

155. Joshipura KJ, Douglas CW, Willett WC. Possible explanations for the tooth loss and cardiovascular disease relationship. Ann Periodontol 1998;3:175–83.

156. Kinane DF. Periodontal diseases' contribution to cardiovascular disease: an overview of potential mechanisms. Ann Periodontol 1998;3:142–50.

157. Lowe GDO. Etiopathogenesis of cardiovascular disease: hemostasis, thrombosis, and vascular medicine. Ann Periodontol 1998;3:121–6.

158. Mealey BL. Influence of periodontal infections on systemic health. Periodontol 2000 1999 [In press].

159. Page RC. The pathobiology of periodontal diseases may affect systemic diseases: inversion of a paradigm. Ann Periodontol 1998;3:108–20.

160. Bader G, Lejeune S, Messner M. Reduction of cyclosporine-induced gingival overgrowth following a change to tacrolimus. A case history involving a liver transplant patient. J Periodontol 1998;69:729–32.

161. Baldwin L, Henderson A, Hickman P. Effect of postoperative low-dose dopamine on renal function after elective major vascular surgery. Ann Intern Med 1994;120:744–7.

162. Mattsson T, Arvidson K, Heimdahl A, et al. Alterations in test acuity associated with allogeneic bone marrow transplantation. J Oral Pathol Med 1992;21:33–7.

163. Niehaus CS, Meiller TF, Peterson DE, Overholser CD. Oral complications in children during cancer therapy. Cancer Nurs 1987;10:15–20.

164. Bressman E, Decter JA, Chasens AI, Sackler RS. Acute myeloblastic leukemia with oral manifestations. Report of a case. Oral Surg Oral Med Oral Pathol 1982;54:401–3.

165. Brown AT, Shupe JA, Sims RE, et al. *In vitro* effect of chlorhexidine and amikacin on oral gram-negative bacilli from bone marrow transplant recipients. Oral Surg Oral Med Oral Pathol 1990;70:715–9.

166. Brown AT, Sims RE, Raybould TP, et al. Oral gram-negative bacilli in bone marrow transplant patients given chlorhexidine rinses. J Dent Res 1989;68:1199–204.

167. Peters E, Monopoli M, Woo SB, Sonis S. Assessment of the need for treatment of postendodontic asymptomatic periapical radiolucencies in bone marrow transplant recipients. Oral Surg Oral Med Oral Pathol 1993;76:45–8.

168. Bartold PM. Cyclosporine and gingival overgrowth. J Oral Pathol 1988;16:463–8.

169. Ferretti GA, Ash RC, Brown AT, et al. Chlorhexidine for prophylaxis against oral infections and associated complications in patients receiving bone marrow transplants. J Am Dent Assoc 1987;114:461–7.

170. Ferretti GA, Hansen IA, Whittenburg K, et al. Therapeutic use of chlorhexidine in bone marrow transplant patients: case studies. Oral Surg Oral Med Oral Pathol 1987;63:683–7.

171. Flaitz CM, Hammond HL. The immunoperoxidase method for the rapid diagnosis of intraoral herpes simplex virus infection in patients receiving bone marrow transplants. Spec Care Dent 1988;8:82–5.

172. Fleming P. Dental management of the pediatric oncology patient. Curr Opin Dent 1991;1:577–82.

173. Montgomery MT, Redding SW, LeMaistre CF. The incidence of oral herpes simplex virus infection in patients undergoing cancer chemotherapy. Oral Surg Oral Med Oral Pathol 1986;61:238–42.

174. Poland J. Prevention and treatment of oral complications in the cancer patient. Oncology 1991;5: 45–50,52,57,61–2.

175. Attal M, Harousseau JL, Stoppa AM, et al. A prospective, randomized trial of autologous bone marrow transplantation and chemotherapy in multiple myeloma. N Engl J Med 1996;335:91–7.

176. Berkowitz RJ, Strandjord S, Jones P, et al. Stomatologic complications of bone marrow transplantation in a pediatric population. Pediatric Dent 1987;9:105–10.

177. Cooper B. New concepts in management of acute leukemia. BUMC Proc 1990;3:31–3.

178. Devine SM, Larson RA. Acute leukemia in adults: recent developments in diagnosis and treatment. CA Cancer J Clin 1994;44:326–52.

179. Greenberg MS, Garfunkel A. Hematologic disease. In: Lynch MA, Brightman VJ, Greenbert MS, editors. Burket's Oral medicine 9th ed. Philadelphia: J.B. Lippincott Co.; 1994. p. 510–8.

180. Lazarchik DA, Filler SJ, Winkler MP. Dental evaluation in bone marrow transplantation. Gen Dent 1995;43: 369–71.

181. Vose JM, Kennedy BC, Bierman PJ, et al. Long-term sequelae of autologous bone marrow or peripheral stem cell transplantation for lymphoid malignancies. Cancer 1992;69:784–9.

182. Armitage JO. Bone marrow transplantation. In: Fauci AS, Braunwald E, Wilson JO, et al, editors. Harrison's Principles of internal medicine, 14th ed. New York: McGraw-Hill Co.; 1998. p. 724–30.

183. Collins RH, Miller GW, Fay JW. Autologous bone marrow transplantation: a review. BUMC Proc 1991;4:3–12.

184. Rhodus NL, Little JW. Dental management of the bone marrow transplant patient. Comp Cont Educ Dent 1992;13:1042–50.

185. Dahllöf G, Heimdahl A, Modéer T, et al. Oral mucous membrane lesions in children treated with bone marrow transplantation. Scand J Dent Res 1989;97:268–77.

186. Seto BG, Kim M, Wolinsky L, et al. Oral mucositis in patients undergoing bone marrow transplantation. Oral Surg Oral Med Oral Pathol 1985;60:493–507.

187. Wescott WB. Dental management of patients being treated for oral cancer. CDA J 1985;13:42–7.

188. American Dental Association. Patients receiving cancer chemotherapy. Chicago: American Dental Association; 1989.

189. Birek C, Patterson B, Maximiw WC, Minden MD. EBV and HSV infections in a patient who had undergone bone marrow transplantation: oral manifestations and diagnosis by in situ nucleic acid hybridization. Oral Surg Oral Med Oral Pathol 1989;68:612–7.

190. Childers NK, Stinnett EA, Wheeler P, et al. Oral complications in children with cancer. Oral Surg Oral Med Oral Pathol 1993;75:41–7.

191. Barasch A, Mosier KM, D'Ambrosio JA, et al. Postextraction osteomyelitis in a bone marrow transplant recipient. Oral Surg Oral Med Oral Pathol 1993;75:391–6.

192. Barrett AP, Schifter M. Antibiotic strategy in orofacial/head and neck infections in severe neutropenia. Oral Surg Oral Med Oral Pathol 1994;77:350–5.

193. Cutler LS. Evaluation and management of the dental patient with cancer. I. Complications associated with chemotherapy or bone marrow transplantation. J Conn State Dent Assoc 1987;61:236–8.

194. Epstein JB, Sherlock CH, Page JL, et al. Clinical study of herpes simplex virus infection in leukemia. Oral Surg Oral Med Oral Pathol 1990;70: 38–43.

195. Kolbinson DA, Schubert MM, Flournoy N, Truelove EL. Early oral changes following bone marrow transplantation. Oral Surg Oral Med Oral Pathol 1988;66:130–8.

196. Mattsson T, Heimdahl A, Dahllöf G, et al. Oral and nutritional status in allogeneic marrow recipients treated with T-cell depletion or cyclosporine combined with methotrexate to prevent graft-versus-host disease. Oral Surg Oral Med Oral Pathol 1992;74:34–40.

197. Nikoskelainen J. Oral infections related to radiation and immunosuppressive therapy. J Clin Periodontol 1990;17:504–7.

198. Peterson DE, Minah GE, Overholser CD, et al. Microbiology of acute periodontal infection in myelosuppressed cancer patients. J Clin Oncol 1987;5:1461–8.

199. Redding SW, Montgomery MT. Acyclovir prophylaxis for oral herpes simplex virus infection in patients with bone marrow transplants. Oral Surg Oral Med Oral Pathol 1989;67:680–3.

200. Schubert MM, Peterson DE, Flournoy N, et al. Oral and pharyngeal herpes simplex virus infection after allogeneic bone marrow transplantation: analysis of factors associated with infection. Oral Surg Oral Med Oral Pathol 1990;70:286–93.

201. Schuchter LM, Wingard JR, Piantadosi S, et al. Herpes zoster infection after autologous bone marrow transplantation. Blood 1989;74:1424–7.

202. Shearer BH, Hay KD. Hard and soft tissue oral changes following bone marrow transplantation. N Z Dent J 1987;83:103–4.

203. Thurmond JM, Brown AT, Sims RE, et al. Oral *Candida albicans* in bone marrow transplant patients given chlorhexidine rinses: occurrence and susceptibilities to the agent. Oral Surg Oral Med Oral Pathol 1991;72:291–5.

204. Wade JC, Newton B, McLaren C, et al. Intravenous acyclovir to treat mucocutaneous herpes simplex virus infection after marrow transplantation: a double blind study. Ann Intern Med 1982;96:265–9.

205. Dahllöf G, Barr M, Bolme P, et al. Disturbances in dental development after total body irradiation in bone marrow transplant recipients. Oral Surg Oral Med Oral Pathol 1988;65:41–4.

206. Dahllöf G, Forsberg CM, Ringdén O, et al. Facial growth and morphology in long-term survivors after bone marrow transplantation. Eur J Orthod 1989;11:332–40.

207. Dahllöf G, Krekmanova L, Kopp S, et al. Craniomandibular dysfunction in children treated with total-body irradiation and bone marrow transplantation. Acta Odontol Scand 1994;52:99–105.

208. Dahllöf G, Modéer T, Bolme P, et al. Oral health in children treated with bone marrow transplantation: a one-year follow-up. ASDC J Dent Child 1988;55:196–200.

209. Dahllöf G, Rozell B, Forsberg CM, Borgström B. Histologic changes in dental morphology induced by high dose chemotherapy and total body irradiation. Oral Surg Oral Med Oral Pathol 1994;77:56–60.

210. Epstein JB, Sherlock CH, Wolber RA. Hairy leukoplakia after bone marrow transplantation. Oral Surg Oral Med Oral Pathol 1993;75:690–5.

211. Ellegaard B, Bergmann OJ, Ellegaard J. Effect of plaque removal on patients with acute leukemia. J Oral Pathol Med 1989;18:54–8.

212. Epstein JB, Vickars L, Spinelli J, Reece D. Efficacy of chlorhexidine and nystatin rinses in prevention of oral complications in leukemia and bone marrow transplantation. Oral Surg Oral Med Oral Pathol 1992;73:682–9.

213. Raether D, Walker PO, Bostrum B, Weisdorf D. Effectiveness of oral chlorhexidine for reducing

stomatitis in a pediatric bone marrow transplant population. Pediatr Dent 1989;11:37–42.

214. Eggleston TI, Ziccardi VB, Lumerman H. Graft-versus-host disease: case report and discussion. Oral Surg Oral Med Oral Pathol Oral Radiol Endod 1998;86:692–6.

215. LeVeque FG. An unusual presentation of chronic graft-versus-host disease in an unrelated bone marrow transplantation. Oral Surg Oral Med Oral Pathol 1990;69:581–4.

216. Williams MC, Lee GT. Childhood leukemia and dental considerations. J Clin Pediatr Dent 1991;15:160–4.

217. Williamson LM. Transfusion associated graft versus host disease and its prevention [editorial]. Heart 1998;80:211–2.

218. Curtis JW Jr, Caughman GB. An apparent unusual relationship between rampant caries and graft-versus-host disease. Oral Surg Oral Med Oral Pathol 1994;78:267–72.

219. Heimdahl A, Johnson G, Danielsson KH, et al. Oral condition of patients with leukemia and severe aplastic anemia. Follow-up one year after bone marrow transplantation. Oral Surg Oral Med Oral Pathol 1985;60:498–504.

220. Woo S-B, Lee SJ, Schubert MM. Graft-vs-host disease. Crit Rev Oral Biol Med 1997;8:201–16.

221. LeVeque FG, Ratanatharathorn V, Danielsson KH, et al. Oral cytomegalovirus infection in an unrelated bone marrow transplantation with possible mediation by graft-versus-host disease and the use of cyclosporine A. Oral Surg Oral Med Oral Pathol 1994;77:248–53.

222. Barrett AP. Graft-versus-host disease. A clinico-pathologic review. Ann Dent 1987;46:7–11.

223. Heimdahl A, Mattsson T, Dahllöf G, et al. The oral cavity as a port of entry for early infections in patients treated with bone marrow transplantation. Oral Surg Oral Med Oral Pathol 1989;68:711–6.

224. Hiroki A, Nakamura S, Shinohara M, Oka M. Significance of oral examination in chronic graft-versus-host disease. J Oral Pathol Med 1994;23: 209–15.

225. Johnson ML, Farmer ER. Graft-versus-host reactions in dermatology. J Am Acad Dermatol 1998;38:369–92.

226. Allen CM, Kapoor N. Verruciform xanthoma in a bone marrow transplant recipient. Oral Surg Oral Med Oral Pathol 1993;75:591–4.

227. Barrett AP. Gingival lesions in leukemia. A classification. J Periodontol 1984;55:585–8.

228. Jones LR, Toth BB, Keene HJ. Effects of total body irradiation on salivary gland function and caries-associated oral microflora in bone marrow transplant patients. Oral Surg Oral Med Oral Pathol 1992;73:670–6.

229. Wandera A, Walker PO. Bilateral pyogenic granuloma of the tongue in graft-versus-host disease: report of a case. ASDC J Dent Child 1994;61: 401–3.

230. Lee L, Miller PA, Maxymiw WG, et al. Intraoral pyogenic granuloma after allogeneic bone marrow transplant. Report of three cases. Oral Surg Oral Med Oral Pathol 1994;78:607–10.

231. Redding SW, Callander NS, Haveman CW, Leonard DL. Treatment of oral chronic graft-versus-host disease with PUVA therapy: case report and literature review. Oral Surg Oral Med Oral Pathol Oral Radiol Endod 1998;86:183–7.

232. Lefkoff MA, Beck FM, Horton JE. The effectiveness of a disposable tooth cleansing device on plaque. J Periodontol 1995;66:218–21.

233. Wingard JR, Niehaus CS, Peterson DE, et al. Oral mucositis after bone marrow transplantation. A marker of treatment toxicity and predictor of hepatic veno-occlusive disease. Oral Surg Oral Med Oral Pathol 1991;72:419–24.

234. Borowski B, Benhamou E, Pico JL, et al. Prevention of oral mucositis in patients treated with high-dose chemotherapy and bone marrow transplantation: a randomized controlled trial comparing two protocols of dental care. Eur J Cancer B Oral Oncol 1994;30B:93–7.

235. Fay JT, O'Neal R. Dental responsibility for the medically compromised patient. J Oral Med 1984;39:148–56.

236. National Institutes of Health. National Institutes of Health consensus development conference statement: oral complications of cancer therapies: diagnosis, prevention, and treatment. J Am Dent Assoc 1989;119:179–83.

237. Rosenberg SW. Oral care of chemotherapy patients. Dent Clin N Am 1990;34:239–50.

238. Carl W. Managing the oral manifestations of cancer therapy. Part II. Chemotherapy. Comp Cont Educ Dent 1988;9:376–86.

239. Cheatham BD, Henry RJ. A dental complication involving *Pseudomonas* during chemotherapy for acute lymphoblastic leukemia. J Clin Pediatr Dent 1994;18:215–7.

240. O'Sullivan EA, Duggal MS, Bailey CC, et al. Changes in the oral microflora during cytotoxic chemotherapy in children being treated for acute leukemia. Oral Surg Oral Med Oral Pathol 1993;76:161–8.

CHAPTER 14

BLEEDING DISORDERS

Spencer W. Redding, DDS, MEd
Carl W. Haveman, DDS, MS

The tissues of the oral cavity are supported by a rich and varied blood supply. Therefore, it is common for abnormalities of the hemostatic system to present with manifestations in the oral cavity. Multiple oral manipulations including periodontal surgery, scaling and root planing, extractions, and biopsies require an intact coagulation system for normal hemostasis. Patients with gingivitis and periodontal disease are particularly vulnerable to bleeding disorders because of the increased vascularity associated with inflammation. Certainly, surgical procedures in these patients subject them to bleeding problems; however, spontaneous bleeding can also occur in sites of significant tissue inflammation. Therefore, it is necessary for the periodontist to have a good working knowledge of the hemostatic mechanism and be prepared to manage locally and, when necessary, systemically patients with diseases of hemostasis. This chapter will discuss the most common causes of oral bleeding and will include material on the appropriate management of these patients.

NORMAL HEMOSTASIS

The evaluation and treatment of patients with bleeding disorders or of patients who present with abnormal bleeding require a basic understanding of the normal physiology of hemostasis. This process is quite complex, involving numerous blood and tissue products, but all activity can be divided into three phases: the vascular phase, the platelet phase, and the coagulation phase. These three phases must work together to achieve adequate clot formation.

The vascular phase is initiated immediately following injury to a blood vessel. Mediation by the autonomic nervous system results in direct vasoconstriction in the area of the injured vessel. Adjacent vessels are also involved in this vasoconstriction process. Blood flow to the area is slowed, resulting in a reduction of blood loss following injury.[1,2]

The platelet phase is also initiated after trauma to blood vessels and results in the circulating platelets attaching to the site of injury in a process termed "platelet adhesion." Other substances that contribute to this process of platelet adhesion include subendothelial collagen, platelet receptors, fibronectin, thrombospondin, and Factor VIII von Willebrand's. Platelet adhesion initiates a process whereby more circulating platelets clump to the initial group of platelets. This process, termed "platelet aggregation," requires substances both internal and external to the functioning platelet. These substances include thromboxane A2, adenosinediphosphate (ADP), and thrombin. The platelet phase is extremely critical in stopping bleeding from small vessels as these small platelet plugs formed in this process can occlude vessels up to 50 microns in diameter.[1,2]

The coagulation phase is the final and most involved of the three phases. It, too, is initiated by the process of vascular injury and results in multiple blood proteins or factors being activated. These factors then activate other factors in a process that is termed the "coagulation cascade." Thrombin is formed as a result of this cascade, and fibrin is formed from the combination of thrombin and fibrinogen. Fibrin is the substance that makes up the stabilized clot at the end of the coagulation process. Prothrombin is converted to thrombin by activated Factor X which results from two different pathways. The intrinsic pathway involves components contained within the blood itself and includes factors XII, XI, IX, and VIII. The extrinsic pathway is activated by substances that are external to the blood, called tissue thromboplastins and includes factor VII. Integrity of both pathways is necessary for normal clot formation. After a clot is formed and stabilized, it is broken down over a period of time. This process, called "fibrinolysis," is initiated even while the clot is being formed. A substance from the blood vessel endothelium, called tissue plasminogen activator (TPA), stimulates the release of plasmin, which dissolves the clot. Both circu-lating factors and plasmin are inactivated by proteins and removed from the circulation by the reticuloendothelial system. This process limits clot formation and lysis to the site of the injury. Figure 14–1 provides a systematic representation of the multiple processes and how they interrelate for normal hemostasis. Even though the three phases of hemostasis are described here as

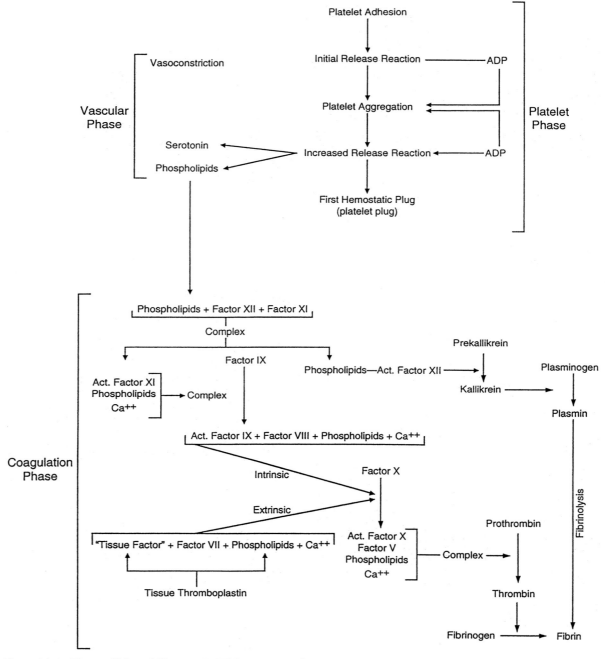

Figure 14–1. Phases of Normal Hemostasis. With permission from Montgomery MT, Redding SW, editors. Oral-facial emergencies. Chicago: Federation of Special Care Organizations in Dentistry; 1994.

separate processes for ease of understanding, it is still imperative to realize that there is multiple interrelation of these three phases. For example, phospholipids released from the platelet phase are necessary for the normal activation of factors in the coagulation phase, and thrombin is required for the smooth functioning of platelet aggregation. All three phases and their interrelation are necessary for normal clot formation.

BLEEDING DISORDERS

Vascular Disorders

Any disruption in the three phases of hemostasis or in their interaction can result in a significant bleeding disorder.[1,2] Vascular disorders other than from trauma are relatively rare. However, the possibility of abnormal and prolonged bleeding must be considered in a person whose hemostatic system is normal but in whom a large vessel has been inadvertently traumatized leading to copious bleeding. Vascular wall abnormalities do occur and include hereditary hemorrhagic telangiectasia and certain deficiency diseases. Hereditary hemorrhagic telangiectasia is an autosomal-dominant inherited disorder characterized by multiple small vascular malformations found on epithelial surfaces (Figure 14–2). When traumatized, these lesions may bleed. Treatment focuses on topical control of the hemorrhage. Steroid therapy may reduce the incidence of bleeding.

Long-term systemic steroid use can induce vascular friability. Also, elderly individuals may manifest senile purpura as a result of a loss of protective fat from the cutaneous vascular bed. Many healthy women, especially in the older age group, will complain of easy bruising.[2]

Platelet Disorders

Platelet disorders can be divided into primary and secondary forms. Primary diseases include idiopathic thrombocytopenic purpura (ITP), thrombotic thrombocytopenic purpura (TTP), and thrombasthenia.

Idiopathic thrombocytopenic purpura presents as a chronic disease characterized by autoimmune platelet destruction. Over 50% of all cases of ITP are without known cause, but ultimately it is determined that many patients have underlying autoimmune diseases such as systemic lupus erythematosus. It has also been recognized increasing-

ly as a complication of HIV infection. In adults, ITP is a chronic disease that waxes and wanes. However, in children, the disease has an acute and usually self-limiting course. It frequently follows minor viral infections. The onset of bleeding problems in patients with ITP may be either insidious or abrupt. These patients present with a reduced platelet count and easy bleeding. Treatment for ITP usually includes prednisone therapy. Splenectomy is performed in patients who fail to respond after 2 to 3 weeks. Another treatment available for ITP is intravenous immune globulin.[3,4]

Thrombotic thrombocytopenic purpura is a relatively rare form of thrombocytopenia, which results in a decreased platelet number and paradoxically widespread platelet thrombi that form in the microcirculation. Some cases involve infectious, genetic or immunologic etiologies, but the cause in most cases is unknown. Major clinical manifestations include thrombocytopenia which may result in severe bleeding, microangiopathic hemolytic anemia, neurologic signs and symptoms including headache, disorientation, seizures, coma, and focal neurologic signs, renal abnormalities including proteinuria and hematuria, and fever. In addition to thrombocytopenia, diagnosis of this disease can be made by looking for microscopic clots in vessels from a gingival biopsy. Unlike ITP, the prognosis for TTP is poor, with up to 50% mortality. Therapy has been highly unpredictable. Initially, prednisone therapy is started, followed by plasmaphoresis with plasma exchange or infusion of fresh frozen plasma. Second-line treatments may

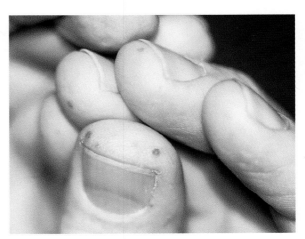

Figure 14–2. Photograph of vascular lesions on fingers associated with hereditary hemorrhagic telangiectasia. With permission from Montgomery MT, Redding SW, editors. Oral-facial emergencies. Chicago: Federation of Special Care Organizations in Dentistry; 1994.

include heparin, aspirin, vincristine, and splenectomy. Platelet transfusions are contraindicated since they may exacerbate the thrombotic component.[4,5]

Primary functional platelet abnormalities are rare. Thrombasthenia, or Glanzmann's thrombasthenia, is an unusual autosomal recessive disease, which shows platelet abnormalities characterized by a structural loss of platelet membrane substances. Platelet count and morphology are normal in this disorder. Treatment of thrombasthenia is often not necessary. However, any platelet-inhibiting drugs, including aspirin, should be avoided. Treatment for severe bleeding involves transfusion of normal platelets.[4,6]

Secondary causes of platelet abnormalities, especially thrombocytopenia, are much more common than primary abnormalities. Any process or condition that either depresses bone marrow function or increases platelet destruction may produce thrombocytopenia. Causes of these abnormalities include antineoplastic chemotherapy, severe liver and renal disease, and nonsteroidal anti-inflammatory drugs. Antineoplastic chemotherapy is toxic to normal bone marrow function; thus, megakaryocyte production is decreased, resulting in lowered platelet counts (Figure 14–3). Patients with severe end-stage liver disease and severe end-stage kidney disease present with both qualitative and quantitative platelet defects. Platelet function is affected by continuous ingestion of high amounts of ethanol in chronic alcoholics and by circulating toxins sec-

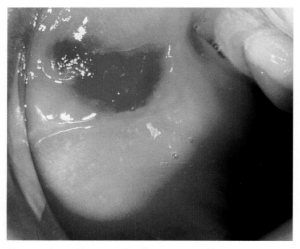

Figure 14–3. Photograph of hematoma of buccal mucosa in a patient who is severely thrombocytopenic from cancer chemotherapy. With permission from Montgomery MT, Redding SW, editors. Oral-facial emergencies. Chicago: Federation of Special Care Organizations in Dentistry; 1994.

ondary to liver or kidney failure. Hypersplenism as a result of portal hypertension secondary to alcoholic cirrhosis results in increased splenic sequestration and a drop in platelet count. Nonsteroidal anti-inflammatory drugs, such as aspirin and ibuprofen, block the conversion of arachidonic acid to thromboxane. Thromboxane accelerates the platelets' release of ADP, which is needed for platelet aggregation; therefore, blocking the formation of thromboxane will reduce the release of ADP and impair platelet aggregation. Nonsteroidal anti-inflammatory drugs thus prolong the bleeding time. It is important to note that aspirin's effect will be exerted on the platelet for its entire lifespan. However, the effect of drugs such as ibuprofen is only for the duration of drug therapy.[4,7]

Coagulation Disorders

Hemophilias

Three disorders account for more than 95% of congenital disorders of blood coagulation. These include the two sex-linked disorders, hemophilia A or factor VIII deficiency and hemophilia B or factor IX deficiency, and the autosomal von Willebrand disease.

Hemophilia A is caused by a deficiency of factor VIII. The diagnosis of hemophilia A is often made from observance of clinical bleeding and a prolonged partial thromboplastin time (PTT) and then an abnormal factor VIII assay. Hemarthrosis is the most characteristic disabling hemorrhage in these patients. Multiple hemarthroses tend to lead to joint swelling and ultimately joint collapse, with marked limitation or complete loss of motion. The disease is characterized by clinical bleeding, which is classified as severe, moderate, or mild, depending on the frequency of hemorrhage and the severity. The severity is usually related to the plasma level of factor VIII. Severely affected individuals tend to have two or three bleeding episodes per month which may be profuse unless treated (Figure 14–4). Moderately affected individuals tend to bleed five to six times per year and may have prolonged periods of free bleeding. Mildly affected individuals may rarely bleed at all, except with significant trauma or surgical stress. Generally, severe hemophiliacs have less than 1% of normal factor VIII, moderate hemophiliacs have between 1 and 5%, and mild hemophiliacs have between 5 and 30%. Inhibitors to factor VIII develop in up to 20% of patients treated with factor VIII. The presence of inhibitors may make it very difficult to treat patients who have bleeds or to provide prophylaxis to patients who are being treated surgically. Inhibitors can often be suppressed but if they are high, patients may not respond to any replacement therapy, making clinical bleeding truly life threatening.[8,9,10]

Hemophilia B—factor IX deficiency or Christmas disease—also results in an increased PTT and a reduced factor IX assay. Types and complications of hemorrhages in hemophilia B are similar to those in hemophilia A. As in factor VIII disease, level of factor IX is indicative of severity of disease, and disease is also described as mild, moderate, or severe.[8,11]

Von Willebrand disease is probably the most commonly diagnosed inherited bleeding disorder in adults because its manifestations are less severe than factor VIII or factor IX disease and often would not have been previously diagnosed. It is an autosomal disease (autosomal dominant in the most common forms but autosomal recessive in the most severe form) and is characterized by reduced levels of factor VIII along with qualitative platelet abnormalities. There are several different molecules related to factor VIII that are important in the understanding of von Willebrand disease. These include factor VIII (VIII), factor VIII von Willebrand's (vWf), and factor VIII von Willebrand antigen (vWf:Ag). Factor VIII von Willebrand's circulates in plasma as a complex with factor VIII. It acts as a carrier for factor VIII and helps promote adhesion of the platelets to the subendothelium and to one another. Therefore, in addition to its role in coagulation, vWf plays a significant part in primary hemostasis or the platelet phase. Therefore, von Willebrand disease will be marked by an increased PTT and a prolonged bleeding time. Von Willebrand disease is divided into three different types, on the basis of the presence of different levels of factor VIII, vWf, and vWf:Ag. (The blood levels of these molecules can vary over time in the same patient. Therefore, testing patients may be needed on more than one occasion to make an accurate diagnosis.) Type I is the most common form of the disease, where patients have reduced levels of all three of the above molecules. Type II variants are marked by differing combinations of normal and reduced levels of these molecules. Bleeding in types I and II is usually much less severe than with severe factor VIII disease. Bleeding from mucous membranes, including from the nasal, intestinal and uterine mucosa, is common as is bruising following minor trauma. Bleeding typically follows minor injury or surgery. Therefore, this disease may be first diagnosed in an adult who has had a minor surgical procedure such as dental surgery. In type

III disease, factor VIII levels are below 10% of normal, and both vWf and vWf:Ag are absent. Type III is the most severe of the von Willebrand types clinically and may involve bleeding into joints and soft tissue.[8,12]

Factor XI disease, or hemophilia C, is an inherited autosomal recessive disease and is usually found in individuals of Jewish ancestry. In these patients, PTT is prolonged and diagnosis is made with a factor XI assay. Most patients are asymptomatic throughout their lives and are diagnosed following postoperative bleeding. Bleeding after tooth extraction is a common first presenting symptom.[8,13]

Management of patients with inherited coagulation disorders will be discussed under "Treatment."

Anticoagulation

The number of patients receiving anticoagulation, especially with Coumadin (warfarin sodium), has increased dramatically in recent years. These patients include those with prosthetic heart valves, chronic atrial fibrillation, or a past history of deep vein thrombosis, transient ischemic attacks, or stroke. Coumadin anticoagulation is an effective and convenient therapy because it can be given orally. Coumadin acts by inhibiting the vitamin-K-dependent carboxylation of factors II, VII, IX, and X (the so-called vitamin-K-dependent factors). Carboxylation of these factors is needed because without this activation, these factors are left out of the coagulation process. As will be explained later

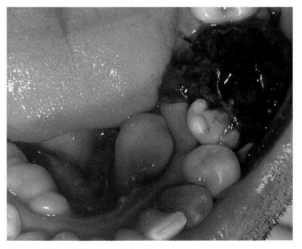

Figure 14–4. Photograph of liver clot after tooth extraction in a patient with hemophilia A. With permission from Montgomery MT, Redding SW, editors. Oral-facial emergencies. Chicago: Federation of Special Care Organizations in Dentistry; 1994.

under the section on treatment, Coumadin anticoagulation is evaluated by prothrombin time (PT) and international normalized ratio (INR). With the increasing number of patients on Coumadin anticoagulation, the potential complication of abnormal bleeding is significant. Patients respond differently to the same dose of Coumadin and must be monitored routinely to ensure that their PT and INR are within the appropriate range. Patients on Coumadin who present to emergency rooms with abnormal intraoral bleeding secondary to an extraction or chronic periodontal disease are among the most difficult of patients to manage. Patients often do not understand the potential side effects of the drugs they are taking. Therefore, Coumadin anticoagulation problems should be considered in any patient that reports with abnormal bleeding.[1,8,14]

Heparin anticoagulation is commonly used in the inpatient setting. Heparin acts by accelerating antithrombin III, which inhibits coagulation factors throughout the cascade in both the intrinsic and extrinsic pathways. Heparin is administered subcutaneously or intravenously and is monitored by PTT.[1]

Liver Disease

The liver is the site of production of fibrinogen, factors II, VII, VIII, IX, X, XII, and XIII as well as antithrombin III. Severe liver disease may result in reduced synthesis of any or all of these factors. Diseases such as alcoholic cirrhosis, chronic hepatitis (especially hepatitis C), and others can result in a significant decrease in these clotting factors. These diseases will be marked by an increase in PT and PTT. The vitamin-K-dependent factors (II, VII, IX, and X) are the most sensitive to liver disease and may be the only abnormalities in mild early hepatic disease. Conversely, factors V and VIII are the most resistant to hepatocellular disease and are only decreased in fulminant hepatitis and severe liver failure. Therefore, a decreased level of factor VIII is an ominous sign.[1,8]

Hemorrhage in patients with severe liver disease can be overwhelming. Bleeding can occur spontaneously from mucous membranes, skin, and other sites. Complications of chronic liver disease, such as varices and gastritis, may become life threatening when complicated by abnormalities of hemostasis. Because of coagulation defects and platelet abnormalities, patients with severe liver disease can be the most difficult to manage with regard to bleeding associated with surgical procedures. In patients with the most severe end-stage liver disease, liver transplantation becomes the only viable therapy. Table 14–1 provides a quick reference for the appropriate characteristics of bleeding disorders.

PATIENT EVALUATION

History

The most important factor in identifying patients with potential defects in hemostasis is patient history. Patients should be asked, through questionnaires and interviews, about any past abnormal bleeding. Any patient that presents with abnormal bleeding should be investigated further to try to determine any past history or any incident that is suspicious. Table 14–2 is a group of appropriate questions to ask the patient who presents with abnormal bleeding.[1]

Laboratory Evaluation

Four screening laboratory tests are commonly used to evaluate patients with suspicion of abnormal hemostasis: PT, PTT, the platelet count, and bleeding time.

Prothrombin time and partial thromboplastin time are commonly ordered together and both evaluate the coagulation phase of hemostasis. Prothrombin time evaluates the extrinsic pathway and is commonly elevated in patients taking Coumadin anticoagulant medication. Platelet phospholipid is added to the patient's blood, and the time is recorded until clotting occurs. Prothrombin time has been standardized in the United States by use of INR, which will be discussed in more detail under "Treatment." The normal value for PT is usually 11 to 14 seconds and is compared with a standard control. Partial thromboplastin time assesses the intrinsic pathway and is elevated with hemophilia A, B, C, and von Willebrand disease. Tissue phospholipid is added to the patient's blood, and time is recorded until clotting occurs. The normal range for this test is between 25 and 35 seconds, and the results are also reported in comparison with a standard control. As mentioned earlier, patients who are taking heparin anticoagulation are often evaluated with PTT.[1,2]

The platelet count evaluates the platelet phase of coagulation and indicates the number of platelets present. It does not evaluate qualitative platelet defects but only quantitative ones. Often, a platelet evaluation will be included with a complete blood count (CBC) but not a specific platelet

TABLE 14–1. Characteristics of Bleeding Disorders

Disorders	Dysfunction — Platelets Number	Function	Coagulation Intrinsic	Extrinsic	Signs and Symptoms Petechiae	Ecchymosis	Epistaxis	Gingival Bleeding	Hemarthrosis	Laboratory Tests BT	PC	PT	PTT
Platelets													
ITP	+	−	−	−	+	+	+	+	−	+	+	−	−
TTP	+	−	−	−	+	+	+	+	−	+	+	−	−
Thrombasthenia	−	+	−	−	+	+	+	+	−	+	−	−	−
NSAIDs/Aspirin	−	+	−	−	+	±	+	+	−	+	−	−	−
Secondary TP	+	−	−	−	+	+	+	+	−	+	+	−	−
Coagulation													
Hemophilia A	−	−	+	−	−	+	±	±	+	−	−	−	+
Hemophilia B	−	−	+	−	−	+	±	±	+	−	−	−	+
Coumadin	−	−	−	+	−	+	±	±	−	−	−	+	−
Heparin	−	−	+	−	−	+	±	±	−	−	−	−	+
Coagulation and Platelets													
von Willebrand disease	−	+	+	−	+	+	+	+	−	+	−	−	+
Alcoholism	+	+	+	−	+	+	+	+	−	+	+	−	+

ITP = idiopathic thrombocytopenic purpura; TTP = thrombotic thrombocytopenic purpura; NSAIDs = nonsteroidal anti-inflammatory drugs; TP = thrombocytopenic purpura; BT = bleeding time; PC = platelet count; PT = prothrombin time; PTT = partial thromboplastin time; + = affected by disorder; − = not affected by disorder
With permission from Montgomery MT, Redding SW. Oral-facial emergencies. Chicago: Federation of Special Care Organizations in Dentistry; 1994.

count. Therefore, this may need to be ordered separately from the CBC. The normal platelet count is between 150,000 and 400,000/mm^3.[1,2]

The bleeding time test evaluates the platelet phase of hemostasis and also the vascular phase. This test evaluates the platelet's ability to clot small vessels up to 50 microns in diameter. Therefore, when it is combined with the platelet count, questions concerning the platelet phase of hemostasis can be answered. This test is performed by making a standardized incision, 1 mm deep and 9 mm long, on the flexor surface of the forearm, distal to a blood pressure cuff on the arm inflated to 40 mm of mercury. Because of the standardization of this test, only smaller vessels are affected. These incisions are blotted every 30 seconds until no blood is absorbed. The normal range of the bleeding time is 3 to 9 minutes, and bleeding is normally stopped after 20 minutes if it persists. Bleeding times between 9 and 20 minutes would be prolonged, though functional. Beyond 20 minutes, the platelet phase of hemostasis would be considered incompetent.[1,2] In recent years, some authors have questioned the value of the bleeding time in predicting clinically significant bleeding.[15] However, it remains the only screening test for disorders of platelet function and vascular disorders.

If patients present with a history of abnormal bleeding, and the screening tests described above are abnormal, more specific tests need to be ordered to make the diagnosis of the bleeding problem. An abnormal PTT or PT may lead to a further evaluation of levels of coagulation factors using specific factor assays to determine which factor is responsible. The normal range of individual factor assays is between 50 to 150% of normal and the most commonly ordered factor is factor VIII.[1,2]

Patients who develop inhibitors to factor VIII are evaluated by the Bethesda assay with the Bethesda Unit (BU) being the standard unit of measurement. Patients with inhibitors are divided into low responders (those who will always have inhibitor levels of less than 20 BU) and high responders (those who will have an inhibitor level of greater than 20 BU at least once). Low responders make up 25% of inhibitor patients, with high responders making up 75%.[10]

TABLE 14–2. Hemostasis Questionnaire

1. Have any of the following members of your family ever had a problem with prolonged or unusual bleeding: parents, brothers and sisters, children, grandparents, great grandparents?
2. Have you ever had marked bleeding for up to 24 hours after a surgical procedure (ie, tooth extraction or tonsillectomy)?
3. Have you ever required a blood transfusion after surgery?
4. Women: Do you feel that you have abnormal bleeding during menstruation?
5. Do you get bruises larger than the size of a quarter for which you cannot remember the injury?
6. Do you experience numerous and severe nose bleeds for up to several hours?
7. Do your gums often bleed not related to trauma or brushing?
8. Are you taking any blood thinner (anticoagulant)?
9. Have you taken any medication, such as pills, powders, or liquids, in the last week?
10. Have you had or do you have any liver disease such as hepatitis or alcoholic cirrhosis?

With permission from Montgomery MT, Redding SW. Oral-facial emergencies. Chicago: Federation of Special Care Organizations in Dentistry; 1994.

TREATMENT

Prevention of untoward bleeding is the best form of "treatment." Obtaining a good history is the best single screening procedure to identify a patient with a bleeding or clotting disorder. Comprehensive extraoral and intraoral examinations are likewise important in discovering clinical signs of an occult bleeding or clotting disorder. No surgical procedures should be performed on a patient suspected of having a coagulation disorder. Such patients should be referred to a physician for screening laboratory tests and final diagnosis. When a patient is known to have a bleeding or clotting disorder, it is essential that their hematologist be consulted concerning appropriate medical management prior to performing any procedures that could result in bleeding. When periodontal surgical procedures are anticipated, the surgeon must take into consideration the fact that the mucoperiosteal flaps on the lingual aspect of the mandible may open up fascial planes into which blood can accumulate and endanger the airway.

A person with an occult coagulation disorder may not have any subjective or objective findings suggestive of the condition. The first indication of the problem may be prolonged bleeding following a dental procedure. During any episode of prolonged bleeding, local measures are the first line of defense to control hemorrhage. These local measures include pressure, topical agents, and stents.[1]

Pressure

Prior to attempting any local measures, it is critical to visualize the source of the bleeding in a clear field with a good intraoral light source. Once the source and severity of the bleeding have been identified, firm manual pressure should be applied with a moist gauze sponge pack for a minimum of 5 minutes. It is imperative that the pressure be applied to the actual bleeding site and that the size of the gauze pack correspond to the size of the bleeding site. Proper pressure is essential to controlling abnormal bleeding. Slowing of the blood flow greatly enhances the process of platelet aggregation and the formation of a platelet plug. Placing sutures across wound margins or across extraction sites may assist in maintaining hemostasis by stabilizing and providing pressure to the tissue responsible for the bleeding. If the bleeding is controlled with pressure, it is advisable to observe the patient for an additional 5 to 10 minutes to confirm hemostasis. Patients should be given both verbal and written postoperative instructions concerning prevention of recurrent bleeding. They should also be supplied with extra gauze packs and instructed on the proper placement and use of the packs.

Topical Agents

Clinicians who treat patients with bleeding disorders need to have sufficient local hemostatic agents available to treat the anticipated bleeding and be prepared to deal with any unexpected complications. When local pressure is inadequate to control bleeding, topical hemostatic agents should be employed to augment the pressure. Oxidized cellulose (Oxycel®, Surgicel®) is one such agent. Its mechanism of action is unclear; however, it physically absorbs blood and promotes clot formation. It should be applied dry and loosely placed, not packed, into the bleeding site and held in place with sterile gauze for 1 to 8 minutes. It is an absorbable hemostatic agent available as a woven fabric that resorbs in 7 to 14 days. It is also bactericidal in vitro against a variety of both gram-positive and gram-negative organisms. It should be noted that according to some authors the acidic nature of oxidized cellulose agents may result in postoperative pain.[16]

Another routinely used topical agent is absorbable gelatin sponge (Gelfoam®). It is a water-insoluble, porous, pliable sponge material prepared from purified pig skin. Its hemostatic action occurs because it absorbs the blood and provides an increased area for clot formation. It can be applied dry or moistened with normal saline and it should be pressed into place with finger pressure and held for 1 to 2 minutes. It is absorbed within 6 weeks. Gelatin sponge does not possess bacteriostatic properties and has been reported to act as a nidus for infection and therefore should not be used in the presence of infection. If it is used in an infected extraction site, impregnating it with tetracycline powder may be beneficial.

Additional topical agents consist of absorbable purified bovine collagen. Hemostatic activity is an inherent property of collagen. When it comes into contact with blood, platelets aggregate in large numbers on the collagen and release coagulation factors enabling the formation of fibrin. Several physical forms of purified bovine collagen are available. One such product is Avitene®, which is a microfibrillar collagen available as an off-white, fluffy, finely fibrous, water-insoluble material with a highly open structure. It can be applied directly to the bleeding surface with dry cotton forceps, then pressed and held in place with a sterile sponge. As soon as it comes into contact with blood, it attracts platelets, which triggers further platelet aggregation and initiates the formation of a platelet plug. It is absorbed in 4 to 6 weeks.

Other absorbable purified bovine collagen products available specifically for dental surgery are CollaTape®, CollaCote®, and CollaPlug®. These are soft, white, pliable, nonfriable sponges. They retain their structural integrity even when wet and their application to wounds is easily controlled. They are highly absorbent, holding blood or solution that is many times their own weight. The sponge structure provides a three-dimensional matrix for additional strength of the blood clot. A piece of CollaTape® or CollaCote® large enough to cover the bleeding wound surface should be held in place for 2 to 5 minutes and subsequently can be removed or left in place. If desired, a periodontal packing can be used to hold it in place. A CollaPlug® is bullet shaped and designed to be placed into an extraction site. It can be held in place with gentle pressure using a sterile Q-tip. These products should not be used on infected wounds. They are, however, very valuable for controlling persistent bleeding from tooth sockets.

Another useful topical agent is thrombin (Thrombogen®), supplied as a sterile powder. The powder also contains calcium chloride and comes with a vial of isotonic saline for use as a diluent. Thrombin requires no intermediate physiologic agent for its action. It converts the fibrinogen of the blood directly into fibrin. Its failure to clot blood occurs in the rare case where the primary clotting defect is due to the absence of fibrinogen itself. The speed with which topical thrombin clots blood depends upon its concentration. The desired strength for dental applications is 100 to 1000 U/mL. It is useful wherever any oozing from small vessels is accessible. It can be applied topically either in its powder form or diluted in isotonic saline or sterile water after the bleeding surface has been sponged or blotted free of blood. It must never be injected or otherwise allowed to enter large blood vessels. Wiping or suctioning the treated surface should be avoided in order that the clot remain securely in place.

Thrombin may also be used in conjunction with Gelfoam® or the Colla® products either in the powder or liquid form. When used as a powder, the Gelfoam® or Colla® product should be moistened with sterile saline or water and then touched to the powder to pick up a light coating of the particles. When used in the diluted form, the Gelfoam® or Colla® product should be saturated with the thrombin solution. With either method, the combination is then applied to the bleeding area and held in place for about 15 seconds with a sterile Q-tip or a small gauze sponge. Thrombin should not be used with oxidized cellulose since its acidity will render the topical thrombin ineffective.

Suturing with a resorbable material may also be very beneficial to controlling hemorrhage. Primary closure should be achieved, if possible. Even without primary closure, sutures place slight pressure on the tissue and may assist in keeping topical agents in place, especially when placed as a figure-of-eight suture across an extraction site into which Gelfoam® or a CollaPlug® has been placed. Another local measure to aid in controlling hemostasis is the injection of a local anesthetic with a vasoconstrictor such as lidocaine 2% with 1:100,000 or 1:50,000 epinephrine. However, caution must be exercised while using this technique as bleeding may resume when the effects of the vasoconstrictor end.

Custom-fabricated acrylic or plastic stents or latex mouthguard appliances may also prove helpful in controlling hemorrhage and in preventing the mechanical displacement of the clot.[1] Care is required during stent construction to avoid excessive pressure on soft tissues, which could result in necrosis. An acrylic or plastic stent can be used to retain CollaTape® or Surgicel® in place over a palatal wound, such as a free gingival or connective tissue graft donor site, while at the same time providing protection of the wound from trauma. When the patient has a known bleeding diathesis, a prefabricated soft latex mouthguard type of appliance may be used to apply a topical agent. Avitene® may be delivered in this type of appliance when generalized bleeding from the gum tissue or gingival sulcus is anticipated. Such an appliance can also be used to hold CollaTape® in place on bleeding sites. These appliances combine the light pressure from the appliance with the hemostatic effects of the topical agents. They should be worn until hemostasis has been maintained for several hours and subsequently only if needed; however, they require cleaning at least once each day because they can promote sepsis.

The choice of a topical agent is somewhat dependent upon the type of bleeding abnormality. Surgicel®, Gelfoam®, and thrombin are useful in most patients with persistent bleeding whereas the absorbable collagen products are more effective for those patients who have a platelet dysfunction or deficiency. It should be noted that many patients are on aspirin anticoagulation therapy, especially those having suffered a heart attack or stroke. Aspirin therapy alone is not usually associated with serious prolonged oral bleeding. In the vast majority of cases, a bleeding tendency from aspirin therapy can be controlled with the local measures cited. If a topical agent is necessary, one of the collagen products should be chosen. A listing of the above topical agents, a source for procurement, and the approximate cost for each can be found in Table 14–3.

Anticoagulants

Anticoagulants are needed to prevent thrombosis and embolism. By far the most widely used is warfarin sodium (Coumadin). A consultation with the patient's physician is essential in the dental management of patients on anticoagulant therapy. Information needed from the physician includes verification of the information obtained from the patient, recent dose modifications, planned duration of anticoagulant therapy, and current laboratory values. Since the early 1940s, prothrombin time (PT) developed by Quick has been the primary means of monitoring the level of oral anticoagulation control. Hematologists have recommended that the level of anticoagulation be one

and a half to three times the control value to prevent thrombosis. The ratio of the patient's PT to a laboratory control PT is termed the prothrombin time ratio or (PTR). Because of the variations in dose response in individual patients during the course of anticoagulant therapy, their dosage must be monitored closely to prevent overdosing or underdosing. In the 1970s, it was found that there were wide differences in the PTR from one laboratory to another. These differences occurred because of the variation in sensitivity of the thromboplastin reagents the laboratories used to perform PT. This meant that some patients were being anticoagulated to a greater extent than others and were prone to having more significant bleeding complications. Because of these variations, the World Health Organization recommended that the PTR be standardized using the International Normalized Ratio (INR) that is based on the sensitivity of different thromboplastin reagents (International Sensitivity Index [ISI]). The INR=PTR^{ISI} results in the INR being essentially the same, regardless of which thromboplastin reagent a laboratory uses.[17] Clinical research supports using the INR over the PTR and it is currently recommended that the INR be used to monitor the level of anticoagulation. Table 14–4 gives the recommended therapeutic range for oral anticoagulation therapy using INR values.[18,19]

Patients receiving oral anticoagulation therapy may present challenging management situations. The American Medical Association and the American Dental Association previously recommended a PT of between 1.5 and 2.5 times the control PT before performing a surgical procedure. Presently, the literature is undecided on the acceptable INR level to perform extractions. Values between 1.5 and 4.0 have been recommended.[19,20] There is concern that reduction or elimination of anticoagulant therapy places the patient at an unacceptable risk of thromboembolism. In assessing risk, clinicians need to weigh the probability of embolism occurring if anticoagulant therapy is reduced. Subtherapeutic anticoagulation levels in patients with a mechanical valve prosthesis entails a significant risk of valve thrombosis.[19] Withdrawal of anticoagulant therapy is not needed for most patients to safely undergo most dental procedures. Dental treatment planning dividing full arch procedures into multiple smaller procedures, using infiltration, periodontal ligament, or intraosseous injections in place of block anesthesia, when practical, and using local hemostatic measures can significantly reduce the risk to the patient by avoiding

TABLE 14–3. Topical and Antifibrinolytic Hemostatic Agents

Agent	Source	Approximate Cost (US dollars)
Surgicel®	Johnson and Johnson Medical Inc. Arlington, TX 76004-3130 (800-255-2500)	$133.00/box of 12 (0.5 × 2.0 inch)
Gelfoam®	Pharmacia & Upjohn Kalamazoo, MI 49001 (800-253-8600)	$23.00/Jar (15 Squares)
Avitene®	Med Chem Products Inc. Subsidiary of C.R. Bard Inc. Woburn, MA 01801 (800-451-4716)	$43.00/0.5 gram pack
CollaPlug® CollaTape® CollaCote®	Calcitek\ Sulzer Medica 2320 Faraday Avenue Carlsbad, CA 92008 (800-854-7019)	$ 63.00/package of 10 $110.00/package of 10 $ 71.00/package of 10
Thrombogen®	Johnson and Johnson Medical Inc. Arlington, TX 76004-3130 (800-255-2500)	$46.00/box (10,000 units)
Amicar®	Immunex 51 University Street Seattle, WA 98101 (800-334-6273)	$ 345.00/480 mL bottle
Cyclokapron®	Pharmacia & Upjohn Kalamazoo, MI 49001 (800-442-4348)	$225.00/10 ampules (10mL/100 mg/mL)

anticoagulation therapy modification. Table 14–5 gives our recommendations with regard to dental treatment and degree of anticoagulation as measured by INR values.

A variety of medications can affect anticoagulant therapy (Table 14–6). Salicylates and nonsteroidal anti-inflammatory drugs should be avoided entirely in patients on anticoagulant therapy. Even acetaminophen should be used with caution. A recent study found a highly significant dose-response relationship between acetaminophen and Coumadin's effect. For patients who reported taking at least four 325-mg tablets per day for longer than 1 week, the odds of having an INR greater than 6.0 were increased tenfold compared with those taking no acetaminophen.[21] Although some antibiotics can adversely affect Coumadin therapy, antibiotic prophylaxis against infective endocarditis is unlikely to affect the patient's anticoagulation status.[19]

Patients in whom the risk of thromboembolism is less of a problem and who need to have their INR values lowered can be managed by discontinuation of their Coumadin dose approximately 48 hours prior to the surgery and restarting it on the day of surgery. The INR should always be checked on the morning of the surgery to ensure it is within an acceptable range. For patients at high risk of thromboembolism, an alternative approach is to discontinue Coumadin and introduce heparin to achieve a PTT of 1.5 to 2.0 times the control, midway between injections. Heparin prevents the conversion of prothrombin to thrombin. It has a short half-life of approximately 90 minutes but its duration of action is dose dependent.[22] It should be discontinued for 4 to 6 hours before surgery and resumed 12 to 24 hours after surgery. Coumadin is resumed on the day of surgery and is continued

TABLE 14–4. Recommended Therapeutic Ranges Using INR Values[18,19,20]

Indication	INR Range
Prophylaxis of venous thrombosis	2.0 to 3.0
Treatment of venous thrombosis	2.0 to 3.0
Prevention of systemic embolism	2.0 to 3.0
Treatment of pulmonary embolism	2.0 to 3.0
Mechanical prosthetic heart valves	2.5 to 3.5

until the INR returns to an optimal range. This method usually requires hospitalization and is very expensive. Because heparin can only be administered parenterally, it is unlikely that patients on heparin therapy will be encountered in other than a hospital-based dental practice.

Of note are the new low-molecular-weight heparins (LMWHs), including ardeparin dalteparin, and enoxaparin, which represent an important therapeutic advance in the treatment of patients with venous thromboembolism. They have a lower incidence of heparin-induced thrombocytopenia, greater bioavailability, longer half-life, and a more predictable anticoagulant response compared with standard heparin.[23] Because of these benefits, these drugs can be used subcutaneously (patient administered), without laboratory monitoring, to treat select patients with venous thromboembolism in the outpatient setting. Periodontists may encounter medically compromised patients in their practices. Because of the predictable anticoagulant response to these drugs, the medical management of these patients to prevent potential bleeding problems should be less complicated compared with patients on Coumadin therapy. Low-molecular-weight heparins are given once or twice daily. If currently used for venous thromboembolism, it would appear reasonable to discontinue the dose prior to any dental surgery and then have the patient resume the next scheduled dose. This should be confirmed with the patient's physician.

Factor Enhancement

Patients with inherited coagulation defects may require factor replacement to prevent postoperative bleeding complications. Therapies to promote coagulation carry significant risks and should be carried out by the patient's hematologist. The type of replacement therapy employed will depend upon the type and severity of factor deficiency. Mild hemophilia A (5 to 25% factor VIII), hemophilia B or von Willebrand disease (type 1) can usually be managed with local measures alone (topical agents plus antifibrinolytic agents, discussed in the next section). In addition to local measures, moderate hemophilia A (1 to 5% factor VIII) or moderate von Willebrand disease (type II) may be managed with desmopressin 1-deamino-8-D-arginine vasopressin (DDAVP).

Desmopressin is a synthetic analog of vasopressin which causes an increased release of endogenous factor VIII and vWf levels by approximately fourfold. This mimics replacement therapy with blood products. Desmopressin can be given via nasal spray, subcutaneous injection, or IV infusion. A dose of 0.3 to 0.5 µg/kg intravenously produces peak factor levels at 30 to 60 minutes, which tapers to baseline at 24 hours. It is also available for subcutaneous or intranasal use. The optimal intranasal dose is 300 µg for adults and 150 µg for children. After intranasal or subcutaneous administration, factor levels peak at 60 to 90 minutes. The above doses can be repeated at 12-hour intervals up to three or four times. Common side effects are facial flushing and headache. In addition, it is a potent antidiuretic and causes the release of the plasminogen activator. Because of the latter effect, adjunctive use of topical tranexamic acid (discussed in the next section) is beneficial. It should be noted that DDAVP does not usually shorten the bleeding time in patients with severe von Willebrand factor deficiency (type III) or dysfunctional von Willebrand factor (type II variant).

TABLE 14–5. Managing Patients as Related to Their INR

INR Value	Recommendations Concerning Invasive Treatment*
4.0 or greater	No surgical treatment until the INR is reduced.
3.5–4.0	Emergency minor surgical procedures only, simple extraction, incision and drainage. Avoid block anesthesia injections; use local measures for hemostasis.
3.0–3.4	Minor surgical procedures, simple extraction, gingivoplasty; block anesthesia not recommended; use local measures for hemostasis.
2.5–2.9	Multiple extractions, single bony impaction, quadrant periodontal flap surgery or scaling and root planing; avoid block anesthesia, if possible, and use local measures for hemostasis.
1.5–2.4	Full-mouth extractions, multiple bony impactions, gingivectomy, multiple quadrant flap surgery; avoid block anesthesia, if possible, and use local measures for hemostasis.

*Local factors such as periodontitis/gingival inflammation or medications the patient is taking can increase the severity of bleeding. Risk assessment must include all applicable factors.

TABLE 14–6. Medications Affecting Coumadin Therapy[18,19,22]

Potentiating effect	Acetaminophen (underappreciated), cephalosporins, chloral hydrate, cimetidine, ciprofloxacin, corticosteroids, diflunisal, erythromycin, fluconazole, fluoroquinolones, indomethacin, ketoconazole, metronidazole, nonsteriodal anti-inflammatory drugs, penicillins, propoxyphene, salicylates, tetracyclines, trimethoprim/sulfamethoxazole.
Opposing effect	Ascorbic acid, barbiturates, carbamazepine, dicloxacillin, nafcillin, penicillin.

Severe factor deficiencies usually require concentrated forms of replacement therapy such as factor VIII concentrate or cryoprecipitate for hemophilia A and some forms of von Willebrand disease (types II and III) and factor IX complex for hemophilia B. For severe hemophilia A (1% or less factor VIII), the therapeutic goal for replacement is 50% of normal. A normal factor VIII level is one unit of factor VIII per one milliliter of blood. To avoid possible hematomas leading to airway obstruction, block injections should not be employed unless at least a 30% level can be achieved.[24] The formula for determining the quantity of replacement factor needed is the desired factor VIII level minus the patient's factor VIII level times the plasma volume (approximately 41 mL/kg of body weight).[1] For example, a patient with 2% of normal factor VIII has 0.02 units/mL. If the patient weighs 70 kg, the patient has a plasma volume of approximately 2870 mL. In order to raise the patient's factor VIII level to 30%, the patient should receive approximately 804 units of factor VIII ([0.30 to 0.02] x 2870). Factor VIII has an 8 to 12-hour half-life unless the patient has developed antibodies to it (5 to 20% of patients). It should be given 10 to 30 minutes prior to surgery. All necessary surgery should be performed at one sitting to minimize the number of times replacement therapy is needed. Patients with inhibitors to factor VIII can be treated with increased doses of factor concentrate if their inhibitor level is low (below 20 BU). With high inhibitor levels, prothrombin complex concentrates (contains factors II, VII, IX, and X) may be used, but the response is highly variable. This product is thought to bypass the factor VIII inhibitor. Unfortunately, some patients with high inhibitor levels will not respond to any form of replacement therapy. All efforts must be made to prevent bleeding episodes in these patients.[10]

In patients with hemophilia B, a moderate factor IX deficiency can be managed with local measures alone or in combination with fresh frozen plasma. For patients with severe hemophilia B, the therapeutic goal for factor IX replacement is 25% of normal. This can be attained by giving an initial dose of 50 units/kg of factor IX complex intravenously followed by 20 units/kg every 12 to 24 hours. Factor IX has a half-life of up to 2 days.

Factor XI deficiency (hemophilia C) can be successfully managed using fresh frozen plasma and local hemostatic measures. The periodontal surgeon must be aware that factor replacement products are very expensive and may carry the risk of transmission of infectious diseases. It is imperative that they be used appropriately and only when needed. Patients requiring these products are best managed by a hematologist.

Antifibrinolysis

In addition to the use of local measures and increasing coagulation action, maintenance of clot stability following formation is critical to prevent rebleeding. This can be accomplished via antifibrinolysis agents such as Amicar (epsilon-aminocaproic acid [EACA]) and Cyclokapron (tranexamic acid). These antifibrinolytics are useful in patients with a broad range of bleeding disorders especially when the bleeding involves mucosal sites. Both these agents block the binding of plasminogen to fibrin and its activation and transformation to plasmin. This results in increased clot stability. Tranexamic acid is about 10 times more potent than aminocaproic acid and has a longer half-life. The half-life of EACA is 4 hours, and it may be given as a tablet or an elixir. The elixir is preferred for oral bleeding because of potential topical effects (plasmin is found on the oral mucosa and in saliva). The recommended oral dose of aminocaproic acid is 50 to 60 mg/kg every 4 hours.[25] However, systemic treatment with antifibrinolytic agents is prohibited in patients using anticoagulant medication because of the risk of thromboembolism.

Tranexamic acid is preferred over aminocaproic acid as a topical agent. The use of tranexamic acid in conjunction with other local measures will significantly decrease postoperative bleeding in patients with hemophilia or those who are on anticoagulation therapy.[16,25,26] Saliva has fibrinolytic qualities, which may contribute to postoperative bleeding in the oral cavity. The topical use of tranexamic acid appears to neutralize the fibrinolytic effects of saliva and stabilize the fibrin structure. It has proven effectiveness in eliminating postoperative complications in patients on anticoagulation therapy who have undergone surgical procedures without lowering their anticoagulant therapy.[16,26] Additionally, topical antifibrinolytic therapy does not increase the risk of thromboembolism. A 1- to 2-minute preoperative rinse with 10 cc of a solution diluted to 50 mg/mL of tranexamic acid, followed by identical rinses four times per day for 4 to 7 days, is usually effective. Its concentration in saliva remains high enough to suppress fibrinolysis for several hours after use. Extraction sites can also be irrigated with the solution during surgery, and postoperative bleeding sites can be treated by pressing with gauze soaked in tranexamic acid. The Colla® products, Gelfoam® and Surgicel® can also be soaked in the agent prior to use. A listing of the above antifibrinolytic agents, a source for procurement, and the approximate cost for each can be found in Table 14–3.

Platelet Transfusions

Postoperative bleeding in patients with mild to moderate thrombocytopenia usually can be managed with local measures alone. However, in addition to local measures, platelet transfusion must be considered for severely thrombocytopenic patients (< 20,000 platelets/mm^3). Regional block anesthetic injections should be avoided when the platelet count is < 30,000/mm^3. The goal for these patients is to raise their platelet count to at least 50,000 platelets/mm^3 prior to a surgical procedure. This should be increased to 75,000 platelets/mm^3 for multiple extractions, multiple quadrants of periodontal surgery, or a bony impaction. Platelet transfusions are usually performed in a hospital setting. One unit of platelets will raise the average patient's count by 10,000 platelets/mm^3 unless the patient has platelet antibodies. At least 30% of transfusions result in complications, and the incidence of patients developing antibodies to platelets after repeated transfusions is approximately 75%; therefore, they should be given judiciously. They are usually given six units at a time at a cost of approximately US $300. Platelet transfusions should be done about 30 minutes prior to the surgical procedure because platelets are rapidly sequestered. If the patient has antibodies to platelets, a continuous transfusion of platelets will probably be required during the surgical procedure. This can only be

accomplished in a hospital environment. Platelet transfusions also carry the risk of infectious diseases.

CONCLUSION

Dental management of patients with a bleeding or clotting diathesis should be accomplished in consultation with the patient's physician. Most patients with mild to moderate bleeding or clotting problems can be safely treated in the dental office using local measures, provided there is proper planning, preparation, and a judicious surgical technique. Hospitalization is reserved for those patients with severe defects. Aspirin and other nonsteroidal anti-inflammatory agents used as postoperative analgesics should be avoided or used only with extreme caution in these patients. Mild narcotics such as codeine or hydrocodone and acetaminophen are safer analgesics. Additional hemostatic agents and recombinant products are being investigated as to their effectiveness.

Early human clinical trials involving interleukin-11, recombinant human thrombopoietin, or polyethylene glycol conjugated recombinant human megakaryocyte growth and development factor have shown promise in increasing platelet production in bone marrow suppressed patients.[27] Recombinant factor VIII, factor IX and activated factor VII are available (Factor VII only in Europe) and are being studied. Clinical studies of recombinant von Willebrand factor are also due to begin.[25]

Fibrin tissue adhesives (fibrin sealants) have also been used clinically with good success.[28] These sealants mimic the last phase of blood clotting by means of the conversion of fibrinogen to fibrin. They consist of two components; (1) fibrinogen and plasma proteins, and (2) thrombin and calcium chloride. When the two components are mixed, thrombin converts fibrinogen into fibrin, and the mixture solidifies. These topical agents have not been recommended because objective data on their efficacy and safety are limited.[25] Undoubtedly, with all these new agents, there will be continued efforts to advance the clinical management and treatment of patients with bleeding and clotting disorders.

REFERENCES

1. Redding SW. Oral bleeding. In: Montgomery MT, Redding SW, editors. Oral-facial emergencies. Chicago: Federation of Special Care Organizations in Dentistry; 1994.p.103.

2. Olive JA. Disorders of hemostasis. In Tullman MJ, Redding SW, editors. Systemic disease in dental treatment. New York: Appleton Century Crofts; 1982.p.195.

3. Bussel J, Cines D. Immune thrombocytopenic purpura, neonatal alloimmune thrombocytopenia, and post-transfusion purpura. In: Hoffman R, Benj EJ, Shattil SJ, et al., editors. Hematology basic principles and practice. 2nd ed. New York: Churchill Livingstone; 1995.p.1849.

4. Schafer A. Thrombocytopenia and disorders of platelet function. In: Stein JH, editor. Internal medicine. 5th ed. Philadelphia: CV Mosby Co.; 1998.p.610.

5. Moake JL. Thrombotic thrombocytopenic purpura and the hemolytic uremic syndrome. In: Hoffman R, Benj EJ, Shattil SJ, et al., editors. Hematology basic principles and practice. 2nd ed. New York: Churchill Livingstone; 1995.p.1879.

6. Bennett JS. Hereditary disorders of platelet function. In: Hoffman R, Benj EJ, Shattil SJ, et al, editors. Hematology basic principles and practice. 2nd ed. New York: Churchill Livingstone; 1995.p.1909.

7. George JN, Shattil SJ. Acquired disorders of platelet function. In: Hoffman R, Benj EJ, Shattil SJ, et al, editors. Hematology basic principles and practice. 2nd ed. New York: Churchill Livingstone; 1995.p.1926.

8. White G. Disorders of blood coagulation. In: Stein JH, editor. Internal medicine, 5th ed. Philadelphia: CV Mosby Co.; 1998.p.617.

9. Brettler DB, Kraus EM, Levine PH. Clinical aspects of and therapy for hemophilia. In: Hoffman R, Benj EJ, Shattil SJ, et al, editors. Hematology basic principles and practice. 2nd ed. New York: Churchill Livingstone; 1995.p.1648.

10. Redding SW, Stiegler KE. Dental management of the classic hemophiliac with inhibitors. Oral Surg Oral Med Oral Pathol 1983;56 (1);145–8.

11. Roberts HR, Gray TF. Clinical aspects of and therapy for hemophilia B. In: Hoffman R, Benj EJ, Shattil SJ, et al, editors. Hematology basic principles and practice. 2nd ed. New York: Churchill Livingstone; 1995.p.1678.

12. White GC, Montgomery RR. Clinical aspects of and therapy for von Willebrand disease. In: Hoffman R, Benj EJ, Shattil SJ, et al, editors. Hematology basic principles and practice. 2nd ed. New York: Churchill Livingstone; 1995.p.1725.

13. Roberts HR, Gray TF. Factor XI and other clotting factor deficiencies. In: Hoffman R, Benj EJ, Shattil SJ, et al, editors. Hematology basic principles and practice. 2nd ed. New York: Churchill Livingstone; 1995.p.1691.

14. Furie B. Oral anticoagulant therapy. In: Hoffman R, Benj EJ, Shattil SJ, et al, editors. Hematology basic principles and practice. 2nd ed. New York: Churchill Livingstone; 1995.p.1795.

15. De Rossi SS, Glick M. Bleeding time: an unreliable predictor of clinical hemostasis. J Oral Maxillofac Surg 1996;54:1119–20.

16. Gaspar R, Brenner B, Ardekian L, et al. Use of tranexamic acid mouthwash to prevent postoperative bleeding in oral surgery patients on oral anticoagulant medication. Quintessence Int 1997;18:375–9.

17. Meehan S, Schmidt MC, Mitchell PF. The international normalized ratio as a measure of anticoagulation: significance for the management of the dental outpatient. Special Care in Dentistry 1997;17(3):94–6.

18. Hirsh J, Dalen DE, Deykin D, Poller L. Oral anticoagulant mechanism of action, clinical effectiveness, and optimal therapeutic range. Chest 1992;102(Suppl):312S–26S.

19. Herman W, Konzelman J Jr, Sutley S. Current perspectives on dental patients receiving coumadin anticoagulant therapy. J Am Dent Assoc 1997; 128:327–35.

20. Beirne OR, Koehler JR. Surgical management of patients on warfarin sodium. J Oral Maxillofac Surg 1996;54:1115–8.

21. Hylek EM, Heiman H, Skates SJ, et al. Acetaminophen and other risk factors for excessive warfarin anticoagulation. J Am Med Assoc 1998; 279:657–62.

22. Gage TW, Pickett FA. Dental drug reference. 4th ed. Philadelphia: CV Mosby Co., 1999.p.700.

23. Litin SC, Heit JA, Mees KA. Use of low-molecular-weight heparin in the treatment of venous thromboembolic disease: answers to frequently asked questions. Mayo Clin Proc 1998;73:545–51.

24. Scully C, Cawson RA. Medical problems in dentistry. 4th ed. Oxford, England: Butterworth-Heinemann; 1998.p.82.

25. Mannucci PM. Hemostatic drugs. N Engl J Med 1998;339(4):245–53.

26. Brandrowshy T, Vorono A, Borris T, Marcantoni H. Amoxicillin-related postextraction bleeding in an anticoagulated patient with tranexamic acid rinses. Oral Surg Oral Med Oral Pathol Oral Radiol Endod 1996;82:610–2.

27. Kaushansky K. Thrombopoietin. N Engl J Med 1998;339(11):746–54.

28. Bodner L, Weinstein JM, Baumgarten AK. Efficacy of fibrin sealant in patients on various levels of oral anticoagulant undergoing oral surgery. Oral Surg Oral Med Oral Pathol Oral Radiol Endod 1998;86(4):421–4.

CHAPTER 15

PHARMACOTHERAPY

Sebastian G. Ciancio, DDS

Drugs were first used to treat disease when Paul Ehrlich treated syphilis with salvarsan, an organic chemical. Much later, in 1936, sulfonamides were introduced for treating infections and antibiotics became clinically available in 1941. Since then, numerous antibiotics have become available and new antibiotics are constantly being evaluated.

Antimicrobial agents either suppress the growth of microorganisms or destroy them. They are divided into three categories: antibiotics, antiseptics, and sulfonamides. In dentistry, antibiotics and antiseptics are most frequently used.

Pharmacotherapeutic agents of value as adjuncts to periodontal therapy can be classified into agents which are useful for their antimicrobial properties and those which are useful for their ability to improve "host resistance." In the former category are antibiotics and antiseptics, and in the latter category are anticollagenase and antiprostaglandin agents.

A sub-antimicrobial dose of doxycyline hyclate has recently become available for use an as adjunct to mechanical methods of periodontal therapy. This agent arrests the progress of periodontal disease and results in probing depth reduction and attachment gain.[1] It produces its effect by reducing the release and activity of matrix metalloproteinases such as collagenase and gelatinase by polymorphonuclear leukocytes. These effects occur without the side effects associated with systemic antibiotic therapy, including the development of bacterial resistance.

ANTIBIOTICS

Antibiotics, which are chemical substances originally produced by microorganisms, either retard the growth of microorganisms or result in their death. Now, some antibiotics are chemically synthesized.

An ideal antibiotic should: (1) be selective and effective against microorganisms without injuring the host; (2) destroy microorganisms (bactericidal action) rather than retard their growth (bacteriostatic action); (3) not become ineffective as a result of bacterial resistance; (4) not be inactivated by enzymes, plasma proteins, or body fluids; (5) quickly reach bactericidal levels throughout the body and be maintained for long periods; and (6) have minimal adverse effects.

Depending on the antibiotic, several mechanisms of action are possible. They include: (1) inhibition of bacterial cell wall synthesis, (2) alteration of bacterial cell membrane permeability, (3) alteration of bacterial synthesis of cellular components, and (4) inhibition of bacterial cell metabolism.

Certain basic terms and concepts are important in understanding the pharmacology of antibiotics; they are described below.

Resistance

Microorganisms are sometimes resistant or unaffected by an antibiotic. Resistance can be natural, that is, present before contact with drug, or acquired and develop during exposure to the drug. The development of acquired resistance is genetic, with a change in the microorganism's DNA, and is inherited by each subsequent generation. Once resistance develops to an antibiotic, it persists, and a new antibiotic must be found that will destroy the resistant strain.

Microorganisms resistant to a particular drug frequently are resistant to other chemically related antimicrobial agents. This is referred to as cross-resistance. Occasionally, cross-resistance can also occur between two chemically dissimilar drugs.

Antibiotic resistance usually implies inactivation of the antibiotic by bacterial enzymes and development by the bacteria of alternative metabolic pathways unaffected by the antibiotic, or by biochemical alterations in the bacteria that prevent the uptake or binding of the antibiotic.

Antibiotic effectiveness can be reduced by inadequate therapy. For example, if a drug is given at a late stage of a disease, it may not control the large number of microorganisms that are present.

At other times, no clinical improvement may be seen even when the microorganisms are sensitive to the antibiotic, which may result from too low a dose of antibiotic. This has an additional danger in that low doses only destroy the weaker microorganisms and allow the stronger to survive, multiply, and possibly become drug resistant. The antibiotic thus serves to permit the growth of less susceptible microorganisms without the competition of the more susceptible bacteria that have been destroyed by the antibiotic. This phenomenon is called "selective pressure." The process of selecting increasingly less susceptible or resistant microorganisms occurs in a stepwise manner. Therefore, it is imperative that an antibiotic concentration be reached at the site of the infection to kill these microorganisms. This can also occur if drug therapy is not long enough. In view of this, it is important that patients take all the medication prescribed to them for the duration prescribed. Too often, patients prematurely stop taking an antibiotic because they "feel better." Lastly, antibiotics can be ineffective if they do not reach therapeutic levels at the site of the infection, or if they are antagonized by their interaction with other drugs.

Spectrum of Activity

This term refers to the different types of microorganisms affected by an antibiotic. An antibiotic may affect only a few species of microorganisms and have a limited spectrum of activity or affect a wide variety and have a broad spectrum of activity. Broad-spectrum antibiotics are only necessary if an infection is caused by a variety of microorganisms. Often, an infection caused by one microorganism will even respond more readily to a limited-spectrum antibiotic that is directed toward that microorganism.

Antibiotic therapy may suppress one group of microorganisms while permitting the growth of another group of bacteria that are normally present but do not cause disease. In large numbers, they can produce a superimposed infection, referred to as a "superinfection."

Type of Action

Antibiotics are either bacteriostatic or bactericidal.[2] Bacteriostatic antibiotics inhibit the growth and multiplication of microorganisms while bactericidal antibiotics kill microorganisms. While bacteriostatic antibiotics alter the metabolic pathways or synthesis of cellular components in microorganisms, bactericidal drugs interfere with the synthesis or function of either the cell wall, cell membrane, or both.

When two bactericidal antibiotics are given together, they may exert a greater effect than when each is given alone. This is called "antibiotic synergism." Sometimes, however, when a bacteriostatic and a bactericidal antibiotic are given together, their effectiveness is negated or reduced. This is called "antibiotic antagonism." In the majority of dental infections, combination therapy is not usually necessary. However, in the prophylaxis of patients with a history of rheumatic fever, combination therapy for antibiotic synergism is sometimes indicated.

Inhibition of Oral Contraceptive Effectiveness

Occasionally, contraceptive failures without obvious cause are reported, and some evidence suggests that these events are related to the concurrent use of certain other drugs, including antibiotics.

It has been suggested that with the trend toward lower steroid dosages in oral contraceptive preparations, there is increased frequency of drug interactions that cause lowered efficacy of oral contraceptives.

Ampicillin and other penicillins were the antibiotics most frequently listed as having the potential to inhibit contraceptives; tetracycline, although listed less frequently, was also implicated in several cases. In some cases, a combination of penicillin and a tetracycline was taken.[3]

Contraceptives belong to the steroid class of drugs. Steroid levels in the body are dependent on metabolic action by bacteria in the gastrointestinal (GI) tract. By suppressing the bacterial flora, antibiotics diminish their ability to maintain the required levels of the contraceptive drug in the GI tract. This, in turn, results in less availability of the drug for absorption. Consequently, plasma concentrations of the steroid are abnormally low, and it is cleared more rapidly from the body than under normal circumstances.

If a patient taking an oral contraceptive is in need of antibiotic therapy as part of dental treatment, the patient should be cautioned about drug interaction and advised to use alternative methods of contraception until cessation of antibiotic therapy.

It should be noted that the clinical importance of this drug interaction is currently being questioned, and ongoing studies may prove it not to be a significant clinical concern.

Antibiotics Used in Periodontics

The most common antibiotics used in periodontics are listed in Table 15–1. They are listed according to frequency of use, with the most commonly used listed first. Dosages vary according to the drug used. However, with oral administration, the initial dose should be double the subsequent doses so that high blood levels are rapidly obtained.

Although systemic antibiotics appear to offer only minimal long-term benefit as pharmacotherapy for adult periodontitis, a number of studies have suggested that they are beneficial in rapidly advancing periodontitis, localized juvenile periodontitis, and refractory periodontitis.

Tetracyclines

Tetracyclines are the most widely prescribed adjunctive agents for periodontal therapy.[4] Tetracyclines are broad-spectrum antibiotics that were initially obtained from soil microorganisms.

Types of Tetracyclines. Seven basic types of tetracyclines are currently in use. They are similar chemically and therefore possess similar antibacterial spectra and have cross-hypersensitivity. When resistance or hypersensitivity occurs to one tetracycline, it will also occur to all in the group. Tetracyclines are summarized in Table 15–2.

The first tetracyclines developed were chlortetracycline, oxytetracycline, tetracycline, and demeclocycline. The next group of tetracyclines developed were doxycycline, methacycline, and minocycline. All these agents have a similar spectrum of activity. However, minocycline appears to be the most effective in the treatment of meningococcal infections. The newer tetracyclines can be administered in smaller doses since they are more rapidly absorbed and more slowly excreted. From Table 15–2, it can be noted that most of the tetracyclines are affected by metal ions but doxycycline and minocycline are affected to a lesser extent. This interaction has also been observed with dairy products and antacids because of their calcium content. Tetracyclines bind to the calcium in the GI tract and cannot be absorbed, so minimal therapeutic benefits can be expected. A similar interaction has been reported with products containing iron, magnesium, and aluminum. Therefore, patients should be told to refrain from foods containing these for at least $1^1/_2$ hours prior to or following administration of the medication by the oral route.

Mechanism of action. Tetracyclines are bacteriostatic drugs that retard the growth of susceptible bacteria by inhibiting protein synthesis. Since they all have the same mechanism of action, resistance to one implies resistance to all tetracyclines.

Tetracyclines can block the antibacterial effect of penicillin. Penicillin is most effective on multiplying, growing bacteria while tetracyclines exert their effect by slowing down the rate of bacterial growth and multiplication. Therefore, concomitant administration of these drugs is contraindicated.

Dosage and Forms. The oral forms include tablets, chewable wafers, capsules, liquids, and ointments. The adult dosage for tetracycline, oxytetracycline, and chlortetracycline is 250 to 500 mg given four times per day. The adult dosage for demeclocycline and methacycline is 150 mg four times per day, that for doxycycline 100 mg daily, and minocycline 100 mg twice daily.

Spectrum of Activity. Tetracyclines are broad-spectrum antibiotics that are effective against a number of oral gram-negative and gram-positive cocci and bacilli. They are also effective against a few viruses, *Treponema*, *Mycoplasma*, *Chlamydia*, and *Rickettsia*. Minocycline may be effective against staphylococci that are not susceptible to other tetracyclines.

Metabolism. These drugs are usually administered orally since injections are painful. Peak plasma levels are attained slowly, so the daily recommended dose is doubled the first day of therapy. These antibiotics pass into most body fluids and tissues. They can also pass through the placenta and occur in low doses in breast milk. However, no adverse effects on the newborn have been reported

TABLE 15–1. Antibiotics of Frequent Use in Periodontal Therapy

	Action	
Antibiotic	Bacteriostatic	Bactericidal
Tetracyclines	✓	
Metronidazole	✓	
Amoxicillin		✓
Clindamycin*		✓
Cephalosporins		✓

*depending on dose, may be bacteriostatic or bactericidal

Table 15–2. Various Tetracyclines

Generic Name	Trade Name	Route of Administration	Affected by Metal Ions
Chlortetracycline HCl	Aueromycin	po, IV	+
Demeclocycline HCl	Declomycin	po	+
Doxycycline and salts	Vibramycin	po, IV	−
Methacycline HCl	Rondomycin	po	+
Minocycline HCl	Minocin, Vectrin	po, IV	-
Oxytetracycline and salts	Terramycin	po, IM, IV	+
Tetracycline and salts	Achromycin V, Cyclopar, Panmycin, Robitet, SK-Tetracycline, Tetracyn, Sumycin, Tetrex	po, IM, IV	+

po = per os (by mouth); IV = intravenous; IM = intramuscular

when the child receives low doses in the mother's milk. These antibiotics also pass into the gingival crevicular fluid and are therefore in intimate contact with the plaque in the gingival crevice. They have an affinity for and are found in higher concentrations in rapidly growing and metabolizing tissue such as liver, tumors, bone, and teeth.

Tetracyclines are excreted mainly by the kidneys and can be recovered from the urine in their unchanged form. Treatment with tetracyclines can also adversely alter the normal oral and intestinal flora, resulting in GI problems, such as diarrhea. Some patients have also developed monilial infections of the GI tract, oral cavity, and vagina due to alteration of the flora.

Adverse Effects. The side effects associated with tetracycline therapy are varied. A number of side effects have been related to the use of outdated tetracyclines, and side effects also are more common in pregnant patients (in addition to the fetal tooth-staining problem). These side effects and toxicities are summarized in Table 15–3. As this table indicates, these drugs are contraindicated in all women in the childbearing age group. In these women, the risks involved in therapy are too high to justify their therapeutic value for dental usage.

In one animal study, tetracyclines were found deposited in damaged areas of the heart, particularly regions containing calcified deposits. Whether these agents are contraindicated in humans with a history of a cardiac infarct is questionable. Further investigations to clarify this are needed; however, no additional studies since 1962 have been reported relative to this effort. Although the incidence of allergy is low, allergy to one tetracycline usually means allergy to all other tetracyclines. Unfortunately, there is no diagnostic laboratory test for allergy to tetracycline.

Regarding teratogenesis, the effects of tetracyclines on the formation of fetal hands and limbs is not established. Other side effects associated with tetracycline therapy are rare and include lymphoepithelioma and simulated systemic lupus erythematosus.

Tetracycline Discoloration of Permanent Teeth. It has been reported that long-term therapy with minocycline (as used for patients with acne) may discolor adult teeth and gingival tissue (Figure 15–1).

In reviewing the cases of discoloration of adult teeth, no pattern of discoloration could be found that was common to all. The tooth discoloration, a gray color, was present at the incisal edge in some cases, the midtooth surfaces in some, and the gingival third in others.[5,6] Minocycline used for long periods has also been reported to cause a yellow pigmentation of the skull. Similarly, black discoloration of the thyroid has been observed.[7]

Permanent tooth-staining can be caused when tetracycline or fluoride is administered during the time when teeth are developing in utero or after birth. If the drug is given during the time when the development of the crowns is being completed and they are calcifying, the crowns as well as the roots will be stained. However, in all cases studied, the patients (who ranged in age from 18 to 29 years) were over the age of tooth formation, with the exception of the younger patients, whose third molar roots could have been forming at the time of therapy. It should be noted that since tetracyclines become incorporated into dentin, this is a permanent discoloration that can

TABLE 15–3. Side Effects and Toxicities of Tetracyclines

Blood urea nitrogen	Elevation of blood urea nitrogen occurs mainly in patients taking diuretics or presenting initially with a high blood urea nitrogen. Nausea, vomiting, and their sequelae are associated with this rise
Bone	Possible retardation of growth and development—may be transient
Gastrointestinal tract	Overgrowth with monilial microorganisms has been reported on a number of occasions in conjunction with tetracycline therapy. However, some articles question this statement. Alteration in absorption of vitamin K may occur, leading to inadequate formation of prothrombin and subsequent bleeding problems
Liver	Lethal hepatic toxicity has been reported in conjunction with use in pregnancy and in the nonpregnant state in the presence of renal dysfunction, shock, and sepsis. Abnormal liver function tests have been reported (due to high dose in the presence of renal dysfunction)
Renal	Azotemia. Also, renal disorders have been reported following administration during pregnancy. A Fanconi-type syndrome has been associated with the use of outdated or degraded tetracycline. Nephrogenic diabetes insipidus has been reported in conjunction with administration of demeclocycline
Skin	Photosensitivity (especially with demeclocycline), rash, onycholysis. Seldom seen with chlortetracycline, minocycline, and tetracycline
Teeth	Permanent discoloration and dysgenesis in the offspring due to administration of tetracycline during the last half of pregnancy or the first 6 years of life. Question of discoloration of permanent teeth under study
Teratogenesis	These agents may be potential teratogens and result in malformed hands and limbs. Do not use in females of childbearing age range who have missed one or more menstrual periods

only be corrected by covering the tooth with restorative materials. Varied reports have appeared in the dental literature suggesting that tetracycline-discolored teeth may be partially bleached with long-term concentrated solutions of hydrogen peroxide sometimes preceded by acid-etching and followed by the application of heat. These findings are not well documented but deserve further investigation.

Indications. *Nondental Conditions.* Since their introduction in 1948, tetracyclines have been widely used, particularly in the treatment of acne. This widespread use has led to antibiotic resistance. A number of gram-negative bacilli now carry factors conferring resistance to tetracyclines and to other drugs, thus decreasing their effectiveness.

Several species of *Escherichia coli*, beta hemolytic streptococci, *Streptococcus pneumoniae*, *Neisseria gonorrhoeae*, some *Bacteroides*, *Shigella*, and *Staphylococcus aureus* are resistant to tetracyclines. Since there is evidence that resistance develops in direct proportion to usage, the prevalence of these resistant strains may increase in the future. However, tetracyclines remain the drugs of choice for a variety of rarely occurring nondental infections.

Dental Conditions. Clinical studies on humans indicate that use of tetracyclines results in enhanced bone formation and possibly reattachment. In addition, animal studies have suggested beneficial effects of antibiotics in terms of early crestal bone repair and reversal of a unique periodontal syndrome in the rice rat. They are valuable in that they not only kill oral pathogens but also diminish the pathogenic potential of these microorganisms. Since plaque is dynamic, a bacteriostatic drug would retard the growth of certain microbial components of plaque. Therefore, by reducing these pathogens before and following therapy, an enhanced response can be expected. This hypothesis is supported by studies in our lab-

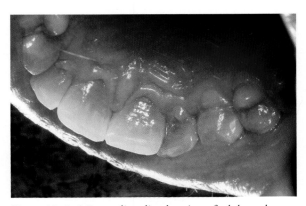

Figure 15–1. Minocycline discoloration of adult teeth.

oratories and elsewhere that have shown the presence of tetracyclines in gingival crevicular fluid following oral administration. Studies comparing tetracycline HCl and minocycline HCl have shown that the minocycline concentration in gingival crevicular fluid is higher than that of tetracycline HCl.[8] Therefore, these antibiotics become an integral part of the crevicular environment and may further exert an effect on plaque and gingival health. They have also been shown to be present in saliva, the level of concentration far below that found in serum.

Although the value of tetracyclines in the treatment of adult periodontitis is questionable, their value is established in the treatment of generalized and localized juvenile periodontitis,[9–11] refractory periodontitis,[12–14] and rapidly progressive periodontitis.[15]

Metronidazole

Metronidazole (Flagyl, Metryl) is a unique antimicrobial agent in that it is effective against anaerobic bacteria and parasites but has little or no effect on facultative and aerobic organisms. It was initially developed in 1959 as an antitrichomonal drug.

Spectrum of Action. Metronidazole is most active against obligate anaerobic gram-negative bacilli (*Bacteroides* sp, *Fusobacterium* sp, *Clostridium* sp) and certain anaerobic protozoal parasites (*Trichomonas, Giardia, Entamoeba*). It is the only antimicrobial agent that consistently exhibits bactericidal activity against *B. fragilis*. It is also effective against obligate anaerobic cocci (*Peptococcus* sp, *Peptostreptococcus* sp). It has minimal efficacy against *Actinobacillus actinomycetemcomitans*.

While metronidazole has no in vitro activity against aerobes, it has been shown to be effective in the treatment of mixed infections. The theory is that susceptible bacteria convert metronidazole to metabolites that are effective against the aerobic organisms in a mixed infection. However, despite the effectiveness of the drug against mixed infections, clinical data supporting its use as the sole agent are lacking; therefore, the drug is often used in combination with other microbial agents in the treatment of periodontal infections.

Contraindications. Its main adverse effect is its interaction with alcoholic beverages, which can result in severe nausea and vomiting, metallic taste, gastric discomfort, and diarrhea.

Indications. In dentistry, metronidazole has been used in the treatment of acute necrotizing ulcerative gingivitis (ANUG), and postextraction anaerobic gram-negative bacteremias and, in combination with other antibiotics (primarily penicillin), in treating severe odontogenic infections.

Although supportive data are weak, metronidazole has been shown to be of benefit in treating severe adult periodontitis when the major outcome evaluated is avoidance of surgery.[16,17] It has also been reported to be of value in treating refractory periodontitis, with or without combining with other antibiotics such as ciprofloxacin, amoxicillin or doxycycline. Although not effective against *A. actinomycetemcomitans*, both metronidazole and its hydroxymetabolite act synergistically with amoxicillin. Metronidazole affects most anaerobes and amoxicillin most facultative and aerobic bacteria, which makes this combination useful to treat many mixed periodontal infections. The recommended dosage for metronidazole is 250 to 500 mg tid for 7 to 10 days.[18]

Amoxicillin

Penicillin, the first antibiotic used in humans, was derived from a number of molds. Although the effect of this derivative from the mold *Penicillium notatum* was discovered as early as 1928 by Sir Alexander Fleming in London, United Kingdom, therapeutic trials did not take place until 1941. This delay mainly resulted from lack of sufficient quantities of the drug for a clinical trial. Difficulties in penicillin production occurred because broth cultures of *Penicillium* could not be produced rapidly.

Amoxicillin is sometimes called a broad-spectrum penicillin and is a derivative of ampicillin. For periodontal therapy, it is often combined with clavulanate, which inhibits β-lactamases produced by some bacteria. It is highly acid stable, and predictable blood levels can be attained following oral administration. Over 90% of the dose administered is absorbed.

Amoxicillin is a bactericidal drug that inhibits the synthesis of bacterial cell walls. The deficient cell walls thus created do not protect bacteria against high osmotic pressure. Fluids enter the cell causing swelling, membrane disruption, and subsequent cell death. The action of the drug also depends on its ability to reach and bind penicillin-binding proteins located in the bacterial cytoplasmic membranes. Because penicillin acts during the synthesis of cell walls, it is most effective against multiplying bacteria. The administration of a bacteriostatic drug in conjunction with penicillin therapy could therefore render the penicillin less effective by slowing down the bacterial growth rate.

Metabolism. Penicillin can be administered orally or parenterally. Since absorption following oral administration is influenced by the presence of food in the stomach, more predictable blood levels can be obtained if the drug is taken on an empty stomach. However, the absorption of amoxicillin from the gastrointestinal tract is not affected by the presence of food and therefore is more predictable following oral administration. Alternatively, predictable blood levels are also possible when the drug is given parenterally.

Once absorbed, penicillin is widely distributed throughout the body, and is found in low levels in the saliva and gingival crevicular fluid. It does not cross the blood-brain barrier in normal persons, but in meningitis it does pass through and may be clinically effective. Penicillin is rapidly eliminated from the plasma by the kidneys; it can cross the placenta and be found in cord blood and amniotic fluid.

Penicillins are excreted in breast milk in low concentrations. Although significant problems in humans have not been documented, a risk-benefit analysis must be done since the drug may lead to sensitization, diarrhea, and candidiasis in nursing mothers.

Adverse Effects. Penicillin toxicity is extremely low, and except for allergic reactions, it is one of the safest drugs known. However, intrathecal injection or topical application during surgery on the brain has resulted in convulsive reactions.

Patients hypersensitive to one penicillin most likely are hypersensitive to all other penicillins. Also, those with a history of hypersensitivity to cephalosporins, griseofulvin, or penicillamine may show a similar response to penicillins.

Indications. Some studies have suggested that amoxicillin is of value in combination with metronidazole (see "Metronidazole") for treatment of localized juvenile periodontitis. In addition, as amoxicillin/clavulanate (Augmentin), in doses of 250 to 500 mg tid, it may be of value in treating refractory periodontitis.[19,20]

Clindamycin

Lincomycin, the predecessor to clindamycin, was discovered in 1962 in soil samples from Lincoln, Nebraska. Although lincomycin is no longer prescribed because of significant adverse effects, its derivative, clindamycin, is still available since it has fewer adverse effects and its antibacterial action is more effective than that of lincomycin.

Mechanism of Action. This antibiotic inhibits bacterial protein synthesis and is usually bacteriostatic but is bactericidal in high doses. The mechanism of action of clindamycin is similar to that of erythromycin and identical to that of chloramphenicol. These drugs bind to a specific subunit of the bacterial ribosomes, thereby inhibiting their protein synthesis.

Spectrum of Activity. Its antibacterial spectrum is similar to that of erythromycin. Because of its ability to penetrate bone, however, it is particularly useful in treating periodontal disease when bacterial invasion of tissue is suspected.

Levels in the crevicular fluid usually are above the minimum inhibitory concentration for periodontal pathogens.[21] It is almost completely absorbed from the GI tract and is excreted in urine, feces, and bile, with the biliary route being the most important. Following oral administration, levels in bone are similar to levels in serum.

Adverse Effects. The main adverse effect of clindamycin is diarrhea and gastric upset if taken on an empty stomach. Therefore, it should be taken with food. Ulcerative colitis has been reported but the frequency of its occurrence is less than that seen with ampicillin or the cephalosporins. When colitis occurs, it is best treated with metronidazole (250 mg qid) or vancomycin (500 mg qid). Since colitis can be fatal, patients must be closely monitored for this condition.

Indications. Clindamycin has been shown to be of value in the treatment of refractory periodontitis, either alone or in combination with amoxicillin/clavulanate (Augmentin).[22–26] The usual dosage is 150 mg tid or qid for 7 to 10 days.

Miscellaneous Antibiotics

Spiramycin. Spiramycin is active against gram-positive organisms and is excreted in high concentrations in saliva. It is used as an adjunct to periodontal treatment in Canada and Europe but is not available in the United States.

This drug has minimal adverse effects. Some studies have suggested its benefit in adult periodontitis but data are not convincing.[27–29]

Ciprofloxacin. Ciprofloxacin is categorized as a fluoroquinolone and was initially developed to treat urinary tract infections. Studies of its value in periodontal therapy are limited, with a possible benefit reported in refractory cases.[30,31] In combination with metronidazole, it is effective against *A. actinomycetemcomitans*.[32] The dosage is 500 mg bid for 8 to 10 days.

Adverse effects include gastrointestinal upset, oral candidiasis, headache, restlessness, insomnia, hypersensitivity, hyperpigmentation, and photosensitivity.

Antibiotic-Associated Pseudomembranous Colitis

Pseudomembranous colitis is a severe diarrheal disease that can result from virtually any orally or parenterally administered antibiotic used in dentistry (Table 15–4), but is most commonly associated with ampicillin, cephalosporins, and clindamycin.

The true incidence of this disease from antibiotic use in dentistry is unknown because definitive diagnosis is based on endoscopic examination of the bowel, and this is rarely performed on patients suffering from diarrhea. However, there are a number of signs and symptoms associated with this disease that should suggest to the dentist that a patient might be suffering from antibiotic-associated pseudomembranous colitis. The majority of patients present with fever, leukocytosis, abundant watery diarrhea, and a crampy abdominal pain beginning on the fourth to ninth day of antibiotic therapy. It is important to note, however, that as many as 40% of these patients do not manifest signs or symptoms until 2 to 10 weeks following the conclusion of antimicrobial therapy.

Etiology

Current data suggest that in the majority of cases the disease is confined to the colon and is caused by a toxin produced by *Clostridium difficile* that is widely distributed in the environment and is a normal inhabitant of the GI tract in approximately 3% of the population. The postulation is that administration of antibiotics alters the normal GI flora, thereby creating an environment more favorable to the growth of *C. difficile* and/or the production and release of its enterotoxin. There is no microbial invasion of the intestinal mucosa, but rather the toxin most likely interacts with the cells lining the lower GI tract, causing cell necrosis and decreased water and electrolyte absorption, and producing a significant diarrhea.

TABLE 15–4. Antibiotics Commonly Used in Dentistry that Are Associated with Pseudomembranous Colitis

Most Common	Less Frequent	Rare
Ampicillin	Amoxicillin	Aminoglycosides
Cephalosporins	Cloxacillin	Metronidazole
Clindamycin	Erythromycin	Tetracyclines
	Penicillin G	
	Penicillin K	

Treatment

Treatment depends on the severity of the disease. If it is mild (as it is in most cases), the most important therapeutic decision is to discontinue the antibiotic (if possible and appropriate) and to rehydrate the patient and replace lost electrolytes. In many patients, this approach usually results in a rapid, complete resolution of symptoms with no further necessary diagnostic tests (endoscopy, or examination of stool to detect *C. difficile* enterotoxin) or treatment regimens. The medication of choice is orally administered vancomycin or metronidazole. It is important to note that under no circumstances should antidiarrheal agents that decrease GI motility be used. They have been implicated in worsening the symptoms and outcome of the disease.

Most patients with pseudomembranous colitis recover without specific therapy, but the mortality rate in seriously ill patients can approach 30%. Because pseudomembranous colitis is associated with antibiotics that are commonly used in dentistry, the practitioner should be aware of this potentially serious adverse reaction. Patients should contact their dentist immediately if diarrhea occurs during or after antibiotic therapy because prompt treatment can produce a rapid symptomatic response with essentially 100% recovery.

Antibiotic Combinations in Periodontal Therapy

An approach using a combination of antibiotics in periodontal therapy has recently been studied by various investigators. Van Winkelhoff and colleagues[33] reported on the concomitant use of metronidazole and amoxicillin in the treatment of *A. actinomycetemcomitans*-associated periodontitis. Their results concluded that this regimen was able to suppress *A. actinomycetemcomitans* (also *Porphyromonas gingivalis*) from being detected from the periodontal pocket for over 1 year. Kornman and colleagues[34] have reported some value in the adjunctive systemic use of metronidazole in combination with amoxicillin or amoxicillin/clavulanate (Augmentin) in the treatment of patients with refractory periodontitis.

Also, Aitken and colleagues[35] indicated that prevention of recurrent periodontitis with metronidazole may be enhanced by previous treatment with doxycycline. The serial use of doxycycline and metronidazole has also been shown to be of value in reducing periodontal pathogens.[36]

A more recent study was designed to compare the effect of short-term systemic administration of a sequential antibiotic treatment therapy using Augmentin and doxycycline with that of a short-term systemically administered doxycycline alone in the treatment of periodontitis caused by *A. actinomycetemcomitans* and *P. gingivalis*.[37] Doxycycline was included in this regimen for both its antibacterial and anticollagenolytic properties.[38]

In a 25-week study, patients were randomly placed in one of two treatment groups: one group (five patients) was to receive doxycycline (200 mg the first day, then 100 mg each day thereafter for a 10-day period); the second group (six patients) received a combination of Augmentin (500 mg tid for 5 days) and doxycycline (200 mg the first day, then 100 mg each day for a total of 5 days). Each patient received one session (approximately 1 to 2 hours) of local therapy via root planing for one half of the mouth; the other half mouth received no local therapy. No attempt was made to alter the patient's oral hygiene regimen.

Clinical and microbiologic measurements were recorded at 0, 4, 12, and 25 weeks as follows: gingival index,[39] plaque index,[40] probing depth and attachment level by using a manual (William's) probe and a controlled-force probe (Interprobe) at eight selected sites in each patient (four sites root planed and another four without root planing), and bleeding upon probing/suppuration.

The results of the study are summarized as follows:

The doxycycline/Augmentin groups produced significant reduction in probing pocket depth (PPD) at 4, 12, and 25 weeks (1.1, 1.3, and 1.1 mm, respectively). The doxycycline group produced a significant reduction in probing depths only at 4 and 12 weeks (both times 0.8 mm) and a significant gain of 0.8 mm in probing attachment level at the same periods; and the doxycycline/Augmentin group in conjunction with root planing produced the most sustained reduction in probing depth and gain in attachment level.

A lower percentage of bleeding sites was noted in the doxycycline/Augmentin group than in the doxycycline group. All sites at 4, 12, and 25 weeks in both groups showed no signs of suppuration, with the exception of one site in the doxycycline group at week 25.

It should be noted that the reductions in probing depths and gains in attachment levels reported were relative to their own baselines and not to each other. When the groups were compared with each other, no intergroup differences were found.

Although there were no significant reductions in the gingival or plaque indexes or the microbial measurements, there was a trend toward reductions in the doxycycline group, which was better than that in the Augmentin/doxycycline group.

LOCALLY DELIVERED MEDICATIONS

Irrigation represents one of the earliest forms of local delivery of a medication. A major limitation of irrigation is the short duration of application of the medication. However, agents with significant substantivity or strong antibacterial properties may show some benefit, particularly in the treatment of gingivitis.

Water and a variety of chemical agents have been shown to be effective as irrigants in reducing gingivitis. Additionally, subgingival irrigation with a variety of antimicrobial agents has been shown to reduce a number of microorganisms associated with the pathogenesis of periodontal disease. Further short-term studies have suggested some reduction of pocket depth; however, long-term studies in this area are needed. It is also noteworthy that irrigants, whether supra- or subgingivally delivered, have been shown to be safe whether applied at home or in the office, and have been well received by patients.

Some representative studies on powered irrigation will be reviewed in this section.

Irrigation with Antimicrobial Agents

A study in the *Journal of Periodontology*[41] evaluated the effect of in-office irrigation with PerioPik® (Teledyne Water Pik) followed by at-home subgingival irrigation with a Pik Pocket® (Teledyne Water Pik) tip and a Water Pik Oral Irrigator® (Teledyne Water Pik). The in-office and at-home irrigant used was Listerine® (Warner Lambert Company).

Included in this study were 50 patients with adult periodontitis and at least four bilateral sites with probing depths between 4 and 5 mm, which bled upon probing. Following baseline examinations, the patients received a half-mouth scaling and prophylaxis and full-mouth subgingival irrigation with either the antimicrobial mouthrinse or control solution professionally delivered. The subjects continued the irrigation at home once daily for 42 days with their assigned rinse delivered via a subgingival delivery system. All sites within the mouth were scored at baseline and at day 42 for supragingival plaque, bleeding on probing, and redness. For the four selected periodontitis sites, probing depth and attachment level were measured at baseline and on day 42; additionally, supragingival plaque and gingival redness were scored on days 7 and 21. Subgingival plaque samples for microbiologic analysis were harvested from the selected periodontal sites at baseline and on days 7, 21, and 42. The samples were analyzed for *Porphyromonas gingivalis, Prevotella intermedia, Fusobacterium* sp, *Capnocytophaga* sp, *Streptococcus sanguis, Porphyromonas loescheii,* and *Treponema denticola.* Microbiologically, irrigation with the antimicrobial mouthrinse resulted in statistically significant reductions compared with control in periodontal pathogens, including black pigmenting species, which persisted at 42 days. Clinically, subgingival irrigation with the antimicrobial mouthrinse produced a significant reduction in supragingival plaque ($p < .001$), bleeding on probing ($p = .019$), and redness ($p = .017$) compared with the control, whether or not a prophylaxis was performed. There were no significant differences between the active and control groups in either probing depth or attachment level ($p > .05$).

The authors concluded that subgingival delivery of an antimicrobial agent with a powered oral irrigation device can play a potential role in the management of chronic periodontitis by virtue of its significant effects on the subgingival periodontopathic microflora and supragingival plaque and gingivitis.

In another study at the University of Minnesota, 74 patients were divided into irrigation and nonirrigation groups.[42] Following a periodontal recall visit, the PerioPik® was used in the office to irrigate all gingival crevices with 1.64% stannous fluoride. Subjects were then given a powered pulsating irrigator with a subgingival delivery tip (the Pik Pocket®) for daily irrigation at home with 200 mL of an iodine-containing solution (tetrahydrazine hydroperiodide) for 8 weeks. In the irrigation group, statistically significant reductions in gingivitis were found compared with the control group and reductions in gingival bleeding compared with baseline. These reductions are noteworthy since the control group was instructed in twice-daily brushing and once daily flossing, following their recall visit. This study also demonstrated the safety of at-home subgingival irrigation using the subgingival tip as well as a high degree of acceptability as shown by an 89% compliance rate.

Supragingival Irrigation

Since patients with gingivitis and/or periodontitis rarely demonstrate optimal oral hygiene even when given oral hygiene information and instruction,

supragingival irrigation with water can be expected to have a therapeutic effect in most patients with periodontal disease (Figure 15–2). In a 6-month assessment of patients with gingivitis who performed daily supragingival irrigation with water, gingival inflammation was shown to be significantly reduced. The therapeutic effects of supragingival irrigation with water corresponded to the effect of twice-daily rinsing with 0.12% chlorhexidine gluconate solution. However, in this study, supragingival irrigation with water influenced neither the supragingival plaque mass nor the composition of the subgingival microflora.[43] Thus, it appears possible that supragingival irrigation reduced gingival inflammation without altering the supra- and subgingival mass. Although the mechanism responsible for this is not exactly known, it can be assumed that through irrigation there is a dilution or removal of bacterial toxins, which leads to an improvement of gingival health. Also, it has been shown that irrigation changes the morphology of bacteria so that, although present, they appear as cells with ruptured membranes.[44]

Following scaling and root planing, daily supragingival irrigation with water for 4 weeks leads to an improvement in gingival health that persists for 1 to 3 months.[45] A 6-month study in the *Journal of Periodontology* evaluated the effect of daily water irrigation in 155 patients receiving maintenance periodontal treatment. The study demonstrated that adjunctive supragingival irrigation with water can provide meaningful clinical outcomes for patients with periodontitis who are being treated in the maintenance phase of periodontal therapy.[46] They also found that irrigation with water was significantly better ($p < .05$) than zinc sulfate irrigation for all parameters measured.

The effect of supragingival irrigation on the subgingival microflora appears to depend on the pocket depth. Supragingival irrigation with water has been shown, in pockets of 5 mm and more, to reduce periodontal pathogenic bacteria, particularly *P. intermedia*, spirochetes, and motile rods.

Further, following supragingival scaling alone, supragingival irrigation with 0.02% stannous fluoride solution as an irrigant resulted in a significant improvement of gingival health, compared with supragingival irrigation with water.[47]

Irrigation with Anti-inflammatory Drugs

Nonsteroidal anti-inflammatory drugs (NSAIDs), such as acetylsalicylic acid, flurbiprofen, naproxen, and others, offer the possibility of limiting the destructive side effects of the immune responses that occur in periodontal disease.

However, the therapeutic effect of irrigation with various concentrations of acetylsalicylic acid solution has not been found to be significantly better than irrigation with water.[48,49] Further studies with more effective anti-inflammatory agents are needed since they are readily absorbed through oral tissues and may offer beneficial effects on the periodontium.

The various irrigants reviewed are summarized in Table 15–5.

Irrigation around Implants

Powered irrigation has also been shown to be of benefit to improve gingival health around implants. A 3-month study was conducted in 24 men and women between the ages of 35 and 75 years to evaluate the effect of irrigation with 0.06% chlorhexidine (PerioGard®) using a powered oral irrigator (Water Pik®) with a special subgingival irrigating tip (Pik Pocket Subgingival Tip®), compared with rinsing with 0.12% chlorhexidine gluconate once daily.[50]

The results of this study showed that irrigation with 0.06% chlorhexidine was significantly better than rinsing with 0.12% chlorhexidine for measures of plaque and health (MGI and PI, $p < .05$) and that the reduction in BI, although not statistically significant, was almost twice as large as that seen in the rinsing group (62% versus 33%). Also, the chlorhexidine-associated stain score was significantly lower in the irrigation group compared with the control ($p = .04$). Further, it was found that the presence of calculus showed a 22% increase in the rinsing group in contrast to a 42% decrease in the irrigation group.

The results of this study show that powered irrigation with a chemotherapeutic agent such as chlorhexidine is supportive of the health of tissues around implants and minimizes calculus and stain associated with the use of chlorhexidine.

LOCAL DELIVERY OF ANTIBIOTICS

The limitations of systemic therapy have prompted research for the development of alternative delivery systems. Recently, advances in delivery technology have resulted in the controlled release of drugs, usually systemically, for certain medical conditions. The oral cavity offers another relatively accessible disease site for localized therapy. The

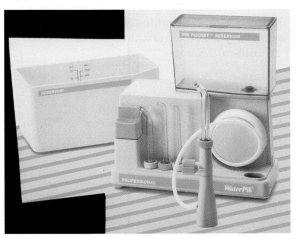

Figure 15–2. Powered irrigation device with both supra- and subgingival applicator tips.

requirements for treating periodontal disease include a means for targeting an antimicrobial agent to sites of infection and for sustaining its localized concentration at effective levels for sufficient lengths of time that, at the same time, evoke minimal or no side effects (Table 15–6).

Tetracycline-Containing Fibers (Actisite®)

The first local delivery product available in the United States and one which has been extensively studied is an ethylene/vinyl acetate copolymer fiber, diameter 0.5 mm, containing tetracycline, 12.7 mg/9 inches (Actisite® tetracycline fiber; manufactured by Alza Corporation, Palo Alto, CA, and distributed by Procter and Gamble Co., Cincinnati, OH) (Figure 15–3). When packed into a periodontal pocket, it is well tolerated by oral tissues, and for 10 days it sustains tetracycline concentrations exceeding 1300 μg/mL, well beyond

TABLE 15–5. Irrigants Showing Benefits as Adjuncts to Periodontal Therapy

	Concentration (%)	Amount (mL)	Application Per Day
Water	N/A	500	1
Chlorhexidine digluconate solution	0.06	200	1
Stannous fluoride solution	0.02	500	1
Listerine®	Undiluted	100	1
Iodine	0.38	200	1

TABLE 15–6. Desirable Characteristics for Locally Delivered Antimicrobials for Periodontal Therapy

Reaches site of disease (base of pocket)
Achieves adequate drug concentrations
Maintains sufficient duration of treatment
Effective against periodontal pathogens
Clinically effective as an adjunctive therapy
Safe for teeth and soft tissues
Minimal adverse side effects
No bacterial resistance
Easy application
Biodegradable

the 32 to 64 µg/mL required to inhibit the growth of pathogens isolated from periodontal pockets.[51,52] In contrast, crevicular fluid concentrations of only 4 to 8 µg/mL are reported following systemic tetracycline administration, 250 mg four times daily for 10 days (total oral dose, 10 g).[53] Thus, controlled site-specific tetracycline delivery can achieve an antibacterial effect at approximately one-thousandth of the dose administered systemically.

Studies demonstrate that the tetracycline fibers, applied with or without scaling and root planing, reduce probing depth, bleeding on probing, and periodontal pathogens and provide gains in clinical attachment level. Such effects are significantly better than those attained with scaling and root planing alone or with placebo fibers. In a 2-month study, compared with scaling and root planing, the fibers used alone have provided over a 60% greater improvement in probing depth and clinical attachment level than scaling alone.[54] The fibers used in conjunction with scaling and root planing have also provided a statistically significant improvement in probing depth reduction and clinical attachment level gain of over 60% and bleeding on probing reductions over scaling and root planing alone at 6 months after therapy.[55]

Among the tested putative periodontal pathogens, no change in antibiotic resistance to tetracycline has been found following tetracycline fiber therapy.[56] Disadvantages of the fiber include the length of time required for placement (10 minutes or more per tooth), the considerable learning curve required to gain proficiency at placement, and the need for a second appointment 10 days after placement for removal of the fiber. Also, placement of fibers around 12 or more teeth has resulted in oral candidiasis.

Another study suggested that rinsing with 0.12% chlorhexidine (Peridex®, Zila Pharmaceuticals, Inc., Phoenix, AZ) following fiber placement had a synergistic effect, enhancing the reduction of bacterial pathogens.[57] It is possible that at-home irrigation with an antimicrobial agent following fiber removal could prolong this synergistic effect.

Evaluation of the effect of tetracycline fibers on root surfaces, using fluorescent light and scanning electron microscopy,[58] showed superficial penetration of tetracycline, with minor penetration into the dental tubules, and a few areas of demineralized root surface. Scanning electron microscopic observations made in this study also revealed reductions in the subgingival microbial flora on the root surfaces of teeth treated with the fibers versus the control specimens. Many of the residual microbes observed in the fiber-treated teeth appeared nonviable, in contrast to the residual microbes found on the root-planed and control specimens.

Subgingival Delivery of Doxycycline (Atridox®)

Atridox® (manufactured by Atrix Laboratories, Fort Collins, CO; licensed for marketing by Block Drug, Inc., Jersey City, NJ) is a gel system that incorporates the antibiotic doxycycline (10%) in a syringeable gel system (Figure 15–4).

A 9-month multicenter study in 180 patients was designed to study the effects of subgingivally placed doxycycline compared with subgingival placement of the vehicle and a herbal agent (sanguinaria). Patients with initial probing depth of > 5 mm in selected sites were included in this study.[59] The patients were instructed in oral hygiene and randomly assigned to one of three groups: vehicle control, 5% sanguinaria in the vehicle control, and 10% doxycycline in the vehicle control. No scaling

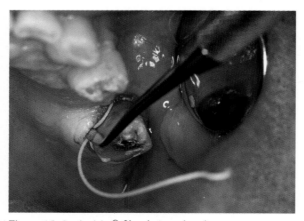

Figure 15–3. Actisite® fiber being placed.

or root planing was performed in any of the groups, and there was no untreated group. Therefore, the study's objective was to evaluate the effect of the various agents, compared with the vehicle when used as a monotherapy.

Treatment with doxycycline was more effective than the other treatments at all time periods with the exception of the 3-month clinical attachment level value. Also, on evaluation of the effect based on initial probing depth, the differential effect in the doxycycline group in comparison with the other two groups was greater as pretreatment probing depth increased. For the doxycycline group, the reduction in clinical attachment level at 9 months showed a gain of 0.4 mm compared with vehicle control, the reduction in probing depth was 0.6 mm greater than vehicle control, and the reduction of bleeding on probing was 0.2 units greater than vehicle control. The differences were small but they were statistically significant. Although resistance was not evaluated in this study, the local application of doxycycline has previously been reported to have shown transient increases in resistance in oral microbes and no overgrowth of foreign pathogens.[60]

Data from two multicenter clinical trials have also been reported, each studying 411 patients with moderate to severe periodontitis.[61] At baseline, patients were randomized to one of four treatment groups: doxycycline, vehicle control, oral hygiene only, and scaling and root planing. Sites with probing depth $\geq$ 5 mm that bled on probing were treated at baseline and then again with the same treatment at 4 months. Clinical assessments were made at months 1, 2, 4, 5, 6, 8, and 9 by measuring clinical attachment level, probing depth, and bleeding on probing. All treatment groups in both studies showed clinical improvements from baseline over the 9-month period. The results for all parameters measured were significantly better in the doxycycline group compared with the vehicle-control and oral-hygiene-only groups. Compared with scaling and root planing, the effects of doxycycline on clinical attachment level gain and probing depth reduction were equivalent. This product has been approved by the FDA for sale in the United States.

Subgingival Delivery System for Minocycline (Dentamycin®, Perio Cline®)

A subgingival delivery system of 2% (w/w) minocycline hydrochloride (Dentamycin®, Perio Cline®; Cyanamid International, Lederle Division,

Wayne, NJ, and SunStar, Osaka, Japan) is available in a number of countries for use as an adjunct to subgingival débridement. This system is a syringeable gel suspension delivery formulation.

In a four-center, double-blind, randomized trial, patients with periodontal pockets at least 5 mm deep were selected, and either 2% minocycline gel or vehicle was applied once every 2 weeks four times.[62] Treatment followed initial subgingival débridement in both treatment groups. Microbiologic assessments were made at baseline and at weeks 2, 4, 6, and 12, with clinical assessments at baseline and weeks 4 and 12. A total of 103 patients were treated and 90 were evaluable for efficacy, of which 48 had been treated with minocycline gel and 42 with vehicle.

A total of 343 teeth (976 sites) were included in the minocycline group with 299 teeth (810 sites) in the control group. The microbiologic analysis in this study focused on three relevant plaque species: *P. gingivalis, P. intermedia* and *A. actinomycetemcomitans.*

Reductions in *P. gingivalis* and *P. intermedia* at weeks 2, 4, 6, and 12 and at weeks 6 and 12 for *A. actinomycetemcomitans* were statistically significant. These results demonstrated the advantages of supplementing standard subgingival débridement with minocycline gel application.

The three primary clinical efficacy variables in this study were probing depth, clinical attachment level, and bleeding index. There was a trend toward clinical improvement in both treatment groups for all three measures, and the reduction in probing depth was significantly greater with minocycline gel.

When sites with probing depth of at least 7 mm and significant bleeding at baseline were considered, the improvements were greater than with 5

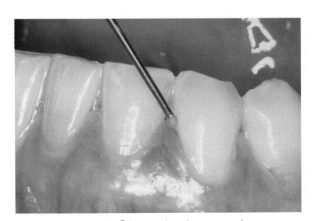

Figure 15–4. Atridox® being placed into a pocket.

mm pockets. The improvements with minocycline were statistically significantly better than the vehicle-control group.

In a 3-month study, 2% minocycline was also evaluated in 30 patients.[63] Patients received oral hygiene education and root planing with local anesthesia. Active or placebo gel was placed subgingivally at planed sites in each subject according to a double-blind protocol, immediately after instrumentation and 2 and 4 weeks later. A periodontal examination was made with a constant force probe before instrumentation and 6 and 12 weeks later. Two subjects failed to complete the study; their pairs were therefore not included in the analysis. Results were tested with an analysis of covariance. The differences between the groups in mean probing depth did not reach statistical significance at any visit, but mean clinical attachment levels were different in favor of the minocycline group ($p < .05$) at both reassessments. There was also a difference in the number of sites that bled after deep probing at 12 weeks, favoring the minocycline group ($p < .05$). This trial showed that adjunctive minocycline gel provided a more advantageous outcome for nonsurgical periodontal treatment in terms of clinical attachment level and bleeding on probing. This product is not available in the United States.

A topical medication (Elyzol®; Dumex, Copenhagen, Denmark) containing an oil-based metronidazole 25% dental gel (glyceryl monooleate and sesame oil) has been tested in a number of studies.[64] It is applied in viscous consistency to the pocket, where it is liquidized by the body heat and then on contact with water hardens again, forming crystals. As a precursor, the preparation contains metronidazole-benzoate, which is converted into the active substance by esterases in the crevicular fluid. Two 25% gel applications at a 1-week interval have been used in clinical studies.[65]

Studies of the metronidazole gel have shown it to be equivalent to scaling and root planing but have not shown adjunctive benefits in conjunction with scaling and root planing. For example, a recent 6-month study in 30 patients showed the following results.[66] The treatment consisted of two applications of the dental gel in two randomly selected quadrants (on days 0 and 7) as well as simultaneous subgingival scaling of the remaining quadrants. Oral hygiene instructions were given on day 21. The average probing depth and the average frequency of bleeding on probing were calculated for all sites with an initial probing depth of 5 mm or more; this was continued at each examination, using the same sites. The statistical analysis showed that both treatments were effective in reducing probing depth and bleeding on probing over the 6-month period. At the end of the follow-up period, the mean reduction in probing depth was 1.3 mm after gel treatment and 1.5 mm after subgingival scaling. Bleeding on probing was reduced by 35% and 42%, respectively. No significant differences between the two treatments were detected. Dark-field microscopy showed a shift toward a seemingly more healthy microflora for both treatment modalities; this effect persisted throughout the 6-month period.

A large multicenter study of 206 subjects investigated two applications of this gel in two randomly selected quadrants versus two quadrants of scaling.[67] As in the study described above, probing depths were reduced by 1.2 mm in the gel and 1.5 mm in the scaling group. At 6 months, the differences between treatments were statistically but not clinically significant. Also, bleeding on probing was reduced by 88% in both treatment groups.

LOCAL DELIVERY OF AN ANTISEPTIC AGENT

Chlorhexidine Delivery System (PerioChip®)

The PerioChip® (manufactured by Perio Products Ltd., Jerusalem, Israel; distributed by Astra USA, Inc., Westborough, MA) is a small chip (4.0 × 5.0 × 0.35 mm) composed of a biodegradable hydrolyzed gelatin matrix, cross-linked with glutaraldehyde and also containing glycerin and water, which has been incorporated into a chip containing 2.5 mg chlorhexidine gluconate (Figure 15–5). It is rounded at one end and inserts easily, in less than a minute, into periodontal pockets that are 5 mm or greater in depth. The PerioChip® releases chlorhexidine and maintains drug concentrations in the gingival crevicular fluid greater than 100 μg/mL for at least 7 days,[68] concentrations well above the tolerance of most oral bacteria.[69] Because the PerioChip® biodegrades in 7 to 10 days, a second appointment for removal is not needed.

Two multicenter, randomized, double-blind, parallel-group, controlled clinical trials of the PerioChip® were conducted in the United States with a total of 447 patients in 10 centers.[70] In these studies, patients received a supragingival prophylaxis for up to 1 hour, followed by scaling and root planing for 1 hour. Chips were placed in target sites with a probing depth 5 to 8 mm at baseline that bled on probing and again at 3 and 6 months if the probing depth remained 5 mm or greater. Sites in control-group subjects received either a placebo chip (inactive) plus scaling and root planing or scaling and root planing alone. Sites in test-group subjects received either a chlorhexidine chip (active) plus scaling and root planing or scaling and root planing alone (to maintain the study blind). Examinations were performed at baseline and at 3, 6, and 9 months.

At 9 months, significant decreases were observed in probing depth from baseline favoring the active chip compared with controls (chlorhexidine chip plus scaling and root planing, −0.95 ± 0.05 mm; placebo chip plus scaling and root planing, −0.69 ± 0.05 mm [$p = .001$]; scaling and root planing alone −0.65 ± 0.05 mm [$p = .00001$]). The proportion of pocket sites with a probing depth reduction of 2 mm or more was increased in the chlorhexidine chip group (30%), compared with scaling and root planing alone (16%), a difference which was statistically significant on a per-patient basis ($p < .0001$). Improvements favoring the chlorhexidine chip compared with controls were also observed for clinical attachment levels at 9 months, improvements which were significant when the data were pooled ($p < .05$). Bleeding on probing was reduced in the active chip group compared with both controls, differences which were significant in one of the two studies ($p < .05$) and also when the data were pooled ($p = .012$). These data indicate that the biodegradable chlorhexidine chip, when used as an adjunct to scaling and root planing, significantly reduces probing depth and maintains clinical attachment levels when compared with scaling and root planing alone.

Another study was reported that evaluated the results of a 6-month clinical trial using the PerioChip®.[68] The study was a randomized, blinded, controlled, split-mouth, multicenter study conducted with 118 patients in three study centers outside the United States. Patients, aged 30 to 65 years, with moderate periodontitis and in good general health were studied. Patients received a full-mouth scaling and root planing. The subgingival instrumentation was performed after baseline measurements were recorded. The two quadrants of the maxillary arch were randomized to the two treatment arms—scaling and root planing alone (control quadrant) or scaling and root planing plus PerioChip® (test quadrant). All remaining maxillary pockets with a probing depth between 5 and 8 mm at the baseline visit were entered into the study. The PerioChip® was inserted into each pocket measuring 5 to 8 mm in the designated quadrant. Clinical measurements, including probing depth, clinical attachment level, and bleeding on probing, as well as gingivitis, plaque, and staining indices, were recorded at baseline and at 1, 3, and 6 months. At the 3-month visit, a full-mouth supragingival prophylaxis was undertaken according to clinical needs, and a chlorhexidine chip was inserted into each test pocket with a remaining depth of 5 to 8 mm.

The average probing depth reduction in the scaling and root planing plus PerioChip®-treated sites was significantly greater than in the sites receiving scaling and root planing alone, at both 3 and 6 months, with a mean difference of 0.42 mm ($p < .01$) at 6 months. Improvement in clinical attachment levels at the treated sites was greater than at sites that received scaling and root planing alone although the difference was statistically significant at the 6th-month visit only ($p < .05$). An analysis of patients with initial probing depths of 7 to 8 mm (n = 56) revealed an even greater improvement in both probing depth and attachment level in those pockets adjunctively treated with PerioChip® compared with scaling and root planing alone, at both 3 and 6 months, suggesting that the deeper the initial probing depth, the greater is the clinical improvement. The mean differences between test and control sites at 6 months for these deeper pockets were 0.71 mm and 0.56 mm for probing depth and clinical attachment levels, respectively.

Relative to bleeding on probing, the scaling and root planing plus PerioChip® sites showed consistently less bleeding on probing than control sites with a significant difference ($p < .05$) between the treatment groups occurring at the 3-month examination. The test quadrants showed a significant decrease ($p < .05$) in gingival index when compared with control quadrants at 3 and 6 months.

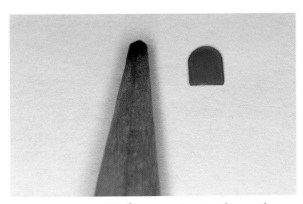

Figure 15–5. PerioChip® compared to tip of a pencil.

No signs of staining were noted in any of the above three studies as a result of the chlorhexidine chip treatment as measured by a stain index. Adverse effects were minimal with a few patients who complained of slight pain and swelling in the first 24 hours after chip placement.

HOST MODULATION

The US Food and Drug Administration recently granted marketing approval for Periostat® for the adjunctive treatment of periodontitis. Periostat®, available as a 20 mg capsule of doxycycline hyclate, is prescribed for use by patients twice daily. The mechanism of action is by suppression of the activity of collagenase, particularly that produced by polymorphonuclear leukocytes. The role of collagenase in the pathogenesis of periodontal disease is illustrated in Figure 15–6. Although this drug is in the antibiotic family, it does not produce any antibacterial effects since the dose of 20 mg twice daily is too low to affect bacteria. As a result, resistance to this medication cannot develop.

Four double-blind clinical multicenter studies in over 650 patients have demonstrated that Periostat® improves the effectiveness of professional periodontal care and slows the progression of the disease process.

The results of the first three studies showed that Periostat® resulted in approximately a 50% improvement in clinical attachment level (CAL) in pockets with probing depths of 4 to 6 mm and a 34% improvement in pockets with probing depths ≥ 7 mm. It was also noted that attachment loss was prevented in sites with normal probing depths (0 to 3 mm) while the placebo groups lost 0.13 mm at 12 months ($p = .05$).[71,72]

The improvement in pocket depth generally paralleled the improvement in CAL after treatment for 12 months. Tooth sites with a baseline pocket probing depth (PPD) of 4 to 6 mm improved by

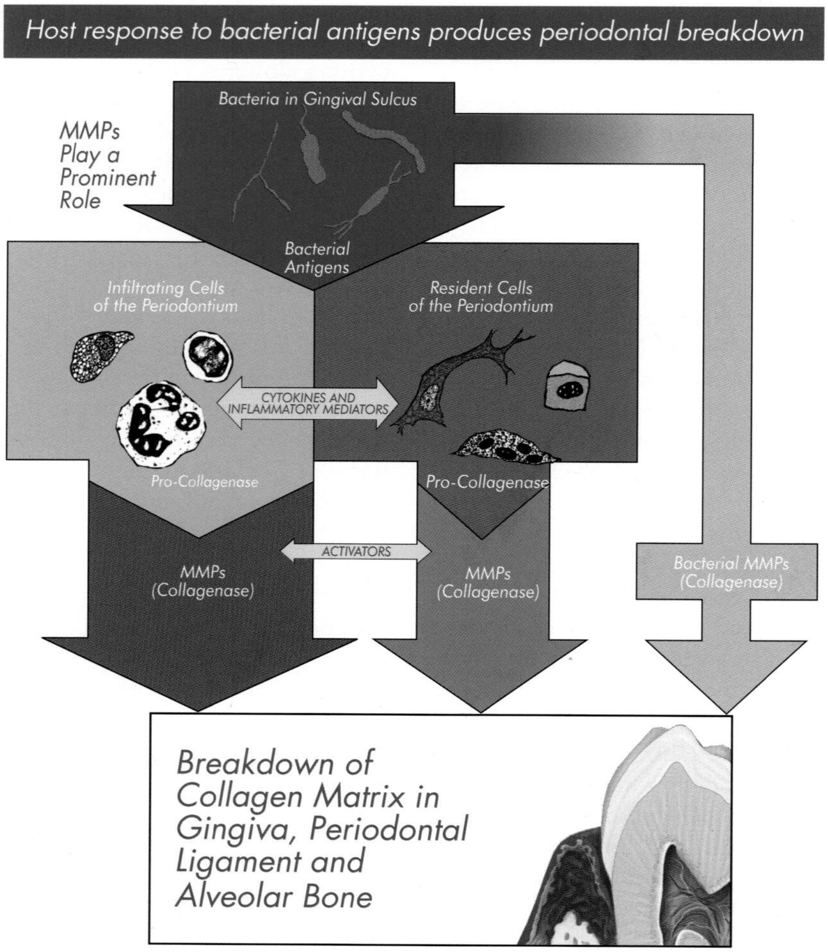

Figure 15–6. Collagenase and the pathogenesis of periodontal disease.

over 50%. Sites with a baseline probing depth ≥ 7 mm, improved by Periostat® by 45%.

Incidences of Rapid Progression

Attachment loss of 3 mm or more occurring during the first 6 months of the three 12-month studies that required interventions by scaling and root planing (SRP) occurred in 52 tooth sites in a total of 9 patients receiving placebo versus 14 tooth sites in a total of 9 patients in the Periostat®-treatment group. Thus, there was a 73% reduction in the incidence of rapid progression of periodontitis associated with Periostat® and scaling treatment. Furthermore, in patients with incidences of rapid progression who received SRP treatment at 6 months, CAL improved by 2.16 mm after treatment with Periostat® plus SRP for an additional 6 months. In comparison, in patients who received placebo plus SRP at 6 months, CAL improved by only 0.78 mm after an additional 6 months ($p = .005$).

Adjunct to Scaling and Root Planing

A fourth study was conducted over a 9-month period in 190 patients who had at least two sites in each of two quadrants with CAL and PPD between 5 mm and 9 mm.[73] The study design was similar to the first three studies with the exception that Periostat® was evaluated as an adjunct to subgingival SRP. All data were analyzed by appropriate statistics as in the previous studies but also included a per-patient analysis of variance (ANOVA).

The results of this study showed that there was a consistent improvement of CAL of approximately 20% (1.03 mm versus 0.86) in patients with a probing depth of 4 to 6 mm ($p < .05$) and approximately 30% (1.55 vs 1.17) in those with probing depths of ≥ 7 mm ($p < .05$). It is also noteworthy that sites with a probing depth of 4 to 6 mm at baseline showed statistically significant improvements in CAL after 3, 6, and 9 months of treatment with Periostat® and SRP ($p < .05$) compared with treatment with SRP and placebo.

Similarly, for sites with a probing depth ≥ 7 mm at baseline, treatment with Periostat® significantly augmented the efficacy of SRP compared with SRP and placebo. Statistically significant improvements in CAL with Periostat® were observed after 3 months ($p < .01$), and after 6 and 9 months ($p < .05$).

Reductions in PPD were similar to those seen for gains in CAL. For sites with a baseline PPD of 4 to 6 mm, a statistically significant reduction was demonstrated after 3, 6, and 9 months in patients receiving Periostat® and SRP compared with patients receiving SRP and placebo ($p < .001$). A mean reduction of 0.96 mm was observed after 9 months of treatment with Periostat® whereas treatment with SRP and placebo resulted in a mean reduction of 0.71 mm ($p < .001$) representing a benefit of over 30%. Likewise, PPD at more severe sites (PPD ≥ 7 mm at baseline) improved significantly after 3 ($p < .001$), 6 ($p < .001$), and 9 months ($p < .01$) of treatment with Periostat® compared with SRP and placebo treatment. A mean reduction of 1.68 mm was seen after 9 months of treatment with Periostat® whereas SRP and placebo treatment resulted in a mean reduction of 1.21 mm ($p < .01$), representing a benefit of almost 40%.

Results of safety studies showed the use of Periostat® 20 mg bid, either with or without mechanical therapy (SRP), did not exert an antimicrobial effect on the periodontal microflora and did not result in a detrimental shift in the normal flora and the colonization or overgrowth of the periodontal pocket by bacteria resistant to doxycycline, tetracycline, minocycline, amoxicillin, erythromycin, or clindamycin. In addition, there was no evidence of any tendency toward the acquisition of multiantibiotic resistance.[74,75]

Although no product is available at this time, host modulation by inhibition of prostaglandins may be of value in the future treatment of periodontal disease. The drugs of interest in this category are the nonsteroidal anti-inflammatory agents.[76]

Agents for Oral Fungal Infections

Oral fungal infections can be expected to increase with an aging population; with increasing age, *Candida albicans*, the agent responsible for these infections, flourishes due to a decrease in salivary flow that may be physiologic, psychological, or medication induced.

Fungal infections may occur as a side effect of antibiotic therapy or during chronic medication with tranquilizers, sedatives, and anticholinergic drugs. If these infections occur in patients wearing full or partial dentures, therapy includes not only medicating the patients but also having them soak their prosthesis in the medication for the duration of the oral therapy. In some cases, the acrylic portions of the appliances must be remade since fungi may be present in its pores. Some common antifungal agents are reviewed below.

Nystatin
Nystatin (eg, Mycostatin) was discovered in 1954 and is an excellent antibiotic for the treatment of

fungal infections. It is most useful in the treatment of both oral and vaginal moniliasis (thrush, candidiasis). This drug binds to the covering membrane of susceptible fungi, altering the permeability of the cell membrane and leading to cell death. It is both fungistatic and fungicidal.

Metabolism. This drug can be given orally but is poorly absorbed from the gastrointestinal tract, and large amounts are found in feces. Also, it is not absorbed from the skin and mucous membranes and is therefore not given parenterally. It exerts its main effect via the topical route in most cases.

Adverse Effects. Adverse effects are rare and include nausea, vomiting, and diarrhea following oral administration. However, no adverse effects have been reported via the topical route. Hypersensitivity reactions have not occurred, nor has resistance. It also appears to be safe for use during pregnancy.

Dosage and Dosage Forms. This antibiotic is available as a tablet or liquid for oral or vaginal use and as an ointment and cream for topical and vaginal use. Since it is not absorbed when swallowed, it has a topical effect in the gastrointestinal tract. For oral candidiasis, a rinse of 400,000 to 600,000 units daily is usually effective. For vaginal conditions, a dose of 100,000 to 200,000 units daily for 2 weeks is indicated.

Ketoconazole

Ketoconazole (Nizoral) is classified as an imidazole, and its oral administration is approved for the treatment of systemic fungal infections. It is also useful for the treatment of oral and vaginal candidiasis (thrush).

Mechanism of Action. Ketoconazole interferes with the synthesis of chemicals needed to form the plasma membrane of fungi, resulting in disorganization of the membrane.

Metabolism. Its absorption from the gastrointestinal tract is better than that of nystatin. It is metabolized in the liver, and only small amounts are found in urine and feces. Since data for its use in pregnancy are lacking, it is not recommended for pregnant women. The presence of the drug in breast milk has been recognized.

Adverse Effects. The most common adverse effects are nausea and pruritus. Headache, dizziness, gastrointestinal problems, nervousness, and liver dysfunction occur less often. Gynecomastia has been reported in 10% of men treated with ketoconazole. Since this medication has some liver toxicity, if it is used for more than 2 weeks, liver function tests should be performed.

Dosage and Dosage Forms. It is available in tablet form in 200 mg doses and also as an ointment. For oral candidiasis, the usual dose is 200 mg daily for 10 days.

Miconazole (Monistat)

This drug is classified as an imidazole and has the same mechanism of action as ketoconazole. However, it is used mainly as an antifungal vaginal preparation and as a skin medication applied topically.

Its main side effects are irritation, burning, or maceration. It is considered safe for use in pregnancy because absorption is less than 1% when applied topically. Studies relative to its use in dentistry are minimal.

Clotrimazole (Lotrimin, Mycelex)

This drug is chemically similar to miconazole. It is available as a topical and systemic agent and is used more widely in Europe than in this country. Since it is more toxic than the other antifungal agents, it should be used when the others have not been successful topically.

Adverse Effects. Its main side effects after topical use are the same as those of miconazole. Also, after topical or systemic use, it may cause hallucinations, gastrointestinal disturbances, and abnormal liver function. Since abnormal liver function has occurred in 15% of patients using the troche, periodic liver function tests are indicated if therapy exceeds 2 weeks.

Dosage and Dosage Forms. A 10-mg troche is available for oral topical use every 3 hours. Studies have shown that if the troche is allowed to dissolve in the mouth for 30 minutes, therapeutic levels can be found in saliva for up to 3 hours. Apparently, this is due to release of the drug from sites in the oral mucosa to which it binds. Since the amount absorbed systemically by this route has not been determined, signs of adverse reactions associated with systemic administration must be monitored. Its safety in pregnancy has not been determined.

Mouthrinses and Dentifrices

Mouthrinses and dentifrices have been shown to be of value mainly in the reduction of plaque and gingivitis. Some of these agents have been shown to have a significant effect in the reduction of gingivitis, and they have received the American Dental Association (ADA) Seal of Acceptance.

Listerine Antiseptic®, Cool Mint Listerine®, FreshBurst Listerine®, chlorhexidine gluconate (Peridex®), and two generic equivalents of Listerine Antiseptic® and triclosan have been granted the

ADA Seal of Acceptance. These antimicrobial mouthrinses provide a standard of comparison for all other available products.

The phenolic compound Listerine® showed a reduction of 20 to 34% in plaque and a reduction of 28 to 44% in gingivitis in two 6-month studies and one 9-month study.[77-79] The bis-biguanide chlorhexidine (0.12%) has also proven effective in the reduction of both plaque and gingivitis.[80] Chlorhexidine, however, has been associated with staining of teeth, altered taste, and increased levels of calculus formation and is available by prescription only. A further consideration is that a patient should rinse and/or irrigate with this preparation at least 30 minutes after brushing because of a decrease in efficacy due to an interaction with the positively charged sodium lauryl sulfate, the detergent component of dentifrices.[81] Similarly, the negatively charged fluoride ion may interact with chlorhexidine and also greatly reduce its efficacy. This cationic nature, however, is the basis for the substantivity of chlorhexidine. This property allows chlorhexidine to bind to negatively charged ions and proteins of the mucous membranes and teeth, and to maintain that contact for some time.[82]

There are several other antimicrobial mouthrinses available that have not yet received the ADA Seal of Acceptance. The quaternary ammonium compounds such as Cepacol®, Scope®, and New Viadent® have some degree of substantivity but less than that of chlorhexidine.[83]

Sanguinaria, an herbal extract, has not been shown to produce significant reductions in plaque and gingivitis in 6-month studies. The recent addition of zinc chloride to the dentifrice and mouthrinse formulations, however, has helped to produce a significant reduction in both plaque and gingivitis.[84] In the United States, the sanguinaria products are available as original formula in Viadent® mouthrinse and toothpaste. To date, however, the ADA Seal of Acceptance has not been awarded to the Viadent® products.

Plax®, a popular prebrushing rinse, has not been shown to reduce plaque and gingivitis extensively enough to receive the ADA Seal of Acceptance. Clinical studies regarding the efficacy of Plax® have yielded equivocal results.[85-92]

Triclosan

Triclosan (2,4,4'-Trichloro-2' – hydroxydiphenyl ether) is a new antiplaque/antigingivitis agent available in dentifrices marketed throughout the world. The addition of a co-polymer (polyvinylmethylether maleic acid [PVM/MA]) has been shown to improve the effectiveness of triclosan by enhancing its retention (substantivity) onto hard and soft oral surfaces. This formula, found in Colgate Total®, has been cleared by the U.S. Food and Drug Administration (FDA) for sale in the United States and is also ADA accepted. Formulas without the co-polymer are not cleared for sale by the FDA. Therefore, formulations by Unilever and Procter & Gamble are only available outside the United States.

The clearance given by the FDA was based on data from two pivotal studies conducted in approximately 600 patients. Both studies were conducted at independent research centers and followed a similar protocol.[93,94] Both these long-term clinical studies provided statistically significant differences ($p < .01$) in gingivitis in favor of the 0.3% triclosan and 2.0% PVM/MA0 co-polymer dentifrice (in a sodium fluoride/silica base). The reduction in gingivitis averaged 24.3%. The Gingivitis Severity Index showed an average reduction of 60.6%. These two pivotal studies provided statistically significant differences ($p < .01$) in supragingival plaque accumulation in favor of the 0.3% triclosan and 2.0% PVM/MA co-polymer dentifrice (in a 0.243% sodium fluoride/silica base) as compared with a placebo dentifrice (in a 0.243% sodium fluoride/silica base). The Quigley-Hein Plaque Index efficacy results showed an average efficacy score of 15%. The Plaque Severity Index results averaged a 19% reduction.

Seven other studies showed a reduction in gingivitis for the Colgate Total® formulation, ranging from 19.7 to 81.5%, with an average reduction of 25.3%. The reduction in Gingivitis Severity was 56%. Reductions in plaque in these studies ranged from 12.7 to 58.9%, with an average reduction of 30.2%. The average reduction in Plaque Severity was 54.9%.[95-101]

In all the studies carried out (in a total of over 1,400 patients), no extrinsic staining was observed, there were no serious adverse effects associated with the triclosan containing dentifrice (Colgate Total®), and there were no complaints of taste alterations or unpleasant taste. Additionally, reductions in calculus averaging 35% have been reported in studies with durations ranging between 3 and 6 months.[102]

A recent study evaluated the effect of a dentifrice containing triclosan/co-polymer on the microflora and clinical signs characteristic of recurrent adult periodontitis.[103] Sixty patients (mean age of 55 years) previously treated for advanced periodontal disease were included in this 36-month study. During a 3- to 5-year period following active therapy, the patients had been enrolled in a supportive periodontal therapy program and were on a 3-month recall interval. All patients who were enrolled had, at various intervals during the preceding 3 to 5 years, exhibited signs of recurrent periodontitis, such as deepened pockets and additional loss of attachment (> 2 mm) and alveolar bone. All subjects presented with moderate gingivitis and exhibited lesions characterized by probing pocket depth of > 5 mm in eight sites (at least two in each quadrant), and loss of interproximal alveolar bone (> 40% of original height), as seen in radiographs. Standardized radiographs were taken at baseline and 36 months. In a subset of 40 patients, the deepest pocket site in each quadrant (ie, four sites per subject) was selected, and samples of the subgingival bacteria were taken. The test group included 30 individuals who used a dentifrice containing triclosan/co-polymer/fluoride, that is, 0.3% triclosan, 2% co-polymer, and 1100 ppm F from 0.243% sodium fluoride. The control group also included 30 subjects who used a dentifrice identical to the one used in the test group but without the triclosan/co-polymer content. No professional subgingival therapy was delivered between the baseline and the 36th-month examinations. The subjects were recalled every 3 months. Re-examinations were performed after 6, 12, 24, and 36 months of the trial.

The clinical results of this study showed that for bleeding on probing (BOP), in both groups between the baseline and the 36th-month examination, there was a small but insignificant decrease in the number of BOP-positive sites (test group 4% and control group 8%). For probing depth, in the test group, the PPD value gradually *decreased* between examinations. The mean reductions in PPD between baseline and the 6th-, 12th-, 24th-, and 36th-month examinations were 0.02 mm, 0.05 mm, 0.03 mm, and 0.14 mm, respectively. In the control group, the mean PPD gradually *increased*, and the corresponding mean PPD increases at the 6th-, 12th-, 24th-, and 36th-month examinations were 0.03 mm, 0.10 mm, 0.17 mm, and 0.19 mm, respectively. The difference in PPD change (mean 0.33 mm) between the test and control groups during the 36th-month interval was statistically significant ($p < .01$). It was also noted that in the test group the frequency of sites with shallow pockets (< 3 mm) *increased* between baseline and 36 months (from 57 to 61%), the medium deep pockets (4 to 5 mm) *decreased* from 31 to 27% while the percentage of sites with deep pockets (6 mm) remained unchanged (12%). In the control group, the frequency of shallow pockets *decreased* with an average of 2% while sites with deep pockets *increased* with an average of 2%. For CAL, the mean value increased between the baseline and the 36th-month. In the test group, the mean additional CAL loss amounted to 0.11 mm (12 months), 0.14 mm (24 months), and 0.18 mm (36 months). The corresponding additional loss in the control group was 0.22 mm (12 months), 0.35 mm (24 months), and 0.52 mm (36 months). The additional loss in probing attachment that occurred between baseline and the 24th- and 36th-month examinations was significantly higher in the control group than in the test group ($p < .05$ and $p < .01$, respectively). In all three intervals (0 to 12 months; 12 to 24 months; 24 to 36 months), the test group exhibited fewer sites with additional attachment loss than did the control group. Thus, between baseline and the 12th month, in the test group, there were 48 loser sites compared with 67 sites in the controls. The corresponding numbers for period 2 (12 to 24 months) were 37 and 59, and for period 3 (24 to 36 months) were 72 and 197.

The microflora analysis showed that the total viable count (TVC) of bacteria decreased in both groups between the baseline examination and the re-examination after 36 months. In the control group, the TVC value was reduced from 15×10^6 to 12×10^6 (not significant). In the test group, the corresponding reduction was more pronounced (from 17×10^6 to 9×10^6) and statistically significant ($p < .05$). It was also noted that for periodontal pathogens, the reductions were greater in the triclosan/co-polymer group than in the control group.

The results of this study suggest that use of a triclosan/co-polymer dentifrice reduced the frequency of deep periodontal pockets and the number of sites that exhibited additional probing attachment and bone loss. This finding may be related to the fact that a number of studies have shown that supragingival plaque reduction has a strong influence on the quantity and quality of the subgingival microflora.[104,105] It has been shown that thorough removal of supragingival plaque results in a reduction in the TVC of subgingival microflora and in the number of periodontal pathogens in shallow (< 3 mm) as well as moderately deep pockets (4 to 6 mm).[106,107]

Triclosan is marketed in Europe as a mouthrinse (Plax®) as well. The European formula differs from the U.S. formula because of the inclusion of triclosan. This triclosan-containing mouthrinse has been shown to significantly reduce plaque and gingivitis with minimal side effects.

EFFECTS OF MEDICATIONS

The Periodontium

Medications can have both beneficial and adverse effects on periodontal tissues. Some of these effects are discussed below.

In terms of their relationship to tissues, medications should be categorized on the basis of the following: alteration of methods in behavior and oral hygiene, alteration of plaque composition, alteration of salivary pH, effect on salivary flow, effect on gingival tissues, effect on alveolar bone, and effect on gingival crevicular fluid. Some effects of medications may increase the risk of dental diseases while some others may actually decrease the risk.

Behavioral Alteration of Oral Hygiene Practice

Patients who are on medications that have a depressant effect on the central nervous system, such as sedatives, tranquilizers, narcotic analgesics, antimetabolites, and antihypertensives, may become careless about their oral hygiene practices; therefore, they have a tendency toward increased plaque formation. The basis for the change in a patient's attitude or behavior must be understood, and an oral hygiene program must be designed on the basis of these changes.

Two of the top 20 prescription drugs in the United States act directly as mood-altering drugs; alprazolam (Xanax) and fluoxetine (Prozac) may make patients more amenable to improving their oral hygiene.[108] However, since drowsiness is a side effect of these medications, motivation may still be a problem. Two other drugs that alter moods as a side effect of their antihypertensive action, enalapril maleate (Vasotec) and captopril (Capoten), may make patients less amenable to following oral hygiene procedures.

Plaque Composition and Salivary pH

Plaque composition and pH as well as salivary pH may be altered by the dosage of medications. Over-the-counter (OTC) medications and liquid pharmaceutical preparations are used daily by some people. Although the active ingredients in these medicines are sometimes necessary for improvement or maintenance of health, some inactive ingredients pose hidden dangers. For example, many liquid or chewable pharmaceutical preparations for children are made palatable by the addition of sucrose, glucose, or fructose as sweeteners. Sugars are the sweetening agents in orally administered antifungal preparations. Since these medications come as lozenges, troches, and oral solutions and are kept in the mouth for extended periods, they may place patients at a significant risk for caries. Antacid tablets also contain large amounts of sugar and, in the older adult, may result in increased caries of root surfaces. The readily fermentable carbohydrates in thick liquid preparations may add significantly to alteration of plaque pH and composition. Although the risk of caries has been shown to increase with the use of these medications,[109] their effects on the periodontal pathogens has not been evaluated.

Sugars, metabolized by bacteria to acid end-products, lower salivary pH as well as the pH within an adherent bacteria-rich plaque that is relatively unavailable to salivary buffering. This lowered pH near the tooth surface can cause ionic dissolution from the hydroxyapatite crystals, increase surface roughness, and enhance the plaque's ability to be more adherent and to initiate caries. It has been shown that human plaque pH decreased significantly after administration of liquid iron supplements[110] and cough syrups.[111]

A controlled clinical study of patients on chronic doses of medication reported a significant increase in both dental caries and gingivitis in a population of children taking liquid or chewable medications continuously for a minimum of 6 months.[112]

The alteration of plaque composition and plaque retention to tooth surfaces may have periodontal implications that must be considered in patients with excess plaque.

Salivary Flow

Adequate salivary flow is critical to the maintenance of the health of oral soft tissues.[113] It has been suggested that "mouthbreathers" have modified plaque accumulations and associated soft-tissue changes. A number of medications that decrease salivary flow (xerostomia) mimic mouthbreathing.[114] For example, a study at our research center evaluated the effect of anticholinergic agents on plaque and oral health in patients who had gastrointestinal ulcers and were receiving such medications.[115] It was found that these patients had a tendency to accumulate more plaque after dental prophylaxis and oral hygiene instructions and had a slower rate of resolution of gingivitis following scaling and root planing. In this short-term study, it was found that a statistically significant reduction occurred in the control patients in all clinical measures of gingival health other than pocket depth, but no significant reductions were observed in the medicated patients. Agents that produce xerostomia include antihypertensives, narcotic analgesics, some tranquilizers, quinolones, antimetabolites, antihistamines, sedatives, and even vitamin D in large doses.[116] In addition to the effect of xerostomia on oral soft tissues, root surface caries may be more prevalent in those taking such medications.[117]

Long-term tranquilizing agents, especially the phenothiazines and meprobamate, have been reported to produce xerostomia and, in some situations, an overgrowth of *C. albicans* in the oral microflora.[118] Patients on long-term phenothiazines have also shown a tendency to developing less calculus.

Gingival Tissue

A number of medications may cause gingival enlargement. Phenytoin (Dilantin) was the first drug reported to produce this effect with the incidence ranging between 3 and 62% (mean 50%). A number of investigations have suggested a causal relationship between inflammation and gingival hyperplasia, the implication being that this hyperplasia could be minimized or prevented if gingival inflammation were eliminated.[119,120] It is possible that, if patients are placed on a strict program of oral hygiene within 10 days of the initiation of therapy with medications promoting gingival enlargement, its occurrence can be minimized.[121,122]

Although the occurrence of gingival enlargement due to phenytoin has been clearly established, its cellular and molecular mechanisms of action for this effect are unclear. A recent study suggests that phenytoin augmented the expression of the gene for platelet-derived growth factor-B (PDGF-B).[123] In this study, the authors also showed that gingival macrophages exposed to phenytoin secrete increased amounts of PDGF. This may increase not only the proliferation of gingival cells but also alveolar bone cells. A recent report suggests that phenytoin has the ability to stimulate bone cell proliferation and differentiation and may mature osteoblastic activities to stimulate bone formation.[124] If so, this may explain the authors' clinical impression of minimal bone loss in patients with phenytoin-induced gingival hyperplasia. The effect on PDGF may also explain an early report in which a patient being medicated with phenytoin underwent orthodontic tooth movement; and with no special rapid movement planned, the teeth moved in half the time with no adverse effects on bone or shortening of the roots.[125] In this case, phenytoin may have favored bone remodeling. It is possible that although phenytoin produces an increased risk factor for gingival enlargement and the associated gin-

givitis, it may result in a decreased risk factor for bone loss found in periodontitis.

Gingival enlargement has also been associated with a number of calcium channel blockers, including nifedipine (Procardia), verapamil (Calan), diltiazem (Cardizem), and isradipine (DynaCirc). Gingival enlargement is seen in 5 to 20% of patients taking these medications.

A proposed mechanism of action relates inflammatory factors within the gingival tissue to gingival enlargement. It has been shown that the histology in a nifedipine patient resembled an inflammatory-type hyperplasia similar to that described for phenytoin, in which numerous inflammatory cells replaced collagen in connective tissue.[126] This paper supports the concept that alteration of the intracellular calcium level in gingival cells by nifedipine in combination with appropriate local inflammatory factors is important in eliciting gingival enlargement.

It has also been shown that if nifedipine could not be discontinued, gingival enlargement did not recur after gingivectomy when thorough plaque control was carried out, again supporting earlier reported findings of the role of inflammation and plaque.[127]

Gingival enlargement has also been reported with cyclosporine, with an incidence of approximately 25%.[128] There are a number of similarities between the clinical and histopathologic changes seen in cyclosporine- and phenytoin-induced gingival enlargement. Also, both drugs are known to have an effect on the immune system, including the induction of lymphoid hyperplasias and lymphomas. For these patients, meticulous plaque control, as a preventive measure upon initiation of and throughout cyclosporine therapy and as a corrective procedure after completion of therapy, may be of value as in the case of patients on phenytoin therapy.[129,130] Also, it has been postulated that cyclosporine alters fibroblastic activity. The role of plaque in this process has not been clearly established, and conflicting results have been reported.

Alveolar Bone

In addition to their antibacterial effects, tetracyclines are now known to inhibit pathologically excessive host-derived matrix metalloproteinase activity during periodontal and other diseases. The discovery of the anticollagenolytic properties of the tetracyclines was made using an animal model of both pathologically excessive collagenase activity in gingival tissues and periodontal breakdown.[131,132]

A recent study showed that treating germ-free and pathogen-reduced rats, inoculated with *Porphyromonas gingivalis*, by the oral administration of a nonantimicrobial dose of a tetracycline (as discussed earlier in this chapter) or a chemically modified nonantimicrobial tetracycline significantly inhibited periodontal bone loss.[133]

Although the mechanisms of this drug effect are not yet clear, tetracyclines can also directly inhibit osteoclast-mediated bone resorption and the production of collagenase and gelatinase.[134] It is not yet known whether this therapeutic effect reflects a direct inhibition of bone resorption longitudinally, the inhibition of episodes of bone resorption in its early stages, or the proanabolic effects on bone formation. These issues as well as others such as the temporal relationship of matrix metalloproteinase (collagenase, gelatinase) induction and bone loss should be addressed in future studies.

Antibiotics have also been shown to be of value in arresting bone loss in special types of periodontal disease, such as rapidly advancing periodontitis, localized juvenile periodontitis, and refractory periodontitis, with the mechanism of action related to the drug's antimicrobial effects.[135]

Nonsteroidal anti-inflammatory drugs (NSAIDs) may reduce bone loss in both animal and human models, with a variety of agents showing some effect.[136] Epidemiologic studies of the periodontium of patients receiving NSAIDs on a long-term basis for arthritis suggested that they had less alveolar bone loss than a similar population not receiving these medications.[137] The mechanism of action of these agents appears to be related to their effect on prostaglandins.

Gingival Crevicular Fluid

An increase in gingival crevicular fluid (GCF) flow may be responsible for more rapid plaque formation. With the increasing severity of gingivitis, the GCF flow also increases, which may contribute to an increased amount of plaque.[138] This relationship was first observed when more plaque was seen to have formed as the gingivitis became more severe. A possible mechanism may be that GCF has higher levels of calcium, which may act as a binding agent favoring bacterial aggregation and precipitation of salivary proteins.[139] Also, it has been noted that plaque wettability increases with disease and that this factor may be affected by GCF. Following this reasoning, since anti-inflammatory drugs decrease gingival inflammation, if an associated decrease in GCF occurs,

one might expect less plaque to be present in these patients. However, in contrast, an earlier study reported that, although GCF flow decreased with topical steroid application of fluocinonide (Sulindac), a systemic nonsteroidal anti-inflammatory drug, this had no plaque-reducing effect.[140] Noting that the same amount of plaque was present in both groups of patients, they concluded that GCF flow may not have an effect on plaque accumulation.

Change in Crevicular Fluid Content

Since GCF is in intimate contact with plaque, alterations in its content and pH deserve investigation. Do anti-inflammatory and other systemic drugs change the pH and composition of this fluid? Are the changes significant to plaque accumulation and metabolism? It has been demonstrated that glucose is present in GCF in levels higher than those found in saliva.[141] An unanswered question is, "Does this level change when oral hypoglycemics or insulin are administered?" Soluble gold salts decrease the number of inflammatory cells in gingival tissues;[142] since metals like gold have antibacterial properties, can their administration improve periodontal health?

Antibiotic Resistance

Since antibiotics have been extensively discussed in this chapter, consideration must be given to the development of resistance to them. Resistance to mouthrinse and dentifrice ingredients or to locally delivered medications has not been demonstrated with one exception. *S. sanguis* resistance to chlorhexidine has been reported after 2 years of use of the drug. However, the clinical significance of this finding is unclear at this time since oral disease has not been associated with *S. sanguis*, although bacterial endocarditis has been caused by this microbe.

However, resistance to systemically administered antibiotics is increasing, and a brief review of this topic follows.

Penicillin was first discovered in 1896 by a French medical student, but at the time the discovery was not evaluated for its true meaning. In 1928, it was rediscovered by Fleming, a Scottish physician. However, penicillin was not mass produced by drug companies until 1943. Shortly after the introduction of penicillin, *Staphylococcus aureus* resistance to it developed, sending manufacturers rushing to produce forms of penicillin that could overcome this resistance.

The development of antibiotic resistance has been dramatic. In 1967, the resistance of *Streptococ-*

cus pneumoniae and Neisseria gonorrhoeae was documented. In 1983, another penicillin-resistant bacterium, Enterococcus fecrisa, developed in hospital settings. Between 1979 and 1987, only 0.02% of pneumococcal strains infecting a large number of patients surveyed by the Centers for Disease Control and Prevention (CDC) were penicillin resistant. The CDC survey included 13 hospitals in 12 states in the United States.[143] Today, 6.6% of pneumococcal strains are resistant.[144] In 1992, 13,300 hospital patients in the United States died of bacterial infections that were resistant to antibiotic treatment.

Although antibiotics themselves do not directly cause resistance, they do create situations that allow an existing variant strain of bacteria to flourish. This results in the development of resistance to the antibiotic. A patient can develop a drug-resistant infection either by contracting a resistant microorganism before treatment or by having a resistant microbe emerge in the body in the course of antibiotic treatment. Drug-resistant infections not only increase the risk of death but are also often associated with prolonged hospital stays and even medical complications. These infections could necessitate removing part of a ravaged lung, or replacing a damaged heart valve.

In another example of the natural development of resistance, erythromycin attacks ribosomes within a cell, enabling it to make proteins. Resistant bacteria have slightly altered ribosomes to which the antibiotic cannot bind. The ribosomal route is also how bacteria become resistant to other antibiotics such as tetracycline, streptomycin, and gentamicin.

Antibiotic resistance can occur in three ways: spontaneous mutations of a bacterium's own genetic material (DNA), acquisition of DNA from another bacterium through transformation, and acquisition via plasmid transmission. Though bacterial antibiotic resistance is a natural process, as outlined above, other factors also contribute to the problem (eg, increased infection transmission coupled with inappropriate antibiotic use).

Today, more people are contracting infections. Sinusitis among adults is on the rise, as are ear infections in children. Nearly 6 million antibiotic prescriptions for sinusitis were written in 1985 and nearly 13 million in 1992. For middle-ear infections, the numbers of prescriptions are 15 million in 1985, and 23.6 million in 1992.

Clearcut reasons for the dramatic rise in infections are not available; however, suggested causes include an increase in communal living situations (day-care centers for children and adults, senior citizen centers, homeless shelters, and nursing homes) and increased use of medications (for immunocompromised patients, transplantation patients, and patients on cancer chemotherapy), which make people more prone to infection. Additionally, the aging of our population is an added risk factor for infection.

ANTIBIOTICS IN POULTRY AND OTHER MEATS

Although the FDA limits the amount of antibiotic residue in meats, the question arises as to whether these foods are a source of low-dose antibiotics, subsequently resulting in resistance. The FDA is also evaluating whether bacterial resistance to quinolone antibiotics can emerge in animals slaughtered for food and consequently cause disease in humans. Although thorough cooking greatly reduces the likelihood of antibiotic-resistant bacteria surviving in meat and infecting a human, the possibility remains. There have been sporadic reports of pathogens resistant to drugs other than fluoroquinolones surviving in cooked meat and infecting a human. For example, in 1983, 18 people in four midwestern states suffered multidrug-resistant Salmonella food poisoning after eating beef from cows fed antibiotics. Eleven of the people were hospitalized and one died.

ANTIBIOTIC RESISTANCE AND HUMAN USE

A study of the development of antibiotic resistance in humans shows that the increase in antibiotic resistance parallels the increase in antibiotic use. This study examined a large group of cancer patients given fluoroquinolones to prevent infection. The patients' white blood cell counts were very low as a result of their cancer treatment, leaving them open to infection. Between 1983 and 1993, the percentage of such patients receiving antibiotics rose from 1.4 to 45%. During these years, researchers isolated Escherichia coli annually from the patients and tested the microbes for resistance to five types of fluoroquinolones. Between 1983 and 1990, all 92 E. coli strains tested were easily killed by the antibiotics. But from 1991 to 1993, 11 of the 40 tested strains (28%) were resistant to all five drugs. Resistance is also occurring to vancomycin, which has been the "last resort" antibiotic for many infections, including Staphylococcus. Vancomycin-resistant enterococci were first reported in England and France in 1987, and appeared in one New York City hospital in 1989. By 1991, 38 hospitals in the United States reported the pathogen. By 1993, 14% of patients with enterococci infections in intensive-care units in some hospitals had vancomycin-resistant strains, a 20-fold increase from 1987. In 1992, a British laboratory observed the transfer of a vancomycin-resistant gene from *Enterococcus* to *Staphylococcus aureus* in the laboratory. The fear now is that if vancomycin-resistant enterococci can transfer their resistance, anti-*Staphylococcus* antibiotics will no longer be of value.

In view of the rapid rise in antibiotic resistance in recent years, all dental prescriptions for antibiotics should be accompanied by careful instructions to the patient regarding proper dosage and taking the full prescription. All antibiotics should be prescribed in situations where their value is well established so that unnecessary prescribing against "normal" bacteria does not occur. These simple safeguards can help us all win the battle against resistant strains.

REFERENCES

1. Ciancio SG. FDA Approves periostat marketing. Biol Ther Dent 1998; 14:21–2.
2. Ciancio SG, Bourgault PC. Clinical pharmacology for dental professionals. 3rd ed. St. Louis (MO): C.V. Mosby Co.; 1989. p.58.
3. Barnett ML. Inhibition of oral contraceptive effectiveness by concurrent antibiotic administration. J Periodontol 1985;56(1):18–21.
4. Preus HR, Lassen J, Aass AM, Christersson LA. Prevention of transmission of resistant bacteria between periodontal sites during subgingival application of antibiotics. J Clin Periodontol 1993;20:299–303.
5. Poliak SC, DiGiovanna JJ, Gross EG, et al. Minocycline-associated tooth discoloration in young adults. JAMA 1985;254:2930–2.
6. Salman RA, Salman DG, Glickman RS, et al. Minocycline-induced pigmentation of the oral cavity. J Oral Med 1985;40:154–7.
7. Attwood HD, Dennett X. A black thyroid and minocycline treatment. Br Med J 1976;2:1109–10.
8. Ciancio SG, Slots J, Reynolds HS, et al. The effect of short-term administration of minocycline HCl on gingival inflammation and subgingival microflora. J Periodontol 1982;9:557–61.
9. Hayes C, Antczak Bouckoms A, Burdick E. Quality assessment and meta-analysis of systemic tetracycline use in chronic adult periodontitis. J Clin Periodontol 1992;19:164–8.
10. Kornman KS, Robertson PB. Clinical and microbiological evaluation of therapy for juvenile periodontitis. J Periodontol 1985;56:443–6.
11. Lindhe J, Liljenberg B. Treatment of localized juvenile periodontitis. Results after 5 years. J Clin Periodontol 1984;11:399–410.
12. Papli R, Lewis JM. Refractory chronic periodontitis: effect of oral tetracycline hydrochloride and root planing. Aust Dent J 1989;34:60–8.
13. Kornman KS, Karl E. The effect of long-term low-dose tetracycline therapy on the subgingival microflora in refractory adult periodontitis. J Periodontol 1982;53:604–10.
14. Shapiro A. Healing potential of periodontal osseous defects treated by scaling and root planing. J Dent Que 1990;27:587–92.
15. Preus H. Treatment of rapidly destructive periodontitis in Papillon-Lefèvre syndrome. Laboratory and clinical observations. J Clin Periodontol 1988;15:639–43.
16. Loesche WH, Schmidt E, Smith BA, et al. Effects of metronidazole on periodontal treatment needs. J Periodontol 1991;62:247–57.
17. Loesche WJ, Giordano JR, Hujoel PP, et al. Metronidazole in periodontitis: reduced need for surgery. J Clin Periodontol 1992;19:103–12.
18. Loesche WJ, Giordano JR. Metronidazole in periodontitis V: debridement should precede medication. Compendium Cont Educ Dent 1994; 25:1198–2001.
19. van Winkelhoff AJ, de Graaff J. Microbiology in the management of destructive periodontal disease. J Clin Periodontol 1991;18:411–20.
20. Collins JG, Offenbacher S, Arnold RR. Effects of a combination therapy to eliminate *Porphyromonas gingivalis* in refractory periodontitis. J Periodontol 1993;64:998–1007.
21. Walker CB, Gordon JM, Cornwall HA, et al. Gingival crevicular fluid levels of clindamycin compared with its minimal inhibitory concentrations for periodontal bacteria. Antimicrob Agents Chemo 1981;19:867–71.
22. Walker CB, Gordon JM, Magnusson I, Clark WB. A role for antibiotics in the treatment of refractory periodontitis. J Periodontol 1993;64:772–81.
23. Magnusson I, Clark WB, Low SB, et al. Effect of non-surgical periodontal therapy combined with adjunctive antibiotics in subjects with "refractory" periodontal disease: I. Clinical results. J Clin Periodontol 1989;16:647–53.
24. Magnusson I, Marks RG, Clark WB, et al. Clinical, microbiological and immunological characteristics of subjects with "refractory" periodontal disease. J Clin Periodontol 1991;18:291–9.

25. Magnusson I, Low SB, McArthur WP, et al. Treatment of subjects with refractory periodontal disease. J Clin Periodontol 1994;21:628–37.

26. Walker C, Gordon J. The effect of clindamycin on the microbiota associated with refractory periodontitis. J Periodontol 1990;61:692–8.

27. Quee TC, Clark C, Lautar-Lemay C, et al. The role of adjunctive Rodogyl therapy in the treatment of advanced periodontal disease. A longitudinal clinical and microbiologic study. J Periodontol 1987;58:594–601.

28. Quee TC, Al-Joburi W, Lautar-Lemay C, et al. Comparison of spiramycin and tetracycline used adjunctively in the treatment of advanced periodontitis. J Antimicrob Chemother 1988;22 (Suppl B):171–7.

29. Bain CA, Beagrie GS, Bourgoin J, et al. The effects of spiramycin and/or scaling on advanced periodontitis in humans. J Can Dent Assoc 1994; 60:209–17.

30. Slots J, Rams TE. Rational use of antibiotics. J Calif Dent Assoc 1990;18:21–3.

31. Slots J, Feik D, Rams TE. In vitro antimicrobial sensitivity of enteric rods and pseudomonads from advanced adult periodontitis. Oral Microbial Immunol 1990;5:298–301.

32. Pavicic M, van Winkelhoff A, de Graaff J. Synergistic effects between amoxicillin, metronidazole, and the hydroxymetabolite of metronidazole against *Actinobacillus actinomycetemcomitans*. Antimicrob Agents Chemother 1991;35:961–6.

33. van Winkelhoff AJ, Rodenberg JP, Goene RJ, et al. Metronidazole plus amoxicillin in the treatment of *Actinobacillus actinomycetemcomitans*-associated periodontitis. J Clin Periodontol 1989;16: 128–31.

34. Kornman KS, Newman MG, Flemmig TF, et al. Treatment of refractory periodontitis with metronidazole plus amoxicillin or Augmentin (Abstract 403). J Dent Res 1989;68(Spec Issue):917.

35. Aitken S, Birek P, Kulkarni GV, et al. Serial doxycycline and metronidazole in prevention of recurrent periodontitis in high-risk patients. J Periodontol 1992;63:97–102.

36. Birek D, Kulkarni GV, Lee WK, et al. Effect of serial doxycycline/metronidazole on recurrent periodontitis pathogens (Abstract 864). J Dent Res 1989;68(Spec Issue):373.

37. Matisko MW, Bissada NF. Short-term sequential administration of amoxicillin/clavulanate potassium and doxycycline in the treatment of recurrent/progressive periodontitis. J Periodontol 1993;64:553–8.

38. Golub LM, Ramamurthy N, McNamara TF, et al. Tetracyclines inhibit tissue collagenase activity. A new mechanism in the treatment of periodontal disease. J Periodontal Res 1984;19:651–5.

39. Löe H, Silness PJ. Periodontal disease in pregnancy. I. Prevalence and severity. Acta Odontol Scand 1953;21:533–51.

40. Silness PJ, Löe H. Periodontal disease in pregnancy. II. Correlation between oral hygiene and periodontal condition. Acta Odontol Scand 1964;22:121–35.

41. Fine JB, Harper DS, Gordon JM, et al. Short-term microbiological and clinical effects of subgingival irrigation with an antimicrobial mouthrinse. J Periodontol 1994;65:30–6.

42. Wolff LF, Bakdash MB, Pihlstrom Bl, et al. The effect of professional and home subgingival irrigation with antimicrobial agents on gingivitis and early periodontitis. J Dent Hygiene 1989;63:222–6.

43. Flemmig TF, Newman MG, Doherty FM, et al. Supragingival irrigation with 0.06% chlorhexidine in naturally occurring gingivitis. I. 6 month clinical observations. J Periodontol 1990;61: 112–7.

44. Cobb CM, Rodgers RL, Killoy WJ. Ultrastructural examination of human periodontal pockets following the use of an oral irrigation device in vivo. J Periodontol 1988; 59:155–9.

45. Aziz-Gandour IA, Newman HN. The effects of a simplified oral hygiene regimen plus supragingival irrigation with chlorhexidine or metronidazole on chronic inflammatory periodontal disease. J Clin Periodontol 1986;13:228–36.

46. Newman MG, Cattabriga M, Etienne D, et al. Effectiveness of adjunctive irrigation in early periodontitis—multicenter evaluation. J Periodontol 1994;65:224–9.

47. Boyd RL, Leggott P, Quinn R, et al. Effect of self-administered daily irrigation with 0.02% SnF$_2$ on periodontal disease activity. J Clin Periodontol 1985;12:420–31.

48. Drisko C, Forgas L, Killoy WJ. Subgingival irrigation with effervescent buffered aspirin solution in gingivitis and periodontitis (Abstract 1257). J Dent Res 1994;73.

49. Flemmig TF, Funkenhauser Z, Epp B, et al. Adjunctive supragingival irrigation in periodontitis treatment (Abstract 554). J Dent Res 1992;72 (Spec Issue):584.

50. Felo A, Shibly O, Ciancio SG, et al. Effects of subgingival chlorhexidine irrigation on peri-implant maintenance. Am J Dent 1997;10: 107–10.

51. Tonetti M, Cugini AM, Goodson JM. Zero order delivery with periodontal placement of tetracy-

cline loaded ethylene vinyl acetate fibers. J Periodontal Res 1990;25:243–7

52. Walker CB, Gordon JM, McQuilkin SJ, et al. Tetracycline: levels achievable in gingival crevice fluid and in vitro effect on subgingival organisms. Part II. Susceptibilities of periodontal bacteria. J Periodontol 1981;52:613–6.

53. Gordon JM, Walker CB, Murphy CJ, et al. Tetracycline: levels achievable in gingival crevice fluid and in vitro effect on subgingival organisms. Part I. Concentrations in crevicular fluid after repeated doses. J Periodontol 1981;52:609–12.

54. Goodson JM, Cugini MA, Kent RL, et al. Multicenter evaluation of tetracycline fiber therapy: II. Clinical response. J Periodontal Res 1991;26:371–9.

55. Newman MG, Kornman KS, Doherty FM. A 6-month multi-center evaluation of adjunctive tetracycline fiber therapy used in conjunction with scaling and root planing in maintenance patients: clinical results. J Periodontol 1994;65:685–91.

56. Goodson JM, Tanner A. Antibiotic resistance of the subgingival microbiota following local tetracycline therapy. Oral Microbiol Immunol 1992;7:113–7.

57. Niederman R, Holborow D, Tonetti M, et al. Reinfection of periodontal sites following tetracycline fiber therapy (Abstract 1345). J Dent Res 1990;69:277.

58. Morrison SL, Cobb CM, Kazakos GM, Killoy WJ. Root surface characteristics associated with subgingival placement of monolithic tetracycline-impregnated fibers. J Periodontol 1992;63:137–43.

59. Polson AM, Garrett S, Stoller NH, et al. Multicenter comparative evaluation of subgingivally delivered sanguinarine and doxycycline in the treatment of periodontitis. II. Clinical results. J Periodontol 1997;68:119–26.

60. Larsen T. Occurrence of doxycycline-resistant bacteria in the oral cavity after local administration of doxycycline in patients with periodontal disease. Scand J Infect Dis 1991;23:89–95.

61. Garrett S, Adams D, Bandt C, et al. Two multicenter clinical trials of subgingival doxycycline in the treatment of periodontitis (Abstract 1113). J Dent Res 1997;76:153.

62. Van Steenberghe D, Bercy P, Kohl J. Subgingival minocycline hydrochloride ointment in moderate to severe chronic adult periodontitis: a randomized, double-blind, vehicle-controlled, multicenter study. J Periodontol 1993;64:637–44.

63. Graca MA, Watts TLP, Wilson RF, Palmer RM. A randomized controlled-trial of a 2% minocycline gel as an adjunct to non-surgical periodontal treatment, using a design with multiple matching criteria. J Clin Periodontol 1997;24:249–53.

64. Ainamo J, Lie T, Ellingsen BH, et al. Clinical responses to subgingival application of a metronidazole 25% gel compared to the effect of subgingival scaling in adult periodontitis. J Clin Periodontol 1992;19 (Part II):723–9.

65. Klinge B, Attström R, Karring T, et al. Three regimens of topical metronidazole compared with subgingival scaling on periodontal pathology in adults. J Clin Periodontol 1992;19 (Part II):708–14.

66. Stelzel M, Flores-de-Jacoby L. Topical metronidazole application compared with subgingival scaling. A clinical and microbiological study on recall patients. J Clin Periodontol 1996;23:24–9.

67. Ainamo J, Lie T, Ellingsen BH, et al. Clinical responses to subgingival application of a metronidazole 25% gel compared to the effect of subgingival scaling in adult periodontitis. J Clin Periodontol 1992;19(Part I):723–9.

68. Soskolne WA, Heasman PA, Stabholz A, et al. Sustained local delivery of chlorhexidine in the treatment of periodontitis: a multi-center study. J Periodontol 1997; 68:32–8.

69. Briner WW, Kayrouz GA, Chanak MX. Comparative antimicrobial effectiveness of a substantive (0.12% chlorhexidine) and a nonsubstantive (phenolic) mouthrinse in vivo and in vitro. Compend Contin Educ Dent 1994;15:1158–68.

70. Jeffcoat M, Bray KS, Ciancio SG, et al. Adjunctive use of a subgingival controlled-release chlorhexidine chip reduces probing depth and improves attachment level compared with scaling and root planing alone. J Periodontol (In press).

71. Caton J, Bleiden T, Adams D, et al. Subantimicrobial doxycycline therapy for periodontitis (Abstract). J Dent Res 1997;76:1307.

72. Ciancio SG, Adams D, Blieden T, et al. Subantimicrobial dose doxycycline: a new adjunctive therapy for adult periodontitis. Presented at the Annual Meeting of The American Academy of Periodontology, Boston, MA, September 1998.

73. Caton JG, Ciancio SG, Crout RJ, et al. Post-treatment effects of adjunctive sub-antimicrobial dose doxycycline therapy. J Periodontology 1999 [Submitted].

74. Walker C, Thomas J. The effect of subantimicrobial doses of doxycycline on the microbial flora and antibiotic resistance in patients with adult periodontitis. Presented at The American Acad-

emy of Periodontology Meeting, Boston, MA, September, 1998.

75. Crout R, Adams D, Blieden T, et al. Safety of doxy-cycline hyclate 20 mg BID in patients with adult periodontitis. Presented at The American Academy of Periodontology Meeting, Boston, MA, September, 1998.

76. Howell TH, Williams RC. Non-steroidal anti-inflammatory drugs as inhibitors of periodontal disease progression. Crit Rev Oral Biol Med 1993;4:177–96.

77. Lamster IB, Alfano MC, Seiger MC, et al. The effect of Listerine antiseptic on reduction of existing plaque and gingivitis. Clin Prev Dent 1983;5:12–6.

78. Gordon JM, Lamster IB, Seiger MC. Efficacy of Listerine antiseptic in inhibiting the development of plaque and gingivitis. J Clin Periodontol 1985;12:697–704.

79. DePaola LG, Overholser CD, Meiller TF, et al. Chemotherapeutic inhibition of supragingival dental plaque and gingivitis development. J Clin Periodont 1989;16:311–5.

80. Löe H, Schiott CR. The effect of mouthrinses and topical application of chlorhexidine on the development of dental plaque and gingivitis in man. J Periodontal Res 1970;5:79–83.

81. Barkvoll P, Rolla G, Svendsen AK. Interaction between chlorhexidine digluconate and sodium lauryl sulfate in vivo. J Clin Periodontol 1989;16:593–5.

82. Mandel ID. Chemotherapeutic agents for controlling plaque and gingivitis. J Clin Periodontol 1988;15:488–98.

83. Davies RM. Rinses to control plaque and gingivitis. Int Dent J 1992;42(Suppl):276–80.

84. Wennstrom J, Lindhe J. Some effects of a sanguinarine-containing mouthrinse on developing plaque and gingivitis. J Clin Periodontol 1985;12:867–72.

85. O'Mahony G, O'Mullane DM. Evaluation of Plax pre-brushing rinse in reducing dental plaque (Abstract). J Dent Res 1990;69:246.

86. Patters MR, Shiloah J. A method for evaluating the effect of a pre-brushing rinse in reducing dental plaque [Abstract]. J Dent Res 1991;70:323.

87. Singh SM. Efficacy of Plax pre-brushing rinse in reducing dental plaque. Am J Dent 1990;3:15–6.

88. Freitas Bastos L, Collaert B, Attström R. Plaque removing efficacy of the pre-brushing rinse Plax [Abstract]. J Dent Res 1991;70:768.

89. Balanyk T, Sharma N, Galustians J. Antiplaque efficacy of Plax pre-brushing rinse: plaque mass/area analysis [Abstract]. J Dent Res 1991;70:374.

90. Rustogi KN, Petrone DM, Singh SM, et al. Clinical study of a pre-brush rinse and a triclosan/co-polymer mouthrinse: effect on plaque formation. Am J Dent 1990;3:S67–9.

91. Cronin MJ, Kohut BE. A two-phase clinical efficacy study of Plax pre-brushing rinse. J Clin Dent 1991;3:19–21.

92. Chung L, Smith SR, Joyston-Bechal S. The effect of using a prebrushing mouthwash (Plax) on oral hygiene in man. J Clin Periodontol 1992;19:679–82.

93. Mankodi S, Walker C, Conforti N, et al. Clinical effect of a triclosan-containing dentifrice on plaque and gingivitis: a six-month study. Clin Prevent Dent 1992;14:4–10.

94. Bolden TE, Zambon JJ, Sowinski J, et al. The clinical effect of a dentifrice containing triclosan and a co-polymer in a sodium fluoride/silica base on plaque formation and gingivitis: a six-month clinical study. J Clin Dent 1992;4:125–31.

95. Garcia-Godoy F, Garcia-Godoy K, DeVizio W, et al. Effect of a triclosan/co-polymer/fluoride dentifrice on plaque formation and gingivitis: a 7-month clinical study. Am J Dent 1990;3:S15–26.

96. Cubells AB, Dalmau L, Petrone ME, et al. The effect of a triclosan/co-polymer/fluoride dentifrice on plaque formation and gingivitis: a six-month clinical study. J Clin Dent 1991;2:63–9.

97. Deasy MJ, Singh SM, Rustogi KN, et al. Effect of a dentifrice containing triclosan and a co-polymer on plaque formation and gingivitis. Clin Prevent Dent 1991;13:12–9.

98. Denepitiya JL, Fine D, Singh SM, et al. Effect upon plaque formation and gingivitis of a triclosan/co-polymer/fluoride dentifrice: a 6-month clinical study. Am J Dent 1992;5:307–31.

99. Palomo F, Wantland L, Sanchez A, et al. The effect of three commercially available dentifrices containing triclosan on supragingival plaque formation and gingivitis: a six-month clinical study. Int Dent J 1994;44 (Suppl 1):S75–81.

100. Triratana T, Tuongratanaphan S, Kraivaphan P, et al. The effect on established plaque formation and gingivitis of a triclosan/co-polymer/fluoride dentifrice: a six-month clinical study. J Dent Assoc Thailand 1993;43:19–28.

101. Lindhe J, Rosling B, Socransky SS, Volpe AR. The effect of a triclosan containing dentifrice on established plaque and gingivitis. J Clin Periodontol 5:327–34.

102. Ciancio SG. Calculus reduction of a triclosan/co-polymer/fluoride dentifrice. Biol Ther Dent 1997;13.

103. Rosling B, Wannfors B, Volpe AR, et al. The use

of a triclosan/co-polymer dentifrice may retard the progression of periodontitis. J Clin Periodontol 1997;24:873–80.

104. Smulow JB, Turesky SS, Hill RG. The effect of supragingival plaque removal on anaerobic bacteria in deep periodontal pockets. J Am Dent Assoc 1983;107:737–42.

105. Hellstrom MK, Ramberg P, Krok L, Lindhe J. The effect of supragingival plaque control on the subgingival microflora in human periodontitis. J Clin Periodontol 1996;23:934–40.

106. Dahlen G, Lindhe J, Sato K, et al. The effect of supragingival plaque control on the subgingival microbiota in subjects with periodontal disease. J Clin Periodontol 1992;19:802–9.

107. McNabb H, Mombelli A, Lang NP. Supragingival cleaning three times a week: the microbiological effects in moderately deep pockets. J Clin Periodontol 1992;19:348–56.

108. Wynn RL. The top 20 medications prescribed in 1993. General Dentistry. 1995; March–April: 114–9.

109. Bosco JA, Pearson RE. Sugar content of selected liquid medicinals. Diabetes 1973;22:776–8.

110. Lokken P, Birkeland JM, Sannes E. pH changes in dental plaque caused by sweetened, iron-containing liquid medicine. Scand J Dent Res 1975;83:279–83.

111. Imfeld TH. Kariogene hustenspezialitaten. Schweiz Mschr Zahnheilk 1977;87:774–7.

112. Roberts IF, Roberts GJ. Relation between medicines sweetened with sucrose and dental disease. Br Med J 1979;2:14–6.

113. Ship JA, Fox PC, Baum BJ. How much saliva is enough? 'Normal' function defined. JADA 1991;122:63–69.

114. Sreebny LM, Schwartz SS. A reference guide to drugs and dry mouth. Gerodontology 1986;5:75–99.

115. Ogle RE, Ciancio SG. The effect of anticholinergic agents on the periodontium. J Periodontol 1971;42:280–2.

116. The United States Pharmacopeia, 21st revision. Rockville, MD: United States Pharmacopeial Convention, Inc.; 1984.

117. Beck R, Kohout FJ, Hunt RJ, et al. Root caries: physical, medical and psychosocial correlates in an elderly population. Gerodontics 1986;3: 242–7.

118. Accepted dental therapeutics. 39th edition. Chicago: American Dental Association; 1982.

119. Ziskin DE, Stowe LR, Zegarelli EV. Dilantin hyperplastic gingivitis. Am J Orthod 1941;27:350.

120. Baden E. Sodium dilantin gingival hyperplasia and conservative treatment: a case report. J Dent Med 1950;5:46.

121. Ciancio SG, Yaffe SJ, Catz CC. Gingival hyperplasia and diphenylhydantoin. J Periodontol 1972; 43:411–14.

122. Hall WB. Prevention of dilantin hyperplasia: a preliminary report. Bull Acad Gen Dent 1969;20.

123. Dill RE, Miller EK, Weil T, et al. Phenytoin increases gene expression for platelet-derived growth factor B chain in macrophages and monocytes. J Periodontol 1993;64:169–73.

124. Nakade O, Baylink DJ, Lau K-HW. Phenytoin at micromolar concentration is an osteogenic agent for human-mandibular-derived bone cells in vitro. J Dent Res 1995;74(1):331–7.

125. Cunat JJ, Ciancio SG. Diphenylhydantoin sodium: gingival hyperplasia and orthodontic treatment. Angle Orthod 1969;3:192–5.

126. Nishikawa SJH, Tada H, Hamasaki A, et al. Nifedipine-induced gingival hyperplasia: a clinical and in vitro study. J Periodontal Res 1991; 52:30–5.

127. Nuki K, Cooper SH. The role of inflammation in the pathogenesis of gingival enlargement during the administration of diphenylhydantoin sodium in cats. J Periodontal Res 1972;78:102–10

128. Stone C, Eshenaur A, Hassell T. Gingival enlargement in cyclosporine treated multiple sclerosis patients. J Dent Res 1989;68:285–9.

129. Seymour RA, Smith DG. The effect of a plaque control program on the incidence and severity of cyclosporine induced gingival changes. J Clin Periodontol 1991;18:107–10.

130. Ciancio SG, Bartz NW, Lauciello FR. Cyclosporine-induced gingival hyperplasia and chlorhexidine: a case report. Int J Periodont Restor Dent 1991; 3:241–5.

131. Golub LM, Lee HM, Lehrer G, et al. Minocycline reduces gingival collagenolytic activity during diabetes: preliminary observations and a proposed new mechanism of action. J Periodontal Res 1983;18:516–26.

132. Golub LM, McNamara TF, D'Angelo G, et al. A non-antimicrobial chemically-modified tetracycline inhibits mammalian collagenase activity. J Dent Res 1987;66:1310–4.

133. Golub LM, Evans RT, McNamara TF, et al. A non-antimicrobial tetracycline inhibits gingival matrix metalloproteinases and bone loss in *Porphyromonas gingivalis*-induced periodontitis in rats. Ann N Y Acad Sci 1994;732:96–110.

134. Delaisse JM, Eeckhout Y, Neff L, et al. (Pro) collagenase (matrix metalloproteinase-1) is present in rodent osteoclasts and in the underlying bone resorbing compartment. J Cell Sci (HNK) 1993;106:1071–82.

135. Ciancio SG, Genco RJ. The use of antibiotics in periodontal disease. Int J Periodont Restor Dent 1990;17:479–93.

136. Williams RC, Jeffcoat MK, Howell TH, et al. Altering the course of human alveolar bone loss with the non-steroidal anti-inflammatory drug flurbiprofen. J Periodontol 1989;60:485–90.

137. Feldman RS, Szeto B, Chauncey HH, Goldhaber P. Non-steroidal anti-inflammatory drugs in the reduction of human alveolar bone loss. J Clin Periodontol 1983;10:131–6.

138. Saxton CA. Scanning electron microscope study of the formation of dental plaque. Caries Res 1973;7:102–19.

139. Hillman DG, Hull PS. The influence of experimental gingivitis on plaque formation. J Clin Periodontol 1976;4:56–61.

140. Vogel RI, Copper SA, Schneider LG, Goteiner D. The effects of topical steroidal and systemic nonsteroidal anti-inflammatory drugs on experimental gingivitis in man. J Periodontol 1984; 55:247–51.

141. Hara K, Löe H. Carbohydrate components of the gingival exudate. J Periodont Res 1969;4:202 –7.

142. Freeman E, Novak MJ, Polson AM. Effects of gold salts on experimental periodontitis. III. Ultrastructural observations. IADR Program Abstracts; 1984.

143. Lewis R. The rise of antibiotic-resistant infections. FDA Consumer 1995;9:11–5.

144. Breiman RF, Butler JC, Tenover FC, et al. Emergence of drug-resistant pneumococcal infections in the United States. JAMA 1994;271:1831–5.

CHAPTER 16

MEDICOLEGAL ISSUES

Edwin J. Zinman, DDS, JD

The dental practitioner has the responsibility to provide patients with treatment that meets the current standards of care. In managing patients with significant systemic conditions or patients whose periodontal disease may adversely affect systemic health, thorough examination and review of relevant medical history are paramount. This chapter reviews important medicolegal issues involving all those that are primarily involved in providing health care: the patient, the physician, and the dental practitioner.

STANDARD OF CARE

Two essential ingredients comprise the standard of care. First, the practitioner must possess that degree of skill and learning ordinarily possessed by prudent practitioners. Second, the practitioner must exercise or use the requisite skill and learning in a reasonably prudent manner.[1]

In recent years, legal standards of care have been influenced by the various specialty organizations that establish parameters of care. Such parameters are peer reviewed, based upon existing scientific literature, and periodically updated. A reasonably prudent practitioner usually adheres to such guidelines. Some organizations include a caveat that parameters of care are not to be equated with the legal standard of care.[2] Nevertheless, an expert witness may reasonably rely upon these parameters in offering expert opinion. Therefore, as a practical matter, a specialty organization's parameters of care are usually consonant with prudent practice, which is also termed "due care."

The standard of care is not average care but rather represents the minimum standards of a reasonably prudent practitioner. Although most practitioners adhere to the standard of care, the median or statistically average practitioner does not exclusively dictate the standard of care. Fifty percent of practitioners do not automatically practice

below the standard of care merely because they render below statistically average care. Nor do fifty percent of practitioners statistically automatically comply with the standard of care merely because they render care above the statistical average.

The standard of care represents what a reasonably prudent practitioner should do under the same or similar circumstances. It is no defense or excuse for a negligent practitioner that other negligent practitioners (even a majority) follow similar negligent practices, or that only a minority of practitioners follow the reasonably prudent approach.

NEGLIGENT CUSTOM

A negligent custom, even if practiced by the majority of practitioners, violates the standard of care. By lay analogy, jaywalking, seatbelt avoidance, speeding, inattention due to car phone use, and going through stop signs are often tolerated traffic violations, except in a court of law, if injury results from such customarily negligent practices.

Examples of negligent dental practice customs include (1) failing to monitor dental unit waterlines for bacterial counts to assure compliance with the American Dental Association's recommended standards of 200 CFU/mL or potable water of 500 CFU;[3] (2) routinely performing endodontics without a rubber dam;[4] (3) failing to record pathologic periodontal probe measurements;[5] (4) prescription periodontics for abutment teeth only while ignoring periodontal disease elsewhere in the mouth;[6] (5) blindly adhering to managed-care guideline restraints which delay, or deny, necessary care and constrain specialty referrals;[7] (6) unnecessary radiation exposure with D-speed film, rather than E-speed film as well as use of short round collimators, rather than long-cone rectangular collimators, for intraoral radiography;[8,9] (7) using a glass-bead or chemiclave sterilizer for terminal sterilization of instruments;[10] and (8) employing cold chemical solution sterilization without adhering to the manufacturer's recommendations for development time, temperature, and dilution.[11]

DUTY TO REFER TO SPECIALIST

While a dental license provides a dentist with the right to perform all dental procedures, few generalists actually possess the knowledge, training, and skill to perform every procedure within the requisite standard of care. Possession of a dental license does not alone prove competency or prudence. For instance, general practice physicians usually lack sufficient training to perform open heart or sophisticated brain surgery. Likewise, general dentists often lack training to perform mandibular fracture reduction, or periodontal regenerative surgery such as membrane grafting or bone augmentation.

A general dentist has the duty to refer a patient to a specialist in situations where other reasonable general dentists would make a referral under similar circumstances.[12] If specialist training and experience are specifically required, the general dentist would be considered negligent for attempting to diagnose or treat and will be held to the specialist's standard of care[12] (ie, what the reasonable and prudent specialist would have done in similar circumstances).

A specialist's treatment failure may be justified as an inherent treatment risk. By contrast, in the case of the general dentist, who does not have adequate training and therefore should not have attempted sophisticated therapy, such failure is considered a negligently caused avoidable risk. Lack of availability of specialists in a certain locality does not justify failure to refer when a referral is indicated. It is the patient's choice whether or not to travel to a distant specialist.

The duty to refer is not limited to general dentists only. Specialists also routinely encounter clinical conditions that are best treated by a more experienced specialist in their discipline or by specialists in another discipline. Competency includes not only knowledge and training but also sufficient experience and mastery. For sophisticated therapies, the standard of care may require mastery even to attempt the therapy.

The referring dentist is not responsible for the treatment results obtained by the specialist, provided the specialist acted independently, without the referring dentist's participation or control. However, the referring dentist may be liable for the specialist's care, if he or she actively participated in or controlled the specialist's treatment. For example, a referring general dentist who prescribes only limited periodontal therapy for a patient who requires comprehensive therapy may be liable if the specialist acquiesces and both the referring dentist and periodontist fail to diagnose and adequately treat all of the patient's periodontal disease.

The referring dentist's chart should reflect a reasonable attempt to determine if the referred patient consulted the specialist and obtained recommended treatment. The chart should also note reminders to the patient about the need to follow through with the referral and the consequences of not doing so. This may be accomplished when the patient returns for a visit to the referring dentist's office. The prudent referring practitioner should check with the patient to ensure that the patient's appointment with the specialist has been kept. Noncompliance, with either consultation or treatment, should be recorded.

UPDATING SKILLS AND LEARNING

The standard of care requires that dentists possess the necessary level of skill and learning ordinarily possessed by prudent practitioners. Most professional negligence suits involve failure by an otherwise qualified practitioner to *maintain* the requisite skill and learning. Experience alone is insufficient to comply with the standard of care. Dentists with many years of experience who only repeat each year the skills and learning present in their first year of practice are likely perpetuating outdated methods.

A prudent practitioner constantly replaces outdated methods with improved and advanced therapies. It is estimated that following graduation, scientific advances surpass even the most up-to-date educational training provided only 5 years earlier.[13] Accordingly, to comply with the standard of care, prudent practitioners should update current knowledge, skill, and learning by subscribing to scientific journals and attending continuing education courses.

The standard of care does not require that every practitioner adopt each and every new technology or device. A prudent practitioner would not incorporate technologic advancements until they are scientifically proven with sufficient studies and are generally accepted in the scientific community. It is not necessary to be the first to adopt the latest technology; nor should a dentist be the last to adopt generally accepted, scientifically proven technologic advances.

GOVERNMENTAL AGENCY STANDARDS VERSUS STANDARDS OF CARE

Merely because a device or drug has received governmental approval, the practitioner who uses, recommends, or prescribes it is not necessarily insulated from liability. Governmental health care agencies, such as the Food and Drug Administration (FDA), set their own minimum standards. Such standards on occasion may still fall short of reasonably prudent practice.

For instance, some newer, unapproved implant devices may be better suited because of their size or maneuverability than some older FDA-approved implant systems, particularly where there is risk of injury to vital structures. Avoiding a permanent injury to a nerve may depend on whether the clinician used a contraindicated FDA-approved implant or an indicated but nonapproved implant. Similarly, manufacturers frequently defend a defective product by underscoring compliance with industry or government standards. However, "compliance with a legislative enactment or an administrative regulation does not prevent a finding of negligence where a reasonable (person) would take additional precautions."[14]

Regulations by the FDA provide that a manufacturer may change an approved drug label before approval if the change is intended to add or strengthen warnings or instructions or delete false or misleading claims for use or effectiveness. The FDA has the authority to take actions that avoid the use of false or misleading labels on drugs. The FDA's Labeling and Nomenclature Committee (LNC) was established to facilitate trademark review for products, as well as the labeling of products that are brought before the FDA for approval.

The FDA does not perform its own drug testing. Instead, the FDA relies on each manufacturer's candor and integrity in submitting drug data both before and after approval. Before being marketed, prescription drugs must be proven safe and effective in double-blinded clinical studies authorized by the FDA (21 United States Code, section 321).

INFORMED CONSENT VERSUS MISREPRESENTATION

The dentist has a duty to disclose all material information to enable the patient to make an informed decision regarding proposed procedures or treatment. This would comprise information that the dentist knows or should know and would be regarded as significant by a reasonable person in the patient's position when deciding to accept or reject a recommended procedure or treatment. The dentist is not bound to discuss the minor risks inherent in common procedures, when such procedures very seldom result in serious ill effects.[15]

The prudent practitioner's goal is to serve and protect the patient's best interests to preserve health. Consequently, a practitioner's fiduciary obligation to his or her patient should not be solely guided by the limitations set by the patient's insurance carrier and by managed care guidelines; nor should the practitioner recommend only the most profitable procedure when reasonably conservative alternative therapies are an option as well.

Honesty is the best policy, which is embodied in the legal obligation of a practitioner to warn patients of inherent, but reasonably unavoidable, therapeutic risks. Before embarking on any procedure that involves the inherent risk of serious injury or death, a practitioner must provide the patient with informed choices of the benefits, risks, and consequences of treatment as well as those of nontreatment, and a similar analysis for reasonable alternative therapies. A practitioner who fails to provide such information to aid informed consent of the patient may be judged negligent.[16,17]

In a failure-to-inform case, the dentist's misconduct is nonfeasance (ie, nonperformance) rather than misfeasance (ie, improper performance). In most states, failure to inform a patient of a material risk constitutes a legal cause for the patient's injury if a reasonably prudent patient, when fully informed of the material risks, would have avoided the risk by not consenting to the proposed therapy. Accordingly, informed consent is tested objectively, ie, what would a reasonably prudent person in the patient's position have decided if adequately informed of all significant perils?[15] Whether a dentist's failure to inform causes injury turns not on biomechanical principles, but rather on human factors measuring reasonable risk avoidance when adequately informed.

Merely because a dentist adequately informs a patient of the material risks of a procedure does not necessarily relieve the dentist of liability if the risk subsequently materializes. Informed consent is not an "affirmative defense" to negligent treatment.[16,17] That is, it is immaterial that the dentist warned the patient of a material risk if the dentist performs negligent treatment. Adequate informed consent avoids liability only when treatment is performed non-negligently, and a previously disclosed material risk subsequently manifests.

If the practitioner intentionally misrepresents known therapeutic goals, limitations, or risks, the practitioner may be subject to a fraud claim for intentionally deceiving the patient. Fraudulent misrepresentations may include intentional overstatement of surgical success while minimizing risks, claiming another's success as one's own, or quoting national success statistics when the quoting practitioner's own success rate is substantially lower.[18,19]

Negligent misrepresentations involve statements that have no reasonable basis (eg, a statement to a 30-year-old patient that her newly placed upper anterior crown should last a lifetime).

Professional liability insurance carriers will defend a suit which claims both negligence and fraud and will indemnify or reimburse the dentist for negligent acts. However, carriers are usually prohibited from indemnifying or reimbursing intentional acts, such as fraud, as contrary to public policy, since liability insurance is intended to cover only unintentional (ie, negligent) conduct (California Insurance Code section 533).[20] The practitioner is generally responsible for payment of any judgments for the portion arising from intentional misdeeds such as fraud.

REFUSAL TO TREAT

Dentists are not obligated to render treatment that is not in the patient's best interest, regardless of the patient's requests. In other words, if the patient requests treatment which the dentist knows to be improper or contraindicated, the practitioner should not accede to a patient's request for negligent care.[16] Rather, the dentist should refuse to treat.

A dentist is also not obligated to treat a patient when there is professional disagreement. When the dentist declines to begin or continue treatment, the patient should be advised in writing and provided with names and addresses of other dentists the patient could go to for treatment. A patient may be discharged after reasonable notice so long as the dentist's refusal to continue treatment does not jeopardize the patient's dental or physical health before the patient's appointment with a new dentist.

A dentist's refusal to treat may not be based on discriminating reasons for protected classes, such as the disabled, or for racial reasons.[21,22]

PHYSICIAN CONSULTATIONS

A dentist should consult the patient's physician whenever the proposed dental procedure or treatment may adversely affect the patient's general health. Discussions with the patient's physician should be documented and confirmed by facsimile or letter.

The dentist who blindly follows the physician's recommendation, even when it conflicts with his own professional judgment, probably violates the standard of reasonable care. Each independent practitioner is ultimately responsible for treatment decisions and should not rely on unreasonable recommendations that are contrary to established specialty parameters of care. When the treatment decisions conflict with each other, allowing the patient to choose is permissible provided that both the dentist's and the physician's treatment recommendations are reasonable.

PERIODONTAL EXAMINATION AND RE-EVALUATION

The American Academy of Periodontology recommends that its Parameters on Comprehensive Periodontal Examination (1995) be regarded as the "standard of care for periodontal examinations."

Periodic re-evaluation following therapy is essential to assess stability or further breakdown. Both host resistance and local factors can affect long-term maintenance. If disease deterioration occurs, the patient must be reassessed for both host resistance and local factors. A practitioner who fails to properly re-evaluate the patient's disease state cannot appreciate whether or not the patient's health is being adequately maintained and therefore fails to make adequate diagnostic or therapeutic decisions. The American Academy of Periodontology Professional Policy Statement on Periodontal Disease Detection states: "Following treatment, the patient must be carefully monitored by the periodontist and the dentist for recurrence of any diseases. Periodic periodontal examinations must be performed, and the records compared to posttreatment recordings. This is essential in order to monitor the effectiveness of therapy during this professional maintenance phase. This maintenance phase is essential to ensure long-term periodontal health and the retention of natural teeth."

If the patient is presently periodontally disease free, the statement also recommends the following long-term care parameters: "All patients must be screened for the presence of periodontal diseases on a regular basis. When periodontal diseases are detected, a comprehensive charting record must be completed and effective treatment should be rendered promptly."

RISK FACTORS

The standard of care requires practitioners to be aware of risk factors and to diagnose the patient's risk susceptibility in order to control or eliminate the risk factor. Failure to do so or to counsel a patient regarding such factors may render the practitioner liable.

Risk factor testing is standard practice since prevention of serious disease is the hallmark of modern medicine. A careful medical history identifies risk factors and the need for a follow-up interview or testing. For example, although the cause of heart disease may be multifactorial (including diet, blood pressure, stress, and myriad other factors), a physician must identify, counsel, and appropriately refer for risk factor reduction, particularly when failure to do so may have fatal complications or cause serious injury. One well-known example involves the relationship between cholesterol level and heart disease. Elevated cholesterol levels have a risk ratio of 2.4.[23] Physician identification, counseling, and public awareness have resulted in changed diets and increased exercise to lower cholesterol levels and thereby reduce the cholesterol risk factor.

This same medical model is increasingly being applied to dentistry, in general, and periodontics, in particular. Many risk factors can be identified and communicated to patients, and their elimination can be incorporated into periodontal therapy. Periodontal disease risk factors may include (1) inherited risk factors (genetic predisposition), (2) systemic risk factors, such as metabolic diseases, (3) acquired risk factors, such as diet or excessive smoking, and (4) local risk factors, such as plaque and calculus. Most acquired and local risk factors can be modified or eliminated after the dentist first assesses a patient's potential risk factors and provides or recommends appropriate counseling and/or therapy.

Statistical associations or risk factors identify at-risk patients who exhibit increased susceptibility to the initiation or progression of periodontitis. Although the standard of care requires the prudent practitioner to both identify and minimize such risk factors, whether the failure to do so actually caused or aggravated periodontitis may be difficult to prove in a legal case. By analogy, not all smokers develop lung cancer. Nor do all hypertensive patients inevitably suffer strokes or myocardial infarcts.

In the 18th century, Benjamin Rush, a Pennsylvania physician and signer of the Declaration of Independence, reported that arthritis sufferers found relief after their infected teeth were extracted. This theory of foci of infection, now abandoned, promoted unnecessary and wholesale teeth extraction for over 100 years.[24] Linkage of oral and systemic disease with anecdotal unscientific research risks unnecessary treatment. For example, attributing systemic illness to dental amalgam is another example of misstated science since, except in the extremely rare instances of mercury allergies, there is no proven connection between dental amalgam, mercury vapors, and systemic disease.[25]

Inherited Risk Factors: Genetic Predisposition

A patient's genetic composition is unchangeable. However, knowledge of genetic predisposition may affect treatment decisions and prognosis. Periodontal disease occurs only in susceptible individuals. Therefore, knowledge of the unchangeable elements of disease susceptibility help the practitioner in determining which factors of host resistance to disease are changeable and which are unchangeable.

According to one study, IL–1–genotype-positive patients have a 6.8-fold increased risk for severe periodontal disease.[23] Awareness of the genetic marker for periodontal disease may allow the practitioner to be aware of susceptibility to severe periodontal disease. Earlier onset and more rapid progression of periodontal pathology are postulated but, to date, it is known only that IL–1–positive subjects have been shown to be at greater risk for severe periodontitis in cross-sectional studies. Longitudinal data to show greater disease progression in genotype-positive subjects are being gathered. Therefore, a genetic risk factor assessment may help the practitioner and patient choose treatment options and determine whether increased frequency of monitoring is warranted. Informed consent reflects the patient's choice after disclosure of material therapeutic risks. The more informed both patient and practitioner become in determining disease prognosis and susceptibility, the more informed they become regarding the level of acceptable risks each is willing to assume in treatment planning. For instance, a practitioner may prudently advise a young genotype-positive patient that a maxillary molar with moderate to severe periodontitis may have a relatively poor prognosis. If that molar required extensive restorative treatment, the patient might elect extraction and replacement with a fixed partial denture. Another useful example of knowledge of genetic predisposition is a young patient with root resorption secondary to orthodontics performed during the patient's teen years. The prognosis will be affected by whether this patient will ever suffer periodontitis since the crown-root ratio is already diminished. Long-term studies extend up to only 15 years.[26] Thus, knowing whether a 25-year-old patient is likely to suffer loss of periodontal attachment after 15 years, at age 40, because of a genetic positive risk factor, would aid prognosis and evaluation.

Genetic testing is an optional diagnostic aid. If improved technology can aid treatment decisions, it is the patient's right to know of newer diagnostic technology in order to make an informed refusal decision or elect such testing. The PST™ test is based on the research premise that 30% of the population has an interleukin-1 gene polymorphism causing such individuals to produce greater IL-1 levels as a host response to bacterial plaque.[27] Not all populations have a similar prevalence of this IL-1 genotype. Genetic testing of a Chinese population group revealed only 2% genopositive rather than the 30% prevalence on which the PST™ test is premised.[28,29]

Genetic testing must be done with the full knowledge and consent of the patient since surreptitious genetic testing, even for experimental reasons, violates the patient's constitutional privacy rights, as well as the fourth amendment protection against illegal searches.[30]

Systemic Risk Factors

Diabetes

Diabetes is a recognized risk factor for periodontal disease progression primarily when metabolic control if poor. Conversely, if the diabetes is controlled, diabetic patients are generally not at risk for increased disease progression.

Findings that periodontal disease adversely affects diabetic control suggest a two-way street between certain metabolic systemic diseases and periodontal disease. Elimination or reduction of oral infection has resulted in improved metabolic control of diabetes.[31] If further studies substantiate these present research studies, both the physician and dentist may reduce the risk for diabetic complications by proper periodontal disease control.

Both the systemic condition and the localized periodontal disease must be controlled for optimal health. Therefore, physicians and dentists need to interact in the overall management of patients to ensure that neither the periodontitis nor the diabetes spirals out of control and adversely affect each other.

Osteoporosis

The linkage between periodontal disease and osteoporosis may represent different aspects of the bone loss process: oral bone loss and systemic bone loss. Postmenopausal patients may demonstrate changed bone density following periodontal disease elimination.[32] Further longitudinal studies are required to explore the extent of the linkage between periodontitis and osteoporosis.

Acquired Risk Factors

Smoking

Smoking and other types of tobacco use are regarded as one of the primary proven risk factors for periodontal disease. Physicians and dentists alike are obligated to counsel patients to curtail or eliminate tobacco use because of the myriad associated health risks. Since tobacco is addictive, counseling patients as close to the onset of the smoking habit as possible is essential.[33]

Excessive smoking is an important consideration in periodontal disease management. The difficulty in controlling this risk factor is due to the patient's addiction, which limits a patient's volitional control. Nevertheless, it is the practitioner's obligation to counsel the patient to discontinue tobacco use and to alert the patient that continued presence of the risk factor may adversely affect treatment outcomes.

Oral Hygiene

Patients with significant pathologic periodontal pockets have demonstrated periodontal disease susceptibility and require constant periodontal maintenance procedures (PMP) at frequent (usually quarterly) intervals. Regular and frequent PMP can maintain the oral health of even patients with less than adequate oral hygiene.[34–37]

Stress

Stress has become an inescapable component of daily life and a periodontal disease risk factor. However, only those patients who are unable to successfully cope with or overcome life's stresses are at increased risk for periodontal disease.[38] Dentists should consider heightened stress levels when assessing risk factors for periodontitis.

Most dentists, however, lack sufficient training to assess a patient's stress level and/or ability for stress management. A referral to a psychotherapist for stress reduction may be appropriate for some patients, for example, in the patient with refractory periodontal disease when disease progression defies conventional local therapy management. A simple screening device (Figure 16–1), incorporated into the health history questionnaire, may assist the dentist in identifying a patient's stress level.

If the patient answers "No" to the coping skills and "Yes" to counseling needs, the practitioner should consider referral to a trained professional in stress management. This will assist in the control of periodontitis, particularly if it is refractory or subject to frequent recurrence as determined at PMP visits.

Cardiovascular Disease

Since cardiovascular disease is the leading cause of death, any reduction in cardiac disease is of vital health care concern. Preliminary research evidence suggests a linkage between periodontal disease and cardiovascular status.[39] Whether a causal relationship exists or there is a predisposed patient group at risk for both periodontal and cardiac disease remains a further research challenge.

Current scientific studies seek to confirm the association between periodontitis and heart disease. Links have been discovered between oral health and systemic medical problems. However, the major issue is distinguishing a causal relationship from a coincidental connection between oral and systemic diseases of a patient susceptible to both diseases. Evidence to date does not conclusively prove a cause-and-effect link between periodontal and cardiovascular diseases. Rather, preliminary research suggests that periodontal disease may increase the risk of cardiovascular disease.[40] However, scientifically, it is premature for a dentist to advise a patient that periodontal disease will lead to a greater risk of stroke and heart attack since the definite causative linkage requires research studies with greater statistical power. Nor can prudent practitioners state that periodontitis is frequently associated with cardiac disease since a definite causal link has not been conclusively established. Rather, periodontal disease may be one of many potential risk factors for cardiovascular disease.

One plausible explanation of the association between cardiovascular and periodontal diseases may be that the same patient group susceptible to heart disease may also be susceptible to periodontal disease, rather than one disease triggering the other disease. Another unproven theory is that periodontal disease may represent an early manifestation of a broader systemic disease component which will continue to progress to the more serious cardiac disease unless the same contributing risk factors are controlled, such as smoking or excessive stress. Further research may determine whether periodontal disease is the prognostic precursor to cardiovascular disease or if periodontitis acts as an aggravating factor in cardiac disease management.

Preterm Birth

The relationship between periodontal disease and preterm low-birth-weight (PLBW) babies deserves further study of the connecting links of this association chain. Preterm birth is frequently considered multifactorial since its causes are multiple and diverse. Risk factors include malnutrition, drug abuse, smoking, and lack of prenatal care. Recent periodontal research preliminarily suggests severe periodontal disease as a risk factor.[45]

Maternal infections predispose to preterm labor, membrane rupture, and spontaneous birth of low-birth-weight babies. Preliminary research with a relatively small case-control study population assessed an added risk of more severe periodontal disease associated with primiparous (first live birth) mothers and small preterm birth (SPB). Whether this is a true interactive risk factor or an independent incident awaits future study of research groups with greater statistical power. Therefore, it is premature to definitively link premature births and periodontal disease; if proven, however, it would mandate counseling pregnant women to control periodontal disease to avoid the risk of SPB.

Identifying a single risk factor and eliminating it does not always reduce disease incidence. For instance, when measuring the effect of eliminating single risk factors, such as malnutrition and prenatal care, on rates of premature birth when studied in isolation, elimination of such single risk factors has not resulted in a decline in preterm birth.[41] Thus, data from multiple trials of single risk factors have provided substantial evidence that controlling only one single factor failed to reduce preterm birth rates.[42]

Controlling preterm delivery and low birth weight has proven an often insurmountable obstet-

		Yes	No
1.	Are you generally able to adequately manage or cope with daily emotional stress?	☐	☐
2.	Do you feel that for the past year you have been unable to adequately manage or cope with daily emotional stress?	☐	☐
3.	Do you desire professional counseling for emotional stress management?	☐	☐

Figure 16–1. A simple screening questionnaire.

rical challenge since the 10% risk of SPB has not changed in the past 40 years despite improved prenatal care.[47] On the other hand, neonatal medicine has improved survival rates of premature births. Further research will establish whether periodontitis disease severity is a marker for a risk factor, which can prognosticate a preterm delivery susceptibility. If proven, clinical periodontal parameters or periodontal gingival crevicular fluid testing may prove to be valuable screening tests for SPB risk assessment.

Local Risk Factors

Bacterial plaque is regarded as the primary causative agent for periodontitis. Nonetheless, not all patients with heavy plaque deposits develop severe periodontitis. Consequently, plaque is a risk factor which only causes periodontal disease manifestation in a susceptible host.

SUBACUTE BACTERIAL ENDOCARDITIS

The mouth is a well-known reservoir of more species of organisms than any other area of the body. Many cases of subacute bacterial endocarditis (SBE) have no known causative precipitating event. However, no studies have shown that procedures such as brushing and flossing can create a bacterial inoculum of sufficient size to establish infective seeding of existing endocardial vegetations. It is therefore scientifically unsound and unproven to recommend that patients at risk for SBE cease or curtail daily oral hygiene procedures to avoid precipitating bacteremias. On the other hand, both the American Dental Association (ADA) and the American Heart Association (AHA) strongly recommend that SBE-susceptible patients maintain impeccable oral hygiene. Elimination or control of periodontal pockets reduces the potential that large numbers of bacteria will invade the bloodstream and thus reduces the potential for periodontal pathogens to contribute to an SBE exacerbation.

The AHA recommends that any dental procedure capable of producing "significant" bleeding has the potential of introducing oral bacteria into the bloodstream and, as such, requires prophylaxis with an appropriate antibiotic for at-risk SBE patients.[43] The AHA notes in its recommendations that the clinician's judgment may supersede a given recommendation. However, unless good cause exists for deviation, the standard of care requires conformance with the AHA guidelines.

Antibacterial mouthrinse products such as chlorhexidine have proven effective in decreasing the overall oral quantity of bacteria and reducing the incidents of bacteremia associated with third molar extractions as well as localized alveolitis.[44–50] Use of these mouthrinse products prior to surgery makes empirical sense and is endorsed by the British antimicrobial societies. However, antibacterial rinses are not proven as an efficacious substitute for administration of systemic antibiotic prophylaxis where otherwise indicated for SBE-at-risk patients.

Mechanical irrigation devices can cause bacteremias, especially in the presence of chronic or acute periodontal infective states associated with poor oral hygiene. These devices have the potential for introducing larger bacteria boluses than brushing or flossing and therefore are not generally recommended for at-risk SBE patients.

The FDA removed from the market Fen (fenfluramine aka Pondimin), as well as the chemically related drug dexfenfluramine (aka Redux) after reports linked these medications to heart valve abnormalities. The benefit of suppressing appetite did not outweigh the risk of valvular heart defects associated with the altered metabolism of serotonin related to these drugs and their off-label prescription.

Both the AHA and the American College of Cardiology (ACC) now recommend that patients who have taken these drugs should undergo a stethoscope examination for heart valvular defects and a follow-up examination in 6 to 8 months. Patients with symptoms of shortness of breath, chest pain, or heart murmurs should have an echocardiographic examination. Asymptomatic patients may have echocardiography depending upon the physician's clinical judgment.

Although the incidence of valvular heart defects appears to be a function of the length of time that the patient takes the medication, the standard of care obligates the dentist to obtain a history of such diet drug usage. A medical consultation is necessary (if not previously obtained) for all patients who have taken diet drugs, including those that are not at risk for SBE.

DRUG SIDE EFFECTS

Prudent periodontics carefully weighs risks against benefits of any prescribed or performed therapy. Newer local delivery drugs enjoy the benefit of sustained local release of the drug over a period of days or weeks, rather than hours. Tetracycline fibers may be impractical in many instances for routine clinical application because it is time consuming to place and maintain the fibers in the pocket during the recommended period of use. On the other hand, second generation delivery agents, such as gels or chips, are both patient and dentist friendly and less time consuming to apply.

Packet inserts for local delivery drugs list contraindications, including allergies. The practitioner may be liable for failure to follow or advise patients of these warnings on drug packet inserts. Liability may also result from failure to follow Physician Desk Reference recommendations. However, these failures alone do not establish violation of the standard of care unless an expert so testifies.[51]

For instance, the packet insert for Periostat (doxycycline hyclate) capsules warns of tetracycline hypersensitivity and possible discoloration of permanent teeth if used during the latter half of pregnancy, or up to age 8 years. Discoloration is more common during long-term use, but may also occur during repeated short-term courses.

The manufacturer of doxycycline warns that the drug may cause harm to the fetus. The manufacturer also advises that "concurrent use of tetracycline may render oral contraceptives less effective." An increased risk of a wrongful life lawsuit (birth of unplanned child) may occur if the patient is prescribed doxycycline but is not adequately advised of any increased risk of unwanted pregnancy and the oral contraceptive dosage is not adjusted or alternative birth-control methods advised.

Since photosensitivity has also been associated with the tetracyclines, patients taking these drugs, including doxycycline, should be cautioned regarding excessive exposure to direct sunlight or any ultraviolet light. Tetracyclines have also been shown to depress plasma prothrombin activity. Thus, patients taking anticoagulant therapy may require a downward adjustment of their anticoagulant dosage.

Although the doxycycline dosage in Periostat is below the concentration required to inhibit periodontitis-associated microorganisms, the lower dosage does not eliminate contraindications, drug interactions, allergies, or potential teratogenic effects. Since the dosage of these newer drugs is lower than the dosage used to treat other infections, the development of resistant strains of microorganisms is reduced. Other local delivery tetracycline drugs, such as minocycline, are in clinical trials and should be marketed in the near future.

Mechanical instrumentation with scaling and root planing has proven effective in the treatment of adult periodontitis. Accordingly, the routine use of local delivery agents with scaling and root planing is usually not justified and is presently an off-label use. Local delivery agents are most often used as adjunctive therapy to conventional care for nonresponding sites with moderate pocket depth or in patients who have recurrent disease despite repeated scaling and root planing. Long-term studies are needed to verify the efficacy of combined therapy even in these instances

Fiberoptic illumination, which provides increased visual access to the subgingival space, increases the effectiveness of calculus removal on root surfaces. Complete removal of subgingival calculus is limited during root planing. Greater pocket depths often result in increased residual calculus due to the increased area of root surface to be scaled and the increased number of irregularities found on the root surface. Deep narrow pockets impede accessibility to root irregularities.

Flap exposure surgery of root surfaces also greatly enhances the effectiveness of scaling and root planing. In one study, an average of 20% of postsurgery surfaces had residual calculus.[52] Nonsurgical pocket distention procedures resulted in approximately 40% of the root surfaces having residual calculus.[57] If flap exposure or pocket distension procedures were not used, 64% of the root surfaces had residual calculus.[57]

Pocket distention following tetracycline fiber removal provides improved visual detection of residual calculus. Thus, a possible added advantage to the use of the tetracycline fiber local delivery system is the increased visual access immediately following fiber removal, which aids root calculus removal.

No studies have addressed the use of local drug delivery in specific types of periodontal bony defects such as intrabony defects or class II furcations. Results from studies assessing local drug delivery systems have not justified extending the time interval between supportive PMP visits by substituting them with local delivery therapies.

Local delivery agents should be used as therapeutic adjunctive aids rather than as monotherapy. Contraindications for using local delivery drugs include using them as (1) a replacement for thorough scaling and root planing, and (2) full-mouth treatment rather than specific local sites.

Efficacious therapies that benefit the patient's health should be the practitioner's first consideration rather than the financial gain from it. Therefore, a third-party insurance carrier's allowance of insurance benefits for local delivery agents should not compromise necessary therapy, nor decrease the frequency of the scaling and root planing procedures. Prudent practitioners are primarily obligated to treat the patient's periodontal pockets rather than comply with the insurance carrier's dictates, or financial pockets.

BURDEN OF PROOF

"Burden of proof" refers to one party's obligation to produce sufficient evidence to prove the fact or contention proffered. "A party has the burden of proof as to each fact, the existence or nonexistence of which is essential to the claim for relief or defense that he is asserting." (California Evidence Code section 500)

In a civil case, the burden of proof must be established by a preponderance of the evidence. Preponderance implies the greater weight of the evidence, ie, a probability (versus a possibility) of truth or an event that is more likely than not to have occurred or be true. Vague, inconclusive, or uncertain evidence fails to meet the burden of proof and is considered conjectural or speculative.

A patient-plaintiff bringing a professional negligence lawsuit generally bears the burden of proving by a preponderance, or greater weight, of the evidence the following elements: (1) negligence, (2) causation, and (3) damages. A defendant-dentist bears the burden of proving by a preponderance of the evidence any affirmative defense, such as lack of adequate oral hygiene, missed maintenance, or refused specialist referral.

Stated otherwise, the patient-plaintiff must prove by at least a 51% or greater likelihood that (1) the defendant-dentist violated the standard of care, (2) that the defendant's negligence caused or aggravated the plaintiff's periodontitis, and (3) injury or damages resulted. For example, the patient-plaintiff may be able to prove that the dentist violated the standard of care by not informing the patient of the potentially deleterious effects of stress on the patient's periodontal health. However, if the patient-plaintiff cannot prove that stress aggravated his periodontitis, the evidence may be speculative that in his individual case the particular risk factor (stress) was the causative culprit. Conversely, if the defendant-dentist contended that the patient-plaintiff was at fault because of his smoking, the defendant bears the burden of proving the plaintiff's smoking aggravated his periodontitis.

As only a minority of the population develop severe pathologic periodontal pockets that cause premature tooth loss, a risk factor of only 15% doubled or tripled still does not reach the 51% or higher proof threshold. It is difficult to prove that a particular risk manifested in any one patient caused severe or worsened periodontitis. Thus, epidemiologic data of increased risk in the general population does not prove individual causation. Accordingly, a practitioner who fails to recognize or reduce the risk factors (thereby violating the standard of care) may yet avoid liability if the patient-plaintiff cannot prove by a preponderance of the evidence that the nonrecognition or nontreatment of a particular risk factor caused or aggravated the particular disease at issue.

If scientific evidence cannot establish the greater weight of evidence in a particular case, the plaintiff may not prevail since the plaintiff will have failed to provide the burden of proof necessary to establish causation despite epidemiologic evidence of the increased disease incidence in the general population.

Epidemiologic research does not establish individual cause and effect but only suggests a potential relationship. Epidemiologic studies best identify very powerful associations, such as in a cohort study in which large groups of people are followed up for a long time. One research study alone does not establish the gold standard of care. The hallmark of science is experimental replication in other independent studies that proves the hypothetical or premised postulate. However, a multicenter study does not always ensure scientific accuracy if a flawed research methodology is repeated at multiple centers.[53–58]

Defense attorneys are particularly skillful in exploring other causes of diseases, which can be multifactorial. Tobacco companies have, for many years, successfully defended lung cancer cases since a particular patient's etiology for lung cancer may be explained by factors other than tobacco, such as environmental, work-related, or idiopathic causes. Tobacco companies also argue that they should not be held accountable for the well-publicized risks of cigarettes which was well-known for years and further argue that there is no fraud to attempt to hide something already known, such as risks of using tobacco.

Similarly, defense counsel defending periodontal negligence actions have been able to establish that risk factors such as smoking, poor oral hygiene, stress, or systemic diseases caused or aggravated a patient's periodontal disease, rather than the dentist-defendant's negligence. Although earlier periodontal literature was equivocal on the role of tobacco and periodontal disease,[59] recent literature has established tobacco's role as one of the most significant risk factors.[60]

Although in some states advising the patient of the greater risk, such as death, absolves the practitioner from failing to advise of the lesser risk, other states (eg, Minnesota) require the practitioner to advise patients of virtually all risks, such as impotence which is a long-term health risk secondary to smoking (88 ALR 3rd 1008). A practitioner should also include long-term risk assessment as part of a patient's comprehensive health care evaluation or re-evaluation. Comprehensive care should include not only diagnosis of existing diseases but also health care warnings of known risk factors as part of a preventive health care measure. Periodontal disease represents a non–life-threatening disease associated with smoking.

After first consulting with the patient's physician, the patient may be cautioned that the smoking is not only beginning to manifest as oral disease, which is one of many predictable diseases associated with smoking, but that continuation can cause other more serious diseases as well since the patient has already demonstrated weakened host resistance and disease susceptibility. Alerting the patient's physician of oral evidence (eg, periodontitis) of the patient's host resistance beginning to break down may serve as an early warning that other more serious systemic diseases may occur in the future. Thus, a prudent practitioner should not only diagnose early warning signs of known diseases but also consider alerting the patient to consult with the patient's physician to determine if the current manifestations of less serious diseases portend the worsening of these diseases and the likely development of more serious diseases linked with the same risk factor.

CIRCUMSTANTIAL EVIDENCE

Evidence is either direct or circumstantial. Direct evidence proves a fact without the need for any inferences. Circumstantial evidence, on the other hand, proves a fact or facts from which an inference of the existence of another fact may be drawn. For example, the fact that a child was taking cookies from the cookie jar can be established if the child was seen taking a cookie from the jar, which is direct evidence. If, on the other hand, the only visual evidence is a half-empty cookie jar, a trail of cookie crumbs to the child's bedroom, and an unhungry child at dinner that night, it is circumstantial evidence which infers the fact that the child took cookies from the cookie jar, even though the act was not seen.

Circumstantial evidence is legally accepted as equally convincing as direct testimony.[61] It is postulated that periodontal disease is episodic and consists of bursts of activities; however, rather than showing linear progression,[62] circumstantial evidence may help establish a causative link with particular risk factors if significant periodontal disease progression coincided with risk factors such as periods of uncontrolled diabetes or excessive smoking, and disease activity ceased when the diabetes was controlled or the smoking eliminated. If the periodontal disease worsened after another bout of uncontrolled diabetes or resumption of smoking, the circumstantial evidence link may reasonably be established as corroborative evidence.

Both the scientific community and the courts accept circumstantial evidence as proof of a postulate.[61] For example, a classic periodontal study demonstrated that dental students developed gingivitis with failure to maintain oral hygiene and that the condition was reversed when oral hygiene measures were restored.[63]

A patient-plaintiff need not prove in a lawsuit that the practitioner's negligence was the sole cause of the patient's disease but, rather, that such negligence was a substantial factor in causing injury.[64] For instance, an expert may testify that defective restorations predispose to bacterial plaque accumulation and resulting periodontal disease.[65] If periodontal disease is confined to the offending plaque retentive restorations, rather than being generalized, such evidence constitutes circumstantial evidence which supports the expert's opinion that the defective plaque-accumulating restoration substantially increased the risk for localized periodontal disease. This opinion is particularly apt if it is clear that the patient's natural host resistance prevented periodontal disease elsewhere in the mouth where the patient had similar types of restorations that were not defective. Such comparative evidence constitutes strong circumstantial evidence that restorative deficiencies caused the localized periodontal disease.

RESEARCH EVIDENCE

Scientific research is the basis for evidence-based parameters of care. Traditionally, most dental clinical decisions were based on the clinician's experience. In an evidence-based approach, however, all scientific evidence is not accorded the same weight. The stronger the scientific supporting evidence, the stronger is the supporting recommendation.[66] An evidence-based approach places greater weight on analytic methods that determine both statistical and clinical significance as well as measure both risks and benefits. Scientific standards include (1) double-blind, placebo-controlled clinical trial to reduce potential bias, and (2) longitudinal studies to evaluate the long-term effects of treatment altering the natural history of a disease.

Under federal law, scientific evidence concerning health care has to meet scientific standards of proof before being admitted into evidence for the jury's consideration. Four factors that must be evaluated to determine if a scientific theory or technique is reliable are:

- whether it has been, or can be, tested;
- whether it has been subjected to peer review or publication;
- its known or potential rate of error; and
- whether it is generally accepted by the relevant scientific community.[67,68]

Emerging and changing technologies offer great benefit to patient care but challenge the prudent practitioner to carefully evaluate manufacturer-supported studies for biased interpretation or inadequate research. Due to political pressures, governmental agencies have shortened the review time as well as the review process for approval. Manufacturers frequently argue that governmental approval delays are due to governmental bureaucracy rather than the adequacy of research data. However, it is important to realize that the pressures to rush a new product to market may also bring about conclusions that have not stood the test of time with long-term clinical studies.

Manufacturer-subsidized researchers use governmental agency approval (such as FDA approval) in their claim for efficacy or superiority. Instead of blindly accepting all advertising claims, prudent practitioners must independently assess the validity of the research claims as biased research or disingenuous data create untrustworthy research conclusions and interpretations.

Governmental approval has not always proven efficacious in the disclosure of risk assessment. The burden of assessing advertised claims has increasingly shifted to the prudent practitioner, who must carefully evaluate the foundation of research conclusions of claimed product efficacy or superiority before wholesale adoption of new devices or therapies and abandonment of the time-tested methods.

Multicenter research studies do not always guarantee statistically valid research conclusions. For instance, the recent FDA approvals of local delivery drugs were based on a 9-month study.[69] The supporting research studies to obtain FDA approval evaluated the therapeutic efficacy of local drug therapy on chronic periodontal disease. Periodontal disease progresses episodically over years, with periods of remission or exacerbation. Yet, the FDA approved for marketing these local delivery drugs with a study that lasted only three-quarters of a year.

The manufacturer also made claims that pocket reduction and clinical attachment levels, when combined with scaling and root planing, were superior to or at least equalled scaling and root planing alone. Reading the study's research protocol reveals that the so-called combined therapy group of the experimental drug, when combined with scaling and root planing, only existed at baseline. Thereafter, scaling and root planing were not repeated at 3 months, 6 months, or at the conclusion of the 9-month period studied. Patients with moderate periodontal disease consisting of 5- to 6-mm pockets with bleeding on probing who were studied in the research group should have been generally maintained with periodontal procedures on a quarterly basis. General practitioners would likely have performed subgingival débridement at (minimal) 6-month intervals. Consequently, the study evaluated what occurred in those that may be regarded as poorly maintained patients, ie, who were maintained solely on the locally delivered drug rather than with quarterly subgingival débridement as is common practice. This is but one of many examples where a prudent practitioner should carefully evaluate advertised conclusions before blindly adopting them.

Drug manufacturers are liable if their sales personnel promote an FDA-approved drug with misleading statements, if the manufacturer is aware of such marketing abuses.[70] The individual practitioner need not abide by FDA-approved uses only and may prescribe a drug for uses unapproved by the FDA but the practitioner who strays beyond the FDA-approved line risks engaging in experimental medicine. Prescribing a drug for unapproved use may be based only on empirical anecdotal evidence rather than controlled careful research studies.

Diet drugs, such as Pondimin and Redux, are a case in point. Although the FDA approved each drug individually by specific labelled use, the FDA never approved the combination of fenfluramine and Phentermine for birth control. Consequently, risks of heart valve damage, which would likely have manifested with long-term clinical testing in a research controlled environment with sufficient numbers of patients, were undetected before mass prescription of the potentially dangerous drug combination occurred.*

Long-term clinical trials with vast numbers of studied patients are often regarded as the ideal validity test group for clinical research. Different patient population groups need to be evaluated to avoid erroneous diagnoses. Nevertheless, such platinum-standard protocols may be tarnished if control groups are not matched with the studied groups for similar variables. Data inaccuracy results when there is misclassification between subgroups, which may affect the research trial outcome.[71]

In order to have predictably valid results, elimination of heterogeneity between trial groups is necessary. Discrepancies occur within clinical research trial groups so that the concept of comparison of similar homogeneous groups is often a myth, considering the variable treatment responses of different persons, populations, and protocols. If the different groups studied have different risks, a fair comparison cannot be established. This may explain the reason for inconsistent results among various studies. Although a greater number of patients provides greater statistical power, size alone does not compensate for research methodologic flaws. As one research team concluded:

> Periodontal research often confuses lack of significance in a clinical trial designed for superiority for equivalence between different therapies. Acceptable mean differences in equivalency trials should be determined based not only on statistical considerations, but also on clinical relevance of the proposed differences.
>
> Equivalency trial has some concepts that are very different from those in a superiority design. It can be difficult distinguishing between the items that are similar between the two designs and those that are different. Equivalency designs require larger sample sizes than their superiority counterparts.

Scientific research continues to guide the prudent practitioner through the ever burgeoning world of science. The long history of randomized,

but controlled, trials, has resulted in improved preventive measures, such as vaccines and disease screening, as well as more efficacious therapies.

In applying diagnostic algorithms, objective probability estimates should be grounded in data from well-designed studies to minimize the effect of numerous biases that potentially cloud diagnostic analysis. Studies that compare patients with severe disease with normal, healthy volunteers, may overestimate the usefulness of diagnostic testing.[72]

Statistical validity is a critical issue to measure quality that explains a substantial variation in research results, including tentative or uncertain results.

Case reports describe a single case with clear benefits. The degree of benefit derived from the new treatment is often greater in single case reports than in large cohort studies of patients entered into a trial study.

To obtain FDA approval, two well-controlled clinical trials are needed. Before prudent practitioners accept evidence for a new drug therapy, they must ensure that it is based on a high proportion of double-blind, randomized, placebo-controlled clinical trials rather than on empirical conclusions. The standard-of-care, evidence-based approach can then integrate scientific research into clinical practice. When scientific evidence is disputed, the court can appoint its own independent expert or panel of experts. For instance, a federal judge in Alabama established a scientific panel to help the court evaluate evidence in 8,600 nationwide breast implant cases.[73] The scientific panel set up under the Federal Rules of Evidence concluded that there was "no evidence that silicone breast implants precipitate novel immune responses or induce systemic inflammation." The independent panel also criticized other studies as "methodologically inadequate," including flawed comparison subjects, "unorthodox data analyses," and other problems. Also, "inconsistent results in studies purporting to evaluate the same immunologic parameters are common."

COMPARATIVE NEGLIGENCE

The U.S. legal system is based in part on the maxim, "No one can take advantage of his own wrong." (California Civil Code section 3517) Regardless of how negligent the practitioner may have been, a patient's own negligence (termed contributory negligence) may partially offset, or eliminate, any liability.

---

*A Texas class action against American Home Products, seller of the diet drugs fenfluramine and dexfenfluramine, seeks medical screening for all Texans who took the drugs for 60 days or more at a cost of around $500 for each test. Class action certification of a Washington state case is expected soon.

In those states that recognize pure comparative negligence, the patient's negligence, if any, is compared with the practitioner's negligence, and any recovery by the patient is offset by the proportion of the patient's negligence. For example, if the patient is held to have been 25% negligent, any recovery for the patient is reduced by 25%. In other states, if the patient's negligence exceeds 51% of the total negligent conduct of both plaintiff and defendant, the plaintiff-patient may be completely denied from any recovery.

Comparative negligence should be distinguished from failure to mitigate (minimize) damages. Comparative negligence assumes that the patient contributed to the cause or aggravation of the injury by the offending practitioner. If, after the injury occurred, the patient fails to obtain recommended treatment from subsequent practitioners, the patient is held responsible for failing to minimize further damages. For example, in a case alleging failure to diagnose and treat periodontal disease, the patient's failure to maintain adequate oral hygiene and attend recommended quarterly periodontal maintenance procedure appointments while under the care of the defendant-practitioner may constitute comparative negligence. The patient's failure to also do so under the care of a subsequent practitioner may constitute a failure to mitigate or reduce further damages.

Patients advised to curtail or quit smoking but who fail to do so may arguably be held to be comparatively negligent. However, if the patient is advised to restrict smoking after he or she has become addicted to smoking, the volitional element is substantially reduced or eliminated since the success of smoking cessation programs frequently does not exceed 6%.[74] Conversely, the reasonably prudent patient may argue that the majority of patients in a similar situation cannot overcome smoking addiction. Accordingly, it is not the patient's fault but, rather, the cigarette manufacturer whose advertisements led to the addictive incurable smoking habit before the patient realized the pernicious effects of smoking. Smokers > age 25 years only constitute 5% of addicted smokers.[83] A practitioner's advice to quit smoking is likely given to an addicted patient. The frustratingly small success rates of smoking cessation programs are therefore not surprising.

CONCLUSION

The guiding principle of the ancient Hippocratic Oath for medical practitioners is "primum non nocere," meaning "First, do no harm." This principle remains the bedrock foundation on which modern medicine provides optimum patient care.

Dentists are ethically obligated to adhere to the patient's best dental health interest. The Hippocratic Oath principles are embodied in the following:

> ". . . I understand and accept that my *primary responsibility* is to my patients, and I shall dedicate myself to render, to the best of my ability, the highest standard of oral health care and to maintain a relationship of respect and confidence. Therefore, let all come to me safe in the knowledge that their total health and well-being are *my first considerations.* . . ." [emphasis added.] (ADA Dentist's Pledge, 1991)

Dentists are legally obligated to protect and preserve the patient's health interests as foremost since the dentist-patient relationship is fiduciary.

In the new millennium, periodontics recognizes the obligation to protect and preserve the patient's total health care. Dentists and physicians are now able to see more clearly in the light of evidence-based periodontics. This new insight illuminates the inter-relationship between oral and systemic health rather than the tunnel vision of earlier views which separated the periodontium from the body's general health system.

REFERENCES

1. California Book of Approved Civil Jury Instructions (BAJI), BAJI No. 6.00.1. 1999.
2. California Dental Association Peer Review Manual, page 1 (1995).
3. American Dental Association Statement on Dental Unit Waterlines (1995).
4. Simpson vs. Davis, 219 Kansas 584, 549 P.2d 950 (1976).
5. American Academy of Periodontology. Parameters of Comprehensive Periodontal Examination (1995).
6. American Academy of Periodontology. Parameters of Comprehensive Periodontal Examination (1995).
7. Jury Award (120 Million) Against HMO is Biggest Ever. Pittsburgh Post Gazette; January 22, 1999. p. A17.
8. Brown R, Hadley JN, Chambers DW. An evaluation of ektaspeed film versus ultraspeed film for endodontic working length determination. J Endo 1988;24:(1):54–6.
9. Hadley J. Dental radiology quality of care: the dentist makes the difference. J Calif Dent Assoc 1995;23(5):17–20.

10. Kolstead RA. How well does the chemiclave sterilize handpieces? JADA 1998;129(7):985–91.

11. Burke FJI, Coulter WA, Cheung SW, Pallemk MS. Autoclave performance and practitioner knowledge of autoclave use. A survey of selected UK practices. Quintessence Intl 1998;29(4):231–8.

12. California Book of Approved Civil Jury Instructions (BAJI), BAJI Nos. 6.01, 6.04. 1999.

13. Fry RJ, Grosovsky A, Hanawalt PC, et al. The impact of biology on risk assessment. Workshop of the National Research Council's Board on Radiation Effects Research. July 21–22, 1997. Radiation Research 1998;150(6):695–705.

14. Carlin vs. Superior Court. 13 Cal. 4th 1004, 920 P.2d 1347, citing Restatement Second of Torts section 402A (1996).

15. California Book of Approved Civil Jury Instructions (BAJI), BAJI No. 6.11. 1999.

16. Sfikas PM. Informed consent and the law. JADA 1998;129:1613–4.

17. Waller vs. Aggarwal. 116 Ohio App.3d 355, 688 N.E. 2d 274 (1996).

18. Hales vs. Pittman 118 Ariz. 305, 576 P.2d 493 (1978).

19. Shelter vs. Rochelle. 2 Ariz. App. 370, 409 P.2d 86 (1965).

20. Quan vs. Truck Insurance Exchange. 67 Cal. App.4th 583, 79 Cal. Rptr.2d 134 (1998).

21. Abbott vs. Bragdon. (1st Cir) 118 S. Ct. 2196 (1998).

22. State vs. Clausen. (Minn. Ct. App.) 491 N.W.2d 662 (1992).

23. Newman M. Genetic, environmental and behavioral influence on periodontal infections. Compendium 1998;19:25–31.

24. Ehrmann EH. Focal infection: the endodontic point of view. Oral Surg 1977;44:628.

25. Anonymous. Dental amalgam: update on safety concerns. JADA 1998;129(4):494–503.

26. Remington DN, Joondeph AJ. Long term evaluation of root resorption occurring during orthodontic treatment. Am J Orth Dent Fac Ortho P 1989;96:43–6.

27. Kornman KS, Crane A, Wong H-Y, et al. The interleukin-1 genotype as a severity factor in adult periodontal disease. J Clin Periodontol 1997;24:72.

28. Piper S. Gary Armitage searches for new ways to diagnose and treat periodontal disease. UCSF Oracal 1998;12:11. Armitage G. Submitted for publication J. Perio.

29. Armitage G, Wu Y, Wang HY, et al. Low prevalence of a periodontitis associated interleukin 1 composite genotype in individuals of Chinese heritage. J Periodontol 1999. [Forthcoming]

30. Norman-Bloodshaw vs. Lawrence Berkeley Laboratory. 9th Cir. 135 F.3d 1260 (1998).

31. Aldridge JP, Lester V, Watts TLP, et al. Single-blind studies on the effects of improved periodontal health on metabolic control in type 2 diabetes mellitus. J Periodontol 1996;67:166–76.

32. Cohen DW, Rose LF. The periodontal-medical risk relationship. Compendium 1998;19:11–24.

33. Severson HH, Andrews JH, Lichtenstein E, et al. Using the hygiene visit to deliver a tobacco cessation program: results of a randomized clinical trial. JADA 1998;129:993–9.

34. Ramjford SP. Maintenance care and supportive periodontal therapy. Quintessence Int 1993;24:465–71.

35. Haffajee AD, Socransky SS, Dzink JL, et al. Clinical, microbiological and immunological features of subjects with destructive periodontal diseases. J Clin Periodontol 1988;15:240–6.

36. Grossi SG, Genco RJ, Machtel EE. Assessment of risk for periodontal disease. II: Risk indicators for alveolar bone loss. J Periodontol 1995;66:23–9.

37. Grossi SG, Zambon JJ, Jo AW. Assessment of risk for periodontal disease. I: Risk indicators for alveolar bone loss. J Periodontol 1994;65:260–7.

38. Moss ME, Beck JD, Kaplan BH, et al. Exploratory case-control analysis of psychosocial factors and adult periodontitis. J Periodontol 1996;67:1060–9.

39. Klokkevold PR. Periodontal medicine: assessment of risk factors for disease. Calif Dent Assoc J 1999;27:135.

40. Offenbacker S, Beck J. Periodontitis: a potential risk factor for spontaneous preterm birth. Compendium 1998;19:32.

41. Gibbs RS, Ronero R, Hiller SL, et al. A review of premature birth and subclinical infection. Am J Obstet Gynecol 1992;166:1515.

42. Iams J. Prevention of Preterm Birth. New Engl J Med 1998;338(1):54–6.

43. Dajani AS, Taubert KA, Wilson W, et al. Prevention of bacterial endocarditis: recommendations by the American Heart Association. JAMA 1997;277:1794–1801.

44. Larson PE. The effect of a chlorhexidine rinse on the incidence of alveolar osteitis following the surgical removal of impacted mandibular third molars. J Oral Maxillofac Surg 1991; 49:932–7.

45. Ragno JR Jr, Szkutnkik AJ. Evaluation of 0.12% chlorhexidine rinse on the prevention of alveolar osteitis. Oral Surg Oral Med Oral Pathol 1991;72:524–6.

46. Bonine FI. Effect of chlorhexidine rinse on the incidence of dry socket in impacted mandibular

third molar extraction sites. Oral Surg Oral Med Oral Pathol 1995;79:154.

47. American Association of Oral and Maxillofacial Surgeons. Report of a workshop on the management of patients with third molar teeth. J Oral Maxillofac Surg 1994;52:1102–12.

48. Rechmann P, Seewald M, Strassburg M, Naumann P. Incidence of bacteremia following extractions—a double blind study on local disinfection using chlorhexidine. Dtsch Zahnarztl A 1989;44:622–4.

49. Rahn R, Schneider S, Diehl O, et al. Preventing post-treatment bacteremia: comparing topical povidone-iodine and chlorhexidine [comment]. J Am Dent Assoc 1995;126:1474.

50. Albandar JM, Gjermo P, Preus HR. Chlorhexidine use after two decades of over-the-counter availability. J Periodontol 1994;65:109.

51. Morlino vs. Medical Ctr. of Orange County. 706 A.2d 721 (1998).

52. Shen EC, Maddalozzo D, Robinson PJ, Geivelis M. Root planing following short term pocket distension. J Periodontol 1997;68:632–5.

53. LeLorier J, Grègoire G, Benhaddad A, et al. Discrepancies between meta-analysis and subsequent large randomized controlled trials. N Engl J Med 1997;337:536–42.

54. Capelleri JC, Ioannidis JP, Schmid CH, et al. Large trials vs. meta-analysis of smaller trials: how do their results compare? JAMA 1996;276:1332–8.

55. Villar J, Carroli G, Belizan JM. Predictive ability of meta-analyses of randomised controlled trials. Lancet 1995;345:772–6.

56. Ioannidis JP, Cappelleri JC, Sacks HS, Lau J. The relationship between study design, results and reporting of randomized clinical trials of HIV infection. Control Clin Trials 1997;18:431–44.

57. Horowitz RI, Singer BH, Makuch RW, Viscoli CM. Can treatment that is helpful on average be harmful to some patients? A study of the conflicting information needs of clinical inquiry and drug regulation. J Clin Epidemiol 1996;49:395–400.

58. Monmaney T. AMA fires editor over publishing sex survey. Los Angeles Times, p. A16 (16 January 1999).

59. Reilly J. Tobacco use assessment is a new vital sign in dentistry. J Mass Dent Soc 1997;46:25–32.

60. Page RC, Beck JD. Risk assessment for periodontal diseases. Int Dent J 1997;47:61.

61. California Book of Approved Civil Jury Instructions (BAJI), BAJI No. 2.0.

62. Williams RC. Periodontal disease: the emergence of a new paradigm. Compendium 1998;19:4.

63. Loe H, Theilade E, Jensen SB. Experimental gingivitis in man. J Periodontol 1965;36:177.

64. California Book of Approved Civil Jury Instructions (BAJI), BAJI No. 3.76.

65. Peumans M, Van Meerbeek B, Lambrechts P, et al. The influence of direct composite additions for the correction of the tooth form and/or position on periodontal health. A retrospective study. J Periodontol 1998;69:422–7.

66. Jeffcoat MK, McGuire M, Newman MG. Evidence-based periodontal treatment. Highlights from the 1996 World Workshop in Periodontics. JADA 1997;128:713–24.

67. Daubert vs. Merrell Dow Pharmaceuticals, Inc. 509 U.S. 579 (1993).

68. Kumho Tire Co. vs. Carmichael. 119 S.Ct. 1167 (1999).

69. Jeffcoat MK, Bray KS, Ciancio SG. Adjunctive use of a subgingival controlled-release chlorhexidine chip reduces probing depth and improves attachment level compared with scaling and root planing alone. J Periodontol 1998;69:989–97.

70. Toole vs. Richardson-Merrill Inc. 251 Cal. App.3d 689; 60 Cal.Rptr. 398 (1967). 21 Code of Federal Regulations, section 801.4 (intended use may be shown by oral statements of manufacturer's representatives).

71. Woods KL. Mega-trials and management of acute myocardial infarction. Lancet 1995;346:611–4.

72. Ransohoff DF, Feinstein AR. Problems of spectrum and bias in evaluating the efficacy of diagnostic tests. N Engl J Med 1978;299:926.

73. Fewer implant cases seen on wake of scientific findings. San Francisco Daily Journal 1998 Dec 2; Sect. C:1.

74. Severson HH, Andrews JH, Lichtenstein E, et al. Using the hygiene visit to deliver a tobacco cessation program: results of a randomized clinical trial. JADA 1998;129:993–9.

INDEX

Neutrophils, 38
Nicotine, 101
  action of, 103
  addiction, 104
  cardiovascular system and, 104
  effects on fibroblasts, 101
  nonpharmacologic agents, 111
  replacement agents, *109*
  withdrawal, 104, 109
Nicotine dependency, 103–114
Nicotine gum, 107, 109–110
  contraindications for, 110
  with patch, 111
Nicotine nasal spray, 110
  contraindications for, 110
Nicotine patches, 109
  contraindications for, 110
  with gum, 111
Nifedipine (Procardia), 23
Night sweats, 64
Nitrendipine, 23
Non-Hodgkin's lymphoma, in AIDS
  patients, 17
Non-Mendelian disorders, 47
Nonfeasance, 275
Nonsteroidal anti-inflammatories,
  206
Nystatin, 259

Occlusion, as risk factor, 25
Optimum treatment, 57
Oral hygiene, and risk, 24
Oral lichen planus, 186
Oropharyngeal cancer, 7–8
  risk factors for, 8
Osler's nodes, 64
Osteoclasts, activation of, 12
Osteogenesis imperfecta, 20
Osteopenia, 167–182
  oral bone and, 171–173
  as risk factor, 18–19
  as risk indicator, 15
Osteoporosis, 169–182, 278
  causes, 171
  classification, 170
  definition, 169
  diet, 177
  future research, 179
  genetics, 177
  high turnover, 174
  involutional, 170
  in liver disease, 213
  pathophysiology, 171
  and periodontal disease, 172–179
  postmenopausal, 170
  as risk indicator, 15, *25*
  as risk factor, 18–19
  risk factors for, 173
  secondary, 170
  smoking and, 175–177

treatment, 178–179
Oxidant stress, 133

Pancreatic transplantation, 214
Panic disorder, 65
Pantomographic index, 73
Papillon-Lefèvre syndrome, 18
  as risk indicator, 15
Partial thromboplastin time (PTT),
  42, 232, 237
  normal range, *41*
Patient evaluation, 35–38
  reasons for, 35
Patient monitoring, 276
Penicillin, 68. *See also* Amoxicillin
  allergy, 68
  with contraceptives, 244
  resistance, 68
Periapical lesions, as risk factor, 25
Periapical pathosis, 199
PerioChip, 256–258
Periodontal disease, 1–9, 279
  background factors, 14–15
  diabetes and, 132–136
  etiology of, 11
  genetics of, 46, 49–62
  glycemic control and, 135–136
  heart disease and, 11
  pathogenesis of, 12
  pre-existing, 24–25
  pregnancy and, 153–155
  presentation, 46
  risk assessment, 12–15, 60, 173,
    283
  as risk factor for COPD, 90
  second-hand smoke, 99
  smoking-associated, 100, *101*
  stroke and, 76–78
  systemic disease and, 1–9, 15–22
  untreated, 91
Periodontal ligament, 2, 4, 5–6, *7*
Periodontitis, 45
  bleeding disorders and, 227
  diabetes and, 135–136
  in diabetics, 132
  early-onset, 46, 49
  etiology of, 56
  HIV associated, 184–191
  in leukemia, 198
  measurement of, 13
  rapidly progressive, 190–191
  recurrence of, 12
  stroke and, *77*, 78
Periodontium, 2–6
  diabetic influence on, 133–135
  medications and, 262–263
  smoking and, 100
Peritonitis, 209
Peroxetine, 153
Petechiae, oral, 64

Pharmacogenomics, 57
Phenytoin (sodium
  5,5-phenylhydantoin), 22–23, 213,
  263–264
  side effects, 22, 263
Physician Desk Reference, 281
Pierre-Robin syndrome, 21
Pigmentation, 23
Plaque, 56
  accumulation, 45
  composition, 262–263
  during pregnancy, 155, *156*, 157
  medications and, 262–263
  respiratory disease and, 87–89
  as risk factor, 24, 280
  types of, 45–46
Plasminogen, 72
Plasminogen activator inhibitor, 155
Platelet count, 41
Platelet disorders, 229–230
  aspirin and, 230
Platelet dysfunction, 196
Platelet transfusions, 240
Platelet-derived growth factor, 129,
  133, 263
Pneumonia, 83–89
  prevention, 92–93
Pocket, 3, *6*
Polymyxin B, 92
Porphyromonas gingivalis, 9, *73*
  heat-shock protein, 78
  as risk factor, 23, *25*
Povidone iodine, 68, 187
Pregnancy, 153–161
  antibiotics, *160*, 162
  breast feeding, 161, *162*
  dental treatment, 158–161
  diet, *158*
  emergency treatments, 158–159
  fetal risk, *159*, 279
  gingivitis, 153
  immunoresponse, 155, *156*
  local anesthetics/analgesics, *160*,
    162
  management, 157–158
  medications, 159
  nicotine replacement during, 110
  nutrition, 157
  perimylolysis, 157
  plaque composition, 155, *156*
  prenatal fluoride, 158
  preterm low-birth-weight births,
    156–157, 279
  radiography, 159
  sedatives, *160*, *162*
  supine hypotensive syndrome, 158
Pregnancy tumors, 154–155, *157*,
  158
Preleukemic syndrome, 18
Premenstrual syndrome, 153